Atlas of
Parasitic Pathology

Dedicated to
Prof. H. M. Seitz, MD and **Prof. U. Pfeifer**, MD,
University of Bonn, Germany,
whose help in completing this atlas is very much appreciated

Current Histopathology

Consultant Editor
Professor G. Austin Gresham, TD, ScD, MD, FRCPath.
Professor of Morbid Anatomy and Histology, University of Cambridge

Volume Twenty

ATLAS OF
PARASITIC
PATHOLOGY

By
K. SALFELDER
Prof. Titular
Laboratorio de Investigación en Patología
Facultad de Medicina
Universidad de Los Andes, Mérida,
Venezuela SA

Assisted by

T. R. de Liscano
Prof. Titular
and

E. Sauerteig
Profesor Asesor
Laboratorio de Investigación en Patologia
Facultad de Medicina
Universidad de Los Andes, Mérida
Venezuela SA

KLUWER ACADEMIC PUBLISHERS
DORDRECHT / BOSTON / LONDON

Distributors

for the United States and Canada: Kluwer Academic
Publishers, PO Box 358, Accord Station, Hingham,
MA 02018-0358, USA
for all other countries: Kluwer Academic Publishers
Group, Distribution Center, PO Box 322, 3300 AH
Dordrecht, The Netherlands

Published in the United Kingdom by Kluwer Academic
Publishers, PO Box 55, Lancaster, UK.

Kluwer Academic Publishers BV incorporates the
publishing programmes of D. Reidel, Martinus Nijhoff,
Dr W. Junk and MTP Press.

Typeset and originated by Speedlith Photo Litho Ltd.,
Stretford, Manchester M32 0JT
Printed in Great Britain by Redwood Press Ltd.,
Melksham, Wilts.

A catalogue record for this book is available from the
British Library.

ISBN 0-7923-8998-0

**Library of Congress Cataloging in Publication
Data**

Salfelder, Karlhanns, 1919–
    Atlas of parasitic pathology / by K. Salfelder ;
assisted by T.R. de Liscano and E. Sauerteig.
        p.   cm. — (Current histopathology ; v. 20)
    Includes bibliographical references and index.
    ISBN 0-7923-8998-0 (casebound)
    1. Parasitic diseases — Atlases.   2. Parasitic
diseases — Histopathology — Atlases.   I. Liscano,
T. R. de.   II. Sauerteig, Eberhard.   III. Title.
IV. Series.
    [DNLM: 1. Parasitic Diseases — pathology —
atlases.   W1 CU788JBA v. 20 / WC 17 S163ac]
RC119.S24   1992
616.9'607 — dc20
DNLM/DLC
    for Library of Congress   92-49790
                                                      CIP

Contents

Consultant editor's note — 7

Preface — 8

I Parasitic diseases — 9

II Protozoan diseases — 13

Haemoflagellate infections — 13
1 American trypanosomiasis — 13
2 African trypanosomiasis — 23

Leishmaniases — 26
3 Cutaneous leishmaniasis — 27
4 Mucocutaneous leishmaniasis — 27
5 Visceral leishmaniasis — 35

6 Giardiasis — 39
7 Trichomoniasis — 41
8 Amoebiasis — 43
9 Acanthamoebiasis — 49
10 Blastocystis infection — 56
11 Toxoplasmosis — 59
12 Babesiosis — 69
13 Sarcosporidiosis — 72
14 Isosporosis — 73
15 Cryptosporidiosis — 76
16 Malaria — 77
17 Pneumocystosis — 85
18 Balantidiasis — 91
19 Microsporidiosis — 94

III Helminthic diseases — 96

A. Nematodiasis — 96
20 Enterobiasis — 97
21 Ascariasis — 100
22 Trichuriasis — 101
23 Uncinariasis — 106
24 Strongyloidiasis — 109
25 Trichinosis — 112

26 Toxocariasis — 115
27 Anisakiasis — 115
28 Gnathostomiasis — 117
29 Angiostrongylosis — 119
30 Capillariasis — 124
31 Dracunculosis — 124

Filaria infections — 126
32 Filariasis — 126
33 Loiasis — 128
34 Onchocerciasis — 131
35 Dirofilariasis — 135
36 Rare and uncommon nematodiases — 137
37 Larva migrans — 138

B. Cestodiasis — 141
38 Taeniasis — 141
39 Diphyllobothriasis — 143
40 Dipylidiasis — 145
41 Hymenolepiasis — 145
42 Cysticercosis — 147
43 Echinococcosis — 148

C. Trematodiasis — 151
44 Blood fluke infection — 151
45 Lung trematode infection — 160
46 Liver trematode infection — 163
47 Intestinal fluke infections — 169

D. Worm eggs — 171

IV Disorders caused by arthropods — 173

48 Scabies — 173
49 Demodicidosis — 175
50 Tungiasis — 178
51 Myiasis — 181
52 Pentastomiasis — 184

Index — 186

Current Histopathology Series

Already published in this series:

Volume 1 Atlas of Lymph Node Pathology
Volume 2 Atlas of Renal Pathology
Volume 3 Atlas of Pulmonary Pathology
Volume 4 Atlas of Liver Pathology
Volume 5 Atlas of Gynaecological Pathology
Volume 6 Atlas of Gastrointestinal Pathology
Volume 7 Atlas of Breast Pathology
Volume 8 Atlas of Oral Pathology
Volume 9 Atlas of Skeletal Muscle Pathology
Volume 10 Atlas of Male Reproductive Pathology
Volume 11 Atlas of Skin Pathology
Volume 12 Atlas of Cardiovascular Pathology
Volume 13 Atlas of Experimental Toxicological Pathology
Volume 14 Atlas of Serous Fluid Cytopathology
Volume 15 Atlas of Bone Marrow Pathology
Volume 16 Atlas of Ear, Nose and Throat Pathology
Volume 17 Atlas of Fungal Pathology
Volume 18 Atlas of Synovial Fluid Cytopathology
Volume 19 Tumours of the Mediastinum

*Other volumes currently scheduled in this series include
the following titles*

Atlas of AIDS Pathology

Atlas of Bone Tumours

Atlas of Neuropathology

Atlas of Endocrine Pathology

Atlas of Ocular Pathology

Atlas of Renal Transplantation Pathology

Atlas of Soft Tissue Pathology

Biopsy of Bone in Internal Medicine

Paediatric Neoplasia

Consultant Editor's Note

At the present time books on morbid anatomy and histopathology can be divided into two broad groups: extensive textbooks often written primarily for students and monographs on research topics.

This takes no account of the fact that the vast majority of pathologists are involved in an essentially practical field of general diagnostic pathology providing an important service to their clinical colleagues. Many of these pathologist are expected to cover a broad range of disciplines and even those who remain solely within the field of histopathology usually have single and sole responsibility within the hospital for all this work. They may often have no colleagues in the same department. In the field of histopathology, no less than in other medical fields, there have been extensive and recent advances, not only in new histochemical techniques but also in the type of specimen provided by new surgical procedures.

There is a great need for the provision of appropriate information for this group. This need has been defined in the following terms:

1. It should be aimed at the general clinical pathologist or histopathologist with existing practical training, but should have value for the trainee pathologist.

2. It should concentrate on the practical aspects of histopathology taking account of the new techniques which should be within the compass of the worker in a unit with reasonable facilities.

3. New types of material, e.g. those derived from endoscopic biopsy should be covered fully.

4. There should be an adequate number of illustrations on each subject to demonstrate the variation in appearance that is encountered.

5. Colour illustrations should be used wherever they aid recognition.

From time to time histopathologists encounter objects in histological preparations and in cytological smears that may be of parasitic origin. This book is a comprehensive, well illustrated aid to such diagnostic problems.

G. A. Gresham

Preface

One large chapter of this atlas is, in some ways, a second, enlarged and improved, edition of an atlas published some years ago[1]. The *Atlas of Parasitic Pathology* concentrates intentionally on the main features of gross pathology and the histopathology of these diseases.

In the four subchapters of each section on a particular parasite, the text is always arranged in the same order (Introduction, The Parasite, Pathogenesis and Pathology); thus, information can easily be found by the reader. Under 'Introduction', general data are summarized in a few sentences. Under 'Pathology', organ involvement, gross pathology and morphology of the aetiological agent are followed by tissue reaction and differential diagnosis.

Several unpublished data and illustrations, as well as personal observations and ideas, are included because we have not published in journals for the last 15 years.

History, epidemiology, clinical data, therapy etc. are not included. Medical students may find these details in the 10th volume of the GKM[2].

In another atlas in this series, differential diagnosis of micro-organisms and non-living structures in tissues has been focused on extensively[3]. For this reason, differential diagnosis of parasites will be discussed here only briefly.

Since the technical terms will be explained in the text or in footnotes, a glossary was considered superfluous.

This atlas is directed to pathologists and should be used as a bench manual to be kept near their microscopes for immediate consultation. Obviously, physicians and professionals of all natural and paramedical sciences, as well as teachers at all levels, may find it useful.

The first main chapter (I) deals with parasitic diseases in general, and definitions of parasites and parasitic infections. Also, data on hosts and transmission are summarized. The principal characteristics of parasitic disorders, in contrast to other infectious diseases, and all the important pathogenic parasites for men, are listed. The important parasitoses in immunodeficient patients are mentioned.

In the following three main chapters (II–IV), protozoan and helminthic diseases, as well as disorders caused by arthropods, are discussed and illustrated.

Principal worm eggs and arthropods are illustrated. Schematic drawings facilitate the understanding of the life-cycle and evolutional stages of parasites, the portal of entry and pathogenesis.

References

1. In Spanish: Salfelder, K. (1985). *Las Protozoonosis en el Hombre*. Oscar Todtmann, C. A. Caracas/Venezuela, and in English: Salfelder, K. (1987). *Protozoan Infections in Man*. Schwer-Verlag, Stuttgart/FRG
2. Thomas, C. (1990). *Grundlagen der Klinischen Medizin*. Schattauer-Verlag, Stuttgart/FRG
3. Salfelder, K. (1990). *Atlas of Fungal Pathology*. Vol. 17, Current Histopathology. Kluwer Academic Publishers, Lancaster

ACKNOWLEDGEMENTS

I am very grateful to many of my colleagues and friendswho gave me material and photographs to illustrate this atlas. Thanks go first to my friends in Mérida and Venezuela: R. Alvarado, A. D. de Arriaga, K. Brass, E. Carrero, W. Diaz, R. Hernández Pérez, A. L. C. de Tirado, G. Volcán and R. Zabala. My good friends, H. D. Eberhard, M. Okudaira, P. Ravisse, S. Stefanko, C. Thomas, H. Werner, and others have helped in many ways. Professor G. Piekarski of Bonn was kind enough to give permission to use some of his plates of the developmental cycles of parasites.

As always, Oswaldo Juergenson, Mérida was an invaluable help with photography.

The publishers, Oscar Todtmann, C. A. Caracas/Venezuela, Schattauer–Verlag, Stuttgart, FRG and Schwer–Verlag, Stuttgart FRG, have permitted us to reproduce previously published illustrations. We would like to express our special gratitude to them.

The CONICIT (Consejo Nacional de Investigaciones Científicas y Tecnológicas) in Caracas and the CDCHT (Consejo de Desarollo Científico, Humanístico y Tecnológico) of the University of the Andes, Mérida/Venezuela have subsidized several research projects of the authors, partially related to this atlas.

The academic Vice-rector of our University, Prof. Carlos Guillermo Cárdenas MD, helped us to finish this atlas. The ex-rector, Prof. Pedro Rincón Gutiérrez MD, founded our laboratory and gave us support in many ways.

The DAAD (Deutscher Akademischer Austauschdienst) of the FRG helped indirectly to finish both atlases in this series written by us.

Professor H. M. Seitz MD and Professor U. Pfeifer MD from Bonn, Germany assisted, in several ways, the final phases of the drafting of this atlas and therefore it is dedicated to these good friends.

Professor G. Austin Gresham of Cambridge, UK was kind enough to help with the 'German' English. Thank you, indeed, Professor Gresham.

Last, but not least, co-operation with Phil Johnstone, the editor of this atlas, was superb.

Parasitic Diseases

I

A parasite in biology is defined in the *Webster Dictionary* of 1983 as a plant or animal that lives on or within another organism from which it derives sustenance or protection without making compensation.

In the *Encyclopaedia Britannica*, 1962 edition, parasites are considered as organisms which live for all or part of their lives on (ecto-) or in (endoparasites) another living organism (host) from which they derive some benefit, such as food, shelter or protection. Parasites producing damage to the host are referred to as pathogens, and the condition resulting from this damage constitutes disease.

Summarizing, there are obligatory and facultative pathogenic parasites, temporary and stationary, as well as endo- and ectoparasites.

In a broad sense, parasitic diseases, or parasitoses, are produced by any micro-organism (or macro-organism), but conventionally in medicine, they are morbid states due to infection with the animal parasite groups, protozoa and helminths. The unicellular protozoa belong to the protists of the second kingdom, and the helminths belong to the pluricellular metazoa, of the fifth kingdom of the living organisms. We would like to add a third group, arthropods, which also belong to the fifth kingdom of living organisms, since the disorders produced by these organisms, and their role as vectors, are of interest in medicine, especially for pathologists.

Parasitoses must be differentiated from zoonoses. The World Health Organization (WHO) defines the zoonoses as: diseases and infections transmitted in a natural way between vertebrates and men. Toxoplasmosis is one of the zoonoses. Anthropozoonoses and zooanthroponoses are infectious diseases, whose agents are pathogens for men and lower animals, but they differ in their mode of infection.

Disorders caused by parasites are both of general importance and great interest. More than one billion human beings are infested; numerous individuals are considerably affected and die[1-29].

Infection with parasites does not always cause disease. Serological tests may be positive in apparently healthy persons, often confirming that infection occurred a long time ago.

Parasitic infections with serious disease are especially frequent in underdeveloped countries, as well as in tropical and subtropical regions.

Recently, these diseases have become more important all over the world because they are observed with increasing frequency as complications of diseases due to acquired immunologic deficiencies. In this context, toxoplasmosis and pneumocystosis must be mentioned. Some infections of this kind may show exacerbation and also a more severe course in debilitated or immuno-deficient persons than under normal conditions. This occurs in amoebiasis, giardiasis, strongyloidiosis and cryptosporidiosis.

Nowadays, campaigns of eradication of vectors are not performed so regularly and systematically as in former times, partly because many people are concerned, excessively and fanatically, with biological equilibrium. This neglect has caused a recrudescence of infectious diseases which had almost been forgotten, for example malaria, Chagas disease, sleeping disease and leishmaniasis.

Monoxenous parasites occur only in one species, man or one of the lower animals. Heteroxenous parasites, on the other hand, may develop in man and lower animals.

Specific parasitoses (e.g. *Taeniasis solium*) occur only in one host; non-specific parasitoses (e.g. blood-sucking arthropods) may occur in several dead-end hosts. The parasitic specificity may refer also to the intermediate host.

Recommended texts on parasitology can be found in alphabetical order in the references at the end of this chapter.

HOSTS

A **dead-end host** is a host in which the parasite reaches an end point and is unable to continue its life cycle.

A **principal dead-end host**, or **typical host**, is a host in which the parasite is commonly found and in which the parasite can complete its development (or the appropriate phase of its development for subsequent completion of its life cycle).

An **accessory or secondary dead-end host** is one which harbours parasites only occasionally.

An **accidental host** is one in which the parasite is not commonly found; nevertheless, it is suitable for the parasite's development. In some instances (e.g. cysticercosis), the accidental host is a dead-end one because, even though the parasite develops through its appropriate stages, it fails to find a portal of exit, and thus the life cycle is blocked.

An **aberrant host** is one in which the parasite cannot complete its development or the appropriate phase of its development.

A **false host** is a person (man) who harbours a parasite which is usually found only in a determined lower animal species. The parasite cannot leave or reach maturity in this host.

A **reservoir host** is any host (a lower animal or man) in which the parasite remains and is available for transmission to another susceptible host, i.e. it is a constant source of transmission.

Table 1 The principal pathogenic parasites in man

Causative agents	Transmission	Disease
Protozoa		
Mastigophora		
Trypanosoma cruzi	*Triatoma* spp.	American trypanosomias
	Diaplacental	Chagas disease
Trypanosoma brucei gamb.	*Glossina* spp.	African trypanosomiasis
T.brucei rhodesiense		Sleeping sickness
Leishmania tropica major and minor	*Phlebotomus* spp.	Cutaneous leishmaniasis
		Oriental sore
Leishmania braziliensis	*Lutzomyia* spp.	Mucocutaneous leishmaniasis
Leishmania donovani	*Phlebotomus* spp.	Visceral leishmaniasis
	Lutzomyia spp.	Kala-azar
Giardia lamblia	oral	Giardiasis
Trichomonas vaginalis	direct	Trichomoniasis
Rhizopoda		
Entamoeba histolytica	oral	Amoebiasis
Naegleria fowleri	transnasal	Primary meningoencephalitis
Acanthamoeba castellani, A. culbertsoni, A. polyphaga	transnasal	Granulomatous encephalitis
Blastocystis hominis	oral	Blastocystis infection
Sporozoa		
Toxoplasma gondii	*oral, diaplacental, blood transfusion*	Toxoplasmosis
Babesia microti, B. bovis	*Ixodes*	Babesiosis
Sarcocystis suihominis, S. bovihominis	oral	Sarcosporidiosis
Isospora belli	oral	Isosporosis
Cryptosporidium spp.	oral	Cryptosporidiosis
Plasmodium falciparum, P. vivax, P. ovale, P. malariae	*Anopheles* spp.	Malaria
Pneumocystis carinii	inhalation	Pneumocystosis
Ciliophora		
Balantidium coli	oral	Balantidiasis
Cnidosporidia		
Nosema connori etc.	oral(?)	Microsporidiosis
Helminths		
Nematodes		
Enterobius vermicularis	oral	Enterobiasis, oxyuriasis
Ascaris lumbricoides	oral	Ascariasis
Trichuria trichiura	oral	Trichuriasis
Ancylostoma duodenale	transcutaneous	Uncinariasis
Necator americanus	transcutaneous	
Strongyloides stercoralis	transcutaneous	Strongyloidiasis
Trichinella spiralis	oral	Trichinosis
Toxocara canis, T. cati	oral	Toxocariasis
Anisacis marina	oral	Anisakiasis
Gnathostoma spinigerum	oral	Gnathostomiasis
Angiostrongylus cantonensis	oral	Angiostrongylosis
Angiostrongylus costaricensis	oral	Angiostrongylosis
Capillaria hepatica	oral	Capillariasis
Capillaria philippinensis	oral	Capillariasis
Dracunculus medinensis	*Chrysops* spp.	Dracunculosis
Filariae		
Wuchereria bancrofti	*Anopheles* spp.	Filariasis
Brugia malayi, B. timori	Culex, *Aedes*	Elephantiasis
Loa loa	*Chrysops* spp.	Loiasis
Onchocerca volvulus	*Simulium* spp.	Onchocerciasis
Dirofilaria spp.	*Anopheles, Culex*	Dirofilariasis
Cestodes		
Taenia saginata	oral	Taeniasis sag.
Taenia solium	oral	Taeniasis solium
Diphyllobothrium latum	oral	Diphyllobothriasis
Dipylidium caninum	oral	Dipylidiasis
Hymenolepsis nana	oral	Hymenolepiasis
Cysticercus cellulosae	oral	Cysticercosis
Echinococcus alveolaris, E. granulosus (hydatidosis)	oral	Echinococcosis
Trematodes		
Schistosoma haematobium, S. mansoni, S. japonicum, S. mekongi	transcutaneous	Schistosomiasis, bilharziasis
Paragonimus westermani, P. africanus, P. kellicottii	oral	Lung fluke
Fasciola hepatica, Clonorchis sinensis, Opisthorchis felineus	oral	Liver fluke
Fasciolepsis buski	oral	Intestinal fluke

Table 2 The principal arthropods

Scientific denomination	Common name	Diseases caused or transmitted
Pulex irritans, Ctenocephalides canis, C. felis,	Fleas*	Pulicosis
Tunga penetrans	Chigoe flea, jigger	Tungiasis
Cimex lectularis, C. hemipterus, Triatoma spp.	Bugs*	Cimicosis
		Chagas disease
Pediculus corporis, P. capitis, P. vestimentorum,	Lice*	Pediculosis
Phthirius pubis		Phthiriasis
Trombicula autumnalis, T. irritans	Harvest mite, red bug, chiggers*	Itch
Sarcoptes scabiei	Itch mites*	Scabies, scratch, eczema (psora)
Demodex folliculorum, D. brevis	Pimple mites	Demodicidosis of hair follicles or sebacious glands
Ixodida spp.	Hard ticks	Ixodiasis, acariasis, babesiosis and other infectious diseases
Diptera (order of insects)		
Anopheles, Aedes, Culex	Mosquitoes or gnats*	Numerous infectious diseases, e.g. malaria and yellow fever
Simulium spp.	Black flies*	Onchocerciasis, Tularaemia etc.
Phlebotomus spp., Lutzomyia spp.	Sand flies*	Leishmaniases, Oroya fever
Chrysops spp., Tabanus spp.	Tabanid flies*	Chrysosis, Loaloa
Glossina palpalis, G. morsitans	Tsetse flies*	Sleeping sickness
Musca domestica,	House fly	Numerous infectious diseases
Cordylobia anthropophaga,	African tumbu fly	
Dermatobia hominis etc.	Tropical warble fly	Myiasis

* = Blood sucking

TRANSMISSION

Transmission **without an intermediate host** may occur:

1. Directly person to person (e.g. *Trichomonas* by sexual intercourse)

2. Through the oral portal of entry (ova or larvae).

3. Transcutaneously by contact with soil harbouring infectious larvae.

Transmission **with an intermediate host** may occur:

1. By eating raw meat or fish.

2. Through the bites or stings of insects.

In **transport hosts**, parasites do not reproduce, but may go through developmental stages.
    In **true or biological vectors**, transmission is mechanical and a parasitic cycle with multiplication may occur before the parasite is infective to the recipient individual.
    Parasitic diseases show certain **special features** which do not occur commonly in bacterial, viral or mycotic infections:

1. Parasites, in general, are living, but they may remain dead in man for a long time. Certain helminths may act as co-carcinogens. The classical locations of these carcinomas are the bladder and the liver. Parasites may go through a complex cycle of evolution in which other living organisms may participate as vectors or as temporary or terminal hosts. The variable phases of evolution and life cycle stages may lead to very different disease patterns.

2. The portal of entry of parasites is usually the skin or the digestive tract, in contrast to fungi causing deep mycoses, which are mostly inhaled.

3. Geographic and socioeconomic factors play an important role in parasitic infections.

4. Parasites may cause severe foreign body reactions and may, by virtue of their size, obstruct hollow organs.

5. Tissue reaction due to parasites, generally, is slow, mild and scarce. Often eosinophilic infiltrations are present. Granulomatous reactions are usually absent.

7. Parasites, and above all protozoans, do not usually stain histologically with special methods, as, for instance, fungi. An exception is the PAS-positivity of amoebae.

8. Toxicity of parasites is usually lower than that of bacteria. Allergic reactions are less frequent and less severe in parasitic diseases, with a few exceptions (*Ascaris, Echinococcus*).

9. Parasites may cause diminished absorption of food materials and may produce heavy losses of blood or other liquids from the gut.

References

1. Ash, L. R. and Orihel, T. C. (1980). *Atlas of Human Parasitology*. American Society of Clinical Pathologists
2. Boch, J. and Supperer, R. (1983). *Veterinaermedizinische Parasitologie. 3. Aufl.* Paul Parey Verlag
3. Brandis, H. and Otte, H. (1984). *Lehrbuch der medizinischen Mikrobiologie. 5. Aufl.* Gustav Fischer Verlag
4. Desowitz, R. S. (1980). *Ova and Parasites*. Harper and Row
5. Diaz-Ungria, C. (1960). *Parasitología Venezolana*. Vol. 1. Segunda parte. Protozoos en Venezuela. Parasitología y Clínica. Editorial Sucre, Caracas
6. Faust, E. C., Russell, P. F. and Jung, R. C. (1974). *Craig y Faust, Parasitología Clínica*. Versión española de la 8° edición en inglés. Salvat Editores, S.A. Barcelona
7. Granz, W. and Ziegler, K. (1976). *Tropenkrankheiten*. Joh. Ambrosius Barth
8. Gsell, O. (1980). *Importierte Infektionskrankheiten. Epidemiologie und Therapie*. Georg Thieme Verlag
9. Gutierrez, Y. (1990). *Diagnostic Pathology of Parasitic Infections with Clinical Correlations*. Lea & Febiger
10. Harms, G., Zwingenberger, K. and Bienzle, U. (1987). *AIDS in*

Africa: Current Knowledge. Landesinstitut fuerTropenmedizin Berlin

11. Paul D. Hoeprich (ed.) (1983). *Infectious Diseases*, 3rd edn. Harper and Row

12. Katz, M., Despommier, D. D. and Gwadz, R. W. (1982). *Parasitic Diseases*. Springer Verlag

13. Kudo, R. R. (1966). *Protozoology*, 5th edn. Charles C. Thomas, Springfield, Ill

14. Mandell, G. L., Douglas Jr., R. G. and Bennett, J. E. (1990). *Principles and Practice of Infectious Diseases*, 3rd edn. Churchill Livingstone

15. Mehlhorn, H. and Peters, W. (1983). *Diagnose der Parasiten beim Menschen*. Gustav Fischer Verlag

16. Mehlhorn, H. and Piekarski, G. (1981). *Grundriss der Parasitenkunde*. Gustav Fischer Verlag

17. Muller, R. (1975). *Worms and Disease*. William Heinemann Medical Books Limited

18. Mumcuoglu, Y. and Rufli, Th. (1982). *Dermatologische Entomologie*. Perimed Fachbuch Verlagsgesellschaft

19. Nauck, E. G. (1975). *Lehrbuch der Tropenkrankheiten*. Mohr, W., Schuhmacher, H. H. and Weyer, F. (eds.) *4 Aufl*. Georg Thieme Verlag

20. Marcial-Rojas, R. A. (ed.) (1971). *Pathology of Protozoal and Helminthic Diseases*. The Williams and Wilkins Company

21. Binford, C. H. and Connor, D. H. (eds.) (1976). *Pathology of Tropical and Extraordinary Diseases*, Vol. I. Armed Forces Institute of Pathology, Washington, D.C.

22. Peters, W. and Gilles, H. M. (1977). *A Colour Atlas of Tropical Medicine and Parasitology*. Wolfe Medical Publications

23. Piekarski, G. (1989). *Medical Parasitology*. Translation of *Medizinische Parasitologie in Tafeln, 3. Auflage*. Springer Verlag

24. Pifano, F. (1964). *Aspectos de Medicina Tropical en Venezuela*. OBE. UCV., Caracas

25. Tischler, W. (1982). *Grundriss der Humanparasitologie, 3. Aufl.* Gustav Fischer Verlag

26. Spencer, H. (ed.) (1973). *Tropical Pathology*. Handb. Spez. Path. Anat. Bd. 8, Springer Verlag

27. Warren, K. S. and Mahmoud, A. A. (1985). *Tropical and Geographical Medicine*. McGraw-Hill Book Company

28. Westphal, A. (1977). *Zoología Especial. Protozoos*. Ediciones Omega, S.A. Barcelona

29. Whittaker, R. H. (1969). New concepts of kingdoms of organisms. *Science*, **163**, 150

Protozoan Diseases

II

Protozoans are unicellular parasites. Several protozoans, e.g. *Giardia lamblia*, *Trichomonas vaginalis*, *Blastocystis hominis* and *Cryptosporidium* spp., are present in the lumens of hollow organs without invasion of tissues. Only a few of the numerous protozoan species are pathogenic for man.

HAEMOFLAGELLATE INFECTIONS

Trypanosomiasis and leishmaniasis infections are caused by organisms with flagella only in the blood.

The trypanosomiases as autochthonous infections occur in geographically limited regions where causative agents and vectors live side by side. In man, the trypanosomes produce two distinct diseases: the American trypanosomiasis (Chagas disease) and the African trypanosomiasis (sleeping disease). Only in Chagas disease are amastigotes found, i.e. parasites without flagella, also called leishmanial forms, in the tissues of man and lower animals. Leishmaniasis, exists in man in three forms: the cutaneous, the mucocutaneous and the visceral forms. The leishmanias in the three forms are morphologically identical in tissues and structurally resemble amastigotes of *Trypanosoma cruzi*.

1. AMERICAN TRYPANOSOMIASIS

Introduction

This is an important protozoan infection, also called Chagas disease, which affects millions of people in Central and South America[1]. It is geographically limited. Chagas disease is endemic in Venezuela and new infections are coming to light because the vectors have not been totally eradicated[2-7]. During the sixties, new infections were not seen. Autochthonous infections are not found outside the Americas.

Dogs and rodents are reservoir hosts as well as man. More organs are involved in experimentally infected mice than in natural infections in man (Figs. 1.1 and 1.2).

The acute form occurs mainly in children. Often the infection is asymptomatic, or there are many clinical symptoms which depend in each case on the organ or organ system involved. Rarely is an early diagnosis made. In symptomatic cases, the prognosis is bad. The chronic form is observed mostly in older people and chronic myocarditis is one of the most frequent causes of sudden death. Chronic *T. cruzi* infections, however, do not appear to be a public health problem in Venezuela at the moment[8].

Clinical aetiologic diagnosis is not easy. The causative agent should be demonstrated. In the acute form, trypomastigotes should be looked for in the blood; this is done with good results at the University Hospital in Barinas. The search for amastigotes in muscle biopsies may be successful (Fig. 1.3). In the chronic form, xenodiagnosis* may be positive, or the infection may be proved only by serological methods. The indirect immunofluorescent procedure has been developed recently for detecting intact amastigotes and phagocytosed amorphous antigen, both intensely fluorescent in human and mouse myocardia[9].

The parasite

The genus *Trypanosoma* belongs to the family Trypanosomatidae. The species *Trypanosoma cruzi* seems to be the only causative agent of Chagas disease. Lately, *Trypanosoma rangeli* has been discussed as a causative agent too. Numerous people in Venezuela, Colombia and Panama are infected with this other species. However, the parasites have been found only in the blood of man and not in tissues.

The trypomastigote (flagellate form) of *T. cruzi* in the blood is $3 \mu m$ wide and $16-22 \mu m$ long including the flagellum. In fixed smears, it is seen as a (C) or (U) form (Fig. 1.4). Its nucleus is situated in the centre of the parasite, is oval-shaped and stains reddish pink with Giemsa. The kinetoplast, $1 \mu m$ in diameter, is prominent and located in the pointed rear part. It represents a particular form of mitochondria. Near the kinetoplast is the base of the flagellum, called the blepharoplast. This structure cannot be differentiated under a light microscope but it is possible with an electron microscope. The trypomastigotes do not multiply in blood. *T. rangeli* shows only minimal structural differences when compared with *T. cruzi* (Fig. 1.5). The flagellum in the latter is shorter. Furthermore, both species may be differentiated by their sialic acid content[10].

After penetrating the tissue cells, the flagellum cannot be discerned with the light microscope within the cell. The parasite transforms into an amastigote with a rudimentary flagellum visible only under an electron microscope. Under the light microscope, these amastigotes, without flagella, reveal a peripherally localized nucleus, measuring $3-5 \mu m$ in diameter and are arranged in nests or pseudocysts, mostly in muscle and glial cells (Figs. 1.6 and 1.7). These pseudocysts do not have an individual capsule. The amastigotes contain, in addition to the nucleus, a characteristic rod-like kinetoplast, generally darker than the nucleus in the H&E and Giemsa stain. The amastigotes of *T. cruzi* are called also 'leishmanial forms'. Parasites in the amastigote form are also found in tissue culture.

---

*Xenodiagnosis is the confirmation of a causative agent in a (human) patient through the development of the parasite in a non-vertebrate (vector) which has been exposed to the patient. For example, promastigotes of *T. cruzi* are observed in a previously healthy triatomid after it has sucked blood from a patient with Chagas disease.

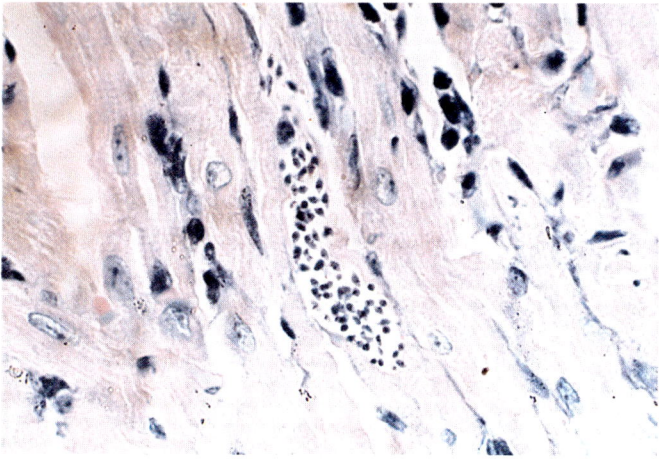

Fig. 1.1 Nest of amastigotes of *Trypanosoma cruzi* in the mycoardium of a mouse inoculated intraperitoneally with the excrement of parasitized vector bugs. H&E

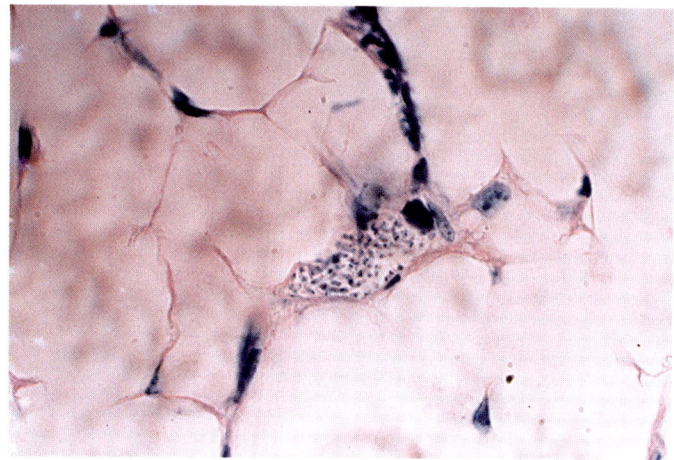

Fig. 1.2 Nest of amastigotes of *Trypanosoma cruzi* in the mediastinal fat tissue of the same mouse as in Fig. 1.1. H&E

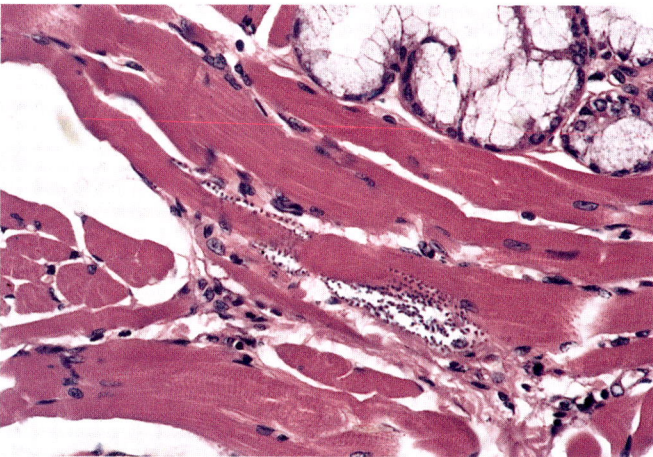

Fig. 1.3 Amastigote nest of *Trypanosoma cruzi* in the muscular fibres of a human tongue. H&E

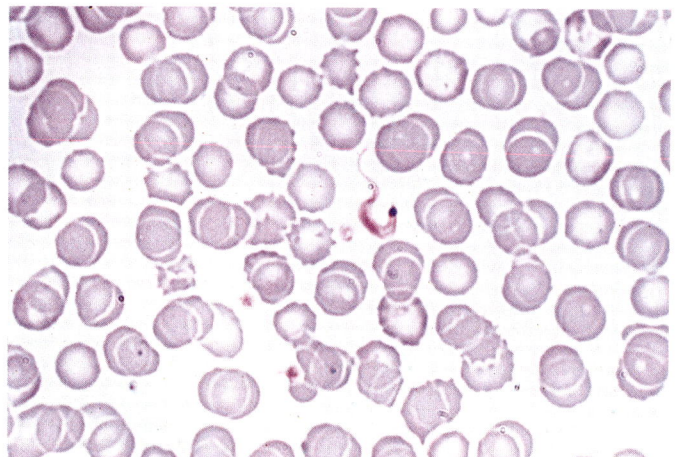

Fig. 1.4 Trypomastigote of *Trypanosoma cruzi* in a blood smear. Giemsa

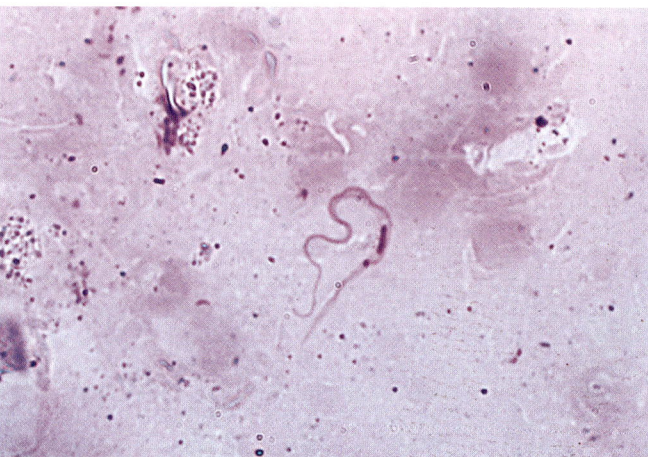

Fig. 1.5 Trypomastigote of *Trypanosoma rangeli* in a blood smear. Giemsa

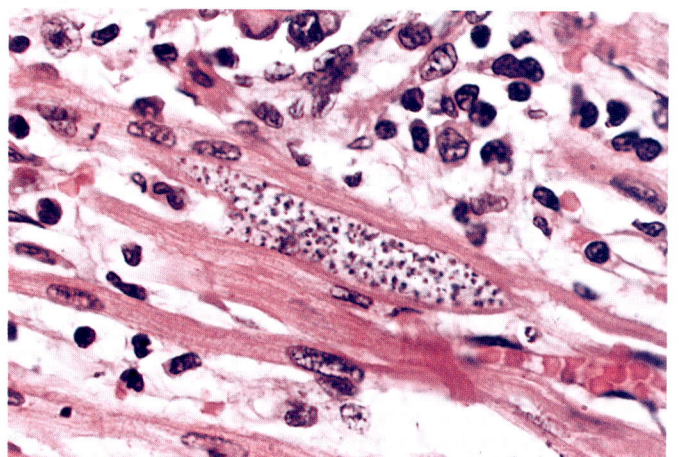

Fig. 1.6 Nest of amastigotes (parasites without flagellum) of *Trypanosoma cruzi* in a muscle fibre of myocardium. H&E

Trypanosoma cruzi may be isolated from human and animal blood relatively easily, as well as from the intestinal tract of the vectors in the culture medium known as NNN (for composition, see the section on Visceral Leishmaniasis). In the culture media, the trypomastigotes of *T. cruzi* are called epimastigotes and are often arranged in a rosette pattern. If preservation of live strains of trypanosomes for a longer period is planned, it is necessary to include intermediate steps in animals and subcultures.

Numerous species of mammals are reservoirs of *T. cruzi*, including, among others, marsupials, bats, rodents, dogs, cats, pigs and monkeys.

Regarding the vectors, 66 species of the genus *Triatoma*, bugs of the family Reduviidae, have been found to be naturally infected with *T. cruzi* (Fig. 1.8). Their habitat extends from sea level to an altitude of 800–1200 m. They are found predominantly in the thatched roofs of rural houses.

Pathogenesis

In the **acute form** of the infection, pathogenesis is easy to understand. Transmission of *T. cruzi* occurs from man to man or animal to man through defecation after the insect bite, more rarely through blood transfusions or, occasionally, diaplacentally. By contrast, transmission of *T. rangeli* takes place directly through an insect bite and not via evacuation.

The metacyclic trypomastigotes, the infectious forms of *T. cruzi* which develop from the epimastigotes in the insect gut contents, enter the host through damaged mucosa or skin. At the conjunctiva, the so-called 'Romaña sign' may be observed (Fig. 1.9). It consists of a unilateral palpebral oedema with conjunctivitis and swelling of the regional lymph nodes. In other cases, a skin nodule may appear at the site of penetration by the parasite, appearing 1–2 weeks after the bite, and is called the 'chagoma of inoculation'. It must be emphasized, however, that, in the majority of cases, the point of entrance cannot be determined. We do not know of any reports of the histological patterns of the portal of entry by biopsy.

Once in the vertebrate host, at the point of entrance, the trypomastigotes enter tissue cells where they lose the flagellum and replicate as rounded amastigotes. Later, they reach the blood stream as trypomastigotes and may thus reach other organs. Here, again, they become amastigotes and produce a tissue reaction; in the heart this takes the form of an acute diffuse myocarditis. The amastigotes reproduce in the intracellular nests until they rupture 2–4 weeks after formation (Fig. 1.10), and the parasites 'disappear'. In reality, they do not disappear; they may return later to the blood stream in the flagellate form (trypomastigotes) and so an endogenous re-infection may take place. In addition, they may be withdrawn from the blood stream by another insect bite. Experimentally, it has been shown recently that, in lower animals, amastigotes are circulating in the blood stream and that they are as infective as trypomastigotes[11].

The pathogenesis of **chronic Chagas myocarditis** remains unknown. This is, in part, due to the difficulty of detecting parasites in the myocardium at this stage of the disease and to the similarities between this and the tissue reaction of so-called idiopathic myocarditis of Fiedler[12]. Several theories of pathogenesis have been proposed[13–15]. The two most favoured hypotheses are the antiheart immune or autoimmune reactions[16,17] and the neurogenic theory of the influence of damage to the vegetative nervous system[18,19]. There are several aspects of the neurogenic theory which deserve comment: the morphological and functional bases of this theory were initially obtained from study of Chagas disease patients at very advanced stages of the disease[20]. More recent clinical[21–23]

and experimental[24,25] studies indicate that myocardial damage may precede the cardiac parasympathetic abnormalities. The reduction in the number of cardiac vagal neurons[26] and the functional disorders of cardiac parasympathetic innervation[27] are also seen in patients with ventricular dilatation who do not have Chagas disease. It seems, then, that the cardiac parasympathetic abnormalities are secondary to the progressive dilatation of the cardiac chambers[28].

We believe that chronic Chagas myocarditis may be due to repeated exogenous and/or endogenous re-infections.

Pathology

The organs which may have intracellular amastigotes of *T. cruzi* in man are those with various types of the musculature cells: smooth muscle cells of the digestive tract as well as skeletal muscle fibres and myocardial muscle fibres. Damage of the latter is of most importance. Furthermore, brain tissue may be affected with amastigote nests in the glial cells; also, the placenta with subsequent congenital trypanosomiasis and, rarely, the testicles. In numerous autopsies performed by the authors, parasites were looked for in the organs of the PMS (lymph nodes, liver, spleen, bone marrow), in other parenchymal organs and in the vegetative nervous system, but were not found[29]. This is in contrast to the findings reported in numerous books. However, in experimentally infected lower animals, amastigotes of *T. cruzi* may be located in cells of numerous viscera.

Gross lesions in the **acute form** of Chagas disease are observed in the heart (Figs. 1.11–1.13), brain and the musculature of the digestive tract, including the tongue. The heart shows hypertrophy and dilatation, the latter developing in the final days with diminished consistency. The myocardium may reveal a fish-flesh or cooked-meat-like aspect or foci of various sizes of a yellowish-white colour are found. In the brain, oedema and multiple petechiae are observed.

In the **chronic form**, hypertrophy and dilatation, mostly of the left ventricle are present. Coronary arteries, even in older patients, are not usually affected. On the surface of the heart, a subepicardial rosary, i.e. a chain of small fibrotic nodules, is seen (Fig. 1.14). Quite often, parietal aneurysms can be observed, in addition to various numbers of whitish scars in the myocardium of variable sizes and shapes. However, none of these lesions is pathognomonic. This means that all these alterations may also appear in cardiopathies with other aetiologies (Fig. 1.15). Aneurysms are mainly located at the apex of the left ventricle; they are thin-walled showing fibrotic tissue and contain thrombi (Fig. 1.16). From these thrombi, arterial embolism often takes place with subsequent infarction in numerous organs.

Regarding **histology**, the parasites appear in tissue sections as amastigotes in intracellular nests, i.e. as parasites without flagella. It must be emphasized that characteristic kinetoplasts in the amastigotes are seen mostly in preparations after recent penetration into tissue cells and when the tissue is removed early and well preserved. This means that these structures are not found in each and every case. In tissue sections of routine autopsies, we only rarely saw the kinetoplasts. We therefore stress that amastigotes are almost never recognized as such, with all the structural details, in tissue sections. They are mostly indistinguishable from other small microorganisms with the H&E stain.

Morphologically, amastigotes are also indistinguishable from species of *Leishmania*. In order to differentiate between these two, we must consider that each of these parasites has particular and specific locations in tissues and the corresponding organs. Small yeast cells are

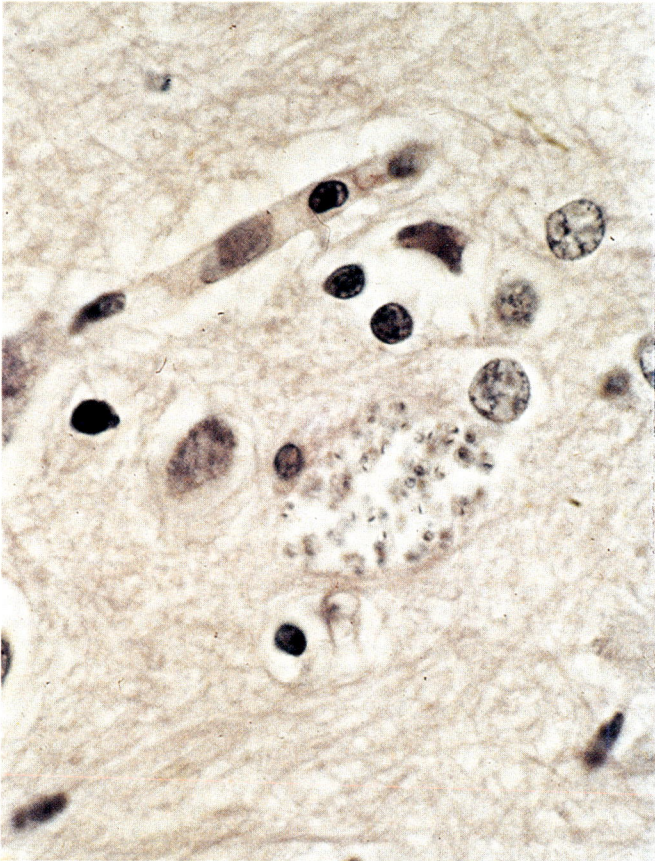

Fig. 1.7 Nest of amastigotes of *Trypanosoma cruzi* in a glial cell (pseudocyst). Rod-like kinetoplasts are visible. H&E

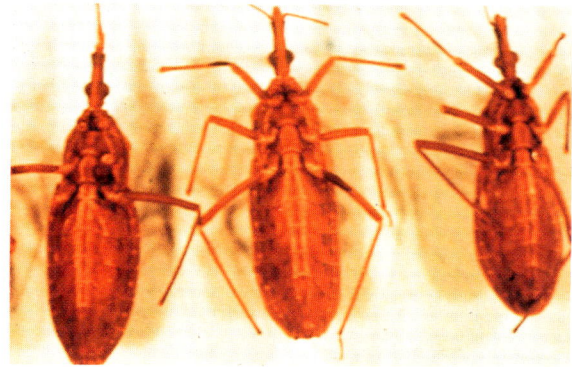

Fig. 1.8 Triatomines (*Rhodnius prolixus*), vectors of Chagas disease

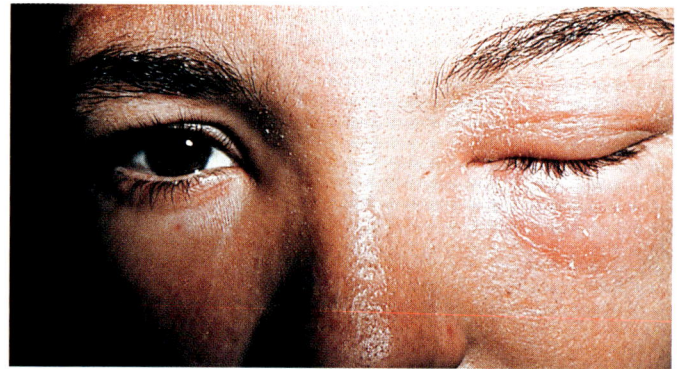

Fig. 1.9 'Romaña's sign' in a *Trypanosoma cruzi* infected patient from Venezuela. This periorbital and unilateral oedema marks the site of entry of the parasite

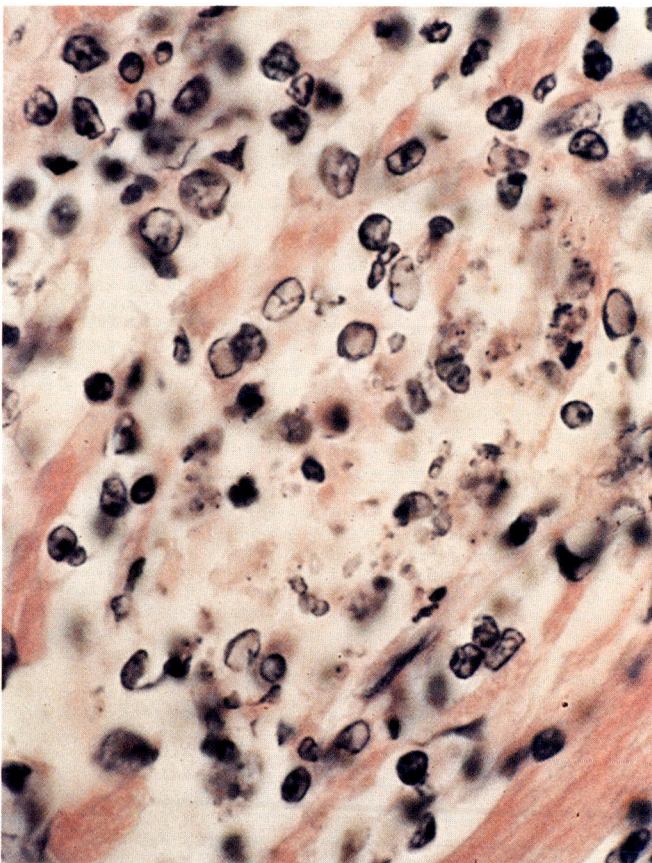

Fig. 1.11 Acute fatal form of Chagas disease with cardiomegaly

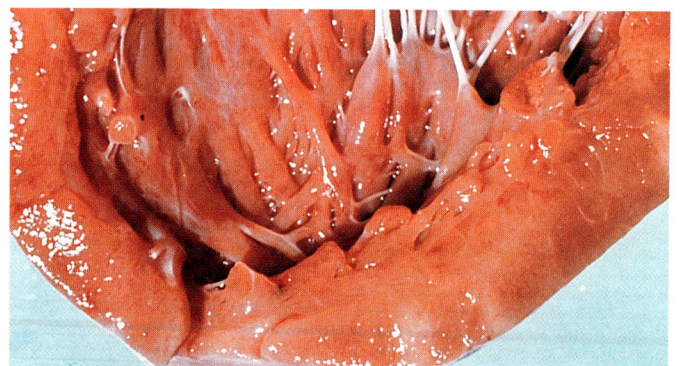

Fig. 1.10 Ruptured nest of *Trypanosoma cruzi* in the acute myocarditis of an infant, one month after becoming ill with fever. H&E

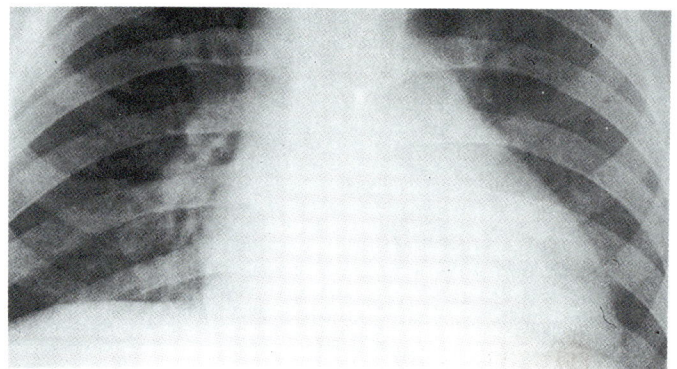

Fig. 1.12 Fish-flesh appearance of the myocardium in acute Chagas myocarditis

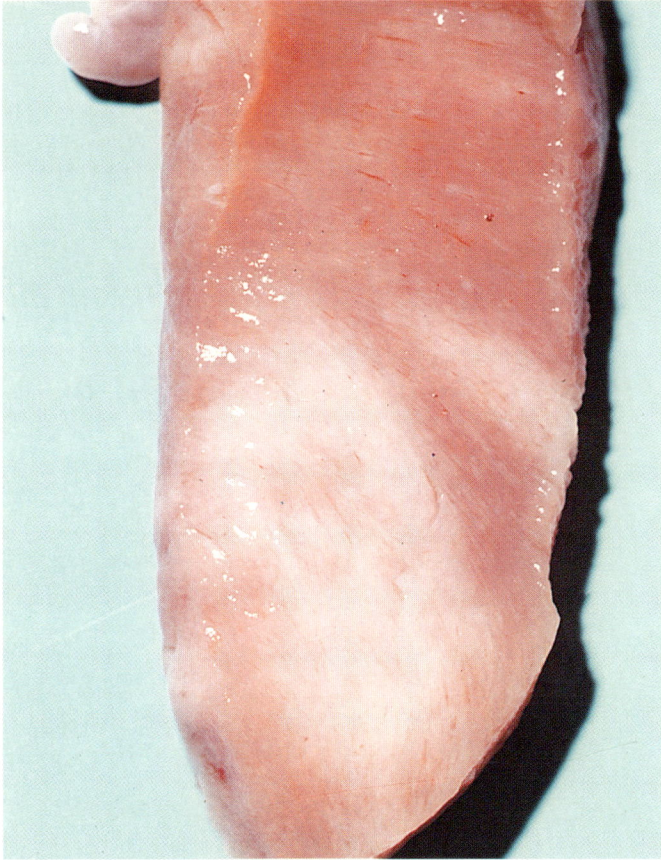

Fig. 1.13 Whitish spots on the cut surface of myocardium in a case of acute Chagas myocarditis

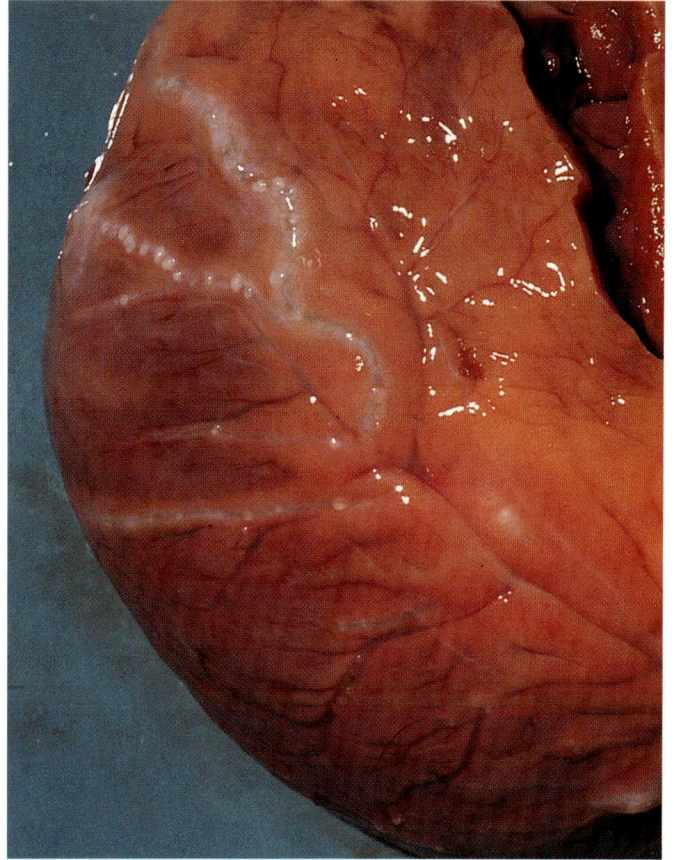

Fig. 1.14 Subepicardial 'rosary' considered typical in cases of chronic Chagas myocarditis

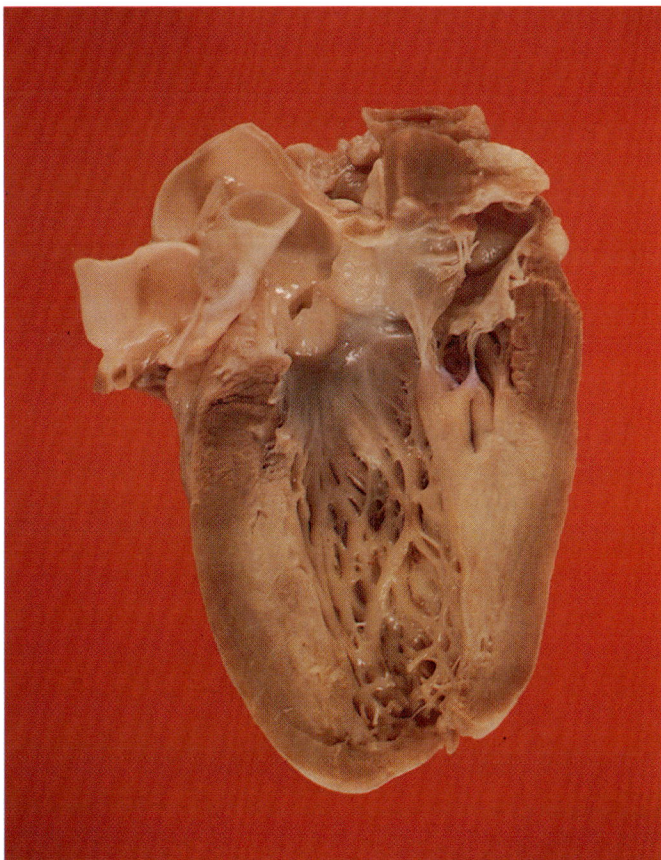

Fig. 1.15 Acute myocarditis in an infant from Mérida. Parasites could not be found in tissues in this case

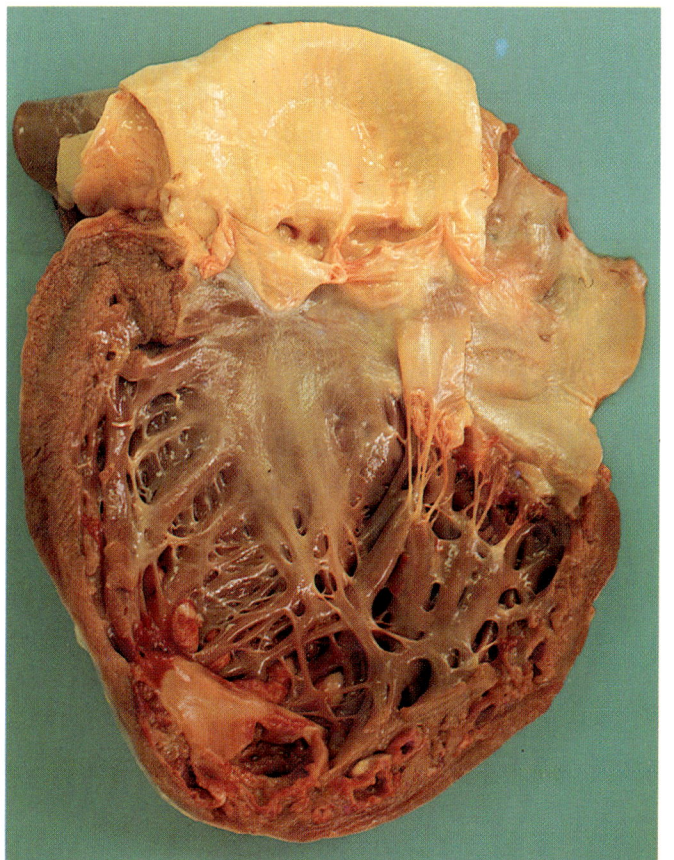

Fig. 1.16 Apical aneurysm of the left ventricle with thrombus in a case of chronic myocarditis

Grocott-positive while small protozoan organisms generally are Grocott-negative. Outside muscle fibres and glial cells, we have never seen parasites in other cells (macrophages or endothelial cells).

The tissue reaction found at the level of myocardium in the **acute form** is a marked cellular infiltration, more or less diffuse (Figs. 1.17 and 1.18), where lymphocytes, histiocytes and plasma cells can be seen while the number of leukocytes is reduced. In wide areas, the muscle fibres disappear because they have been totally replaced by the infiltrates. This is a true myocarditis, apparently as a result of the action of parasites present in variable numbers of intracellular (myocardial fibres) nests. We are, therefore, at a loss to understand why nowadays numerous researchers call this typical inflammatory process of the disease myocardiopathy, instead of myocarditis.

As far as the central nervous system is concerned, the inflammatory process is disseminated and localized in the white and grey matter. In the white matter, there is a diffuse gliosis present. The reaction of the neurocytes is mild and non-specific. The parasitic cells or nests of them are hardly ever surrounded by cellular infiltrates. Notably, the intracellular localizations of amastigotes are seldom recognized as such with a light microscope. There are three main types of lesions:

1. Small granuloma-like cell infiltrates (100–500 μm), often situated near arterioles but also 'free' in the parenchyma, composed of lymphocytes and histiocytes as well as microglial rod-like cells.

2. Cuff-like cellular infiltrates in the perivascular Virchow–Robins' spaces formed by lymphocytes, plasma cells and monocytes.

3. Small glial nodules consisting of astrocytes with rod-like microglial cells. A non-specific meningitis occurs occasionally, in addition to acute Chagas encephalitis. Primary Chagas meningitis has not, to our knowledge, been reported (Figs. 1.19–1.23).

In other organs, the parasites cause a non-specific, often scarce, inflammation, usually of the interstitial type (Figs 1.24–1.28). In Chagas orchitis, parasites are located inside seminiferous tubules, and cellular infiltrates are present in the interstitium (Fig. 1.29).

In the **chronic form**, the heart is the main organ involved. Lesions in the brain are not observed. The chronic myocarditis shows areas of fibrosis of variable size, with and without cellular infiltrates, either totally or partially replacing the muscle tissue (Figs. 1.30–1.34). If exclusive fibrosis is observed, without cellular infiltrates or with only scarce ones, a diagnosis of myocarditis may be questionable.

The cellular infiltrates are made up primarily of lymphocytes, histiocytes, plasma cells and, very rarely, neutrophilic leukocytes. Sometimes, a variable number of eosinophilic leukocytes is observed and, occasionally, myogenous multinuclear giant cells are found. The origin of the myogenous giant cells, i.e. that they grow from muscle fibres, could be corroborated in one case, when lipofuscin pigment was observed in a giant cell (Fig. 1.35). The presence of giant cells does not indicate a granulomatous reaction because of the lack of epithelioid cells. Micronecroses are found occasionally in cases of chronic myocarditis as well as typical acute cardiac infarcts.

In the great majority of all these cases, parasites cannot be found in the tissues in spite of intensive and prolonged search. In practice, therefore the question arises of whether one is faced with myocarditis due to infection with trypanosomes or with the so-called 'chronic idiopathic myocarditis' which occurs all over the world and,

obviously, also in regions of endemic Chagas disease.

Regarding the so-called endomyocardial fibrosis, a well-known entity in Africa and in some way related to African trypanosomiasis, it cannot be ruled out that this cardiopathy in South America has links with the *Trypanosoma cruzi* infection. However, only few cases of this sort have been observed in South America.

So-called mega-organs, mostly reported in Brazil, Argentina and Chile, have not been found in Venezuela.

References

1. Schenone, H. and Rojas, A. (1989). Algunos datos y observaciones pragmáticas en relación a la epidemiolgía de la enfermedad de Chagas. *Bol. Chil. Parasitol.*, **44**, 66
2. Brass, K. (1955). Statistische Untersuchungen über die idiopathische Myokarditis im Raum Valencia, Venezuela. *Frankf. Z. Path.*, **66**, 77
3. Doehnert, H. R. and Motta, G. (1965). Enfermedad de Chagas y miocarditis crónica. *Arch. Venez. Med. Trop. Parasit. Med.*, **5**, 124
4. Maeckelt, G. A. (1965). *El Diagnóstico Parásito-immunológico de la Infección Chagásica.* Universidad Central de Venezuela, Caracas
5. Salfelder, K. (1971). *Pathologisch-anatomische Probleme der Chagas-myokarditis, Krongressber.* II. Tag. Oester. Ges. Tropenmed., IV. Tag. Dtsch. Tropenmed. Ges. Verlags. Kont. H. Scheffler, Luebeck, p. 72
6. Sauerteig, E. (1978). Es todavía la enfermedad de Chagas un problema de salud pública? Hospital "Dr. Luis Razetti", Barinas/Venezeula
7. Novoa Montero, D. A. (1983). Chagas' disease and chronic myocardiopathy: An epidemiologic study of four Venezuelan rural communities. *Doctoral thesis.* The Johns Hopkins School of Hygiene and Public Health, Baltimore
8. Novoa Montero, D. A. (1990). Similar death rates among chagasic and non-chagasic Venezuelan rural adults through a 12-year follow-up study. *XL Conven. An. ASOVAC,* Cumaná/Venezuela
9. Chandler, F. W. and Watts, J. C. (1988). Immunofluorescence as an adjunct to the histopathologic diagnosis of Chagas' disease. *J. Clin. Microbiol.*, **26**, 567
10. Schottelius, J. (1984). Differentiation between Trypanosoma cruzi and Trypanosoma rangeli on the basis of their sialic acid content. *Tropenmed. Parasit.*, **35**, 160
11. Ley, V., Andrews, N. W., Robbins, E. S. and Nussenzweig, V. (1988). Amastigotes of Trypanosoma cruzi sustain an infective cycle in mammalian cells. *J. Exp. Med.*, **168**, 649
12. Fiedler, F. (1899). Festschr. 4. Stadtkrankenhaus Dresden-Friedrichstadt
13. Tanowitz, H. B. *et al.* (1990). Enhanced platelet adherence and aggregation in Chagas' disease: a potential pathogenic mechanism for cardiomyopathy. *Am. J. Trop. Med. Hyg.*, **43**, 274
14. Morris, S. A. *et al.* (1990). Pathophysiological insights into the cardiomyopathy of Chagas' disease. *Circulation*, **82**, 1900
15. Andrade, S. G. (1990). Influence of Trypanosoma cruzi strain on the pathogenesis of chronic myocardiopathy in mice. *Mem. Inst. Oswaldo Cruz*, **85**, 17
16. Jaffé, R. Dominguez, A., Kozma, C. and Gavaller, B. V. (1962). Bemerkungen zur Pathogenese der Chagaskrankheit. *Z. Tropenmed. Parasit.*, **12**, 2
17. Cossio, P. M. *et al.* (1977). Chagasic cardiopathy. Immunopathologic and morphologic studies in myocardial biopsies. *Am. J. Pathol.*, **86**, 533
18. Koeberle, F. (1959). Cardiopathia parasympathicopriva. *Münch. Med. Wschr.*, **101**, 1308
19. Oliveira, J. S. M. (1985). A natural model of intrinsic heart nervous system denervation: Chagas' cardiopathy. *Am. Heart J.*, **110**, 1092
20. Amorim, D. S. *et al.* (1982). Chagas' disease as an experimental model for studies of cardiac autonomic function in man. *Mayo Clin. Proc.*, **57**, 42
21. Davila, D. F. (1988). Heart rate response to atropine and left ventricular function in Chagas' heart disease. *Int. J. Cardiol.*, **21**, 143
22. Fuenmayor, A. J. *et al.* (1988). The Valsalva maneuver, a test of the functional status of cardiac innervation in chagasic myocarditis. *Int. J. Cardiol.*, **18**, 351
23. Casado, J., Davila, D. F. *et al.* (1990). Electrocardiographic abnormalities and left ventricular systolic function in Chagas' heart disease. *Int. J. Cardiol.*, **27**, 55
24. Davila, D. F. (1988). Vagal stimulation and heart rate slowing in

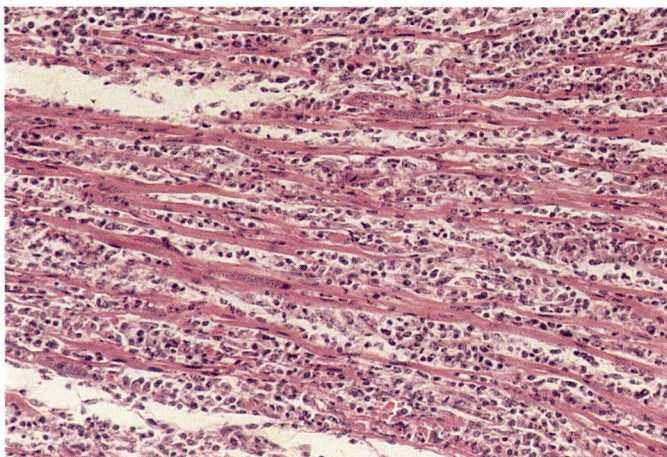

Fig. 1.17 Acute diffuse chagasic myocarditis. Nests of parasites are difficult to discern at this magnification. H&E

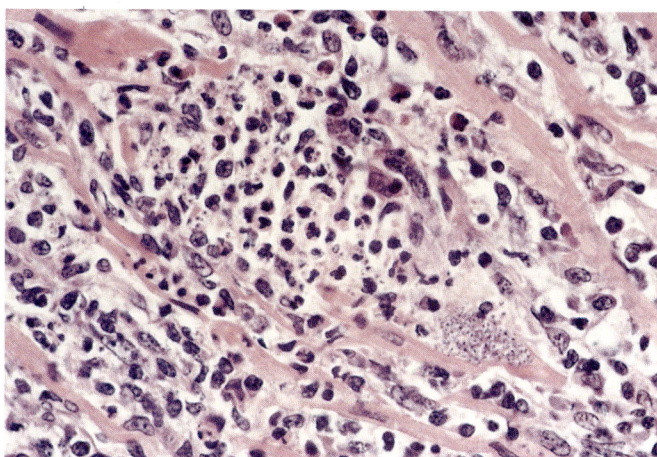

Fig. 1.18 Acute chagasic myocarditis at higher power with muscle fibres replaced by cellular infiltrates and a nest of parasites faintly visible. H&E

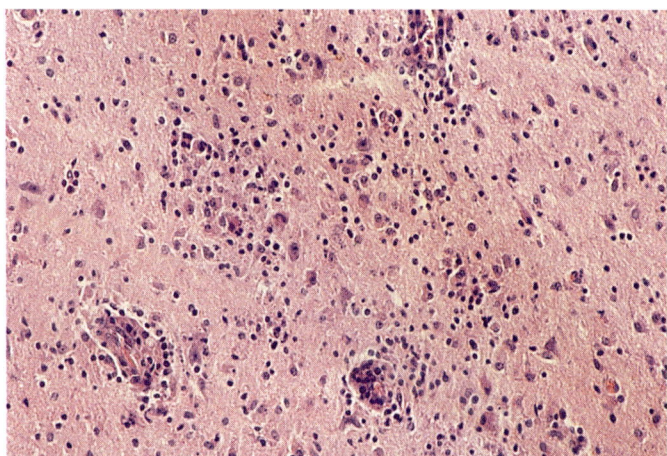

Fig. 1.19 Acute chagasic encephalitis at low power. H&E

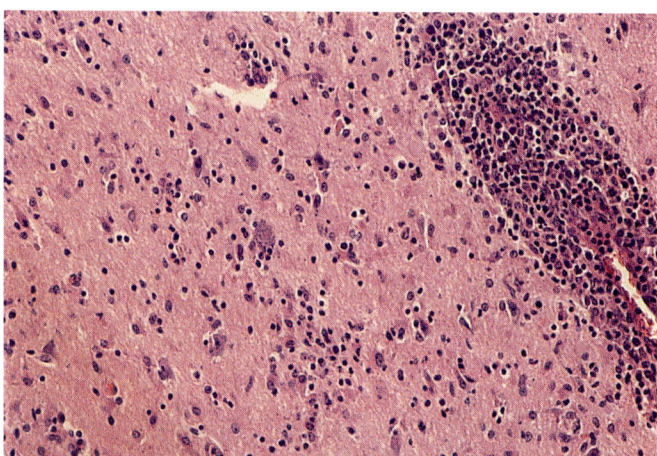

Fig. 1.20 Acute chagasic encephalitis with a marked perivascular cell infiltrate. H&E

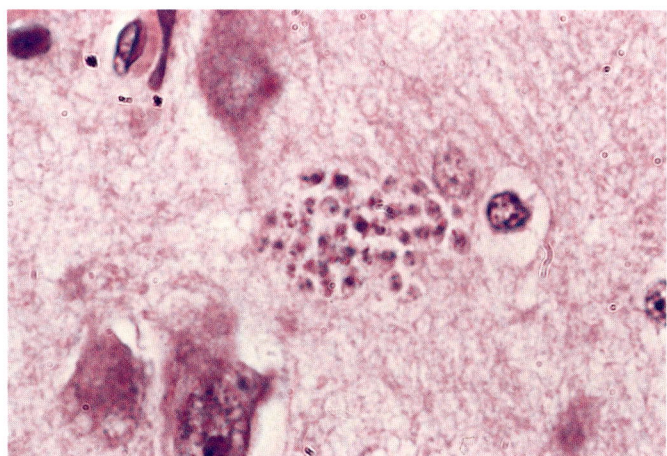

Fig. 1.21 Nest of *Trypanosoma cruzi* amastigotes in the brain without inflammatory reaction. Outlines of a glial cell not visible. H&E

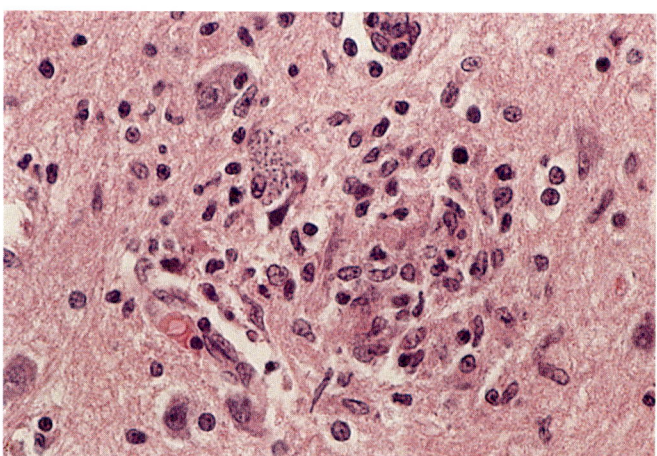

Fig. 1.22 Parasitic nest in the cellular infiltrate of an acute chagasic encephalitis. H&E

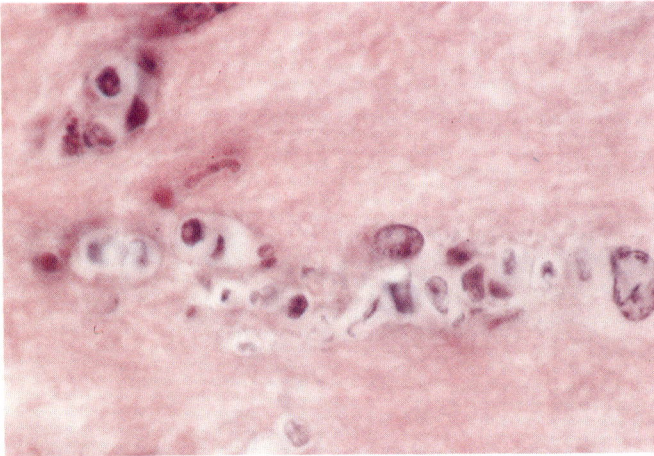

Fig. 1.23 Necrobiotic cells in an acute chagasic encephalitis mimicking parasitic structures. H&E

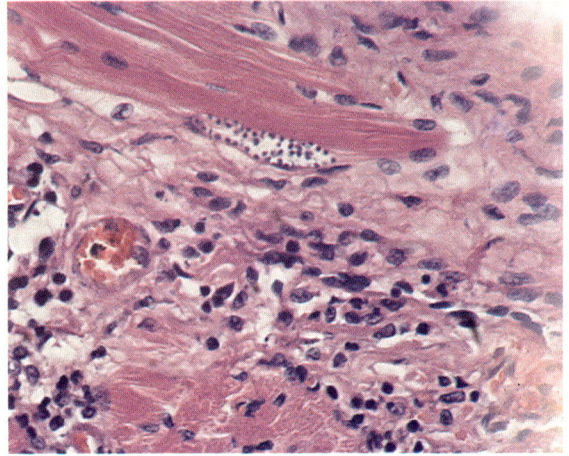

Fig. 1.24 Marked inflammation in acute chagasic oesophagitis. H&E

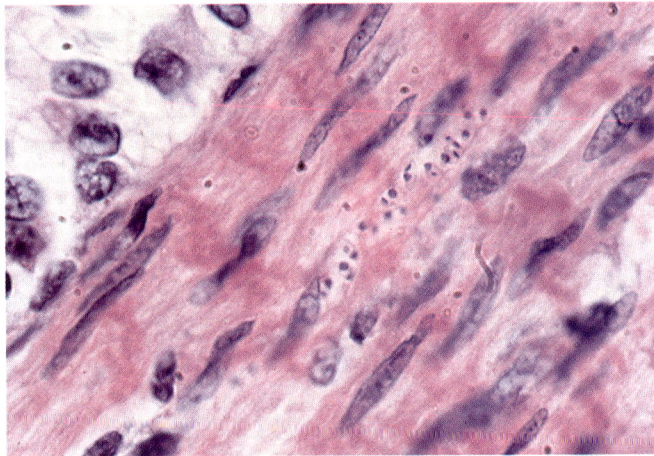

Fig. 1.25 Acute chagasic enteritis. H&E

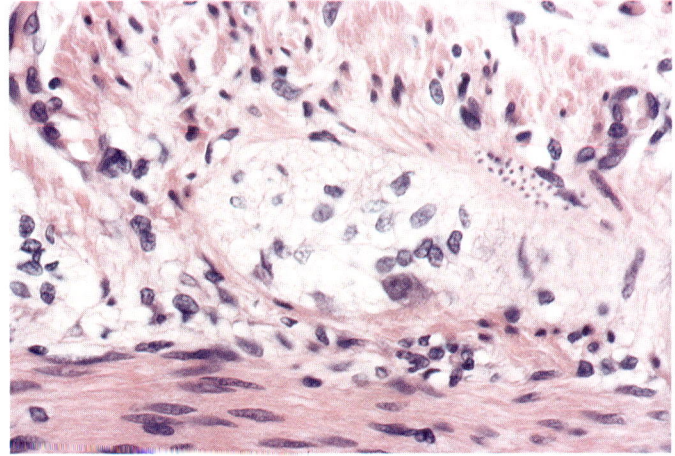

Fig. 1.26 Acute chagasic colitis. Note parasites localized in the digestive tract in muscle cells. H&E

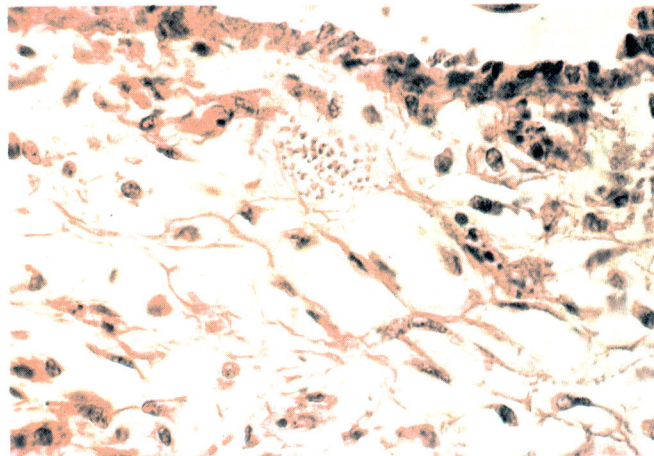

Fig. 1.27 Nest of *Trypanosoma cruzi* amastigotes in placental villus. A case of congenital Chagas infection. H&E

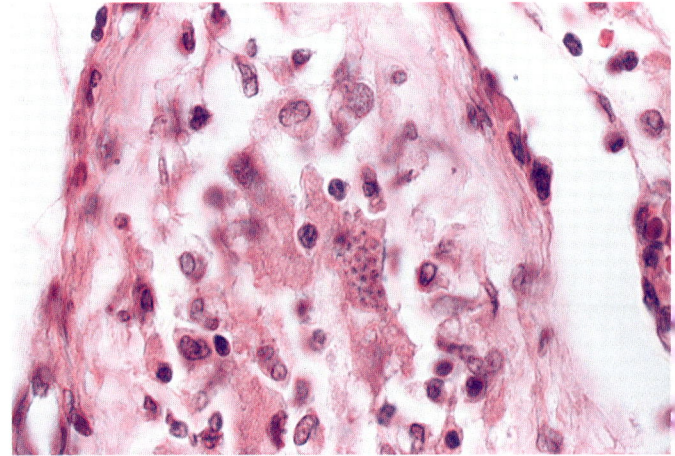

Fig. 1.28 Same case as Fig. 1.27 at higher power. H&E

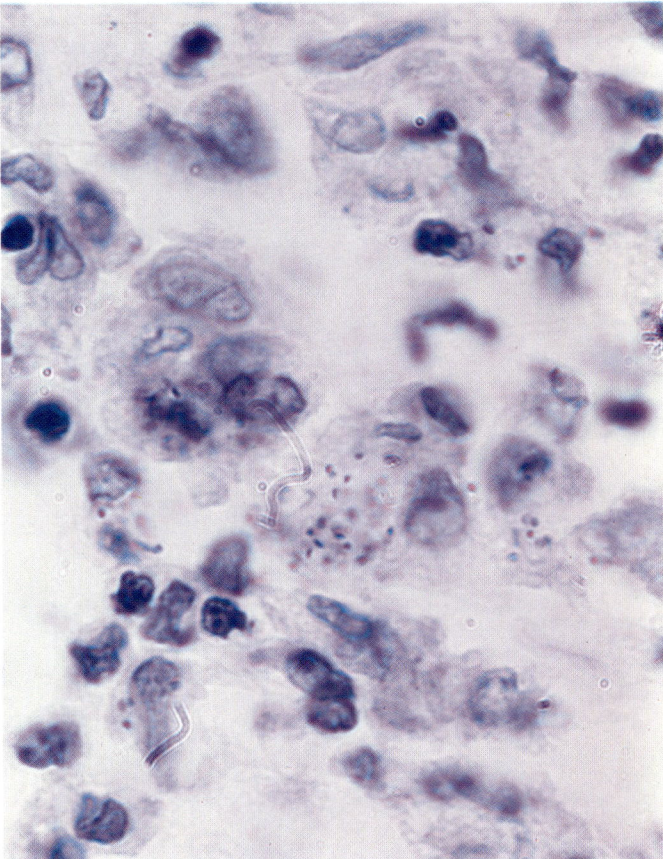

Fig. 1.29 Chagas orchitis with nests of parasites in a seminiferous tubule. Giemsa

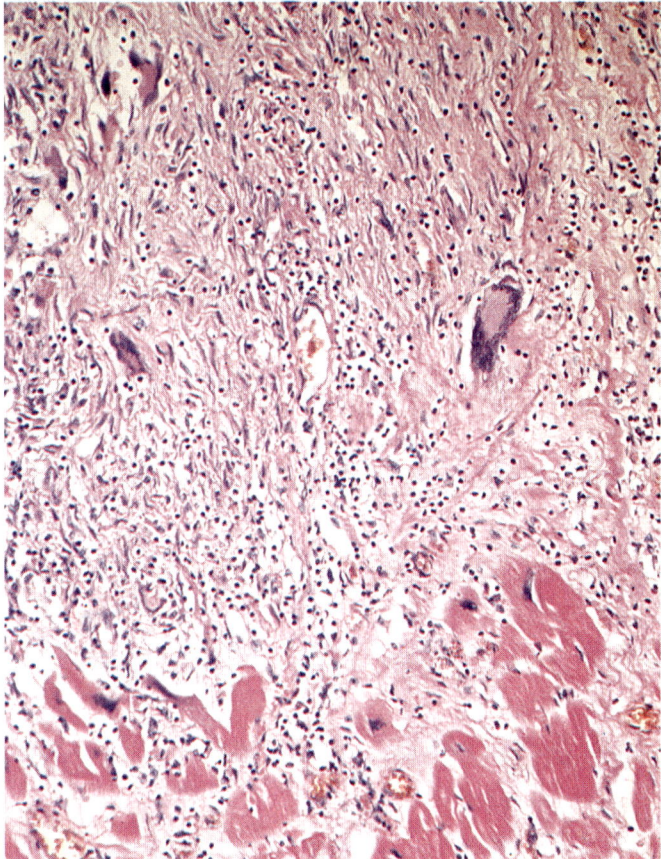

Fig. 1.30 Chronic myocarditis with several myogenous giant cells. H&E

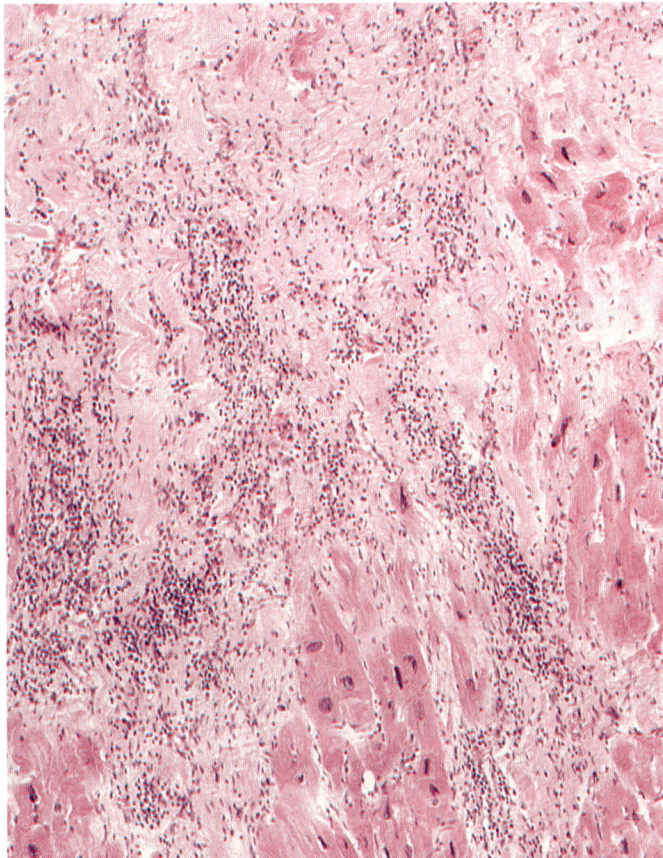

Fig. 1.31 Chronic myocarditis with fibrosis and focal cellular infiltrates. H&E

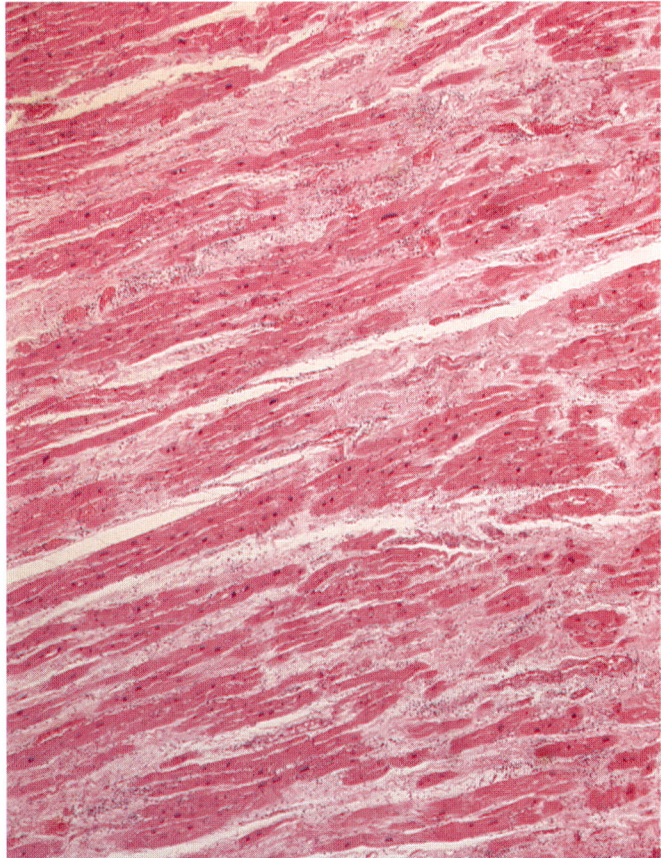

Fig. 1.32 Chronic myocarditis with marked fibrosis and scarce cellular infiltrates. H&E

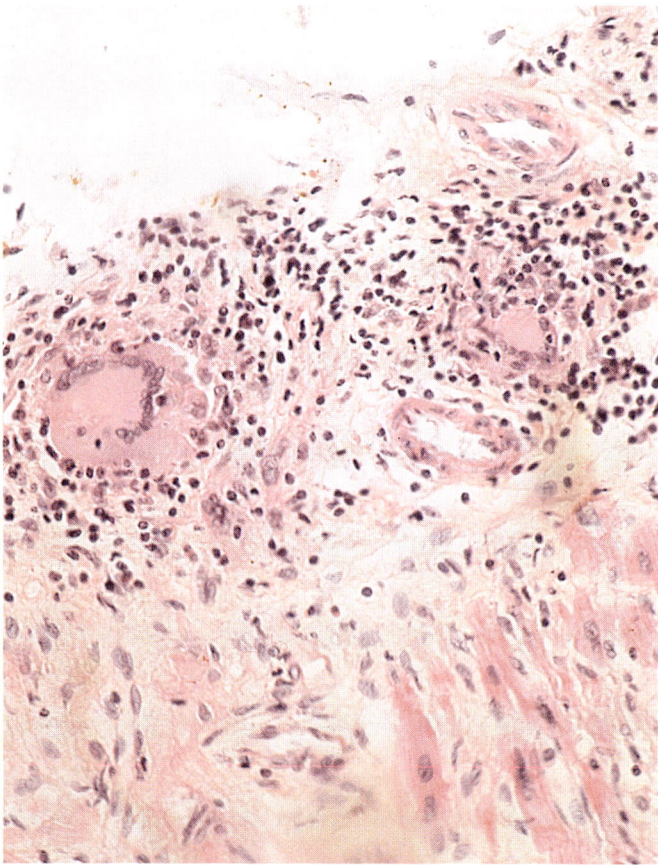

Fig. 1.33 Chronic granulomatous myocarditis of unknown aetiology. H&E

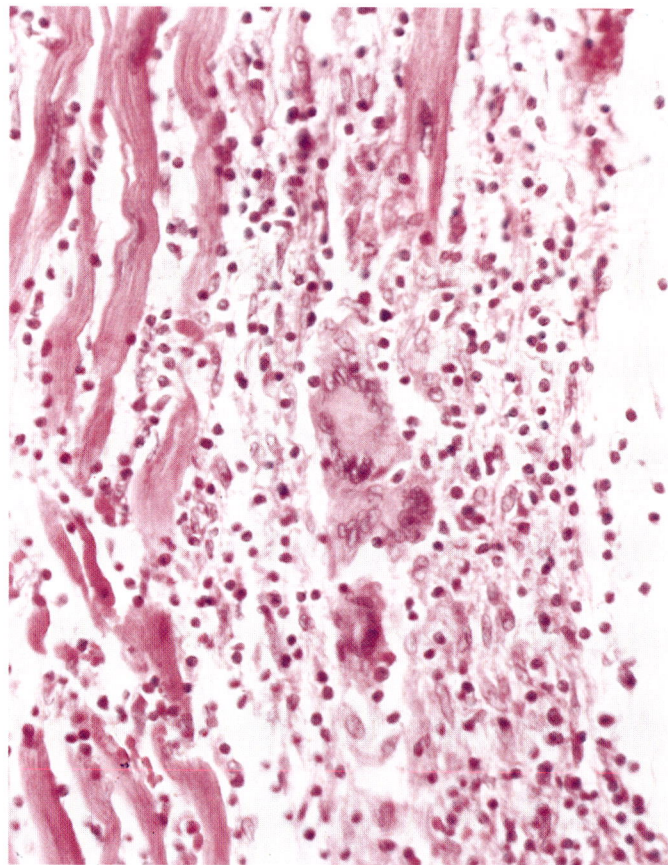

Fig. 1.34 Another case of chronic myocarditis with giant cells and undetermined aetiology. H&E

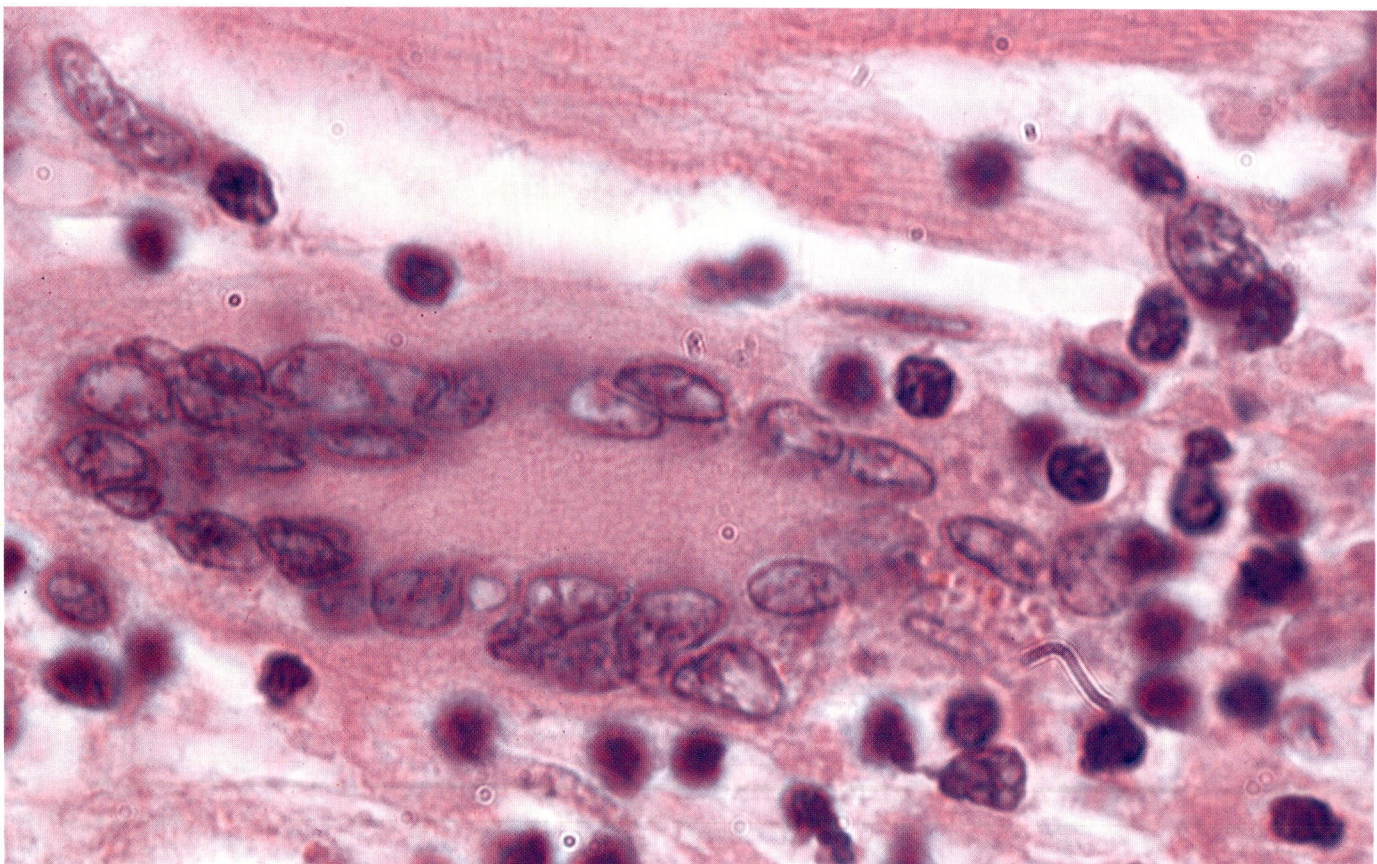

Fig. 1.35 Myogenous giant cell in a case of chronic myocarditis showing granules of lipofuscin pigment, thus revealing the myogenous origin of the giant cell. H&E

acute chagasic myocarditis. *J. Auton. Nerv. Syst.*, **25**, 233

25. Gottberg, C. F. *et al.* (1988). Heart rate changes in acute chagasic myocarditis. *Trans. R. Soc. Trop. Med. Hyg.*, **82**, 851

26. Amorim, D. S. and Olsen, E. G. J. (1982). Assessment of heart neurons in dilated (congestive) cardiomyopathy. *Br. Heart J.*, **47**, 11

27. Amorim, D. S. (1981). Is there autonomic impairment in (congestive) dilated cardiomyopathy. *Lancet*, **1**, 525

28. Davila, D. F. (1989). Cardiac parasympathetic abnormalities. Cause or consequence of Chagas' heart disease? *Parasitol. Today*, **5**, 327

29. Sauerteig, E. (1991). Chagaskrankheit. In *Tropenmedizin in Klinik und Praxis*. Thieme Verlag, Germany (in press)

2. AFRICAN TRYPANOSOMIASIS

Introduction

This infection is also known as sleeping sickness. Epidemics with high mortality rates had depopulated vast regions of Africa. The preventive campaigns of the WHO to control the vectors have had the result of limiting considerably this disease. Also, it has been possible to treat cases with effective drugs. However, eradication of vectors has not been total; still more or less important epidemics occur. WHO experts believe that, in spite of all efforts, complete extermination of this disease will not take place in the near future.

Natural infections occur in domestic and wild animals[1]. The disease may be produced by inoculation into laboratory animals[2-5] (Fig. 2.1).

In African trypanosomiasis, histological preparations do not show the parasites as amastigotes, in contrast to American trypanosomiasis. This must be emphasized as the most important morphological difference between these two parasitoses.

The infection is limited to equatorial Africa. Two forms of the disease may be distinguished: in the western and central parts of this continent, a chronic and relatively benign disease is observed[6]. In the later stages, symptoms of the CNS appear and the outcome may be fatal. In the eastern parts of the continent, on the other hand, the disease takes a more severe course. In untreated patients, death occurs, frequently 1–3 months after infection[7]. Clinical diagnosis in early stages of the disease may be made by observing trypomastigotes in blood smears and smears of puncture fluids taken from the chancre, lymph nodes, body cavities and also of the spinal fluid. Cultures can be made on artificial media[8] or by inoculation of rodents and monkeys.

The parasite

The three species of African trypanosomes belong, like *Trypanosoma cruzi*, to the genus *Trypanosoma* and the family Trypanosomatidae. *Trypanosoma brucei gambiense* is responsible for human infection in the western and central parts of the continent, *Trypanosoma brucei rhodesiense* in eastern parts and *Trypanosoma brucei brucei* is only a pathogen in domestic animals. All three are structurally identical. They differ in their pathogenicity in man and lower animals.

Both *T. gambiense* and *T. rhodesiense* each have a specific group of vectors, live in different geographical regions and have different reservoir hosts. They do infect superior vertebrates, but, in general, do not cause disease; that is, these animals are reservoir hosts and a source of infection for man but do not become ill. On the other hand, domestic animals, such as horses, donkeys, camels, dogs and cats, fall ill when infected by trypanosomes belonging to the species *T. brucei brucei*. The disease is called 'Ngana', which means 'useless' or 'weak' and has a fairly high mortality rate. Some wild animal species, certain domestic animals and man, on the other hand, do not become ill when infected by *T. brucei brucei*.

The three species appear only in the flagellate form (trypomastigotes) and have variable sizes (Fig. 2.2). Trypomastigotes succumb fast: a good fixation is required to preserve them. In stained smears, the trypomastigotes measure 1.5–3.5 μm in width and 15–30 μm in length, including the flagellum. The nucleus stains dark with the Giemsa, Wright and other similar stains and is situated towards the centre.

The trypomastigotes are difficult to recognize in unstained smears because they are colourless, thin and transparent. However, it is possible to detect them when they are alive because of their motility. This type of trypanosome has a small kinetoplast situated near the rear end. The flagellum originates in the blepharoplast near the kinetoplast, which, however, is not identifiable with a light microscope. Trypanosomes of this type may multiply by longitudinal division of the trypomastigote. This is in contrast to *Trypanosoma cruzi* which reproduces only in the amastigote form.

Man is the principal reservoir host for *T. brucei gambiense*, but wild and domestic animals (pigs for example) may act as reservoir hosts. However, wild animals (above all antilopes) and also domestic animals are the principal hosts for *T. rhodesiense*, infection from man to man being less frequent.

The vector for *T. brucei gambiense* and *T. brucei rhodesiense* is the tsetse fly (Fig. 2.3), *Glossina palpalis* and *Glossina morsitans*, respectively. These species do not have important structural differences. Either male or female fly may act as vector.

Pathogenesis

When the non-infected tsetse fly (*Glossina* spp.) bites an infected man or lower animal, it sucks blood and, with it, the trypanosomes, which then reach the intestinal tract of the vector. The parasites multiply in the gut of the fly and three weeks later they reach the salivary glands, in the meantime having become metacyclic and infectious.

Therefore, when an infected fly bites a healthy man, it transmits the trypanosomes. This bite, by the way, is painful. At the site of the bite, which is almost always the cervical region, a skin nodule is produced and inflammation of the regional lymph nodes develops. Both lesions constitute the 'inoculation chancre' of the African trypanosomiasis, also named Winterbottom's symptom (Fig. 2.4). From this focal cutaneous lesion, haematogenous dissemination results, with clinical manifestations of fever, general malaise and splenomegaly. In experiments recently carried out on lower animals, it has been found that the parasites first reach the meninges; encephalitis develops later in addition to the meningitis[2].

Pathology

Both the gross and the microscopic lesions are similar in the two forms of African trypanosomiasis[9]. The CNS, lymph nodes, spleen and heart are all involved and sometimes there are effusions in all corporal cavities. In the central nervous system oedema and petechiae are found as gross lesions. The lymph nodes and the spleen may be enlarged. Apparently, no other gross manifestations have been observed and no specific gross features characteristic for this infection are known.

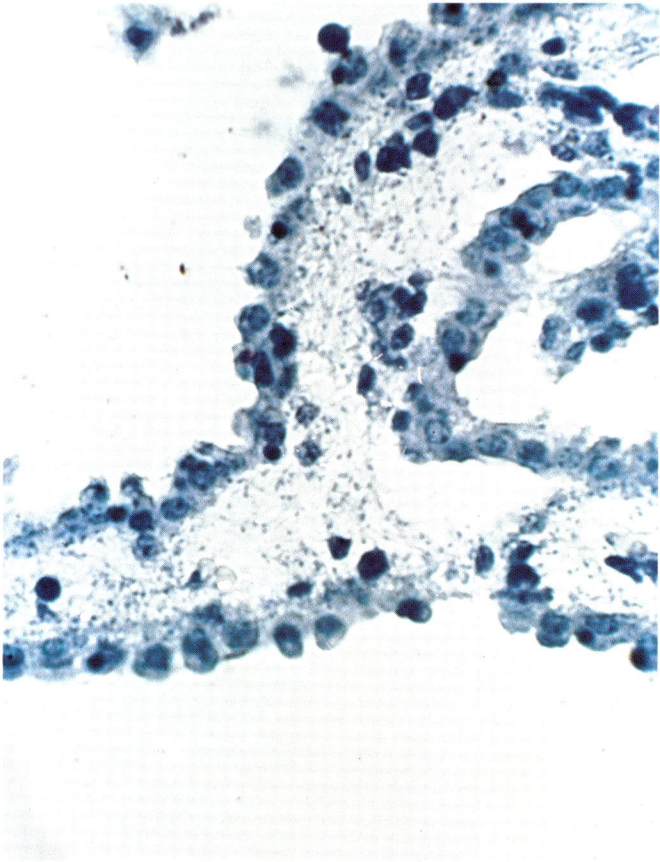

Fig. 2.1 Numerous amastigotes of *Trypanosoma rhodesiense* in a villus of the choroid plexus. Experimental infection of a mouse (H. Schmidt, 1983). Giemsa

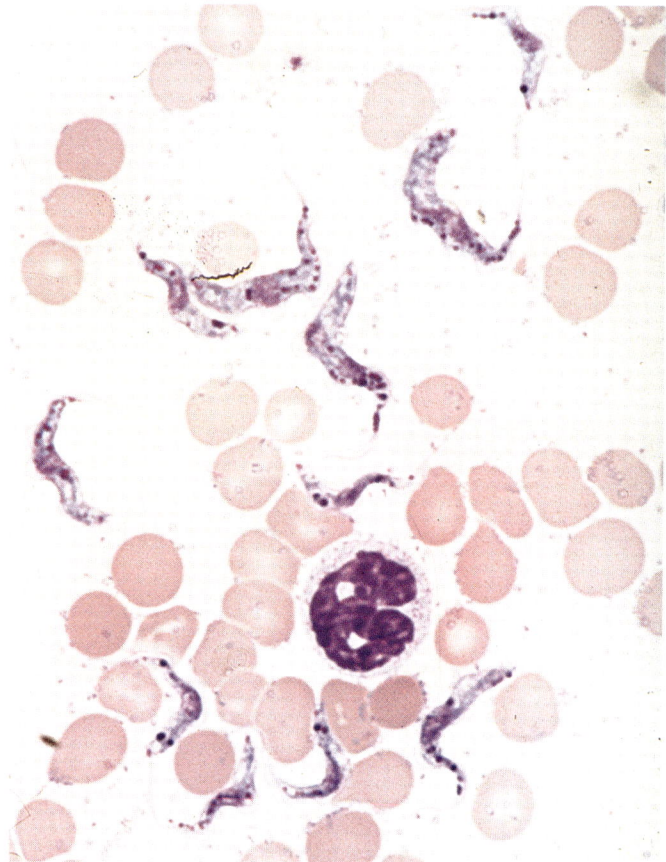

Fig. 2.2 Numerous trypanosomes of *Trypanosoma gambiense* in a blood smear. Giemsa

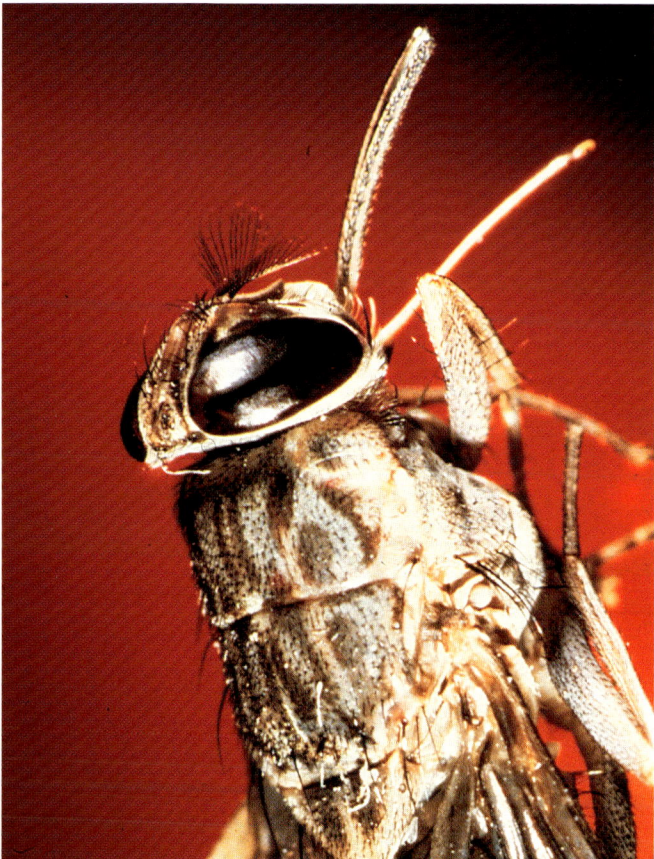

Fig. 2.3 Tsetse fly (*Glossina*), vector of African trypanosomiasis

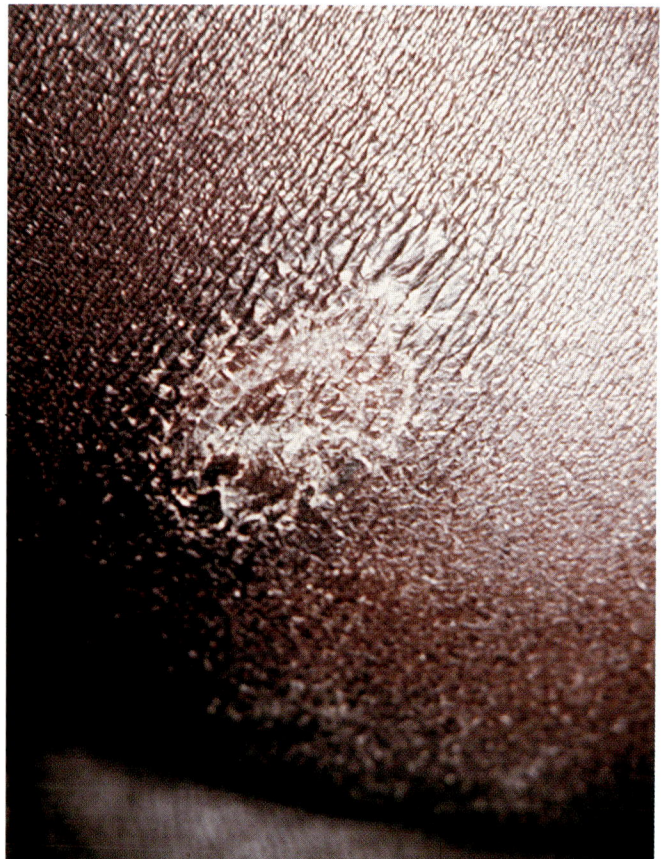

Fig. 2.4 Skin chancre. Residual scar of an infection in African trypanosomiasis

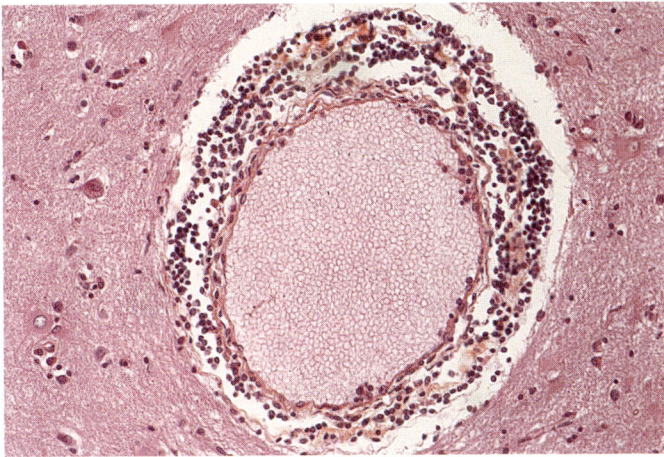

Fig. 2.5 Typical perivascular infiltrates in the encephalitis of sleeping sickness. H&E

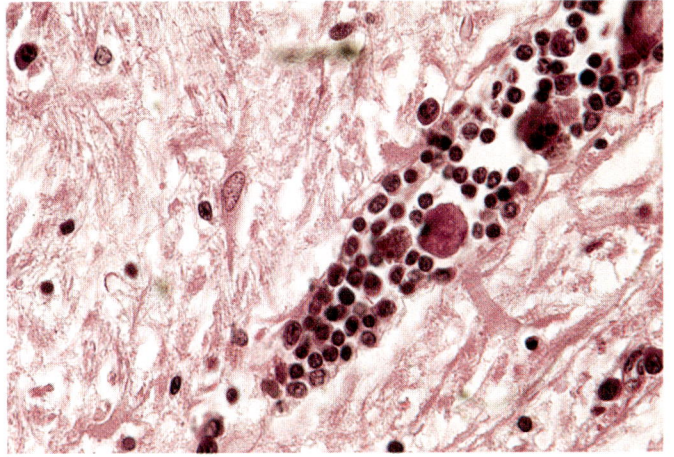

Fig. 2.6 Perivascular infiltrate with a 'morula cell'. H&E

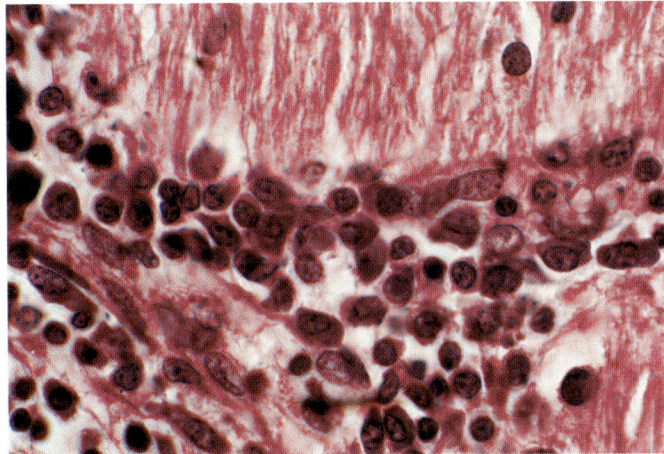

Fig. 2.7 Higher magnification of a perivascular infiltrate in African trypanosomiasis encephalitis. H&E

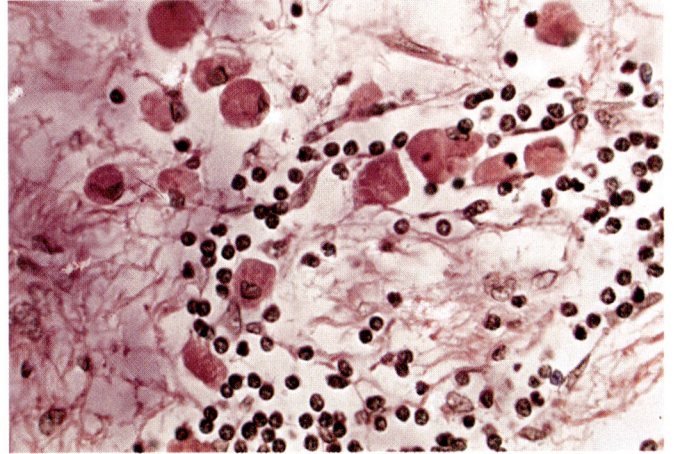

Fig. 2.8 Numerous 'morula cells' in a case of cryptococcosis with brain lesions. H&E

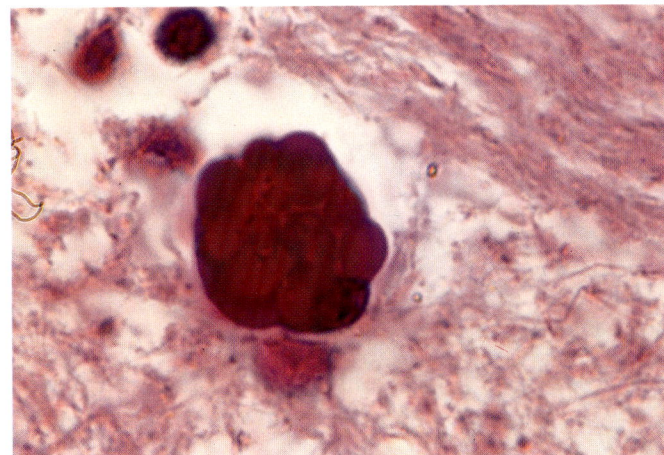

Fig. 2.9 Higher magnification of a 'morula cell' in African trypanosomiasis encephalitis. Note the confluence of the intraplasmatic corpuscles. H&E

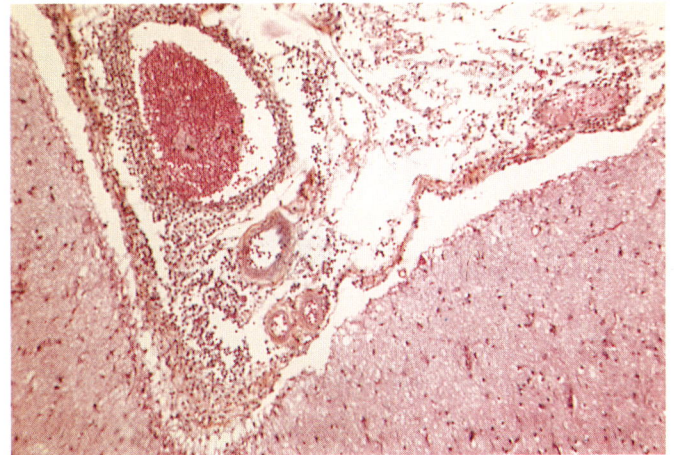

Fig. 2.10 Leptomeningitis in a case of African trypanosomiasis encephalitis

Under the microscope, the causative agent cannot be found in tissue sections as is the case in the acute form of Chagas disease. Only in experimental animals are parasitic elements seen in the tissues, and amastigotes and trypomastigote-like forms have been reported[2].

Regarding tissue reaction, the inflammation is present in the white and grey matter and there are regions with oedema. Here, also, progressive forms of astroglial elements are seen with an homogeneous eosinophilic cytoplasma which is irregularly shaped (gemistocytic transformation). Neurocytes do not show any specific lesions.

In the often-dilated perivascular spaces, cellular infiltrates, consisting of lymphocytes, plasma cells and monocytes are found. In addition, there are many 'corpuscular structures', measuring from 20–30 μm in diameter, which are strongly eosinophilic, spherical or ovoid in shape, and situated in the cellular infiltrates or in the oedematous areas. They consist of small eosinophilic bodies measuring 2–3 μm in diameter, either showing a morula aspect or appearing homogeneous. The latter is due to confluence of the small bodies. These structures represent Russell or Mott bodies and are characteristic of this disease but are also observed in cases of encephalitis due to other aetiologies. We have seen them in encephalitis due to *Cryptococcus neoformans* or *Histoplasma capsulatum* var. *capsulatum*. Mononuclear inflammation is seen also in the pia mater spreading along blood vessels into the cerebral cortex (Figs. 2.5–2.9).

In enlarged lymph nodes and the spleen, a reactive hyperplasia and infiltrates of histiocytes and plasma cells are seen histologically. In the infrequently encountered pancarditis, lymphohistiocytes and plasma cells are observed in infiltrates of the endocardium, myocardium[10] and the pericardium. Occasionally, fibrosis of variable degree is also present at these sites.

Endomyocardial fibrosis, frequently seen in Africa, is usually of undetermined aetiology. Nevertheless, it has been interpreted as a possible residual lesion of pancarditis caused by trypanosomes[11,12].

The authors of this atlas were able to review personally only a limited number of histological preparations of a few cases of sleeping sickness provided by friends. Together with other colleagues, we believe that the absence of causative agents in tissues, as reported in the literature, may be because histology has not been carried out systematically and thoroughly after postmortem examinations.

References

1. Schoening, B. (1989). The dog as reservoir host of Trypanosoma brucei gambiense. *Trop. Med. Parasit.*, **40**, 500
2. Schmidt, H. (1983). The pathogenesis of trypanosomiasis of the CNS. *Virchows Arch. (Pathol. Anat.)*, **399**, 333
3. Sudarto, M. W. (1990). Immunohistochemical demonstration of Trypanosoma evansi in tissues of experimentally infected rats and a naturally infected water buffalo (Bubalus bubalis). *J. Parasitol.*, **76**, 162
4. Emeribe, A. O. *et al.* (1990). Platelet aggregation inhibition in Trypanosoma vivax infection of sheep. *Cent. Afr. J. Med.*, **36**, 1
5. Grootenhuis, J. G. (1990). Susceptibility of African buffalo and Boran cattle to Trypanosoma congolense transmitted by Glossina morsitans centralis. *Vet. Parasitol.*, **35**, 219
6. Sachs, R., Mehlitz, D. and Zillmann, U. (1984). Sleeping sickness in West-Africa: parasitological-epidemiological field studies in Liberia. *Zbl. Bakt. Hyg. A.*, **258**, 384
7. East African Trypanosomiasis Research Organization Report. (1965). Authorities of the East African Common Services Organization
8. Brun, R., Jenni, L., Schoenenberger, M. and Schell, K. F. (1981). In vitro cultivation of bloodstream forms of Trypanosoma brucei, T. rhodesiense, and T. gambiense. *J. Protozool.*, **28**, 470
9. Poltera, A. A., Ows, R. and Cox, J. N. (1977). Pathological aspects of human African trypanosomiasis (HAT) in Uganda. *Virchows Arch. Abt. Path. Anat.*, **373**, 249
10. de Raadt, P. and Koten, J. W. (1968). Myocarditis in Rhodesian trypanosomiasis. *E. Afr. Med. J.*, **45**, 128
11. Brink, A. J. and Weber, H. W. (1966). Endomyocardial fibrosis (EMF) of East, Central and West Africa compared with South African endomyocardiopathies. *S. A. Med. J.*, **40**, 455
12. Poltera, A. A. and Cox, J. N. (1977). Pancarditis with valvulitis in endomyocardial fibrosis (EMF) and in human African trypanosomiasis (HAT). A comparative histological study of four Uganda cases. *Virchows Arch. Abt. A. Path. Anat.*, **275**, 53

LEISHMANIASES

Traditionally, three types of disease are produced by species of the genus *Leishmania*:

1. The cutaneous leishmaniasis or oriental sore, seen in the Old World and caused by *Leishmania tropica* (Wright).

2. The mucocutaneous leishmaniasis, seen in the New World and due to *Leishmania braziliensis* (Vianna).

3. The visceral leishmaniasis or Kala-azar, seen in both the Old and New World, and produced by *Leishmania donovani* (Laveran, Mesnil).

There are arguments against this classification; mainly that skin lesions may be seen in all three types. Nevertheless, it is useful from the geographical point of view and for other practical reasons.

Some features common to the three species of leishmanias must be emphasized:

1. The amastigotes of the three species of *Leishmania* (and of *Trypanosoma cruzi*) are structurally identical and therefore these species cannot be distinguished in tissues.

2. The leishmanias do not show flagellate forms (trypomastigoes) in mammalian blood.

3. The leishmanias (and trypanosomes) may be cultured in the artificial NNN medium. This medium (Nory, McNeal, Nicolle) contains bactoagar, sodium chloride, distilled water and, in addition, defibrinated blood, from diverse animal species, and penicillin.

Many details of the pathogenesis of the different types of leishmaniasis and of the virulence of their causative agents still need to be investigated. The gross and microscopic features of cutaneous and mucocutaneous leishmaniasis are similar. The only difference is that the mucosae may be involved in the latter.

We describe the mucocutaneous leishmaniasis in most detail; our personal experience has been gained studying leishmaniasis in the New World.

3. CUTANEOUS LEISHMANIASIS

Introduction

This infection is called also oriental sore or boil, tropical ulcer, sore of Jericho, Aleppo, Delhi or Biskra, or leishmaniasis of the Old World[1-3].

The disease occurs in the Mediterranean region, Asia Minor, India, China and Africa stretching from east to west between the 10° and 13° of latitude. Natural infections exist in several lower animal species[4]. Rodents may be used for experimental purposes[5,6].

Three types of the disease are considered: the urban type (*L. tropica minor*) which is mostly anthropozoonotic; the rural type (*L. tropica major*) which is zoonotic; and the diffuse cutaneous leishmanias (*L. tropica aethiopica*). The two types first mentioned usually show solitary lesions. The last is characterized by multiple lesions. This is apparently due to an anergic disposition of unknown origin; the Montenegro skin test in this type is negative.

The cutaneous leishmaniasis may heal spontaneously. Clinical diagnosis is made by confirmation of the causing agents in smears or biopsies; also, fine needle aspiration biopsy may be performed[7].

The parasite

Leishmania tropica is encountered in tissues in the amastigote form. The amastigotes are spherical, measure 2–4 μm in diameter and show a kinetoplast. Structurally, the amastigotes of all the *Leishmania* species are identical, not only the species causing the cutaneous, mucocutaneous and visceral leishmaniasis (*L. tropica, L. braziliensis* and *L. donovani*), but also *L. tropica minor, L. tropica major* and *L. tropica aethiopica*. It is therefore difficult to understand why different names were given to the leishmanias producing the different clinical forms of the disease.

The reservoir host for the urban form of *L. tropica* is predominantly man; for the rural form of cutaneous leishmaniasis, however, dogs, cats, rodents and monkeys.

Vectors of the disease are female sand flies of the genus *Phlebotomus*.

Pathogenesis

Infection takes place through the bite of a sand fly (Fig. 3.1), mostly on uncovered parts of the skin. The incubation period varies from 2–8 months. Usually, a solitary skin nodule develops which grows slowly and may later ulcerate and become a scar.

Multiple skin lesions appear to be due to an anergy of unknown origin. There is no satisfactory explanation at present for the differences in localization of the lesions in the two forms of leishmaniasis found in different geographical regions, i.e. why, in case of the cutaneous leishmaniasis, neither mucosae nor internal organs are affected.

Pathology

In the great majority of cases, a single skin lesion is found. The urban type of cutaneous leishmaniasis is characterized by the so-called 'dry' form of the disease, i.e. the skin nodules do not have a tendency to ulcerate. When it relapses, it is called 'lupoid leishmaniasis'. In the rural type, on the other hand, there is a tendency to ulcerate and then it is called the 'humid' form.

While only solitary skin lesions used to be seen in the *L. tropica* infection, recently multiple lesions, mainly in the face, have been described, mostly in certain regions of Africa. This form of the disease which was unknown in the Old World previously, is called diffuse tegumentary, lepromatoid, keloid or tuberculoid leishmaniasis. These cases of leishmaniasis with single or multiple lesions in the skin are practically identical to the leishmaniasis lesions in the New World; lesions are limited to the skin without involvement of the mucosae (Figs. 3.2 and 3.3).

In some reports recently, it was stated that, histologically, the tissue reaction in the American form of leishmaniasis shows special patterns which allow differentiation from the disease in the Old World. However, as yet, these data have not been confirmed.

As we do not have much personal experience of leishmaniasis of the Old World, we shall refrain from giving detailed descriptions of this infection. The few cases we could examine showed infiltrates of numerous plasma cells, a pattern not, perhaps, so pronounced in the mucocutaneous leishmaniasis. In a case of cutaneous leishmaniasis of the Old World, numerous parasites were seen (Fig. 3.4). All the following details of mucocutaneous leishmaniasis also apply to the cutaneous form. Only the data about epidemiology and, of course, all details about the involvement of the mucosae relate solely to the American leishmaniasis.

References

1. Price, E. W. and Fitzherbert, M. (1965). Cutaneous leishmaniasis in Ethiopia. *Med. J.,* **3**, 57
2. Bryceson, A. D. (1969). Diffuse cutaneous leishmaniasis in Ethiopia, I. The clinical and histological features of the disease. *Trans. R. Soc. Trop. Med. Hyg.,* **63**, 708
3. Pringle, G. (1957). Oriental sore in Iraq. Historial and epidemiologic problems. *Bull. Endem. Dis. (Baghdad),* **2**, 41
4. Mutinga, M. J., Kihara, S. M., Lohding, A., Mutero, C. M., Ngatia, T. A. and Karanu, F. (1989). Leishmaniasis in Kenya: description of leishmaniasis of a domestic goat from Transmara, Narok District, Kenya. *Trop. Med. Parasitol.,* **40**, 91
5. Krampitz, H. E. (1981). Primary and secondary skin leishmaniasis in experimental rodent hosts. *Zbl. Bakt. Hyg. I Abt. Orig. A.,* **250**, 191
6. Cillari, E. *et al.* (1990). Rapid quantitative method for measuring phagocytosis of Leishmania promastigotes using a double radiolabelling method. *J. Immunol. Meth.,* **130**, 57
7. Akhtar, M. *et al.* (1991). Diagnosis of cutaneous leishmaniasis by fine needle aspiration biopsy; report of a case. *Diagn. Cytopathol.,* **7**, 172

4. MUCOCUTANEOUS LEISHMANIASIS

Introduction

This disease is also named American tegumentary leishmaniasis or leishmaniasis of the New World and has been confirmed as an autochthonous infection from Northern Argentina to Southern Mexico[1]. The name depends on the particular anatomical locations and the country or region (Mexico, Panama, Peru, the Guianas, Amazonas or Brazil). Some other local names are 'chicleros' ulcers', espundia, buba, uta and pianbois (forest yaws). The disease is well known in Venezuela[2-5]. It is usual to

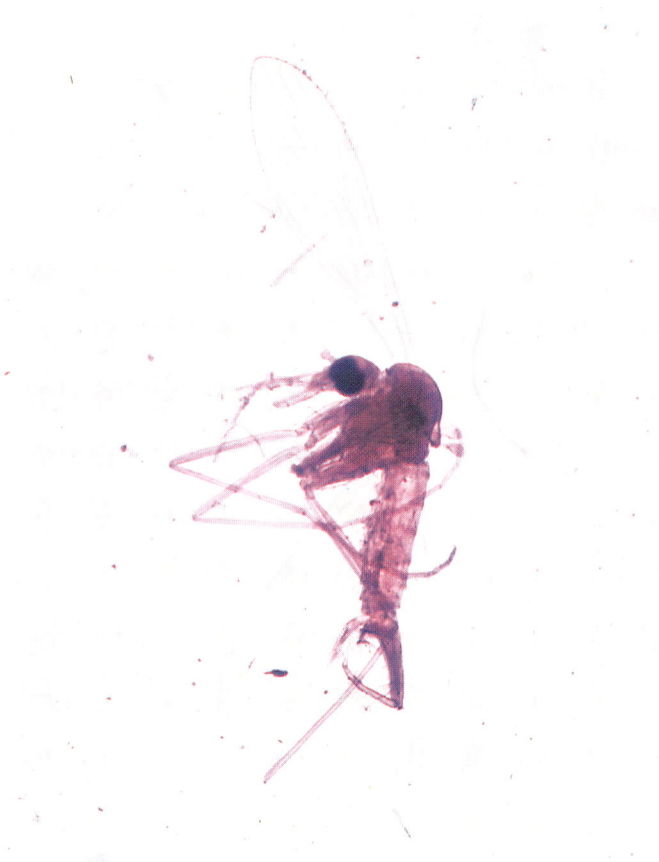

Fig. 3.1 *Phlebotomus*, male. This genus of sand-flies is the vector for all the species of leishmanias. Only the females are vectors

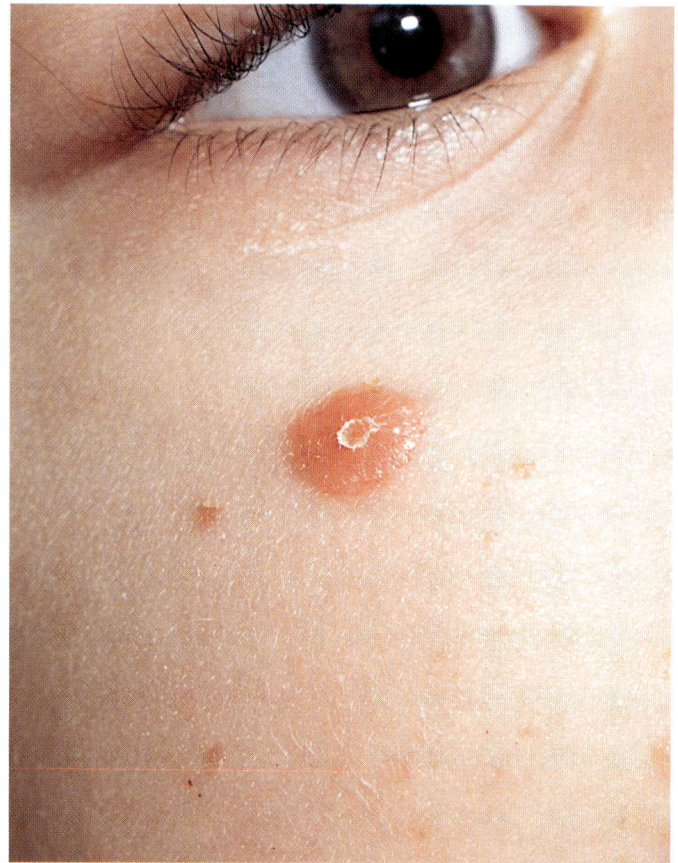

Fig. 3.2 Early stage of leishmanial infection in the Old World

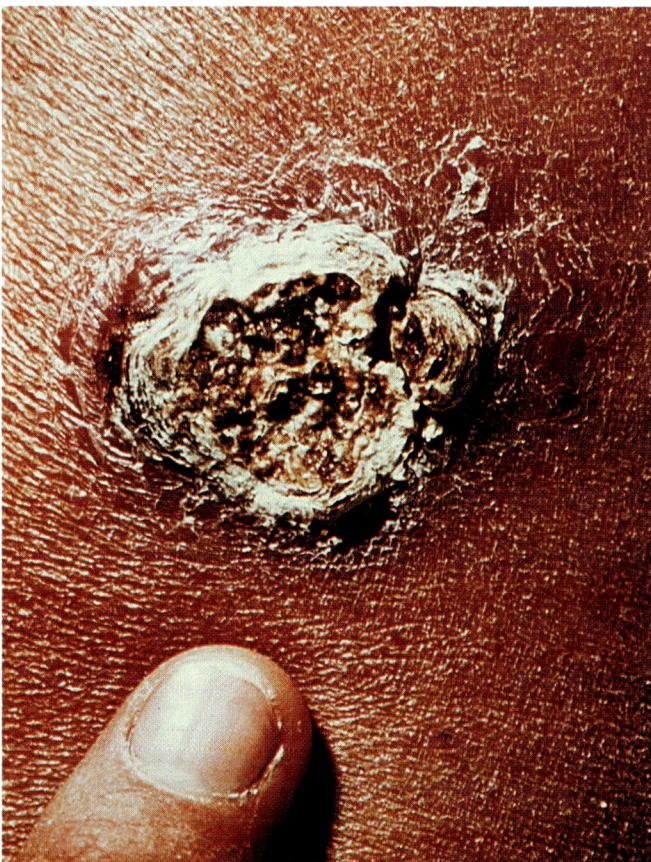

Fig. 3.3 Advanced or chronic stage of oriental sore with a single skin ulcer

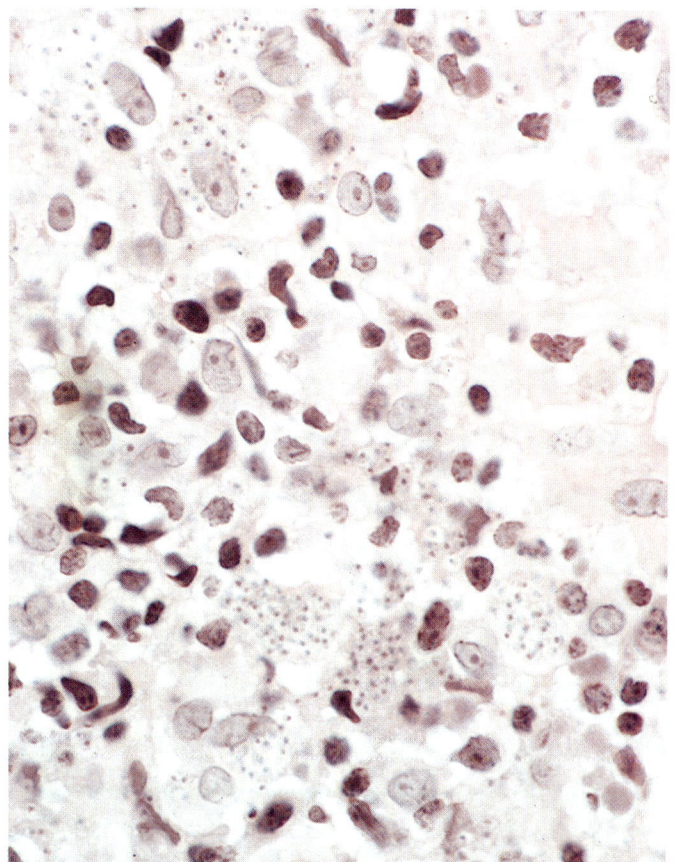

Fig. 3.4 Oriental boil. Case from Afghanistan with numerous parasites in this field. H&E

observe groups of patients with this infection, not single cases, in rural areas with abundant woods and vegetation.

Natural infections occur in dogs and certain wild lower animal species. Experimentally, visceral lesions may be produced in hamsters by inoculation with *L. braziliensis*[6].

Cutaneous lesions are similar to those of the Old World, but usually more extensive and not as easily cured as the latter. The mucosal lesions are located in the oral or nasal cavity and may lead to perforation of the nasal septum or the pharyngeal wall. Prognosis is less favourable than in the cutaneous leishmaniasis of the Old World.

Clinical diagnosis is made by confirmation of the causative agent in biopsies or smears from the surface of ulcerations. The cutaneous test of Montenegro[7] is positive in more than 75%. The immunoperoxide method facilitates diagnosis[8].

The parasite

Leishmania braziliensis is the causative agent of muco-cutaneous leishmaniasis. Other species described as causative agents are apparently only subspecies or variants of *L. braziliensis*. This may be the case, for instance, in the 'new species' isolated in the Venezuelan Andes by Scorza *et al.* in 1978[9]. Also *Leishmania mexicana*[10] will not be considered here since it is of no importance in this context. This species may be differentiated from *L. braziliensis* by using DNA probes[11].

L. braziliensis has one form with (in the vector and in cultures) and one without flagella. The aflagellate forms, leishmanias or amastigotes, measuring $2-3\,\mu m$ in diameter, are found in mammalian tissues (Fig. 4.1). They are slightly smaller than the amastigotes of *Trypanosoma cruzi* and the nucleus is situated on the edge attached to the cellular membrane, which is thin and often not discernible. The rod-like kinetoplast of the amastigotes may be easily seen in well-preserved recently infected tissue, which has been fixed immediately after being removed from the patient. In tissues of routine biopsy material, we have not seen kinetoplasts, but have seen them convincingly in selected cases only.

It must again be emphasized that *Leishmania braziliensis* is structurally identical to *Leishmania tropica* and *Leishmania donovani*, as well as to the amastigotes of *Trypanosoma cruzi*.

Reservoir hosts for *L. braziliensis* are rodents, certain wild animal species and, more rarely, dogs which show cutaneous lesions produced by *L. braziliensis*.

Vectors are females of sand fly species belonging to the genus *Phebotomus* or *Lutzomyia*, for instance *L. longipalpis*. In Venezuela, the most important vector is *Phlebotomus panamensis*.

Pathogenesis

When the females of infected phlebotomes (sand flies) bite healthy men or lower animals, they inject promastigotes into the superficial layers of the dermis. Here, they lose their flagella and penetrate into histiocytes, or are phagocytosed by macrophages. The inflammatory reaction leads to a nodular skin lesion which becomes visible between 2 weeks and 4 months after the bite of the insect.

If a patient has several leishmania lesions, three pathogenic possibilities exist:

1. They are the result of multiple bites,

2. They originated through autoinoculation from a single primary lesion as a result of a single bite, or

3. There was a haematogenous dissemination with the consecutive appearance of multiple skin nodules.

The diffuse tegumentary leishmaniasis starts, apparently, with a single nodule which probably spreads haematogenously, producing multiple skin lesions. This process may take years.

Why and how involvement of the facial mucosae occurs mostly is not clear. Probably, it is due to haematogenous dissemination. However, in the course of parasitaemia, involvement of the internal organs never takes place.

Pathology

Mostly, lesions are found in areas of the skin usually not covered by clothing. Weeks or months after the bite, one or several papules develops or skin nodules appear, reaching variable dimensions. Later, they ulcerate and become chronic lesions; when untreated, there is no tendency to spontaneous healing. On the whole they are difficult to differentiate from skin afflictions due to other causes, especially as they have a chronic evolution (Figs. 4.2–4.9).

The clinical form known as 'diffuse tegumentary leishmaniasis' with multiple skin lesions shows characteristic papulomatous nodules in contrast to the solitary or isolated lesions of the common leishmaniasis (Fig. 4.10). The nodules become confluent and are transformed into cauliflower-like lesions which present a papillomatous appearance with an irregular surface. Characteristically, epidermal ulceration does not occur regularly[12].

The lesions in the mucosae are localized in the nose, oral cavity (Fig. 4.11), pharynx, larynx and trachea, and may or may not be accompanied by cutaneous lesions. In cases without active cutaneous lesions, a scar in the skin may indicate a former primary cutaneous infection by leishmanias. The alterations of the mucosae vary considerably in shape and size and are often tumour-like with ulcerations. Sometimes, they produce stenosis and occlusions in the upper parts of the respiratory and digestive tract which occasionally require surgery.

Exceptionally, the amastigotes are observed histologically in epithelial cells of the epidermis or the mucosae; predominantly they are encountered inside the histiocytes where they reproduce by division and lead to clusters of parasites inside individual tissue cells. The cytoplasm of these tissue cells often shows a clear or vacuolized aspect and, consequently, these cells seem to be 'small cysts'. Numerous histiocytes with clear cytoplasm and many parasites are seen, mainly in acute infections and in diffuse tegumentary leishmaniasis. When the parasitized histiocytes rupture, the liberated amastigotes invade other cells or are phagocytosed by other macrophages. It must be emphasized that the liberated and single amastigotes outside tissue cells are difficult to recognize as such and, therefore, diagnosis cannot be made. The number of leishmanias in each inflammatory focus is very variable. If they are present in great numbers, the intracellular leishmanias are easily recognizable in the 'vacuoles' of histiocytes which, however, are frequently empty due to the loss of parasites during the cutting procedures. On the other hand, if they are scarce or situated extracellularly, or in smears, their visualization may be difficult and often it is impossible to see them. In addition to their intracellular localization in histiocytes with a clear cytoplasm, the borders of necrotic areas should be reviewed in order to detect leishmanias. When the parasites are clearly recognizable, the kinetoplast is not usually well preserved (Fig. 4.12). Some parasitologists insist upon making a diagnosis of leishmanias only when kinetoplasts are visible. We have not often seen kinetoplasts in our material and would like to stress that our experience leads us to make a diagnosis of leishmanias only when organisms are Grocott-negative.

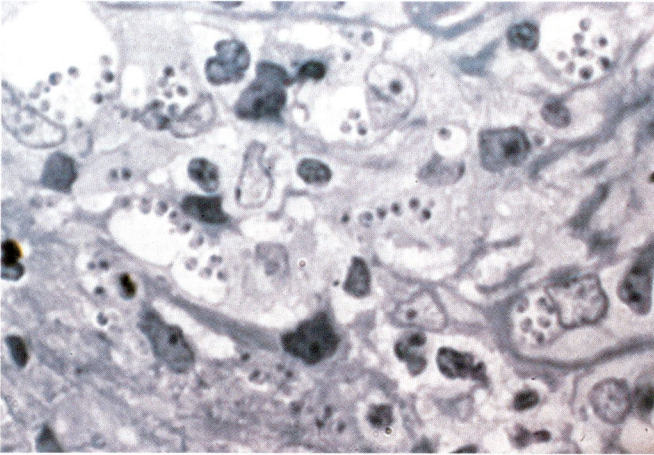

Fig. 4.1   Numerous amastigotes of *Leishmania braziliensis* arranged in clusters. Thick section, Giemsa

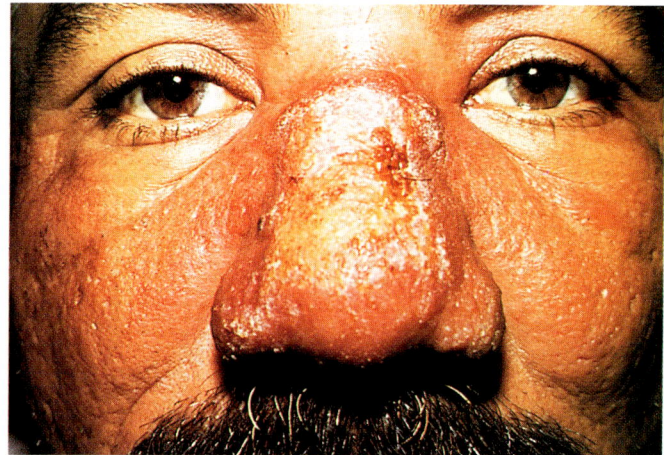

Fig. 4.2   Muco-cutaneous leishmaniasis. Large ulcerative lesion of the nose

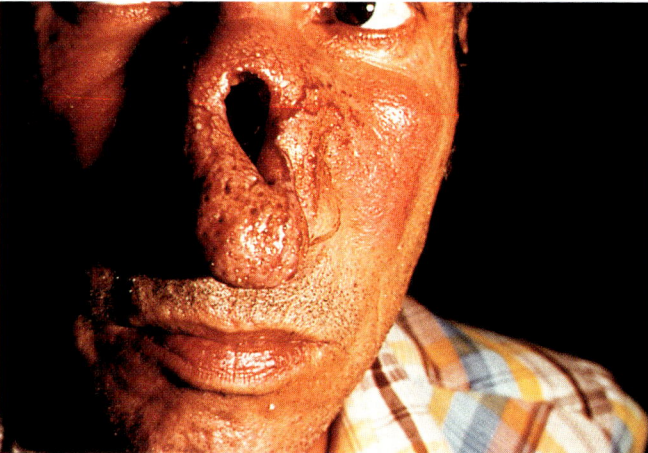

Fig. 4.3   Muco-cutaneous leishmaniasis. Profound ulcer with perforation of the ala nasi

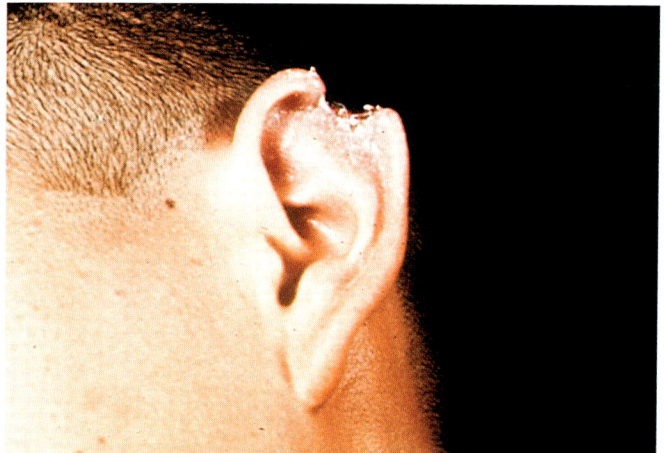

Fig. 4.4   Muco-cutaneous leishmaniasis. Deep skin lesion with defect of the ear lobe

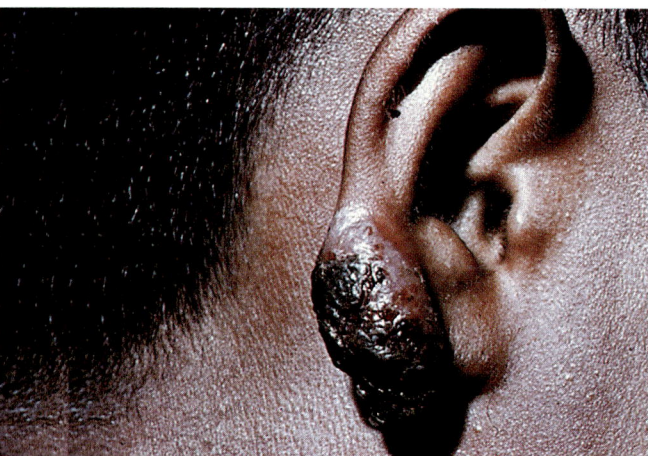

Fig. 4.5   Muco-cutaneous leishmaniasis. Papulomatous lesions with haemorrhages

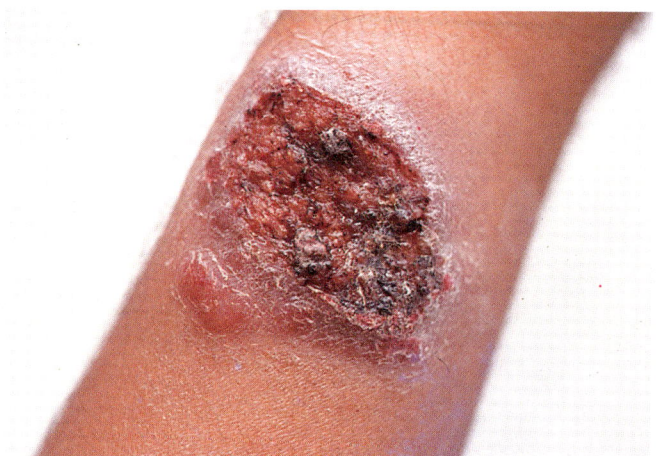

Fig. 4.6   Muco-cutaneous leishmaniasis. Large skin ulcer with a granular ground on an arm

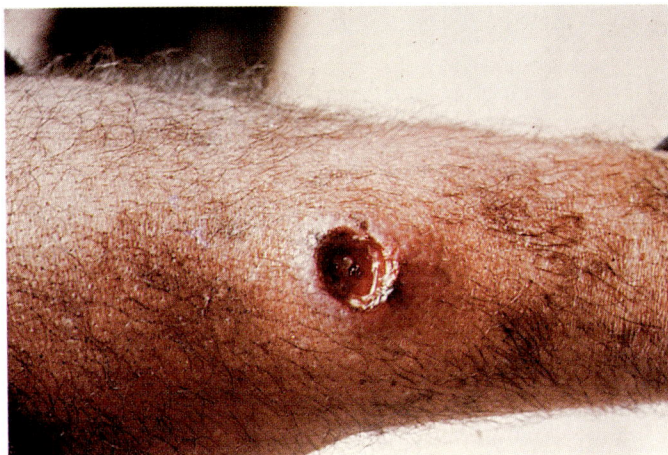

Fig. 4.7 Muco-cutaneous leishmaniasis. Deep skin ulcer with sharp borders on a thigh

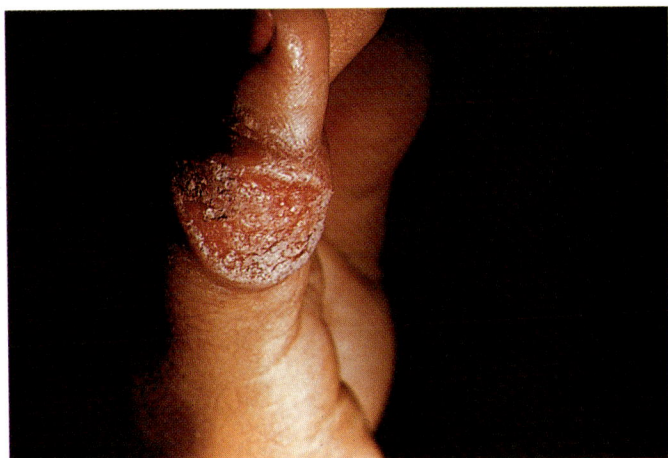

Fig. 4.8 Muco-cutaneous leishmaniasis. Large skin ulcer with thick borders on a finger

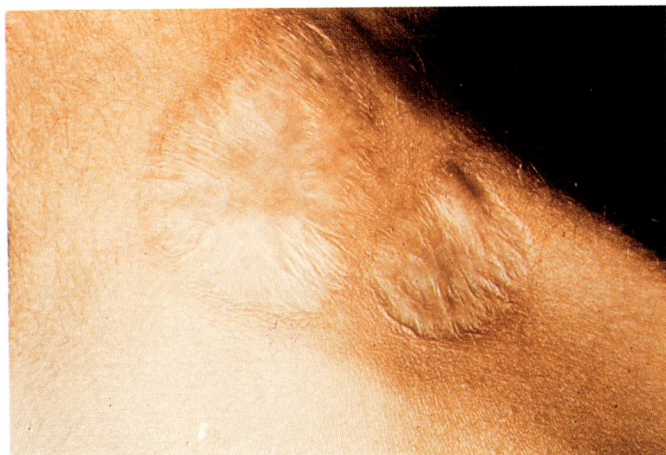

Fig. 4.9 Typical leishmaniatic skin scar

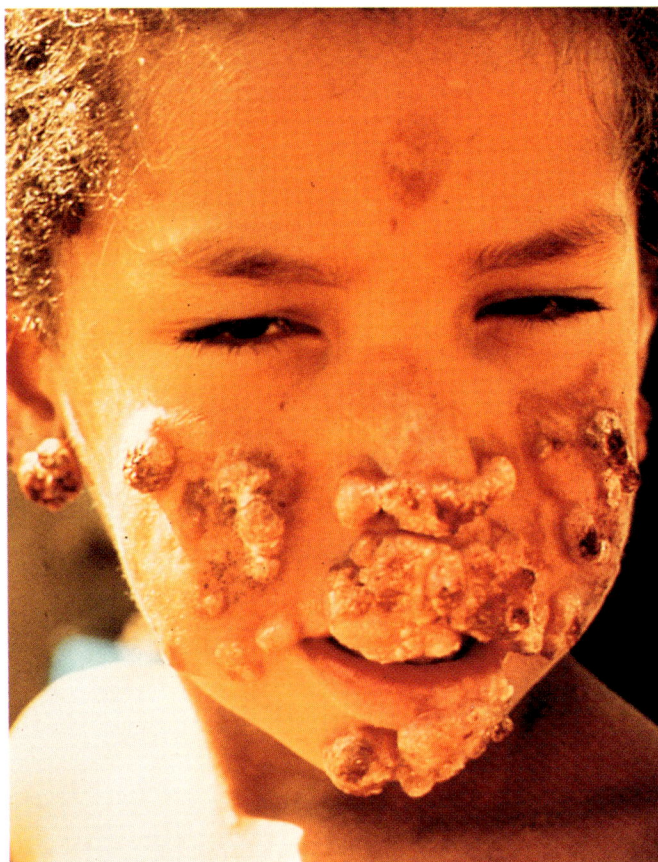

Fig. 4.10 Multiple nodular foci in the face, typical of 'diffuse tegumentary leishmaniasis', also called 'leproid'

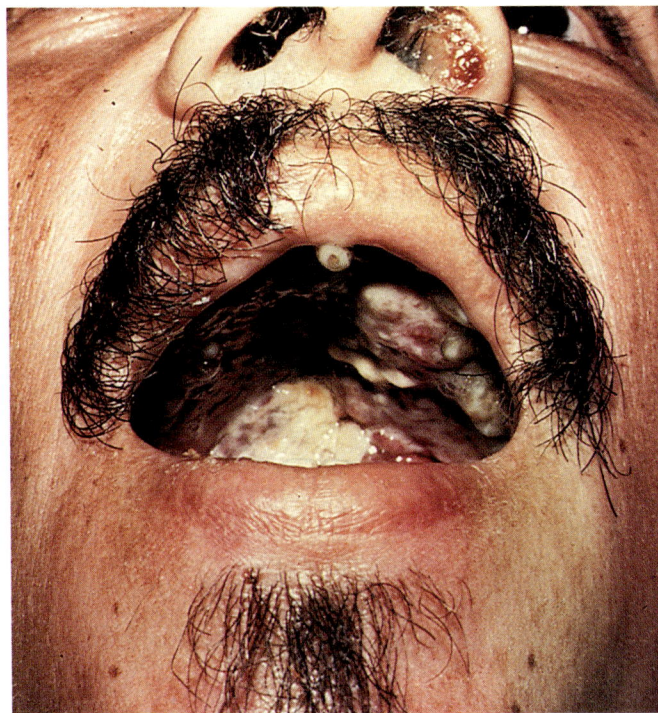

Fig. 4.11 Muco-cutaneous leishmaniasis. Extensive lesions in the mucosa of mouth, pharynx and nose

In our material, parasites have been confirmed in tissue sections in only 50% of all cases of mucocutaneous leishmaniasis[13,14]. Even scarcer were the parasites in other series of routine biopsies[15].

When making a differential diagnosis, histiocytes with clear or vacuolated cytoplasm are commonly observed in skin and mucosa in lesions of leprosy, rhinoscleroma and histoplasmosis capsulati.

In addition, amastigotes of *L. braziliensis* in tissues must be differentiated from amastigotes of leishmanias of other species and *Trypanosoma cruzi*. Furthermore, *Toxoplasma gondii* and small yeast cells, e.g. *Histoplasma capsulatum* var. *vapsulatum*, species of *Candida*, *Torulopsis glabrata* and *Penicillium marneffei* must be distinguished, as well as other small forms of yeast cells in mycoses which normally show large yeast cells in tissues, such as *Coccidioides immitis*, *Blastomyces dermatitidis* and *Paracoccidioides brasiliensis*. Fungus cells may be ruled out when the elements under discussion are Gram-, PAS- and Grocott-negative. Before making a histological diagnosis of leishmaniasis, we always perform the Grocott test[16]. Haematoxylin-positive chromatin particles may also look like leishmanias in tissues (see reference 17, Chapter 23).

Tissue reaction in skin and mucosa lesions is identical. The factors which determine the type of tissue reaction are:

1. The stage of evolution and the duration of the disease,

2. The virulence of the species or strain of the infectious leishmanias,

3. The human organism's immunological status,

4. The presence or lack of a secondary infection, and

5. The action of drugs in cases where the patient receives treatment.

What is usually seen is a diffuse tissue reaction with dense cellular infiltrates composed of a variable number of lympho- or histiocytes, plasma cells and, occasionally, mast cells and/or eosinophilic granulocytes. If there are numerous histiocytes with clear cytoplasm and intracellular parasites, some scientists call the tissue reaction 'histiocytoma'. In a recently observed case with marked infiltrates of histiocytes showing a clear cytoplasm containing numerous amastigotes (Figs. 4.13 and 4.14), a unique (for us) feature was detected: a single multinuclear giant cell contained several tissue cells which harboured amastigotes. This means that there was a double phagocytosis: first, amastigotes were engulfed by histiocytes and later the histiocytes were engulfed by a giant cell (Fig. 4.15).

In addition to diffuse cellular infiltrates, one can also observe granulomatous reactions with epithelioid and giant cells. Epithelioid granulomas sometimes show central necroses, features which are indistinguishable from granulomas caused by *Mycobacterium tuberculosis*. We have not seen as many cases with typical granulomas. Instead, there have been quite numerous instances when the exclusive presence of epithelioid cells leads to the diagnosis of leishmaniasis (Figs. 4.16–4.19).

Pseudoepitheliomatous hyperplasia of the epidermis is typical of chronically ulcerated leishmanial lesions, but this feature is also found in chronic cutaneous lesions of deep mycoses and in other chronic dermatopathies.

Exudation of granulocytes and microabscesses are not common in mucocutaneous leishmaniasis. When granulocytes are found, they are mostly located near the surface of a tissue defect at the base of an ulceration. Microabscesses are the typical lesions in infection due to *Sporothrix schenckii*.

We were never able to confirm the presence of parasites in lymphangitis or regional lymphadenitis which are common in patients with leishmania lesions. This is probably because the patients were not examined at the right time or because these lesions in the lymph nodes were due to secondary bacterial infections. However, experimentally, parasites have been confirmed in regional lymph nodes of lower animals[18]. The differences that exist between the leishmaniases of the Old and New World have not been elucidated. Further studies are needed on this subject.

In the rather rare 'diffuse tegumentary leishmaniasis', tissue reaction shows numerous histiocytes with clear cytoplasm containing many parasites in the inflammatory foci; a granulomatous reaction is never observed.

The lack of parasites in tissues in numerous apparently chronic cases makes it imperative, in practice, to give at least a presumptive histological diagnosis based only on a more or less characteristic tissue reaction.

References

1. Pessoa, S. B. and Barreto, M. P. (1948). *Leishmaniose Tegumentar Americana*. Min. de Educacao e Saude, Rio de Janeiro
2. Pifano, F. and Scorza, J. V. (1960). Aspectos immunológicos de las leishmanias que parasitan al hombre, con especial referencia a la Leishmania brasiliensis Pifano, Medina y Romero, 1957. *Arch. Venez. Med. Trop. Parasit. Med.*, **111**, 16
3. Kerdel-Vegas, F. (1966). Histopatología de la Leishmaniasis americana. *Med. Cutánea*, **3**, 267
4. Convit, J., Rodríguez, G., Henriquez, A. J. and Medina, R. (1968). Histopatología de la Leishmaniasis Tegumentaria Americana. *Derm. Venez.*, **XI**, 475
5. Pons, R., Serano, H. and Marmol Leon, P. (1974). Incidencias de la Leishmaniasis tegumentaria americana en poblaciones del Dtt. Miranda del Edo. Zulia (Venezuela). *Kasmera* (Univ. del Zulia), **5**, 31
6. Kahl, L. P. *et al.* (1991). Leishmania (Viannia) braziliensis: comparative pathology of golden hamsters infected with isolates from cutaneous and mucosal lesions of patients residing in Tres Bracos, Bahia, Brazil. *Am. J. Trop. Med. Hyg.*, **44**, 218
7. Montenegro, J. (1926). A cutis-reaccao na leishmaniose. *Ann. Fac. Med. Sao Paulo*, **1**, 323
8. Salinas, G. *et al.* (1990). Detección de amastigotes en leishmaniasis cutánea y mucocutánea por el método de immunoperoxidasa, usando anticuerpo policlonal: sensibilidad y especifidad comparadas con métodos convencionales de diagnostico. *Mem. Inst. Oswaldo Cruz*, **84**, 53
9. Scorza, J. V., Valera, M., Scorza, C. de, Carnevali, M., Moreno, E. and Lugo-Hernández, A. (1979). A new species of Leishmania parasite from the Venezuelan Andes region. *Trans. R. Soc. Trop. Med. Hyg.*, **73**, 293
10. Piekarski, G. (1987). *Medical Parasitology*. Springer-Verlag
11. Barker, D. C. and Butcher, J. (1983). The use of DNA probes in the identification of leishmanias: discrimination between isolates of the Leishmania mexicana and L. braziliensis complexes. *Trans. R. Soc. Trop. Med. Hyg.*, **77**, 285
12. Goto, H. *et al.* (1990). A case of multiple lesion mucocutaneous leishmaniasis caused by Leishmania (Vianna) braziliensis infection. *J. Trop. Med. Hyg.*, **93**, 48
13. Salfelder, K. (1971). Erfahrungen bei der pathologisch-anatomischen Diagnose von tiefen Mykosen und Parasitosen. *Beitr. Path.*, **143**, 197
14. Arriaga, A. D. de (1977). *Leishmaniasis Muco-cutánea en los Hospitales de Mérida y Barinas*. Trabajo de Ascenso, Fac. de Med. ULA, Mérida
15. Sotto, M. N., Yamashiro Kanashiro, E. H., da Mata, V. L. and de Brito, T. (1989). Cutaneous leishmaniasis of the New World: diagnostic immunopathology and antigen pathways in skin and mucosa. *Acta Trop. Basel.*, **46**, 121
16. Grocott, R. G. (1955). A stain for fungi in tissue sections and smears, using Gomori's methenamine silver nitrate technique. *Am. J. Clin. Path.*, **25**, 975
17. Salfelder, K., Liscano, T. R. de and Sauerteig, E. (1990). *Atlas of Fungal Pathology*. Kluwer Academic Publishers
18. Travi, B., Rey-Ladino, J. and Saravia, N. G. (1988). Behavior of Leishmanias braziliensis s. 1. in golden hamsters: evolution of the infection under different experimental conditions. *J. Parasitol.*, **74**, 1059

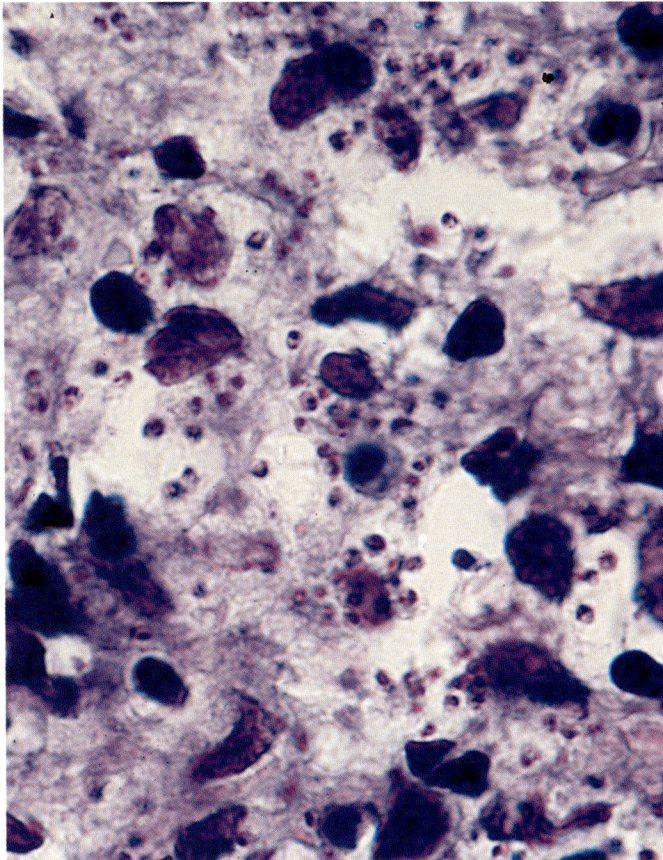

Fig. 4.12 Numerous amastigotes of *Leishmania braziliensis* arranged diffusely and in clusters. Giemsa and Wright

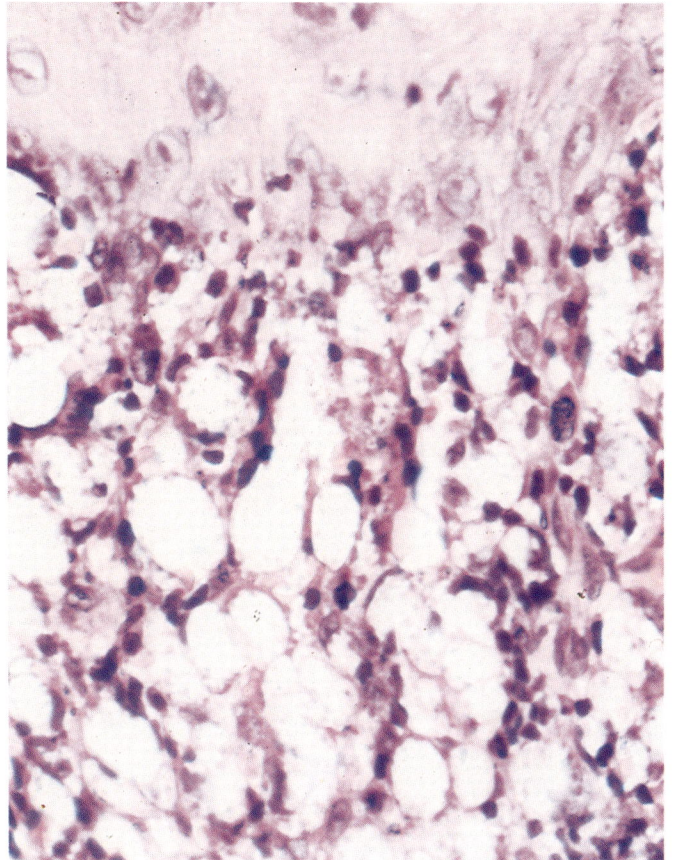

Fig. 4.13 Muco-cutaneous leishmaniasis. Numerous histiocytes with clear or vacuolic cytoplasm. The parasites have fallen out during the process of cutting and staining. H&E

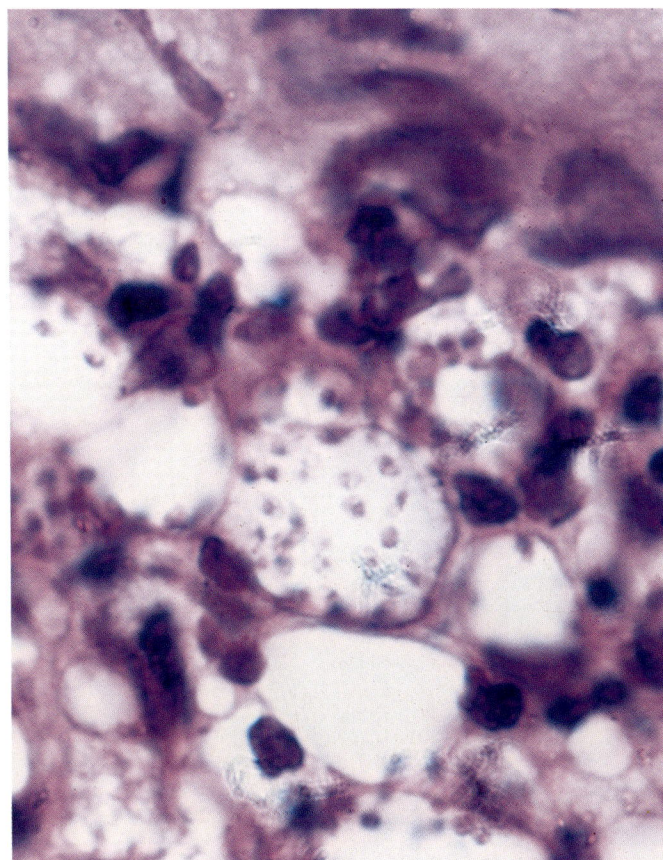

Fig. 4.14 Higher magnification of lesions in Fig. 4.13 with preserved leishmanias in a histiocyte. H&E

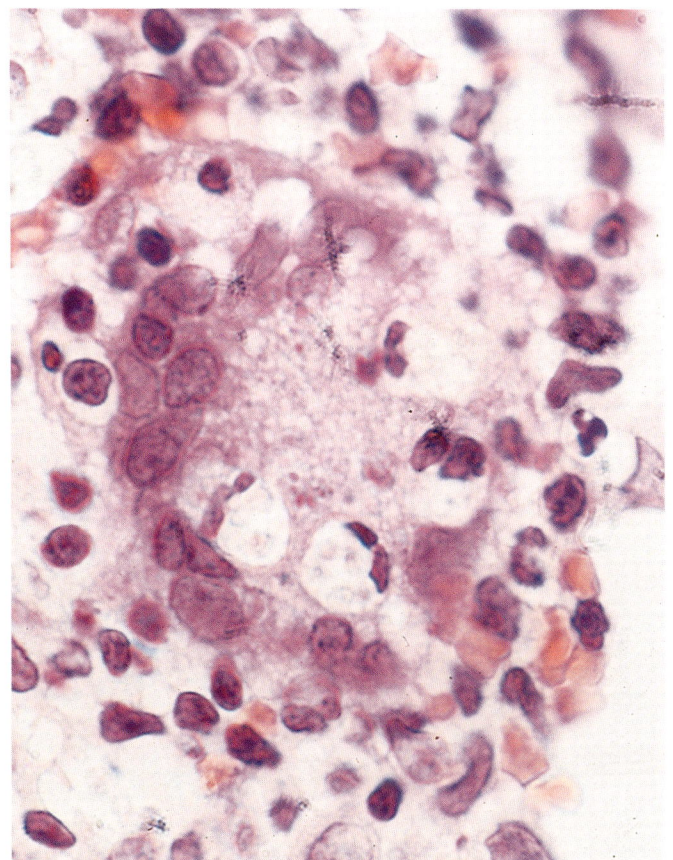

Fig. 4.15 Same case as Figs. 4.13 and 4.14. Giant cell with a 'double phagocytosis'. First, macrophages engulf leishmanias and then the giant cell phagocytoses the leishmania-containing macrophages. H&E

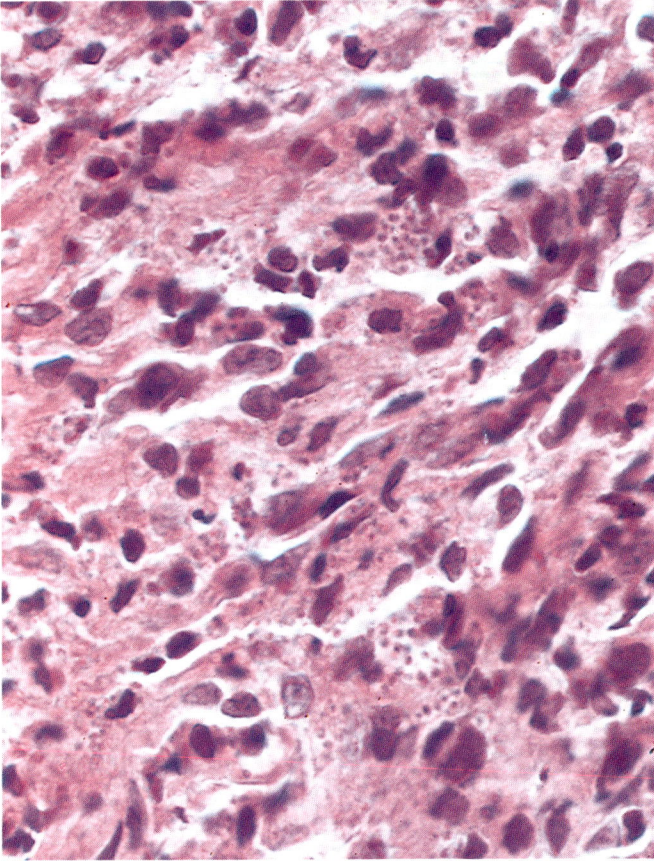

Fig. 4.16 Muco-cutaneous leishmaniasis. Typical epithelioid cell reaction. Furthermore, small nests of parasites (intracellularly located) are seen. H&E

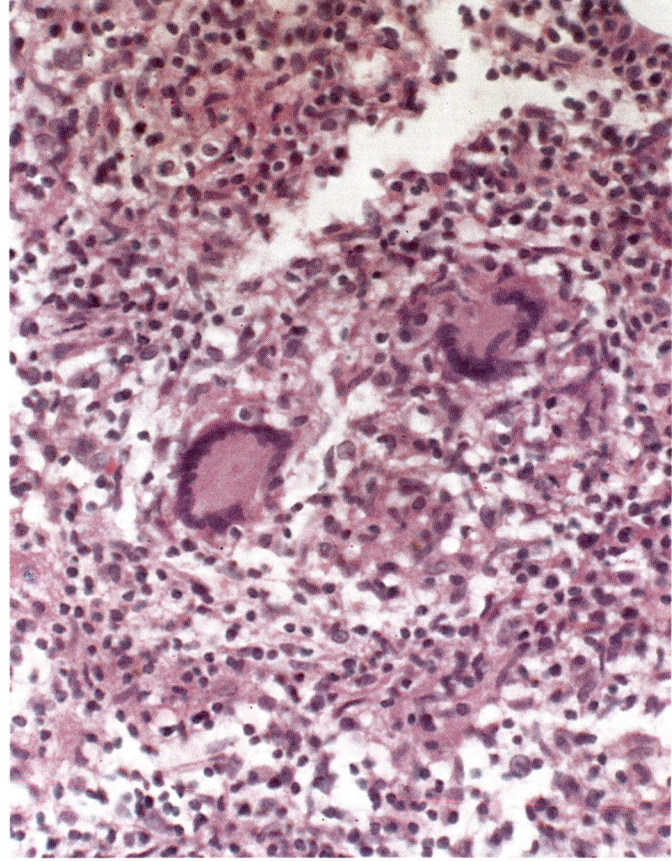

Fig. 4.17 Muco-cutaneous leishmaniasis. Dense cell infiltrates and granulomatous reaction with giant cells. H&E

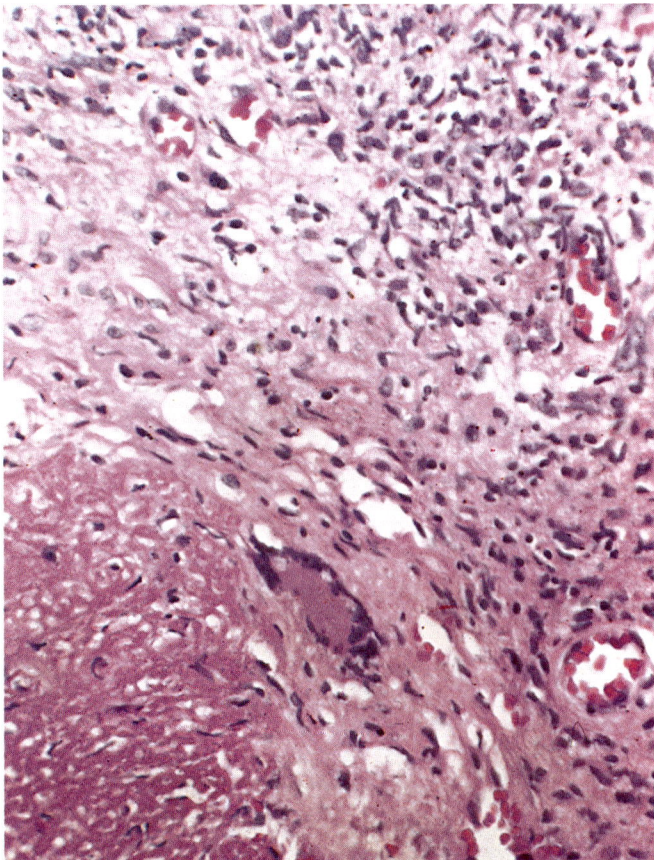

Fig. 4.18 Muco-cutaneous leishmaniasis. Granulomatous reaction with giant cell and necrosis. H&E

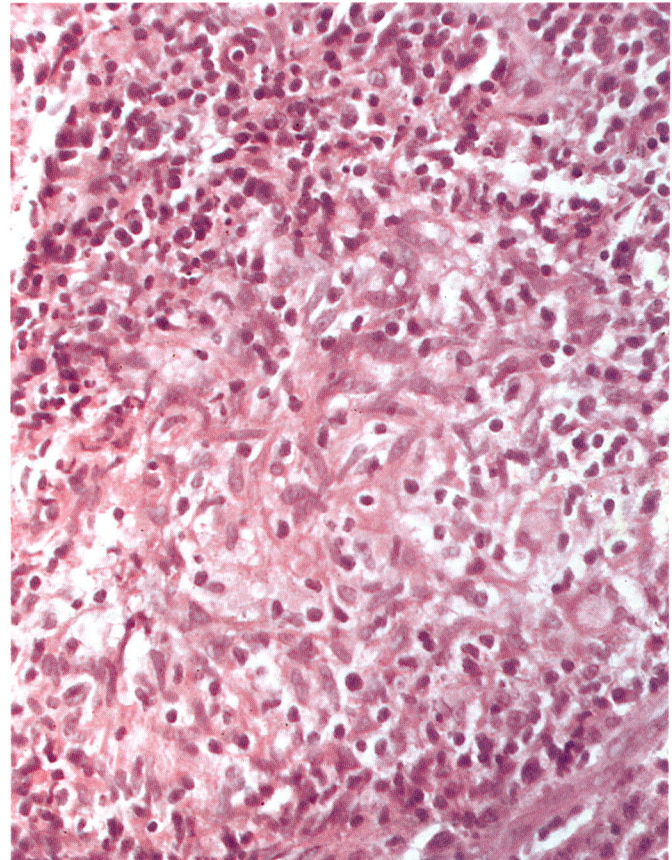

Fig. 4.19 Muco-cutaneous leishmaniasis. Dense cellular infiltrate and numerous 'clear' epithelioid cells. This is a characteristic histological feature of chronic leishmaniasis. Parasites are mostly not visible. H&E

5. VISCERAL LEISHMANIASIS

Introduction

This disease is called also kala-azar, which means black fever, or tropical splenomegaly, as well as 'infantile anaemia with tumour of the spleen'. The prevalence of this infection is low. The vector has been controlled by anti-anopheles campaigns, but has not been totally eradicated.

The infection is endemic in the countries surrounding the Mediterranean Sea, the Middle East, Asia, Africa and South America; only a few cases are reported in Central America and Mexico and human cases of Kala-azar are known in Venezuela[5,6].Mostly, children are affected[1-4].

Dogs, canine species and wild animals (foxes and several rodent species) can be naturally infected[7]. Experimentally, mice, dogs, monkeys, cats, hamsters and other animals may be inoculated[8-10].

Anaemia, increased IgG and marked splenomegaly are the clinical signs. Almost 90% of untreated patients die 1–2 years after the beginning of the disease. With current therapy, almost 90% can be cured. Visceral leishmaniasis has also been found in AIDS patients[11].

Clinical diagnosis is made by confirmation of the causative agent, for instance, in biopsies of the bone marrow, culture and inoculation into laboratory animals.

The parasite

Leishmania donovani is the causal agent of the disease in man and lower animals. The amastigotes of *L. donovani* have the same structure as *L. tropica* and *L. braziliensis* and are called Leishman and Donovan (L-D) bodies*. *L. donovani chagasi* is a new clinical variant of cutaneous leishmaniasis in Honduras[12].

Amastigotes of *L. donovani*, as well as the other species of *Leishmania* stain well in mammalian tissues with H&E and Giemsa and are negative when the methods of Gram, PAS and Grocott are used. They are situated in intracellular clusters inside the histiocytes and phagocytes of the PMS†. They have either a spherical or an oval shape, and measure 1.5–3 μm in diameter (Fig. 5.1). They are slightly smaller than the amastigotes of *Trypanosoma cruzi*, but otherwise cannot be distinguished from the latter. In smears, they appear to be larger than in tissue sections. The nucleus and kinetoplast may be seen in well-preserved material. When kinetoplasts are not detected in the tissue sections, it is due to the age, degeneration or necrobiosis of the amastigotes, or it may be that the tissue was not preserved in time or in the correct manner.

The flagellate forms of *L. donovani*, the promastigotes, are found in cultures at temperatures of 20–30°C. Characteristically, as in other species of leishmanias, flagella are not encountered in the blood of mammals.

Reservoir hosts of *L. donovani* vary according to geographic region: man almost exclusively in India; dogs and other canine species in Mediterranean countries; man and certain wild animals, but not dogs, in Africa. Wild and domestic animals are reservoir hosts in South America. For information about asymptomatic carriers of the disease, see under Pathogenesis below.

Vectors are species of the genus *Phlebotomus* (sand

flies) and, in the New World, mosquitos of the genus *Lutzomyia*.

Pathogenesis

The bite of an infected female sand fly almost always produces the so-called 'leishmanioma', a circumscribed skin nodule which soon disappears. In some cases, this nodule does not appear or is not noted by the patient. General malaise, fever and weakness, signs of generalized disease, appear 2–6 months later.

In man, as well as in lower animals, asymptomatic carriers of kala-azar are known to have parasites in the dermis without visible alterations of the skin. These asymptomatic carriers play an important role in the transmission of the infection.

Pathology

The main organs involved are the spleen, the liver (Fig. 5.2), bone marrow, lymph nodes (Figs. 5.3–5.6) and the lymphatic tissue of the digestive tract (Figs. 5.7 and 5.8). In addition to spleno- and hepatomegaly (the latter less pronounced), there are no characteristic gross features of this infection.

Cutaneous lesions, as manifestations of a late form of kala-azar, have been described in India. This so-called 'cutaneous leishmaniasis post-kala-azar' is sometimes observed 1–2 years after a patient was thought to have been cured. The clinical late form shows spots which slowly enlarge and form nodules of a lepromatous aspect; usually, they do not ulcerate. The 'leishmaniomas' of the skin in the primary infection soon disappear, as noted above.

Clinically a differential diagnosis must be made, especially in infants, with generalized histoplasmosis capsulati. However, the latter is fatal in a very short time, whereas the progression of kala-azar is slower. In any splenomegaly occurring in endemic areas, kala-azar must be considered.

Histologically, parasites (amastigotes of *L. donovani*) are plentiful in the organs of the PMS. They are located in clusters inside histiocytes. Occasionally, they are also located in liver cells; here, they must be looked for with an electron microscope[13]. In the other organs, they are less numerous. It is a 'must' to rule out small yeast cells by application of special fungus stains. With HE, the parasites stain well. With the indirect immunoperoxidase method, they may be marked specifically[14].

Amastigotes of *L. donovani* are scarce in histiocytes in cases of chronic kala-azar (Figs. 5.9–5.11) and in the cutaneous nodules of the late form of the disease. It is most important to make a differential diagnosis with histoplasmosis capsulati in view of the characteristic location of the small yeast cells and the amastigotes inside histiocytes.

Tissue reaction in the visceral leishmaniasis is not characteristic. When numerous parasites are present in tissues, there is practically no tissue response. When parasites are scarce, marked infiltrates of lymphocytes and, above all, plasma cells, are seen with numerous typical Russell bodies (Figs. 5.12 and 5.13).

---

*The so-called Donovani bodies, however, are causal agents of inguinal granuloma, a quite different nosologic entity.

†PMS = phagocytic–mononuclear (cell) system and has replaced RES (reticulo-endothelial system from Aschoff) and RHS (reticulo-histiocytic system).

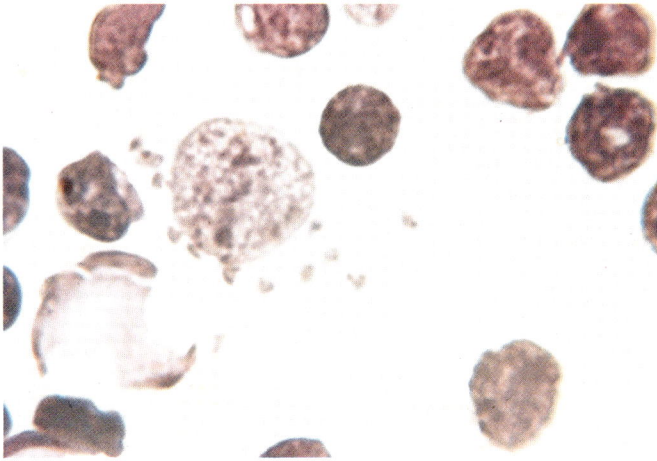

Fig. 5.1 Kala-azar. Numerous leishmanias (*Leishmania donovani*) are seen near a large cell nucleus in the smear of a human bone marrow. Kinetoplasts cannot be recognized. H&E

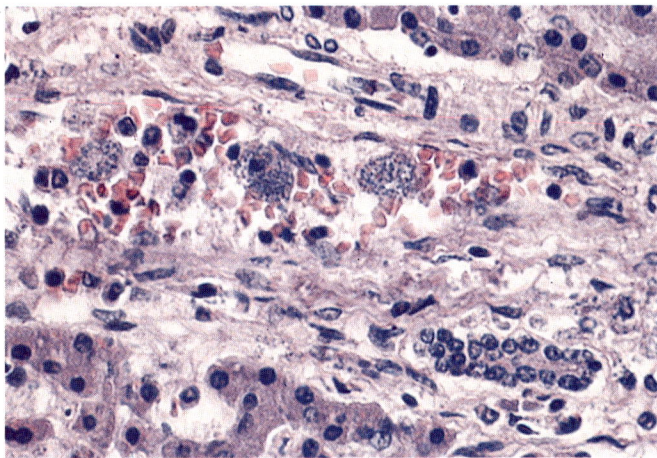

Fig. 5.2 Kala-azar. Nests of leishmanias (*Leishmania donovani*) are seen clearly in macrophages of a portal field in the liver in a case of an acute infection. H&E

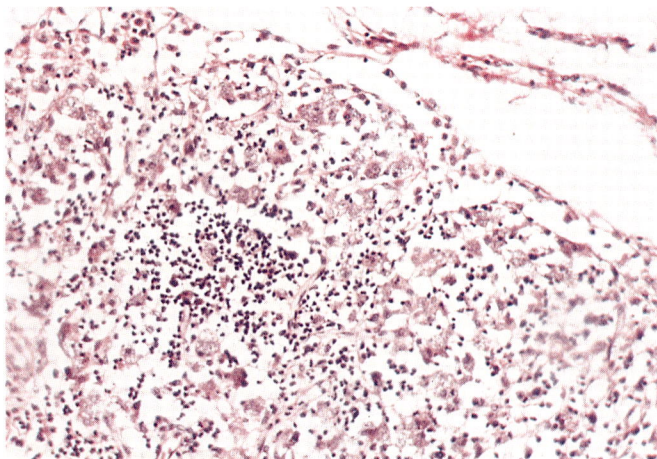

Fig. 5.3 Numerous intracellular nests of leishmanias (*Leishmania donovani*) in mesenteric lymph node of a human case at low power. H&E

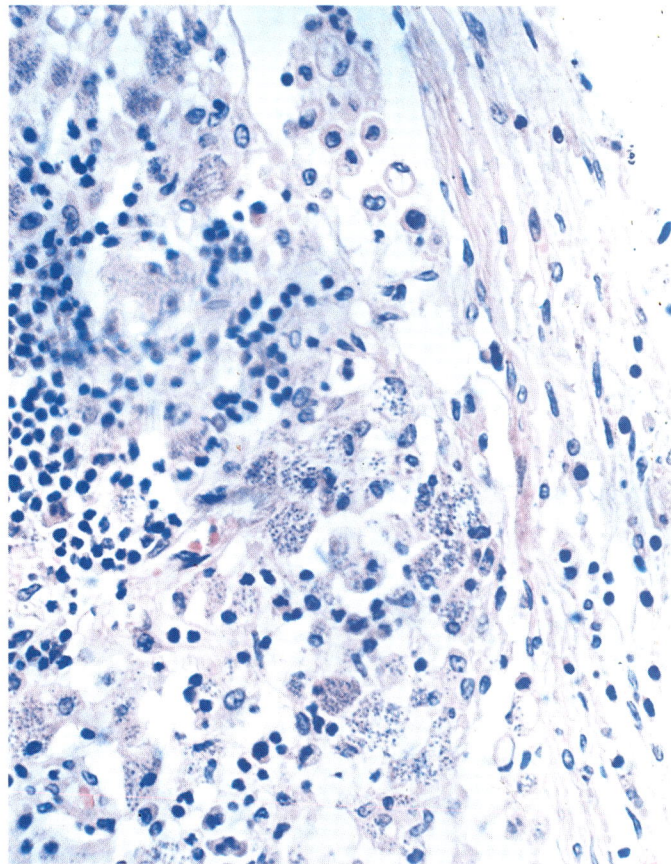

Fig. 5.4 Same case as Fig. 5.3 at higher magnification. H&E

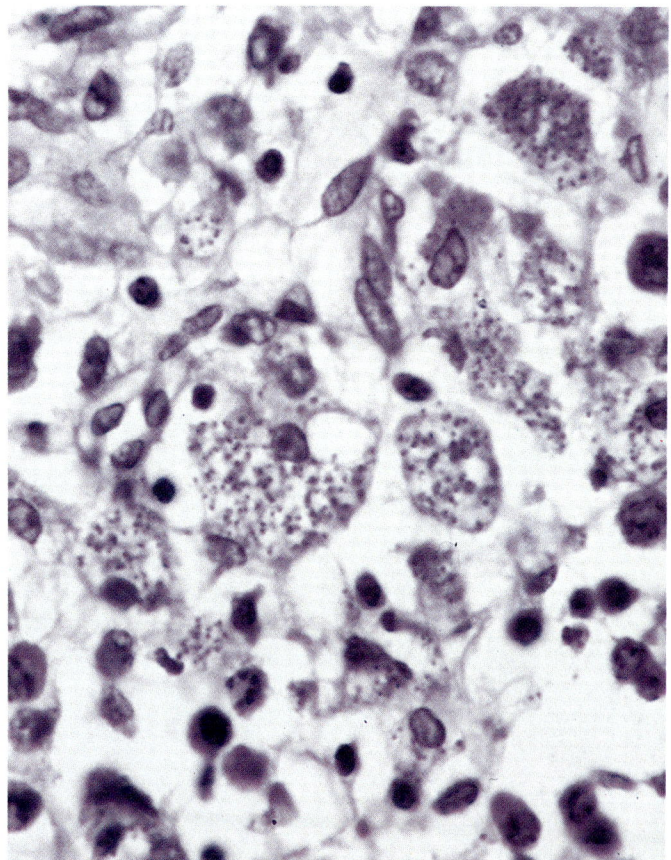

Fig. 5.5 Same case as Figs. 5.3 and 5.4 at higher magnification. H&E

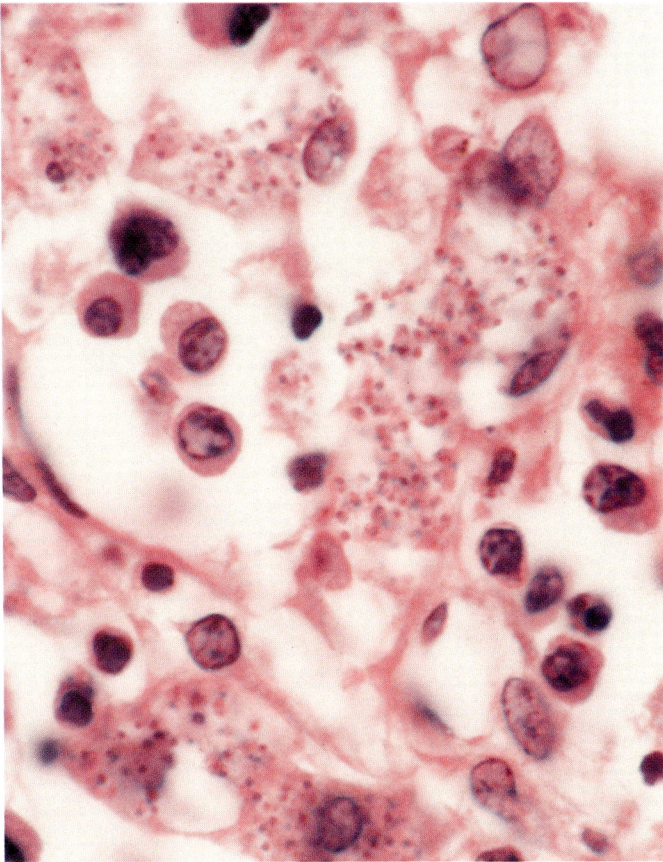

Fig. 5.6 Same case as Figs. 5.3–5.5 at a still higher magnification. Kinetoplasts, however, cannot be detected. H&E

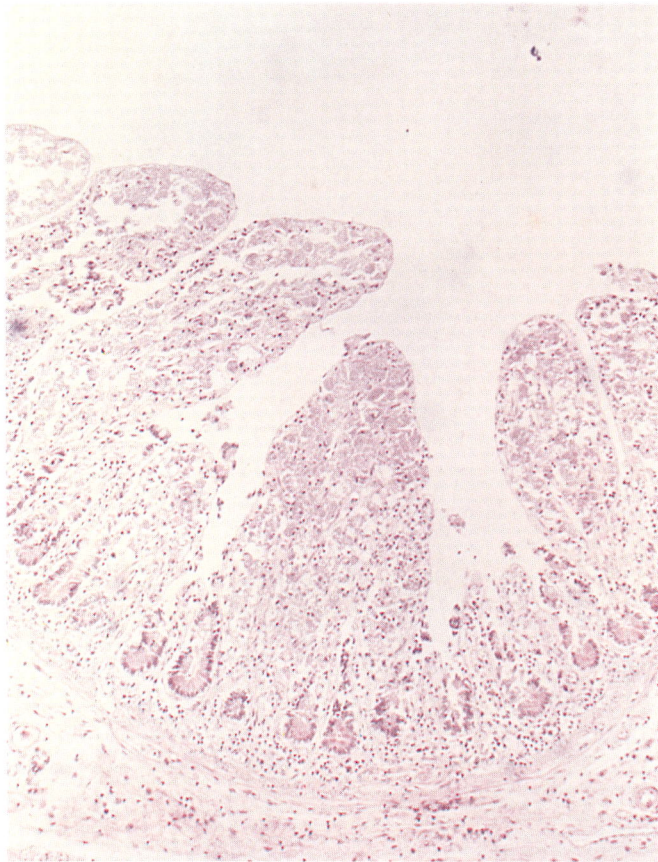

Fig. 5.7 Kala-azar. Human small intestine with thickened villi of the mucosa due to numerous leishmania-containing macrophages. H&E

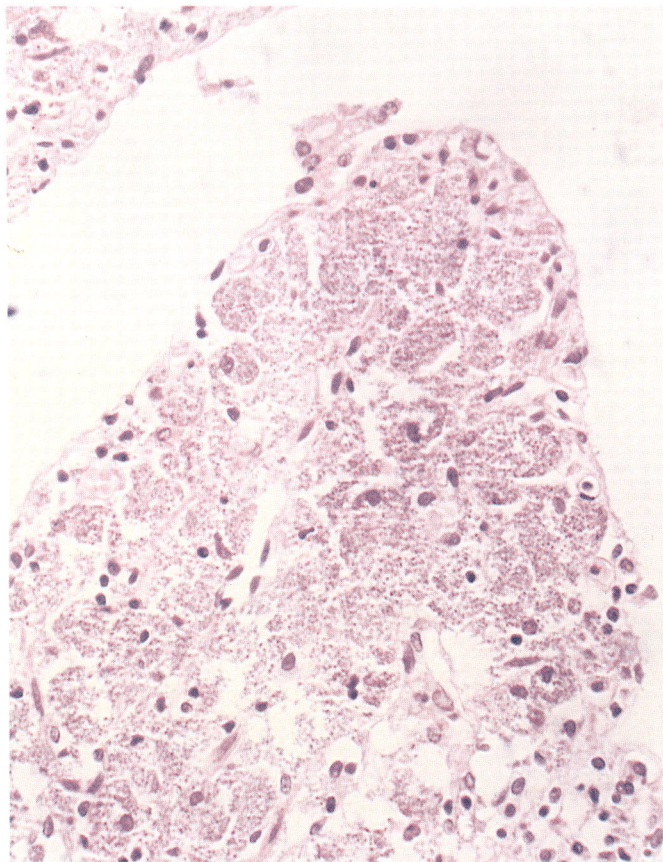

Fig. 5.8 Villus of the mucosa from Fig. 5.7 at higher power. Numerous intracellular organisms of *Leishmania donovani* may be seen. H&E

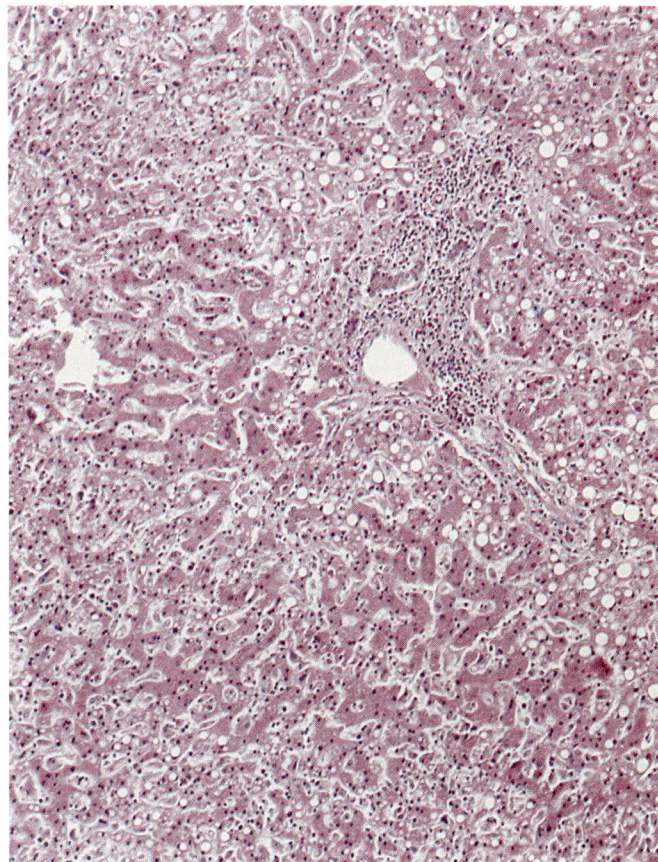

Fig. 5.9 Liver tissue in case of chronic kala-azar at low power. H&E

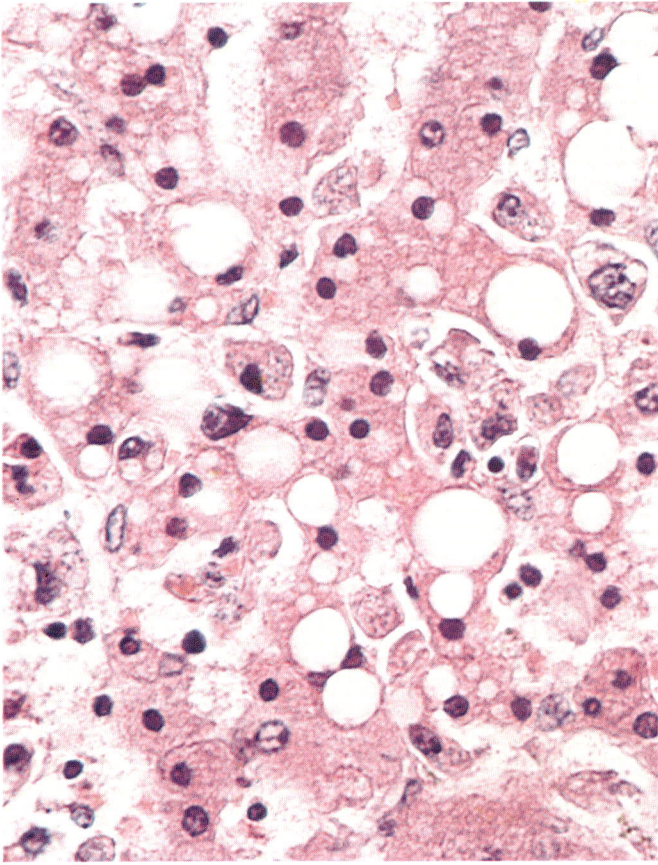

Fig. 5.10 Same case as Fig. 5.9 at higher magnification. Nests of leishmanias (*Leishmania donovani*) may be seen in Kupffer cells. H&E

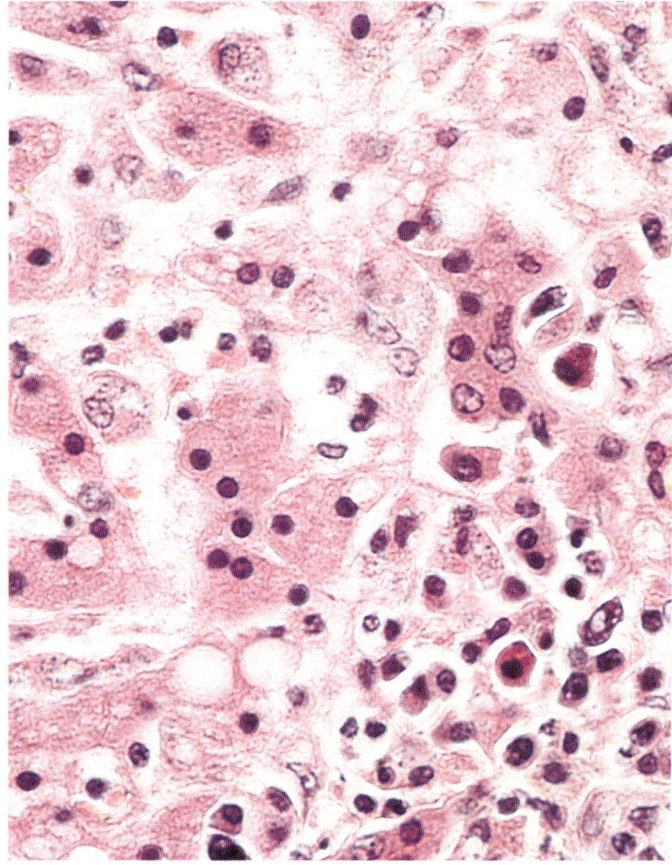

Fig. 5.11 Same case as Figs. 5.10 and 5.11 at a still higher magnification. Parasites and cell infiltrate may be recognized. H&E

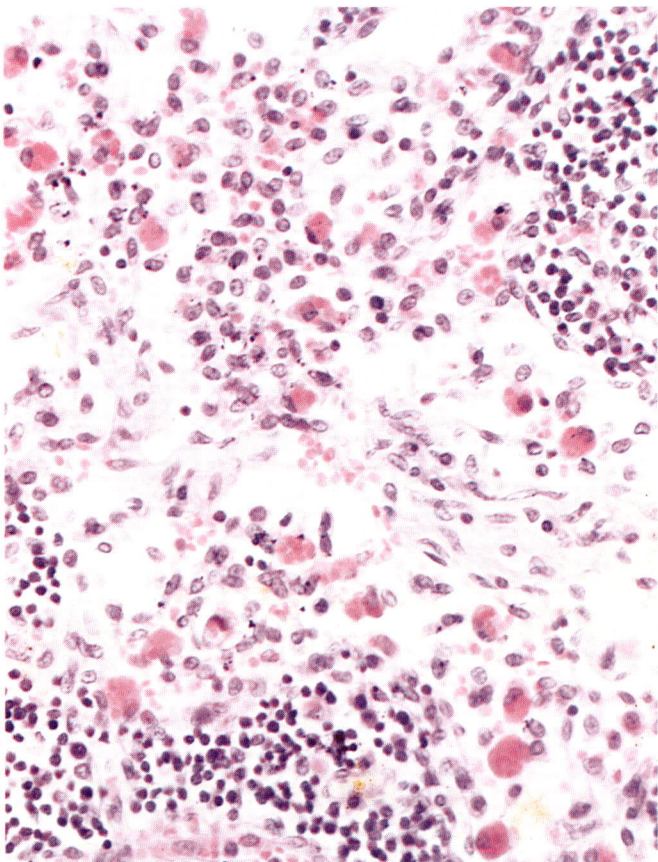

Fig. 5.12 Kala-azar. Human lymph node with numerous Russell bodies. H&E

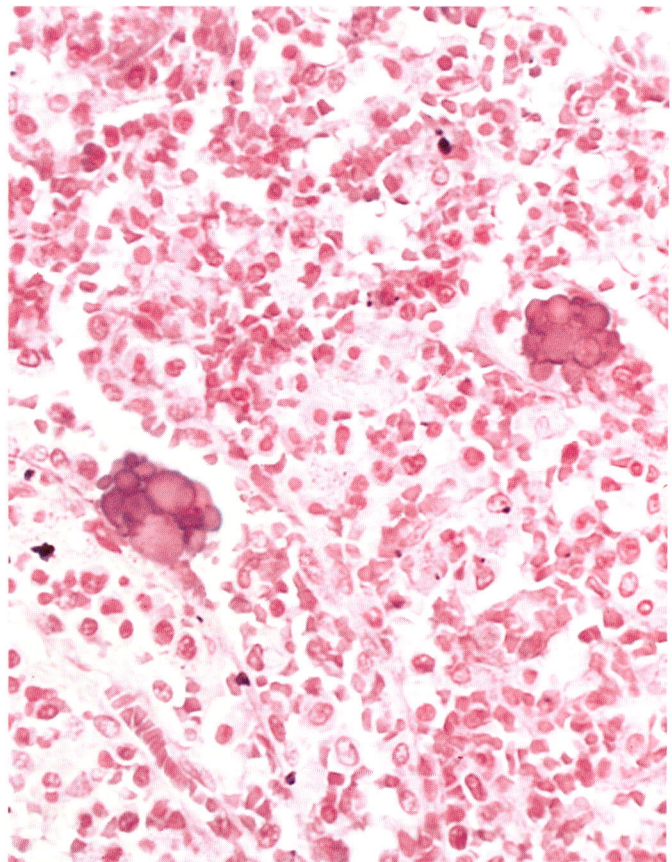

Fig. 5.13 Kala-azar. Human spleen with two large cells (plasma cells) containing Russell bodies. Parasites may not be discerned. Fibrine.

References

1. Heilmann, A., Doehnert, G. and Wohlenberg, A. (1971). Tödlich verlaufende Leishmaniasis visceral bei Mittelmeerurlaubern. *Dtsch. Med. Wschr.*, **96**, 31
2. Loehr, H. and Wolf, H. (1978). Viszerale Kala-azar-Erkrankung beim Kind. *Dtsch. Med. Wschr.*, **103**, 424
3. Alencar, J. E. (1978). Leishmaniose visceral no Brazil. *Rev. Med. Univ. Fed. Ceara*, **17**, 129
4. Gottstein, U., Steiner, K., Hank, H., Klimaschewski, G. and Sedlmeyer, I. (1975). Kala-azar eine wichtige Krankheit nicht nur der Tropen. *Dtsch. Med. Wschr.*, **100**, 2022
5. Martinez, N. A. and Pons, A. R. (1941). Primer caso de Kala-azar en Venezuela. *Gac. Med. Caracas*, **48**, 329
6. Pifano, F. (1954). Estado actual del Kala-azar en Venezuela. *Arch. Venez. Pat. Trop.*, **2**, 213
7. Swenson, C. L., Silverman, J., Stromberg, P. C., Johnson, S. E., Wilkie, D. A., Eaton, K. A. and Kociba, G. J. (1988). Visceral leishmaniasis in an English foxhound from an Ohio research colony. *J. Am. Vet. Med. Assoc.*, **193**, 1089
8. White, M. R., Chapman, W. L. Jr. and Hanson, W. L. (1989). A comparison of experimental visceral leishmaniasis in the opossum, armadillo and ferret. *Lab. Anim. Sci.*, **39**, 47
9. Laurenti, M. D. *et al.* (1990). Experimental visceral leishmaniasis: sequential events of granuloma formation at subcutaneous inoculation site. *Int. J. Exp. Pathol.*, **71**, 791
10. Lujan, R. *et al.* (1990). Leishmania braziliensis in the squirrel monkey: development of primary and satellite lesions and lack of cross-immunity with Leishmania donovani. *J. Parasitol.*, **76**, 594
11. Falk, S., Helm, E. B., Hubner, K. and Stutte, H. J. (1988). Disseminated visceral leishmaniasis (kala-azar) in acquired immunodeficiency syndrome (AIDS). *Pathol. Res. Pract.*, **183**, 253
12. Ponce, C. *et al.* (1991). L. donovani chagasi: new clinical variant of cutaneous leishmaniasis in Honduras. *Lancet*, **337**, 67
13. Duarte, M. I., Mariano, O. N. and Corbett, C. E. (1989). Liver parenchymal cell parasitism in human visceral leishmaniasis. *Virchows Arch. A.*, **415**, 1
14. Ferrer, L., Rabanal, R. M., Domingo, M., Ramos, J. A. and Fondevila, D. (1988). Identification of Leishmania donovani amastigotes in canine tissues by immunoperoxidase staining. *Res. Vet. Sci.*, **44**, 194

6. GIARDIASIS

Introduction

A synonym for this parasitosis is lambliasis. The infection occurs worldwide; 2–10% of the population, mostly children, are infected in countries with a cold or temperate climate. In countries with a warm climate, the percentage goes up to 20–50%[1]. The prevalence among subjects at risk in certain countries is not negligible[2]. In Venezuela this intestinal infection is well known.

Dogs, cats and rodents are carriers of the parasite and may be used for experimental purposes[3,4].

Clinically, diarrhoea with yellowish fetid faeces are observed, occasionally accompanied by abdominal pain and cramps; also steatorrhoea[5] and malabsorption syndrome have been found. Prognosis is always favourable; there are no reports of a fatal outcome. Infection is symptomatic in children but usually asymptomatic in adults[6].

Clinical diagnosis is made by confirmation of mobile trophozoites in the duodenal contents[7]. Cystic forms of giardias are found in faeces. Giardiasis often occurs in combination with another bacterial or viral enteritis.

The parasite

Giardia lamblia or *Lamblia intestinalis* is a flagellated protozoan with vegetative (trophozoites) and cystic forms. The trophozoites are pear-shaped, measure 10–12 μm in length, 5–10 μm in width and are 3–5 μm thick. They possess 2 nuclei and 4 basal corpuscles near the round anterior pole. These 4 corpuscles, found between the two nuclei, are the origin of the 8 filaments which appear as 4 pairs of flagella outside the parasite. On the ventral surface, there is a so-called 'suction disc', visible only with an electron microscope, which corresponds to a circumscribed shallow part used by the parasite to attach itself to the intestinal mucosa.

The cysts of *Giardia lamblia* are oval and have 4 nuclei, situated at one pole. They measure 8–14 μm in length and 6–10 μm in width. In the interior of the cyst, one can see longitudinal filaments which reach beyond the membrane as short flagella. There are between two and four basal corpuscles shaped like a sickle or a banana. The cysts survive in a humid environment for weeks or months[8].

The giardias stain well with the Giemsa, H&E, and iron haematoxylin. They are Grocott-positive (Figs. 6.1–6.5). To see the structural details, fresh live giardias must be used with special methods of fixation and phase contrast.

Pathogenesis

The cystic forms of *G. lamblia* in the faeces of man or animal carriers contaminate water and foods, i.e. transmission occurs from man to man or animal to man directly and orally. Some insects and other small animals may also act as vehicles (seldom).

In the small bowel, cysts become trophozoites which attach themselves by means of the rims of the 'suction discs' to the superficial cells of the microvilli of the mucosa. Here they multiply copiously by fission but do not penetrate into the tissues.

It seems that it is the massive reproduction of giardias, with the resulting microlesions and the production of large amounts of mucoid substances, that leads to the enteritis. Other theories have also been put forward as pathogenic factors[9], e.g. the mechanical prevention of interchange of alimentary substances.

Pathology

The trophozoites of *Giardia lamblia* are found in the duodenum, sometimes in the jejunum and, occasionally, in the upper parts of the ileum. Location at other sites has not been confirmed. The cysts are located in the lower parts of the small intestine, in the large bowel and in formed faeces. Gross intestinal lesions have not been reported.

Histologically, the material obtained routinely in autopsies cannot be used for studying giardias or the lesions caused by these parasites. Biopsies must be performed and the material then examined under an electron microscope[10–12].

The attachment of the giardias to the surface of the mucosa apparently acts as an irritant with the subsequent inflammation. In acute cases, infiltrates of neutrophilic and eosinophilic granulocytes are found in the stroma of the upper parts of the mucosa and, in chronic cases, lymphohistiocytic ones are seen[13].

Ulceration of the mucosa, which is occasionally observed, is not thought to be due to giardias but to other infectious agents, such as bacteria or viruses.

References

1. Faust, E. C. and González-Mugaburu, L. (1965). Parasitological surveys in Cali, Departamento del Valle, Colombia, XI. Intestinal parasites in ward Silva, Cali during four years period. 1956–1960. *Am. J. Trop. Med. Hyg.*, **14**, 276

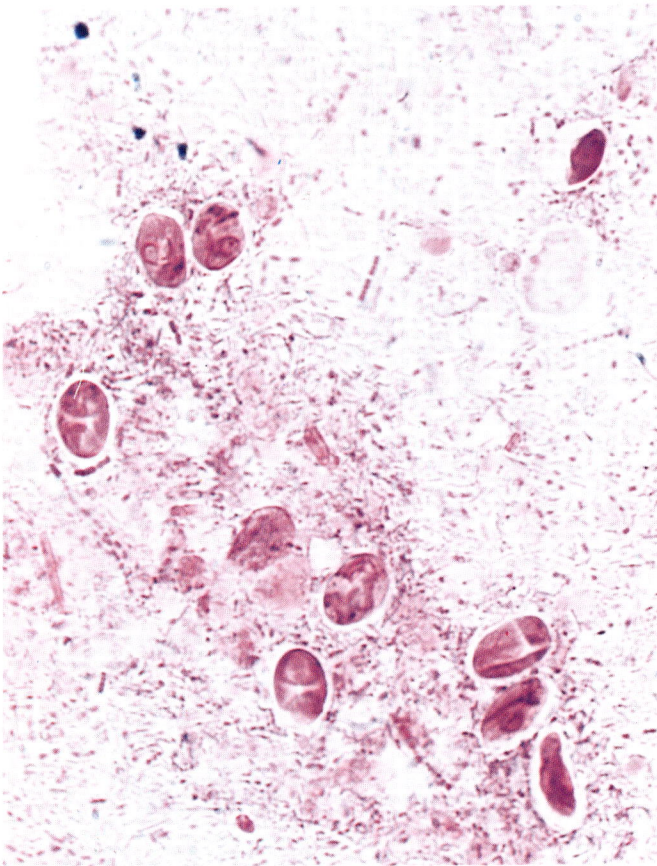

Fig. 6.1 Giardias in faecal smear of an autopsy. H&E

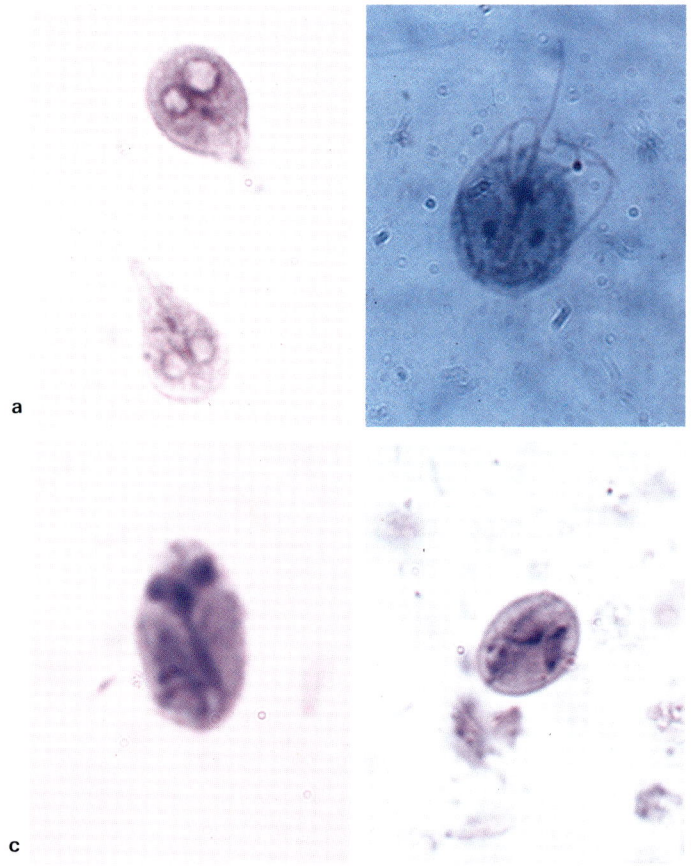

Fig. 6.2 Trophozoites (**a** and **b**) and cysts (**c** and **d**) of *Giardia lamblia*. Giemsa

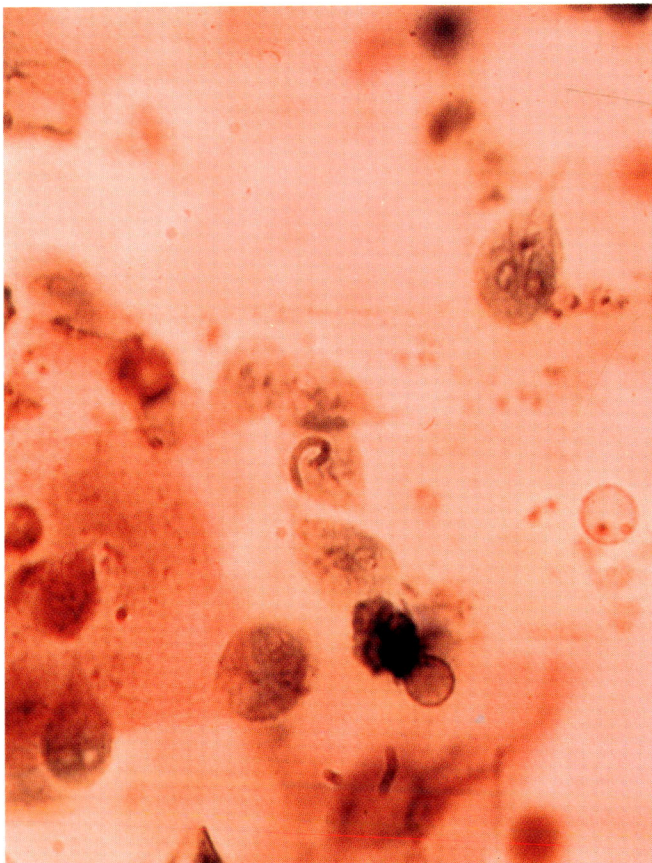

Fig. 6.3 Cluster of *Giardia lamblia* trophozoites in faeces. Trichrom

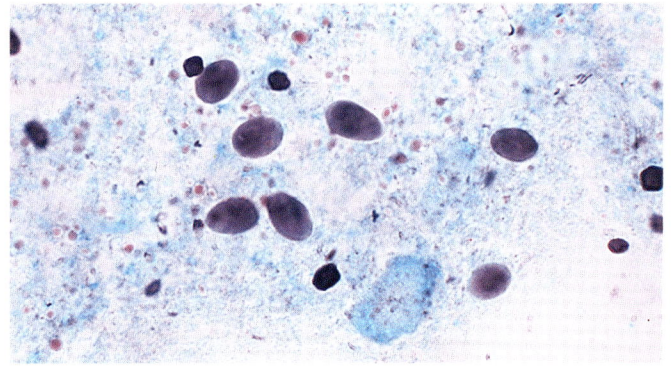

Fig. 6.4 Giardias in a smear of intestinal content. Autopsy material. Grocott

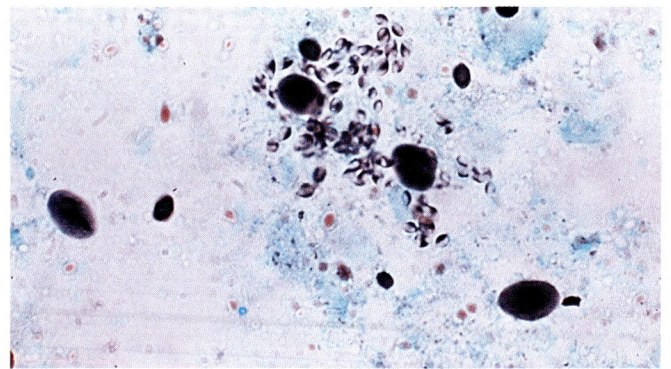

Fig. 6.5 Giardias and yeast cells (of *Candida* sp. ?) in smear of intestinal content. Autopsy material. Grocott

2. Cotte-Roche, C. *et al.* (1991). Role de la giardiase dans la dyspepsie non ulcereuse. *Presse Med.,* **20**, 936
3. Arashima, Y. *et al.* (1990). Studies on the giardiasis as the zoonosis. *Kansenshogaku-Zasshi,* **64**, 295
4. Romia, S. A. *et al.* (1990). Virulence of Giardia lamblia isolates to laboratory mice. *J. Egypt. Soc. Parasitol.,* **20**, 633
5. Amini, F. (1963). Giardiasis and steatorrhea. *J. Trop. Med. Hyg.,* **66**, 190
6. Peterson, H. (1973). Clinical significance of G. lamblia (Lamblia intestinalis). *Acta Hepatogastroenterol. (Stuttg.),* **20**, 449
7. González Carbajal Pascual, M., Cayon, R., Pérez, A. and Sotto, A. (1988). Value of endoscopic smears of the duodenal mucosa in the diagnosis of giardiasis in adults. *Rev. Gastroenterrol. Mex.,* **53**, 37
8. de Regnier, D. P., Cole, L., Schupp, D. G. and Erlandsen, S. L. (1989). Viability of Giardia cysts suspended in lake, river, and tap water. *Appl. Environ. Microbiol.,* **55**, 1223

9. Ament, M. E. and Rubin, C. E. (1972). Relation of giardiasis to abnormal intestinal structure and function in gastrointestinal immunodeficiency. *Gastroenterology,* **62**, 216
10. Takano, J. and Yardley, J. M. (1965). Jejunal lesions in patients with giardiasis and malabsorption. An electron microscopic study. *Bull. Johns Hopkins Hosp.,* **116**, 413
11. Rosekrans, P. C. M., Lindeman, J. and Meijer, C. J. L. M. (1981). Quantitative histological and immunohistochemical findings in jejunal biopsy specimens in giardiasis. *Virchows Archiv. A. (Pathol. Anat.),* **393**, 145
12. Khanna, R. *et al.* (1990). An ultrastructural analysis of changes in surface architecture of intestinal mucosa following Giardia lamblia infection in mice. *Gastroenterol. Jpn.,* **25**, 649
13. Oberhuber, G. and Stolte, M. (1990). Giardiasis: analysis of histological changes in biopsy specimens of 80 patients. *J. Clin. Pathol.,* **43**, 641

7. TRICHOMONIASIS

Introduction

This disease (for which there is no synonym) is endemic all over the world. The infection is observed predominantly in promiscuous females but males may be infected[1]. Trichomoniasis is common in Venezuela.

Trichomonas vaginalis is not found in lower animals, although other species of this genus have been detected in squirrel monkeys[2], and systemic trichomoniasis has been found recently in squabs (young pigeons).

The infection is almost always asymptomatic or latent. Once symptoms appear, the infection remains active for a long time, causing complaints like vaginal flux and marked prurigo. Even with efficient therapy, patients are not always cured by a single treatment as relapses and reinfection are frequent. Clinical exacerbation, common during menstruation and pregnancy, has been ascribed to changes in pH of the vaginal milieu.

Clinical diagnosis may be confirmed by examination of vaginal, cervical or prostate secretions and/or urine; the typical mobile flagellates can be found in fresh specimens. In asymptomatic females, trichomoniasis is often found when cytological examinations (Papanicolaou) are made in order to rule out a carcinoma.

Trichomoniasis is quite often associated with previous bacterial, viral or mycotic infections of the urogenital tract and with carcinoma of cervix. It has been confirmed, however, that this parasitosis is not a carcinogenic risk.

The parasite

Trichomonas vaginalis is the only pathogenic species in this genus. Other flagellates found in the digestive tract and in the oral cavity of man are almost always apathogenic[3].

The parasite is almost always pear-shaped and measured $7-30\,\mu m$ in length (on average $13\,\mu m$). The size varies with the type and strain, and the pH of the medium. At the anterior end, a blepharoplast is seen, and from this, originate 4 anterior flagella and one posterior flagellum with an undulating membrane. The nucleus is situated towards the rear end. In fresh preparations, the parasites can be seen moving with the aid of their flagella and the undulating membrane. They stain well with H&E, iron haematoxylin, Giemsa or the Papanicolaou method (Figs. 7.1 and 7.2). In cultures (Fig. 7.3), the parasites may phagocytose leukocytes, bacteria and red blood cells. Leukocytes and epithelial cells are able to phagocytose parasites[4].

Pathogenesis

An infected male transmits the infection from one female to another through sexual relations. The reservoir host of *Trichomonas vaginalis* is the infected female.

There may also be indirect transmission through sanitary installations or infected underwear. Infection of newborn babies is due to contamination during parturition.

Pathology

In the female, the parasite lives in the vagina, in the cervical channel, in the urethra and, occasionally, in the lower part of the bladder[5]. In males, they have been found in the urethra and the prostate; some observers have also noted them in the seminal vesicles[6]. Invasion of human tissues by *Trichomonas vaginalis* has not been reported. Gross lesions are not known.

The histological alterations which may be produced by these parasites can be summarized in the following manner:

1. The epithelial cells may degenerate and show cytoplasmic vacuolization (Fig. 7.4),

2. Regeneration and endocervical metaplasia of the epithelial cells may occur (Fig. 7.6),

3. Inflammation with lympholeukocytic and plasma cell infiltrates may be seen in the epithelium and in the stroma,

4. Erosions of the surface and mucopurulent exudation may occur (Fig. 7.5).

It is not entirely clear whether these alterations are due to the irritation produced by these parasites or due to a secondary bacterial infection. It has been established, however, that the parasites do not cause endometritis, puerperal infections, sterility, miscarriages or carcinoma.

The parasites may produce some alterations in tissue cells which could be confused with those seen in neoplastic processes. Therefore, if there is infection with this parasite, it must be taken into consideration when cytology and biopsy specimens are examined in order to avoid a false positive diagnosis of malignancy.

Cytologic differential diagnosis of the parasite must consider: artificial particles, as a result of contaminated slides, epithelial cells or their nuclei, and deformed granulocytes, histiocytes or degenerated parabasal cells.

References

1. Feo, L. G. (1944). The incidence and significance of Trichomonas vaginalis infestation in the male. *Am. J. Trop. Med.,* **24**, 195
2. Scimeca, J. M., Culberson, D. E., Abee, C. R. and Gardner, W. A. Jr. (1989). Intestinal trichomonads (Trichomonas mobilensis) in the natural host Saimiri sciureus and Saimiri boliviensis. *Vet. Pathol.,* **26**, 144

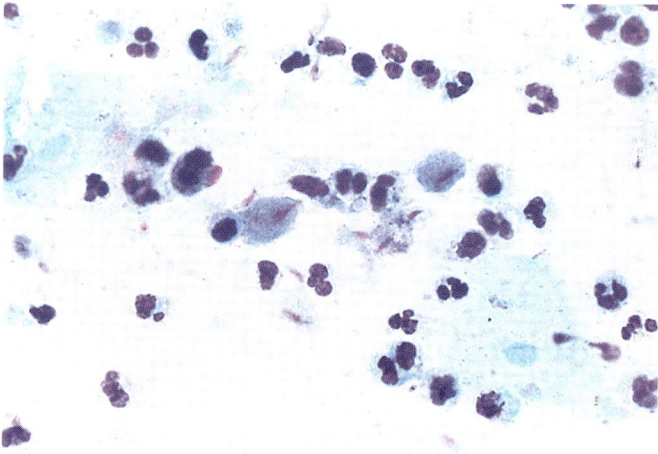

Fig. 7.1 Smear from the uterine cervix. Organisms of *Trichomonas vaginalis* and leukocytes. Papanicolaou

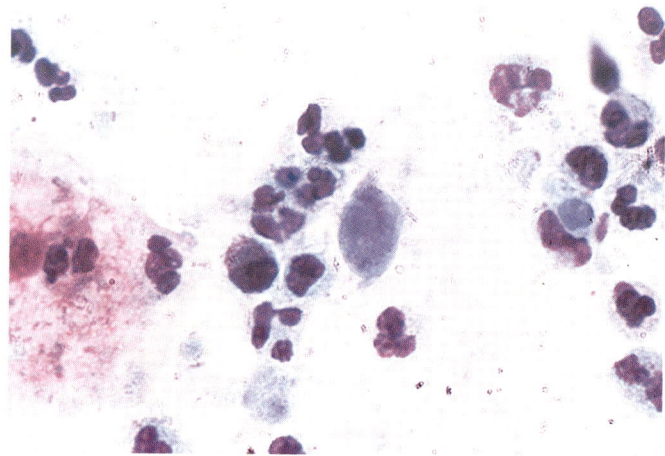

Fig. 7.2 Higher magnification of a smear from uterine cervix. Papanicolaou

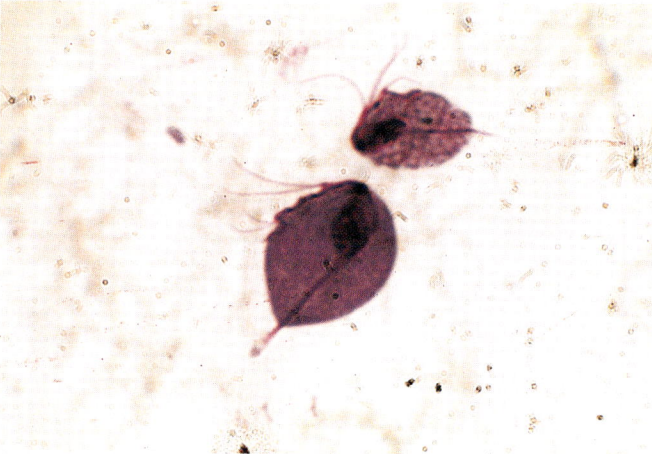

Fig. 7.3 Smear of cultured parasites with visible flagella. Giemsa

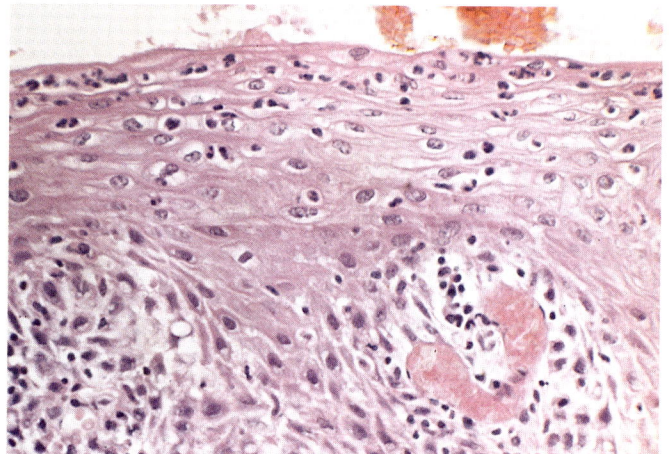

Fig. 7.4 Trichomoniasis. Vacuolic degeneration of epithelial cells and inflammation at epithelium and stroma. H&E

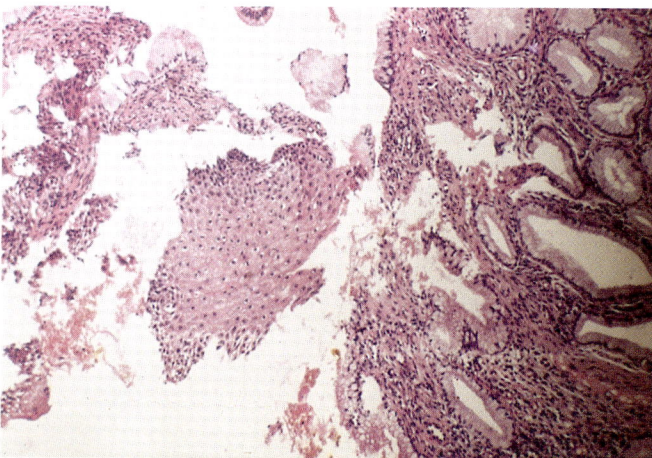

Fig. 7.5 Trichomoniasis. Islet of epithelial metaplasia (detached) at the endocervix. H&E

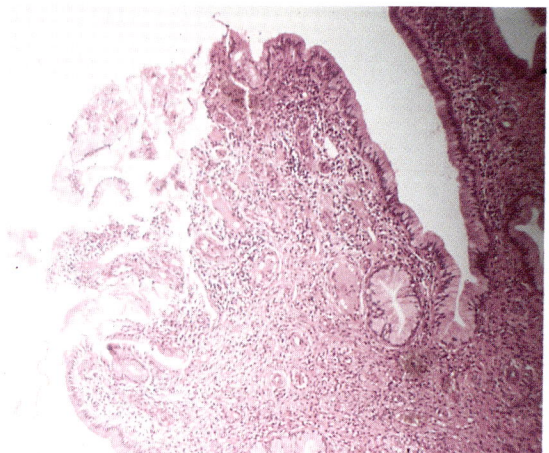

Fig. 7.6 Trichomoniasis. Erosion and marked inflammation at the endocervix. H&E

3. Honigberg, B. M. (1978). Trichomonads of importance in human medicine. In Kreier, J. P. (Hrsg) *Parasitic Protozoan II*. Academic Press: New York London San Francisco
4. Asami, K. (1952). Bacteria-free cultivation of Trichomonas vaginalis. *Kitasato Arch. Exp. Med.*, **25**, 149
5. Heckel, N. J. (1936). A study of the pathologic alterations in the female bladder and urethra resulting from infection with Trichomonas vaginalis. *J. Urol.*, **35**, 520
6. Crowley, E. (1964). Trichomonas prostatis and trichomenorrhea. A new link in the diagnosis and treatment of trichomoniasis. *J. Urol.*, **91**, 302

8.　AMOEBIASIS

Introduction

This disease is also called amoebic dysentery. It is still an important infection, with involvement mainly of the digestive tract. However, it may be treated successfully with modern drugs when an early diagnosis is made. When extraintestinal organs are involved, aetiological diagnosis is not easily made.

The prevalence of amoebiasis is approximately 10% of the world population and it occurs in practically all countries and all social groups[1]. The disease is frequently more severe in tropical and subtropical regions. Amoebiasis is endemic in Venezuela; in the fifties and sixties numerous fatal cases were still observed in Mérida/Venezuela[2,3]. Epidemic outbreaks may occur simultaneously with bacterial dysentery.

Natural *Entamoeba histolytica* infections are found in dogs, rats, pigs and monkeys but they are of no relevance to the human infection. Rats and other laboratory animals may be used as experimental models[4-7].

The dysenteric syndrome is characterized by blood and mucoid substances in the diarrhoeal stools. Relapses, after variable periods of apparent cure, are more frequent than definitive cures of an acute stage.

Clinical diagnosis is made by confirmation of the causative agent. This requires well-trained laboratory personnel since other species of amoebae must be ruled out and not all elements which are mobile in fresh preparations represent amoebae. Also, in biopsies and sections of cell blocks of a semiliquid material, amoebae are sometimes difficult to distinguish from tissue cells and other elements[8,9]. Serological diagnosis is indicated, above all, in patients with liver abscesses[10].

The parasite

Entamoeba histolytica is the only pathogenic species of the intestinal amoebae, i.e. this species may invade tissues. The other four species of intestinal amoebae (*Entamoeba coli, Endolimax nana, Iodamoeba buetschlii, Dientamoeba fragilis*) are non-invasive. Soil amoebae are mentioned in the next section, Acanthamoebiasis.

Two forms of *Entamoeba histolytica* exist, the trophozoites and the cysts. The former can be seen in diarrhoeal stools and in tissues; the latter are found in formed faeces and are able to survive outside the human organism representing an 'enduring form'.

The trophozoite measures 7–35 µm, is irregularly shaped and moves by typical amoeboid pseudopodia in fresh preparations. The nucleus is vesiculous or annular. In the cytoplasm, erythrocytes, fragments of tissue cells or engulfed leukocytes are often present (Fig. 8.1). After the division of trophozoites, cysts develop. These are amoebae with thicker membranes. The cysts are spherical and measure on average 11 µm. A young cyst has one nucleus; a mature one up to four nuclei.

We are more inclined to examine permanent and stained preparations than to look at unstained smears. For smears and tissue sections, the classical stain is iron haematoxylin (Heidenhain) which is somewhat better than haematoxylin–eosin. We prefer a modification of the PAS method[11]

(Fig. 8.2). Amoebae also stain partially with the Grocott method.

Amoebae may be cultured in diverse artificial media. They may harbour HIV-1 but there is no transmission to human cells[12].

Pathogenesis

The amoebic cysts are the infectious elements of *Entamoeba histolytica*. They reach the human digestive tract through water, food or by other means, such as dirty hands or indirect vectors such as flies. The most important source of infection is man; a carrier of cysts is generally asymptomatic and apparently completely healthy. Patients with signs of amoebic dysentery are not the source of infection; they eliminate only trophozoites which die quickly.

When the cysts of *E. histolytica* reach the digestive tract, they transform into trophozoites which are able to penetrate the wall of the large bowel. They migrate through the mucosa and may reach the serosa through all the layers of the intestinal wall. The classical concept is that the vegetative forms (trophozoites) themselves produce proteolytic (cyto- and histolytic) enzymes (as indicated by the name *Entamoeba histolytica*) in order to facilitate the penetration of tissues but this has not been convincingly demonstrated. Be that as it may, the parasitic invasion leads to tissue necrosis. The action or co-action of bacteria, before and after formation of necroses, is also not clear. There is always an associated bacterial infection.

Lately, both in amoebiasis and in other pathological intestinal conditions, the necroses have been interpreted as being lesions similar to infarcts. This means that the necroses can be explained as the result of the formation of thrombi or microthrombi which produce ischaemic processes and consecutive infarcts. However, true thrombi have not been found in our series of cases of amoebic colitis.

The amoebae spread by contiguity, by lymphogenous and haematogenous dissemination from primary intestinal lesions (and from other sites). Haematogenous spread is the most frequent and important, while dissemination by contiguity or contact is less common, and lymphogenous spread is an exception. The large bowel and the liver are the preferential organs for amoebic infections. From the liver, they can also reach other viscera. Frequently, these amoebae are encountered in an organ or organ system distinct from the intestine, appearing to be an 'isolated disease' because the intestinal lesions have recovered and the patients may not even remember the diarrhoeal episodes which possibly occurred only once years ago.

Pathology

Intestinal amoebiasis. The incubation period has not been precisely defined. The superficial necrotic lesions in the mucosa soon detach and multiple large ulcerative areas remain in the mucosa, involving deeper layers of the intestinal wall (Figs. 8.3–8.6). These ulcers in the large intestine are deep crater-like defects with undermined rims and are called 'button-hole' ulcers (Figs. 8.7 and 8.8).

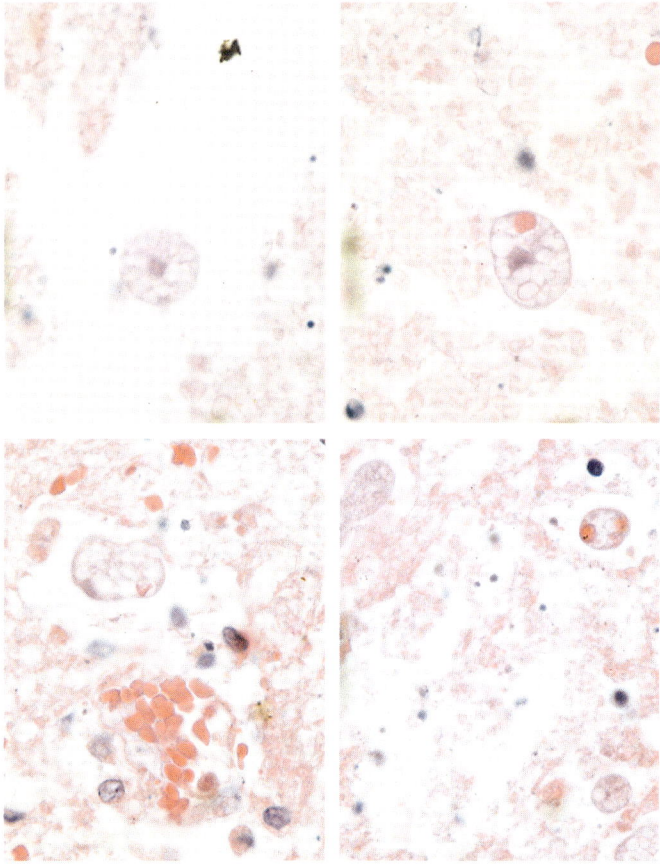

Fig. 8.1 Trophozoites of *Entamoeba histolytica* in tissues. H&E

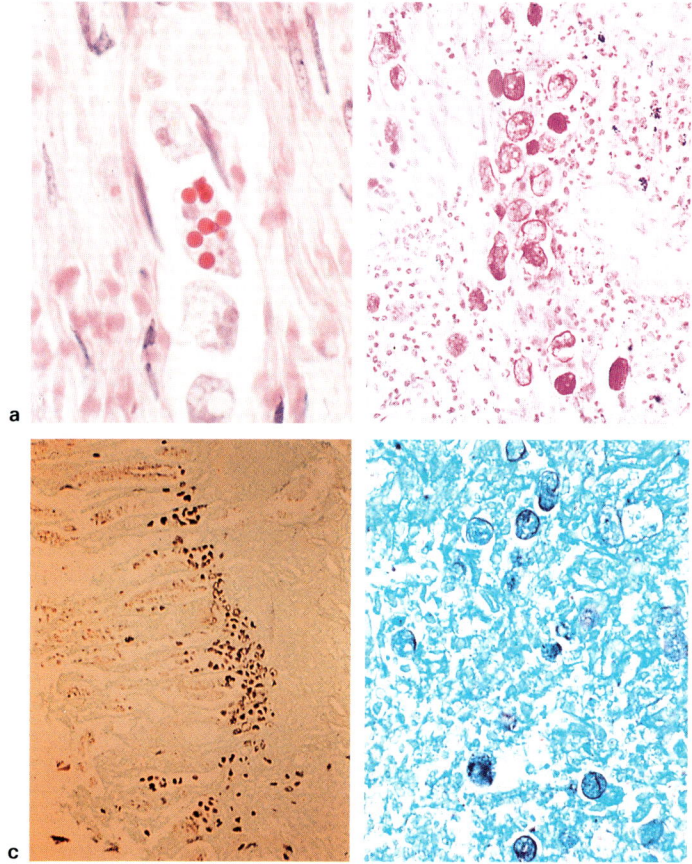

Fig. 8.2 Trophozoites of *Entamoeba histolytica* in tissues:
a. Erythrophagia. H&E
b. Special stain for amoebae. PAS
c. Marked amoebae at intestinal mucosa. Grocott
d. Amoebae. Grocott

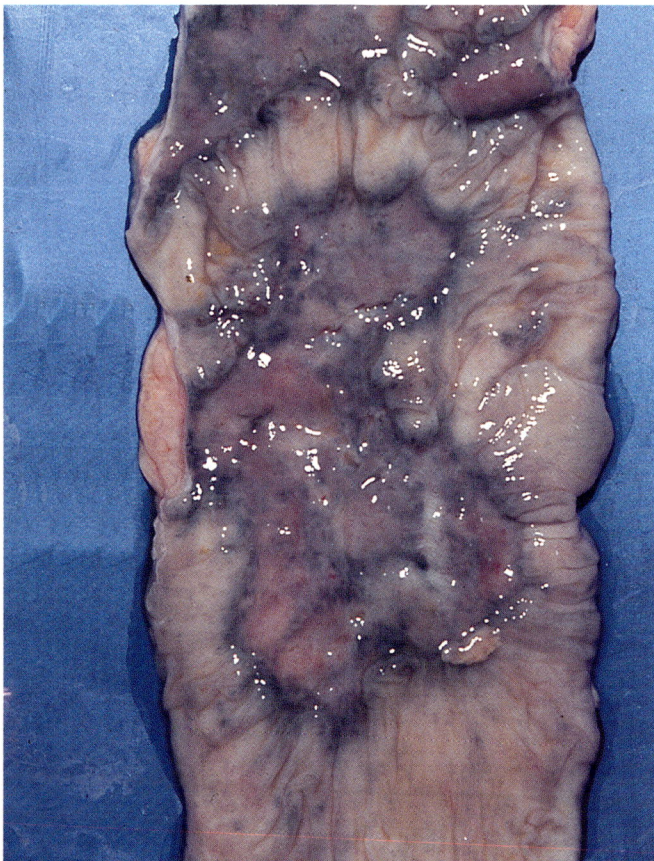

Fig. 8.3 Amoebiasis. Large intestine with deep mucosal ulcer showing thick borders

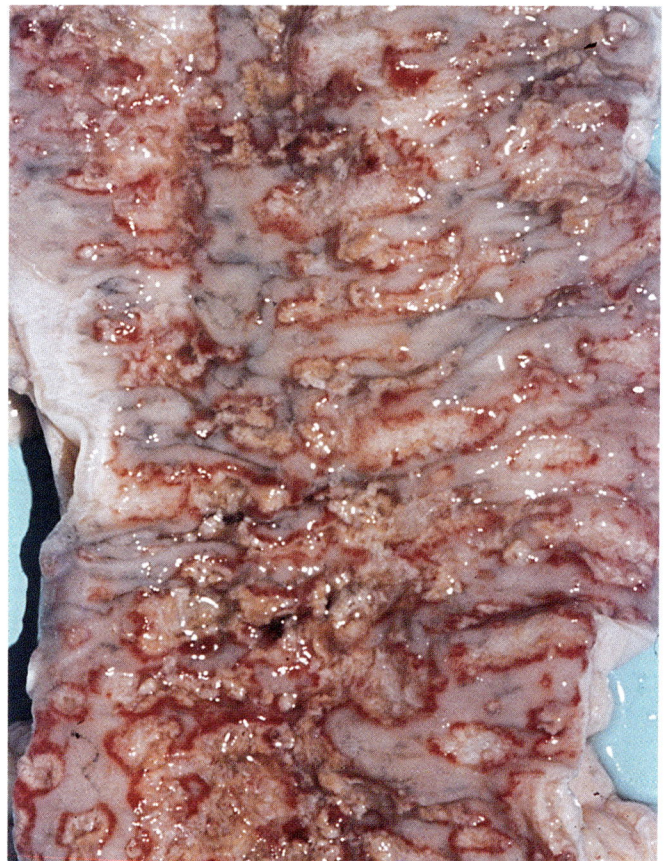

Fig. 8.4 Amoebiasis. Numerous necrotic foci and ulcers in the mucosa of the large intestine

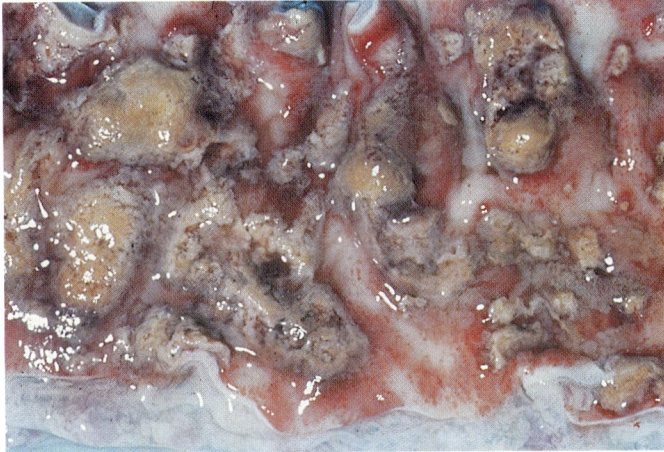

Fig. 8.5 Amoebiasis. Small and large necrotic foci in the mucosa of the large intestine

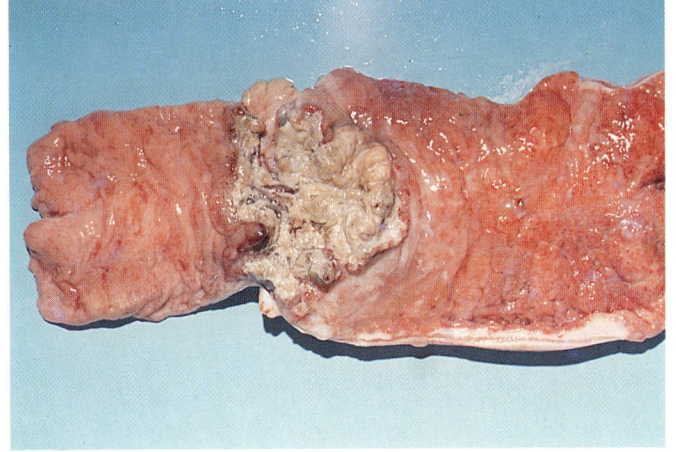

Fig. 8.6 Amoebic colitis with carcinoma of the colon transversum. Under the microscope in this lesion adenocarcinoma in addition to amoebae was found. It was not possible to determine which of these two processes was the initial one

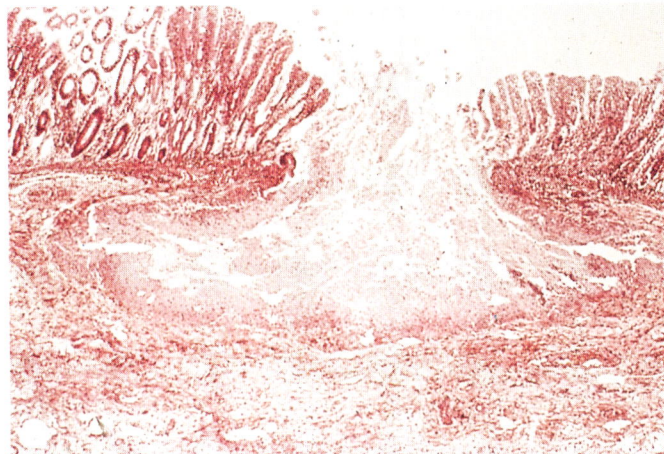

Fig. 8.7 Amoebiasis. A complete, characteristic 'buttonhole ulcer' of the large intestine comprising mucosa and submucosa with the borders of the entire circumference undermined. H&E

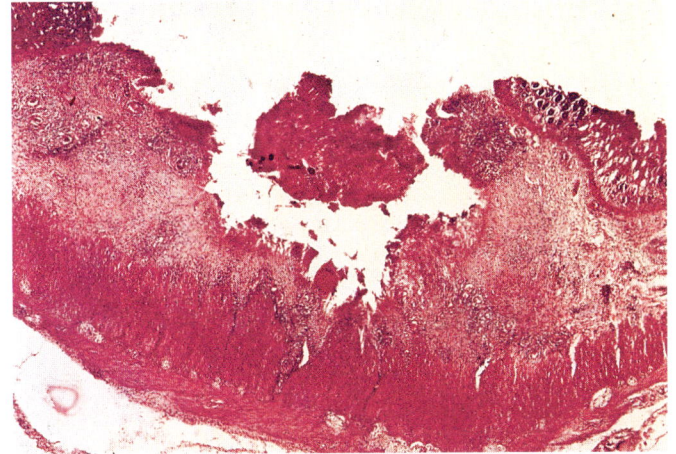

Fig. 8.8 Amoebiasis. A recently formed ulcer involving mucosa and submucosa of the large intestine in the form of a 'buttonhole'. H&E

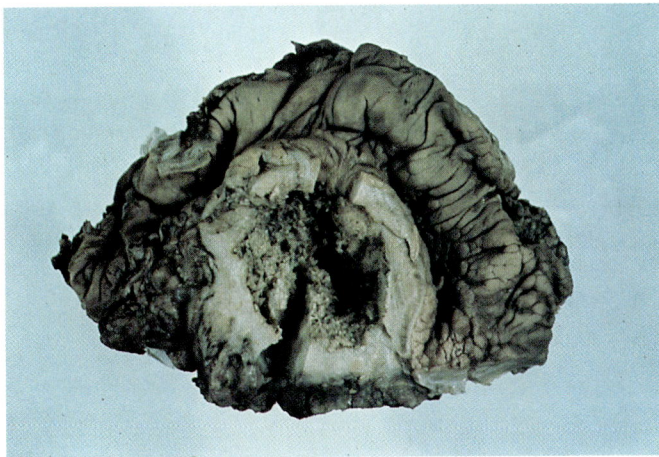

Fig. 8.9 'Amoeboma' of the mesocolon. The opened large intestine presents an enlarged (cut) fistula connecting intestinal lumen with a large 'tumour' which shows a cavity (necrosis) on the central part. The 'tumour' is formed by chronic granulation tissue with numerous amoebae in the mesocolon

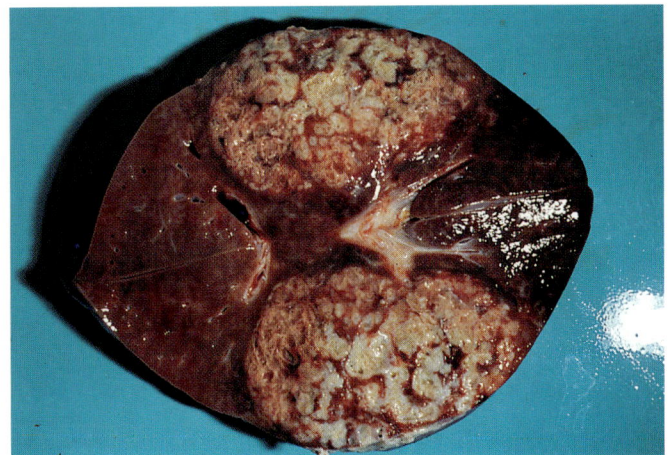

Fig. 8.10 Solitary amoebic liver abscess

However, it must be noted that ulcers with these characteristics are also found in bacterial dysentery and that they do not appear exclusively in amoebiasis. In our material, the ulcers of the amoebic colitis do not occur more frequently at any particular site in the large bowel: they occur in the caecum, both flexurae or in the rectosigmoidal region. Relatively frequently, the appendix showed amoebic lesions, although large grossly detectable lesions were not seen at this site. More frequently, the appendix and part of the ileum were involved, showing, microscopically, more or less extensive necrotic lesions in the intestinal wall, but almost never grossly visible ulcers. Isolated amoebic appendicitis is not common[13]. The amoebic ulcers in the large intestine, which are often deep, may reach the serosa where circumscribed peritonitis is provoked. Perforation of these ulcers with consequent diffuse peritonitis, which used to be a serious complication, is no longer seen, apparently because diagnosis is made earlier and/or therapy is more efficient.

Other important complications are peri-appendicular abscesses and colo-abdominal, colo-gastric or colo-hepatic fistulae. Fistulae between the colon and renal pelvis, rectum or bladder are rarer. Amoebic lesions of the spleen, pancreas and kidneys are formed rarely by contiguity.

In **chronic intestinal amoebiasis**, with or without mucosal ulcers, the mucosa becomes thicker and polypoid tumoral lesions form. These are the basis of the extensive chronic inflammation of the intestinal wall. Many authors believe that strictures, stenosis, scars of the intestinal wall and peritoneal adhesions are the result of chronic lesions caused by amoebae. However, we have looked for this type of sequel for many years in our autopsy and biopsy material and have never been able to attribute them to amoebic infections.

The lesions named 'amoebomas' and 'amoebic granulomas' need a brief discussion: Many cases described as 'amoebomas', 'amoebic granulomas', lesions of an 'X-ray aspect of a large tumour' or an 'inflammatory parasitic pseudotumour' do not merit this denomination. They correspond solely to a circumscribed thickness and/or dilatation of an intestinal segment in an amoebic infection, with the exception of a few cases, e.g. a reported amoeboma really similar to a carcinoma[14].

One of our cases showed amoebic alterations of a tumourous appearance and probably merits a denomination of resemblance to a tumour (see Fig. 8.9). An intestinal segment of the large intestine had been resected with the presurgical clinical diagnosis of carcinoma of the colon. In the surgical specimen, a large chronic paraintestinal abscess in the mesocolon was found which was in contact with the intestinal lumen through a 'not open perforation', i.e. a fistula. The central necrotic masses of this abscess, where numerous amoebae were found, were surrounded by a broad fibrotic shell. The 'large nodule' observed in this case was, in truth, very similar to a tumour or neoplasm and should be called a peri- or para-intestinal amoeboa.

In more than 30 years, only one case of amoebic colitis and an apparently coincident carcinoma of the colon has been seen in our material. However, primary carcinomas at this site are rare in our autopsy and biopsy material in comparison with other countries.

Hepatic amoebiasis. The amoebae reach the liver, usually by means of the portal vein, and there they produce either single (Fig. 8.10) or multiple (Figs. 8.11 and 8.12) pylephlebitic abscesses. The solitary amoebic abscesses previously described as being typical are the exception rather than the rule[15]. The amoebae first cause necrotic foci which may be confused with tumours or tumour metastases. Later, the foci become soft in the central parts and, on the whole, look like abscesses with a semiliquid necrotic content, often similar to chocolate because of massive old haemorrhages. The formation of a liver abscess by contiguity due to amoebiasis of the colon transversum is exceptional. Diagnosis of amoebic liver abscesses may be difficult[15].

Hepatomegaly (Fig. 8.13) in cases of amoebic colitis may occur without amoebic abscesses in the liver. In this case, the enlargement of the liver is due to an infectious–toxic reaction of this organ or a secondary infection, but not necessarily to the parasites. The hepatomegaly has been called 'amoebic hepatitis', but this name does not seem appropriate since, in these cases, amoebae are not present in the liver. The name 'reactive hepatitis' may be more suitable. When amoebae invade hepatic tissue, they produce abscesses but not amoebic hepatitis. Complications which may occur in this type of cases are:

1. Peripherical abscesses may perforate Glisson's capsule and drain towards the abdominal cavity, the stomach, pancreas, spleen or through the abdominal wall (Fig. 8.14).

2. Skin fistulae may originate in the right upper abdominal region.

3. Subdiaphragmatic or subphrenic abscesses may result which may perforate the diaphragm and cause pleural and pulmonary lesions with formation of abscesses or hepato-bronchial fistulae, mostly in the lower lobule of the right lung (Figs. 8.15 and 8.16). Amoebic abscesses in the lower lobule of the left lung are less frequent and are the result of amoebic lesions in the left lobe of the liver.

4. Rarely, amoebic lesions have been found in the pericardium and in the oesophagus.

5. Sometimes, metastatic abscesses resulting from haematogenous dissemination are formed in the lung.

6. Rarely, *E. histolytica* produces brain abscesses (Fig. 8.17). In the two latter instances, the point of departure may have been an amoebic lesion in the large intestine or an amoebic liver abscess.

Rare extraintestinal amoebic lesions. In addition to the relatively frequent extraintestinal lesions mentioned above, the parasites may also cause lesions in less common sites: the lymph nodes; the skin of the perineal region; the uterine cervix; and the penis.

1. Amoebae in the lymph nodes (Figs. 8.18 and 8.19) do not cause important inflammatory reactions. If lymphadenitis is present in cases of amoebiasis, it is usually due to a secondary infection rather than to the amoebae.

2. Amoebic lesions of the rectum may lead to amoebic cutaneous perineal alterations (Figs. 8.20–8.22) which may originate by contiguity and cause recto-cutaneous fistulae and lesions similar to cutaneous tumoral manifestations. This type of lesion naturally heals rapidly when specific anti-amoebic drug treatment is applied. Making a differential diagnosis between cutaneous amoebiasis and Meleney's synergistic gangrene is discussed in reference 17.

3. Sometimes, we have come across amoebic lesions at the exocervix (Figs. 8.23 and 8.24) which resemble cauliflower-like growths and are virtually impossible to differentiate from cervical carcinomas. If, in regions endemic to amoebiasis, these exocervix lesions are seen with extensive necrotic areas and carcinomatous cells are not immediately found, it is recommended that amoebae are looked for using the special staining methods. Amoebae may be found in routine Papanicolaou smears: in one case, in a patient wearing an

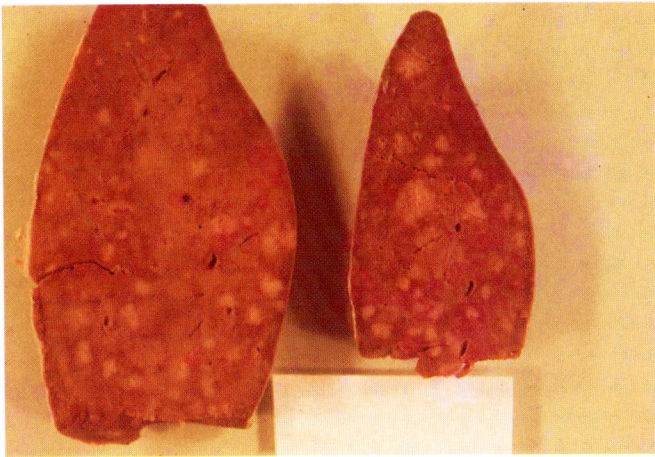

Fig. 8.11 Multiple hepatic abscesses due to amoebic infection in a 4-month-old infant

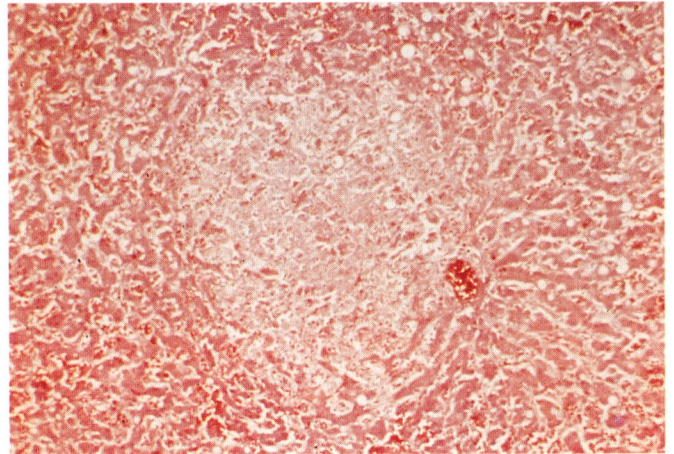

Fig. 8.12 The histological picture of a liver 'abscess' of the case shown in Figure 8.11. Parasites are not seen at this magnification and staining method. H&E

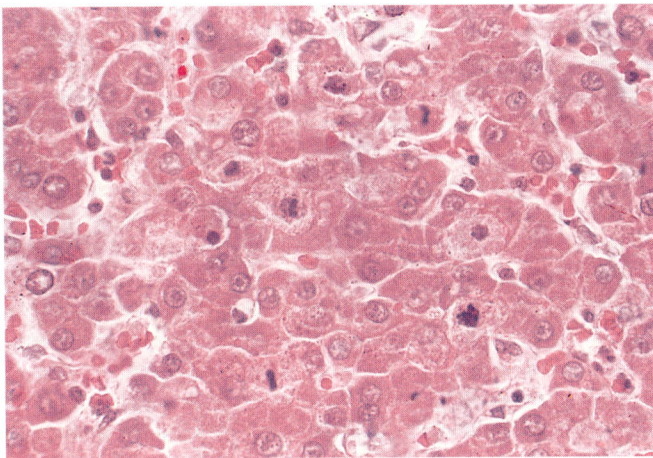

Fig. 8.13 'Reactive hepatitis' with hepatomegaly in an amoebic infection. Numerous mitoses of hepatocytes are seen, but never amoebae. H&E

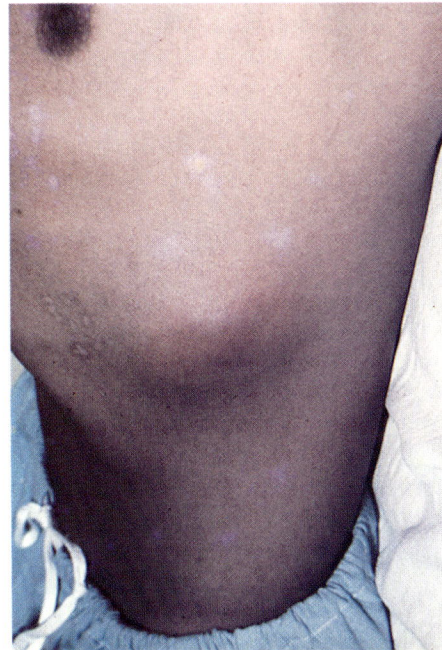

Fig. 8.14 The protuberance seen in the skin of the right-hand upper quadrant of the abdomen is produced by an amoebic liver abscess

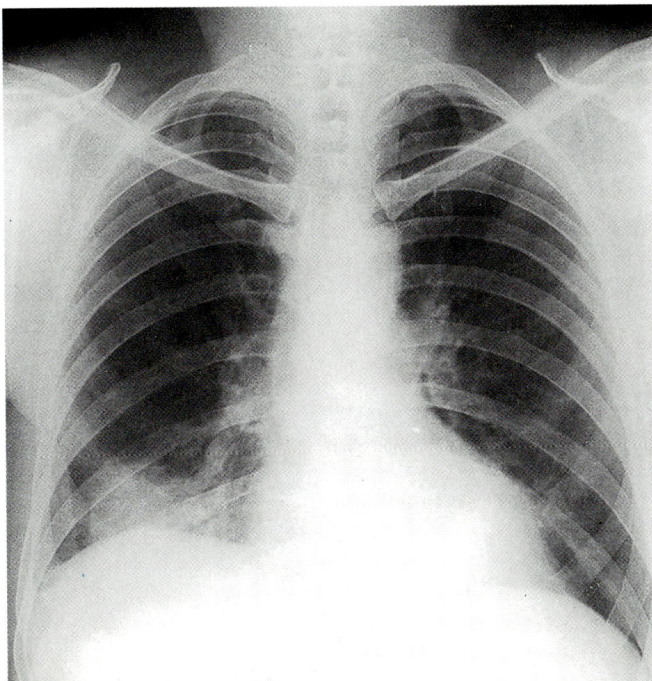

Fig. 8.15 Amoebic abscess in the lower lobule of the right lung

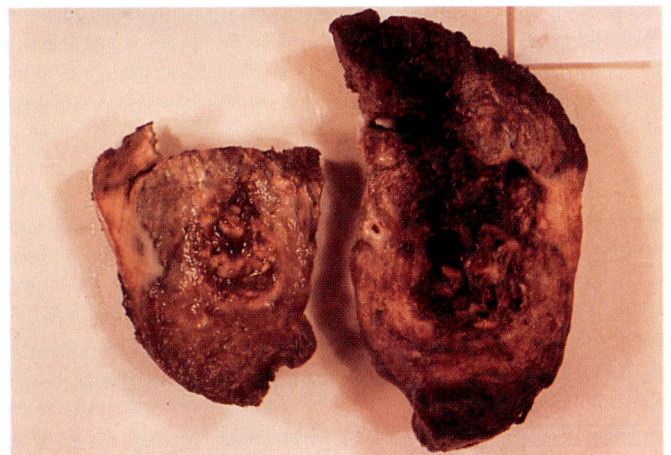

Fig. 8.16 This surgical specimen is the resected lung abscess of Fig. 8.15

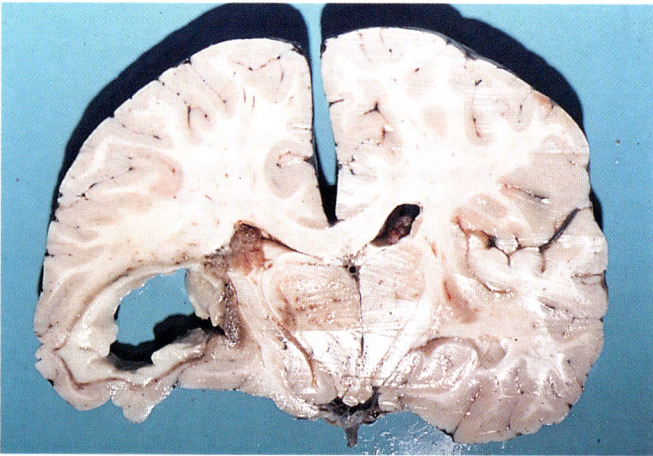

Fig. 8.17 Amoebic brain abscess. The central nervous system is very rarely attacked by *Entamoeba histolytica*

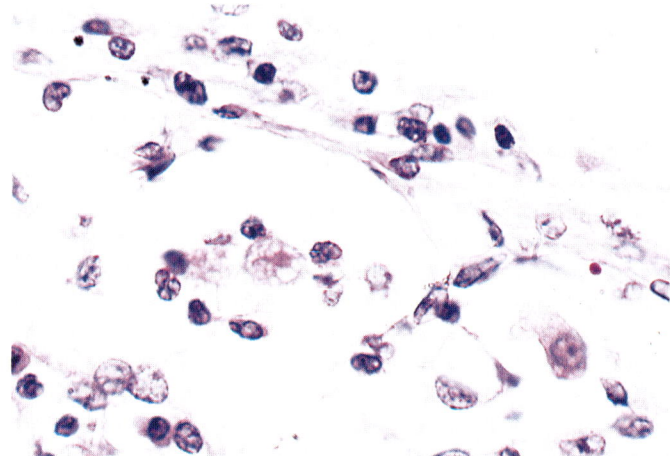

Fig. 8.18 Two structures are seen in the marginal sinus of a mesenteric lymph node which represent amoebae. This organ is rarely invaded by amoebae. H&E

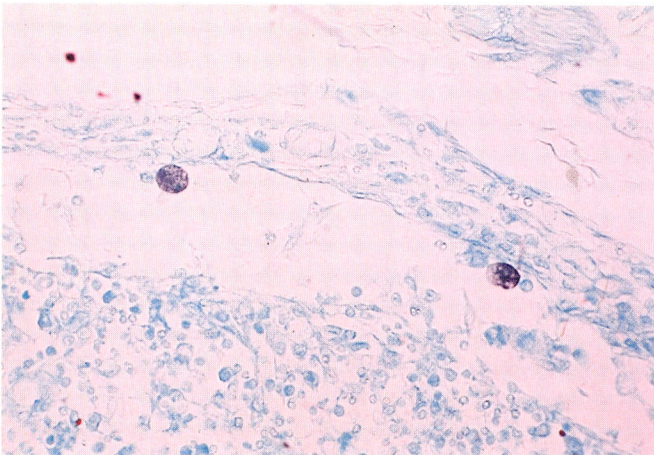

Fig. 8.19 The same lymph node as in Fig. 8.18 with parasites positive in this staining method. Grocott

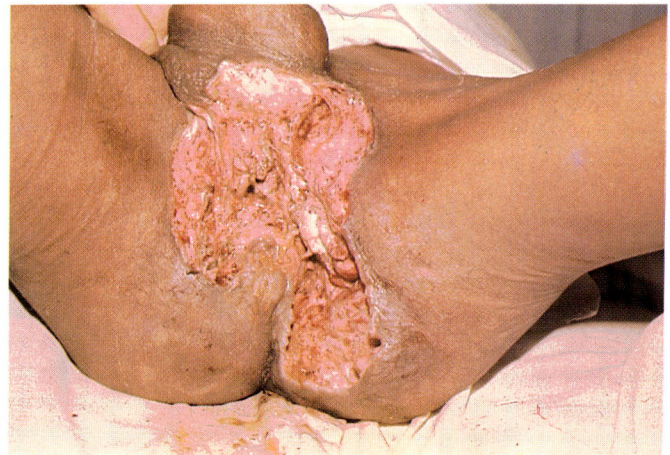

Fig. 8.20 Amoebae were found in the biopsy of this extensively ulcerated perineal region. Cutaneous carcinoma had been the clinical diagnosis previously

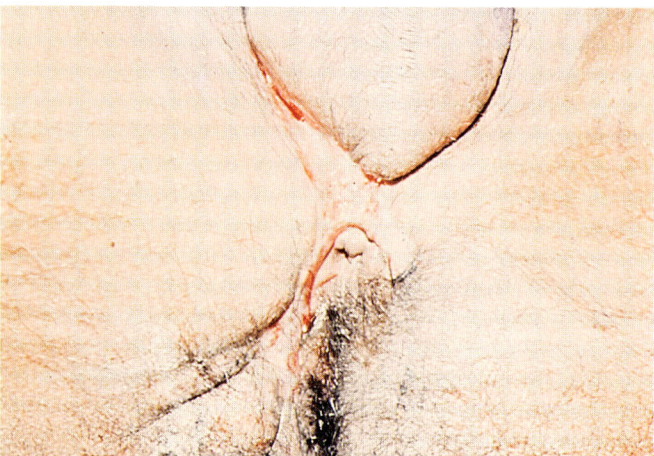

Fig. 8.21 The same case as in Fig. 8.20 three months after specific treatment

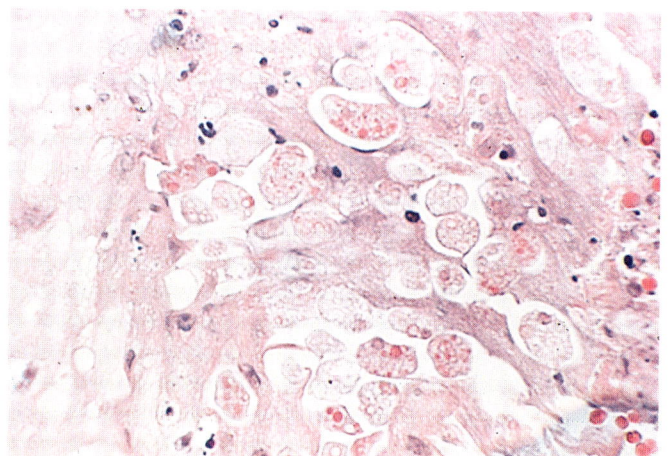

Fig. 8.22 Histology of the case of Fig. 8.20. Numerous organisms of *Entamoeba histolytica* are seen. H&E

intrauterine contraceptive device[18], and, in another, in association with a cervical squamous cell carcinoma[19]. Amoebic infections of the uterine cervix without mucosal defects are an exception.

4. Amoebic lesions of the penis (Fig. 8.25) are rare and originate only from sexual relations with an infected individual.

Histopathology. In order to obtain good results in the diagnosis of the amoebae, it is indispensable to have personal experience. Personnel who have no appropriate training and do not examine this sort of specimen daily run the risk of making too many false positive diagnoses. Histological diagnosis of amoebiasis may be difficult[20]. Figs. 8.26–8.28 show intestinal lesions at low power.

The trophozoites of E. histolytica can be seen in the intestinal content and in the tissues of the intestinal wall at various stages of preservation. If the results of the H&E or iron haematoxylin staining methods are not satisfactory, the PAS and Grocott methods give good results and bring the parasites out clearly, above all in cases with few parasites and in slides with badly preserved ones. Often, amoebae contain red blood cells, a phenomenon called erythrophagia (Fig. 8.2a). Occasionally, numerous amoebae are situated in the lumen of blood or lymphatic vessels, without signs of vasculitis (Fig. 8.29). Sometimes, it is difficult to distinguish amoebae from macrophages or ganglion cells (Fig. 8.30). The problem of differential diagnosis of the different species of amoebae may arise in smears of the intestinal content but does not exist in tissue sections since only E. histolytica is found in tissues.

The amoebae may be present in the cavities of abscesses, in the liver or in other viscera, but, more often, they perish and disappear before being recognized by the pathologist. However, amoebae are more likely to be encountered in the granulation tissue on the periphery of an abscess. Nevertheless, in spite of the use of special staining methods, false negative diagnoses are also possible when pus of liver abscess is obtained by puncture. Recently, we have achieved good diagnostic results by examining sections of cell blocks of this material stained with the PAS method. In these sections, only a few necrobiotic amoebae, difficult to recognize as such, were detected with the H&E stain but they came out clearly with the PAS method (Fig. 8.31).

The tissue reaction consists mainly of lympho-histiocytic infiltrates; occasionally eosinophilic leukocytes are present. Neutrophilic leukocytes and fibrine exudation are scarce or absent and, when they are present, are due to a secondary associated bacterial infection.

In the liver, the so-called abscesses are not true ones because their content consists of semiliquid necrotic material without leukocytes. The above mentioned reactive hepatitis, present in the hepatomegaly of amoebic colitis, shows infiltrates of lympho-histiocytes and a certain number of granulocytes in the hepatic sinus and in periportal spaces. Also, a marked oedema and,

occasionally, numerous hepatocytes showing mitoses can be observed.

'Amoebic granulomas' have been mentioned above when 'amoebomas' were discussed. It must be emphasized that the terms granulomas or granulomatous reactions refer to histological features. Neither granulomas nor granulomatous reactions are found in amoebic infections.

References

1. Miller, M. J., Matthews, W. H. and Moore, D. F. (1968). Amebiasis in Northern Saskatchewan. *Can. Med. Assoc. J.*, **99**, 696
2. Rolfini, R. G. (1965). Enterocolitis grave en el material autópsico de Mérida. *Tesis doctoral*. Universidad de Los Andes, Mérida/Venezuela
3. Liscano, T. R. de (1978). Amibiasis. Revisión del Material Anatomo-Patológico de Mérida. Trabajo de Ascenso, Fac. de Medicina, ULA, Mérida/Venezuela
4. Rigothier, M. C., Vuong, P. N. and Gayral, P. (1989). A new experimental model of cecal amebiasis in rats. *Ann. Parasitol. Hum. Comp.*, **64**, 185
5. Becker, I., Pérez Tamayo, R., Montfort, I., Alvizouri, A. M., Pérez and Montfort, R. (1988). Entamoeba histolytica: role of amebic proteinases and polymorphonuclear leukocytes in acute experimental amebiasis in the rat. *Exp. Parasitol.*, **67**, 268
6. Chadee, K. and Meerovitch, E. (1989). Entamoeba histolytica: diffuse liver inflammation in gerbils (Meriones unguiculatus) with experimentally induced amebic liver abscess. *J. Protozool.*, **36**, 154
7. Yu, Y. and Lian, W. N. (1991). Histopathology of experimental hepatic amebiasis. *Chung-Kuo*, **9**, 35
8. Koppats, K. *et al.* (1990). Colitis ulcerosa oder Amoebenkolitis-ein kasuistischer Bericht. *Z. Ges. Inn. Med.*, **45**, 25
9. Mironov, N. A. and Soskin, Ia M. (1990). A fatal case of amebic dysentery (Russ.). *Med. Parazitol. Mosk.*, **58**, 9
10. Hossain, A., Bolbol, A. S., Chowdhury, M. N. and Bakir, T. M. (1989). Indirect haemagglutination (IHA) test in the serodiagnosis of amoebiasis. *J. Hyg. Epidemiol. Microbiol. Immunol.*, **33**, 91
11. Salfelder, K. (1961) Ueber eine kontrastreiche Anfärbung von Entamoeba histolytica im Gewebe. *Z. Tropenmed. Parasit.*, **12**, 273
12. Brown, M. *et al.* (1991). Detection of HIV-1 in Entamoeba histolytica without evidence of transmission to human cells. *AIDS*, **5** 93
13. Nadler, S. *et al.* (1990). Appendiceal infection by Entamoeba histolytica and Strongyloides stercoralis presenting like acute appendicitis. *Dig. Dis. Sci.*, **35**, 603
14. Spencer, H. (ed.) (1973). *Tropical Pathology*. Handb. Spez. Path. Anat. Bd. 8, Springer Verlag
15. Trautmann, M. *et al.* (1990). Multiple Amöbenleberabszesse: sonographische Diagnostik und ultraschallgezielte Punktion. *Ultraschall Med.*, **11**, 142
16. Disko, R. and Schinkel, T. (1979). Zur Diagnose des Amöben-Leberabszesses. Eine Studie an 107 Fällen. *Münch Med. Wschr.*, **121**, 1536
17. Davson, J., Jones, D. M. and Turner, L. (1988). Diagnosis of Meleney's synergistic gangrene. *Br. J. Surg.*, **75**, 267
18. Arroyo, G. and Quinn, J. A. Jr. (1989). Association of amoebae and actinomyces in an intrauterine contraceptive device user. *Acta Cytol.*, **33**, 298
19. Arroyo, G. and Elgueta, R. (1989). Squamous cell carcinoma associated with cervicitis. Report of a case. *Acta Cytol.*, **33**, 301
20. Konstantinov, G. S. and Blokhin, A. V. (1988). The morphology of amebiasis. *Arkh. Patol.*, **50**, 44

9. ACANTHAMOEBIASIS

Introduction

Free-living 'soil' or 'water' amoebae may cause severe diseases of the central nervous system with meningitis or meningo-encephalitis. Species of the genus *Naegleria* cause primary amoebic meningo-encephalitis (PAME), while *Acanthamoeba* species cause chronic granulomatous amoebic encephalitis (GAE). Keratitis due to acanthamoebae has also been observed[1-5]. *Naegleria* is not an acanthamoeba. Acanthamoebiases are really 'infections due to free-living amoebae'.

In the world literature, no more than 200 cases have

been recorded, mostly in small groups of children or adolescents. They have been found in Australia and New Zealand, in European countries, in the USA and single cases have been observed elsewhere. In Venezuela, we know of three reported cases[6,7].

Spontaneous acanthamoebiasis, to our knowledge, has been reported only exceptionally in lower animals[8]. Experimentally, amoebic infections of this kind may be produced by various routes in mice, rabbits and monkeys. Rhinitis, encephalitis and pneumonia (after direct inoculation) have been achieved in these animals[9-11].

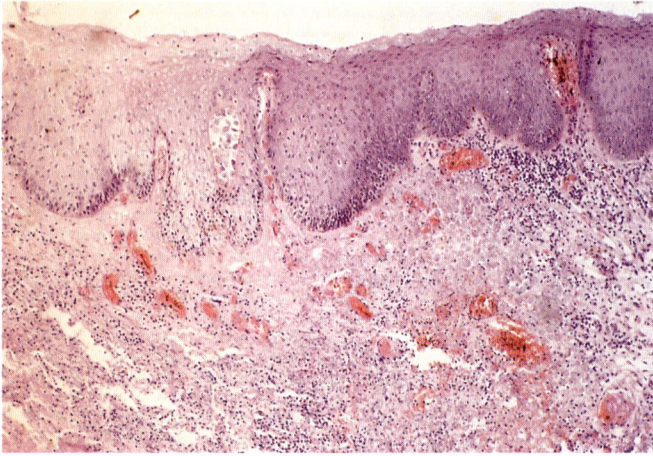

Fig. 8.23 Amoebic cervicitis. Parasites are not seen at this magnification and with this staining method. H&E

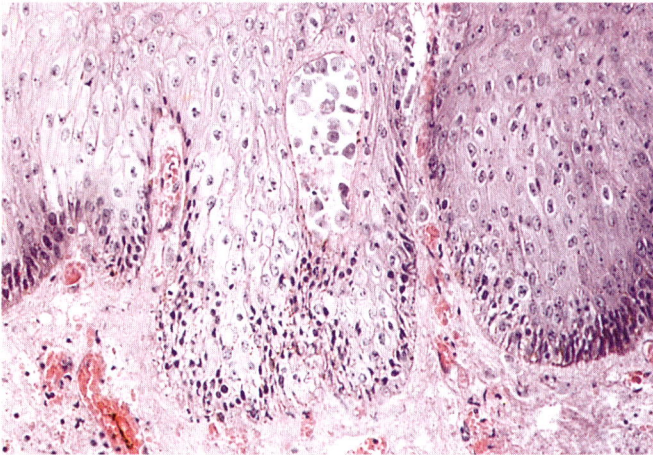

Fig. 8.24 Higher power of Fig. 8.23. A nest of amoebae may be recognized easily in this field. H&E

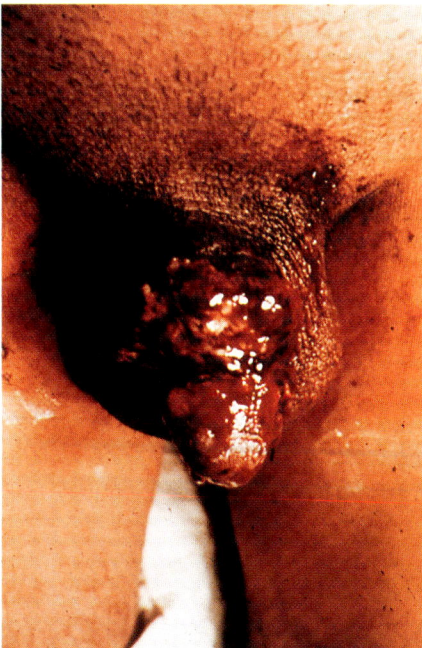

Fig. 8.25 Amoebic lesions of the penis with extensive ulceration and haemorrhages

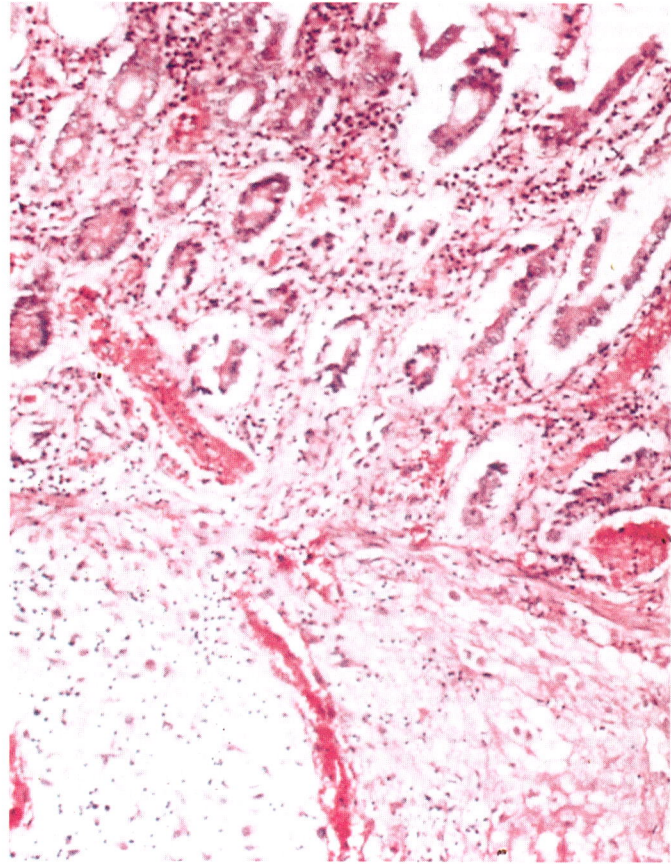

Fig. 8.26 Low power view of early amoebic colitis. H&E

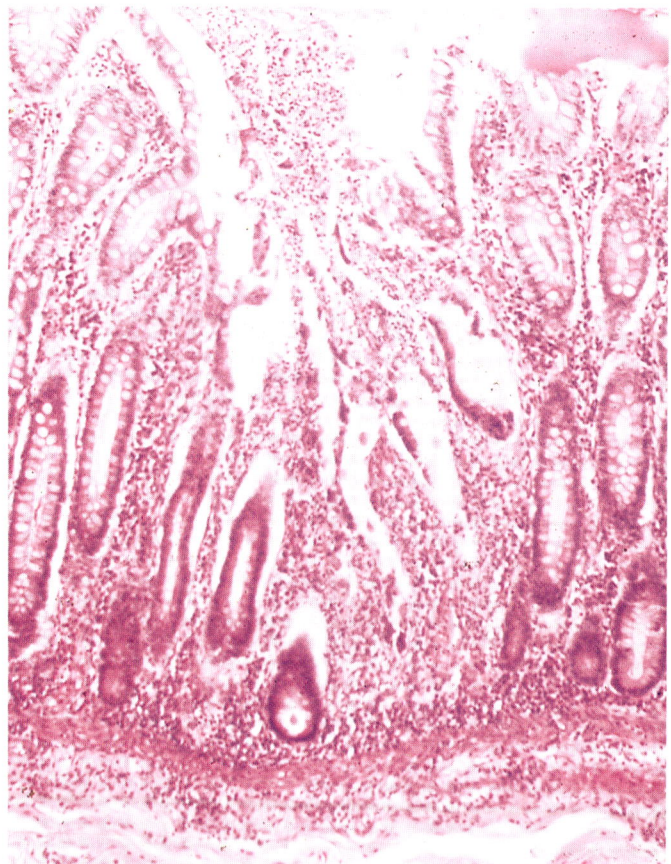

Fig. 8.27 Early circumscribed necrosis of the mucosa of the large intestine due to infection with amoebae. Parasites are not seen at this magnification. H&E

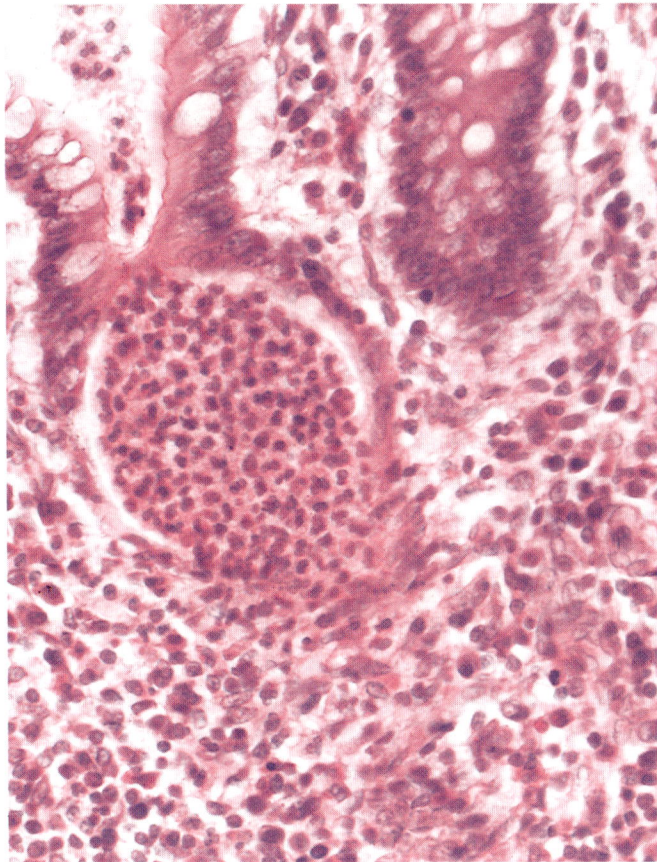

Fig. 8.28 Early lesion of amoebic colitis with an abscess at a crypt. The leukocytic exudate is probably due to secondary bacterial infection. H&E

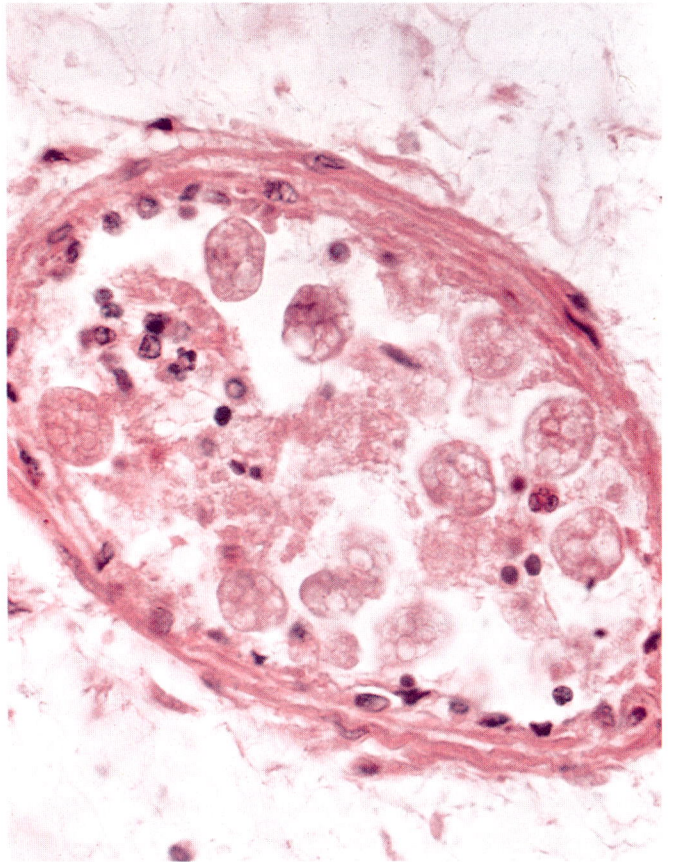

Fig. 8.29 Numerous amoebae present in the lumen of a vein in the submucosa of the large intestine. The wall of the vein is intact. H&E

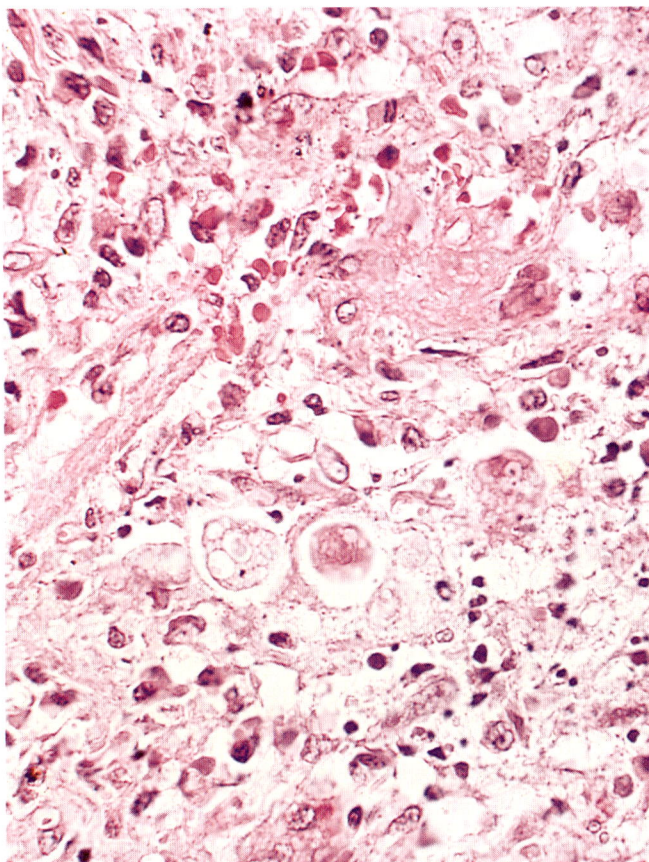

Fig. 8.30 *Entamoeba histolytica* seen in tissues with the routine stain. H&E

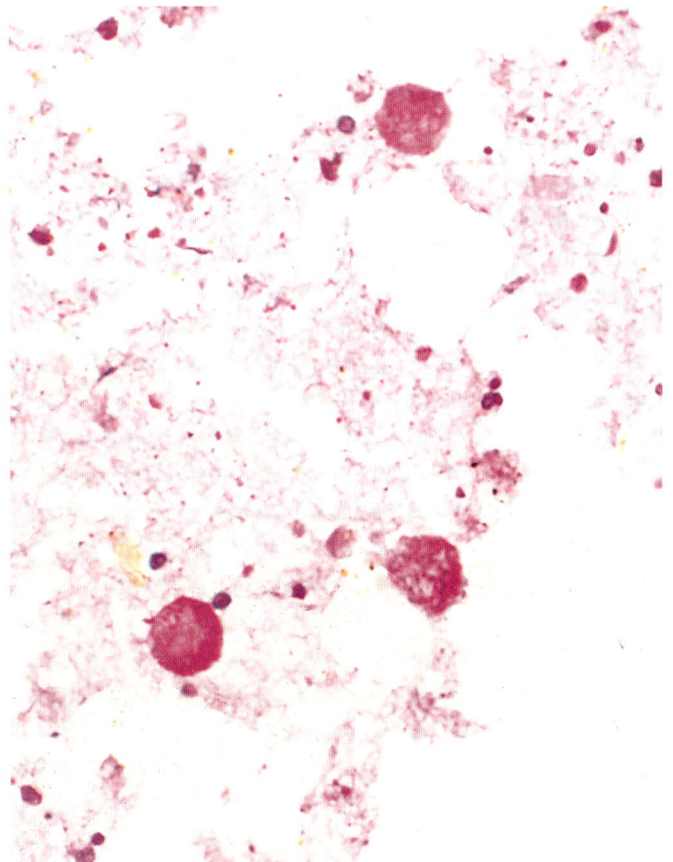

Fig. 8.31 Amoebae in section of a cell block from contents of a liver abscess are seen clearly with this staining method. PAS

The disease produced by *Naegleria* species (PAME) is reported with increased frequency after swimming in pools, lakes and rivers. This form shows an acute fulminating course and is always fatal. In addition, PAME occurs more frequently than GAE.

The amoebic infection caused by *Acanthamoeba* species, on the other hand, occurs as an opportunistic infection[12] in clinically ill or immunosuppressed patients and without contact with water. It has been reported in AIDS patients[13,14] and has a more chronic course but nevertheless, a fatal outcome.

Clinical diagnosis of this disease is made by detecting trophozoites in the spinal fluid (Fig. 9.1) by culture of spinal fluid or tissue specimens of the brain in the NNN medium. Immunofluorescence techniques and the complement fixation test are performed in special research laboratories.

The parasite

The important pathogenic species for man and mouse are *Naegleria fowleri*, *Naegleria australiensis*, *Acanthamoeba castellanii* and *Acanthamoeba culbertsoni*. The terms *Limax* and *Hartmanella* as genera are now obsolete. Non-pathogenic species of soil or water amoebae do exist but will not be described here in detail.

The *Naegleria* and *Acanthamoeba* species measure between 10 and 40 μm. The former are somewhat smaller, about 7–22 μm, and the latter, 15–45 μm. Trophozoites and cysts may be distinguished. Trophozoites are seen in tissues. They are spherically shaped and almost always possess only one nucleus, but, exceptionally, up to three may be present. They stain with H&E, iron haematoxylin and trichromic methods and are PAS- and Grocott-negative. In spinal fluid, trophozoites measure 8–10 μm and are motile.

Cysts (persistent forms) of these amoebae are found ubiquitously, e.g. in dust, water and in the upper respiratory tract of man[15-18]. They are uninuclear and have a thick membrane which may be irregular. Acanthamoeba cysts may show stellate or polyhedral structures; they have been described in tissues by García Tamayo *et al.*[7].

In the presence of bacteria, amoebae may be cultured easily in Nelson medium and also in Bacto agar Difco in horse serum. Axenic cultures have been achieved too. In tissue cultures, soil amoebae have a typical cytopathic effect. In plate cultures *Naegleria* species have 2 flagella.

Pathogenesis

In *Naegleria* infections, the portal of entry of the parasites is probably the nasal mucosa. Here an inflammatory process develops. The amoebae penetrate the mucosa and migrate along blood vessels and nerve fibres (*N. olfactorius*) centripetally, through the cribriform plate of the ethmoid into the subarachnoid space and, from there, into the brain. This movement of amoebae has been shown experimentally after intranasal administration of culture material[19].

By haematogenous dissemination, the amoebae, apparently, reach internal organs and may cause inflammatory processes. However, the parasites soon perish in these viscera and have not been confirmed at these sites. Involvement of lung, kidney, liver, pancreas, lymph nodes and myometrium has been described but without the presence of parasites in these viscera.

Acanthamoeba species may use the upper respiratory tract as portal of entry. The CNS is probably secondarily affected from another active focus, e.g. the lungs or the skin[20].

Pathology

Meninges and brain are affected by species of *Naegleria*, and the brain (occasionally also the meninges) by *Acanthamoeba* species. Further, the cornea may be involved.

In human beings, lesions produced by these species of amoebae have been reported in liver, lungs, kidneys, pancreas, lymph nodes and myometrium, but the parasites themselves have not been described in internal organs outside of the CNS (possibly they perish soon after haematogenous dissemination).

Grossly, the purulent and haemorrhagic necrotizing meningitis and the purulent foci in cortical and subcortical areas of the brain, as well as the keratitis, do not present special or specific features. They may be easily confused with the suppurative meningitis or necrotizing haemorrhagic encephalitis of any other aetiology. Specific gross lesions of internal organs are not known. Circumscribed tumour-like lesions have been observed in the brain in the GAE form of the disease[21].

Histologically, we have seen, personally, only three cases, one from Venezuela, one from Czechoslovakia and one from the USA, all of the PAME variety. The amoebae in the tissues of these cases were almost solely trophozoites. Only a few large parasites seemed to be cysts, some with thin membranes and others with thicker and irregular membranes. García Tamayo *et al.* have illustrated cysts in tissues in an *Acanthamoeba* infection[7]. On an average, the amoebae measured 10 μm and were of a spherical shape, or occasionally amoeboid or polyhedral. The majority of amoebae had one small nucleus, centrally located; only few amoebae had several nuclei, but no more than three nuclei could be seen in one amoeba. Often, the cytoplasm of the amoebae was clear, similar to a vacuole, but inhomogeneous or granular inclusions were also seen in variable amounts in the cytoplasm. The amoebae in these cases stained weakly with the H&E, iron haematoxylin and the Goldner stain (Fig. 9.2) but did not stain at all with the PAS or Grocott methods. Often, large nests of numerous amoebae showed necrobiotic changes of the amoebae themselves. Figs. 9.3–9.5 show brain tissue with soil amoebae at low power, Figs. 9.6 and 9.7 at medium power and Figs. 9.8–9.10 at high power with the H&E stain.

The parasites were mostly located, often in clusters with numerous amoebae, in perivascular clear spaces or in nests, localized in the parenchyma without any alterations or showing clear spaces. This means that there is focal destruction of brain tissue. Frequently, the walls of large blood vessels were invaded by amoebae. Often, parasites situated in dense cell infiltrates, e.g. granulocytes, were recognized only with difficulty. They were seen clearly inside nerve cells (neuronophagy) (Fig. 9.9), a feature which previously had been erroneously interpreted by us as phagocytosis (amoebae engulfed by macrophages). Tissue reaction in these cases consisted of oedema, colliquative necrosis, exudation of fibrin and extensive cellular infiltrates with a predominance of neutrophilic leukocytes. Often, the latter were densely packed with necrobiosis of these cells, i.e. a real suppurative lesion was present. In addition, thromboses of small and medium blood vessels and extensive haemorrhages were observed. Perivascular infiltrates with granulocytes, lymphocytes and plasma cells were found in the parenchyma, without amoebae. In some areas, a marked proliferation of astrocytes was noted.

A granulomatous reaction with giant cells was described in the GAE form[22-24]. We have not seen lesions of this kind personally.

Histological differential diagnosis of amoebae is relatively easy. In tissues, intestinal amoebae (*Entamoeba*

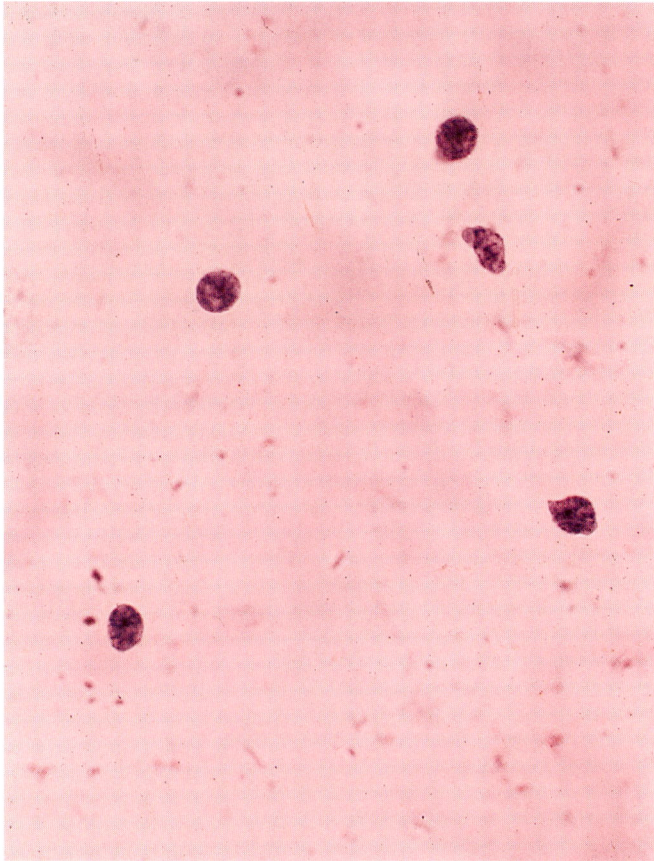

Fig. 9.1 *Naegleria fowleri* in smear of spinal fluid. H&E

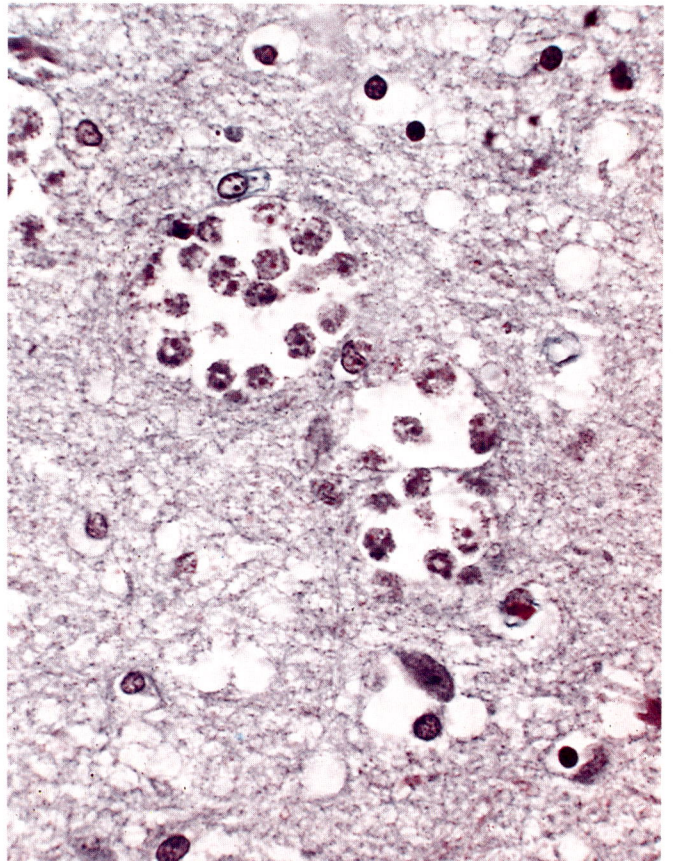

Fig. 9.2 Clusters of soil amoebae in brain. Goldner

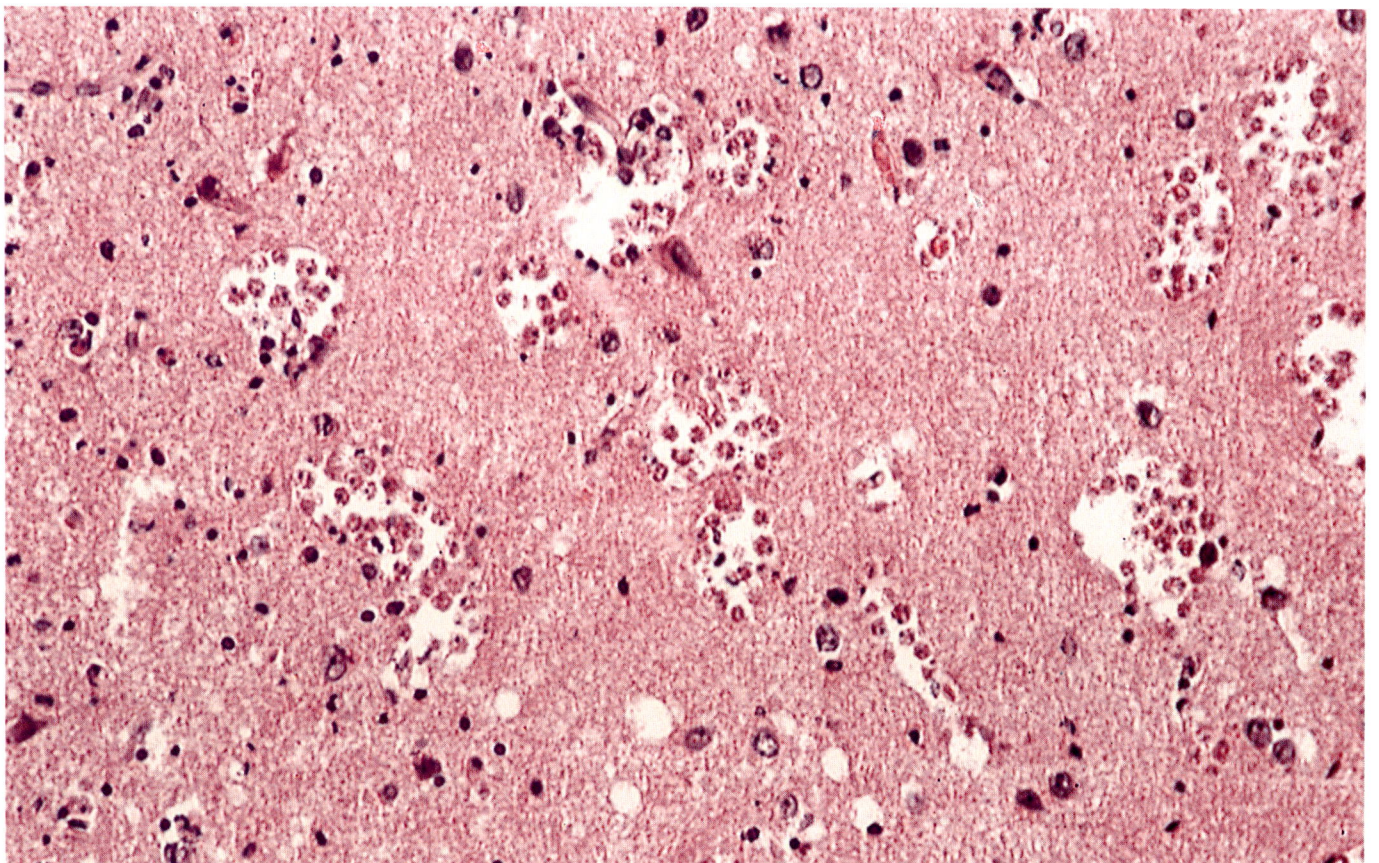

Fig. 9.3 Low power view of brain tissue with numerous clusters of soil amoebae. H&E

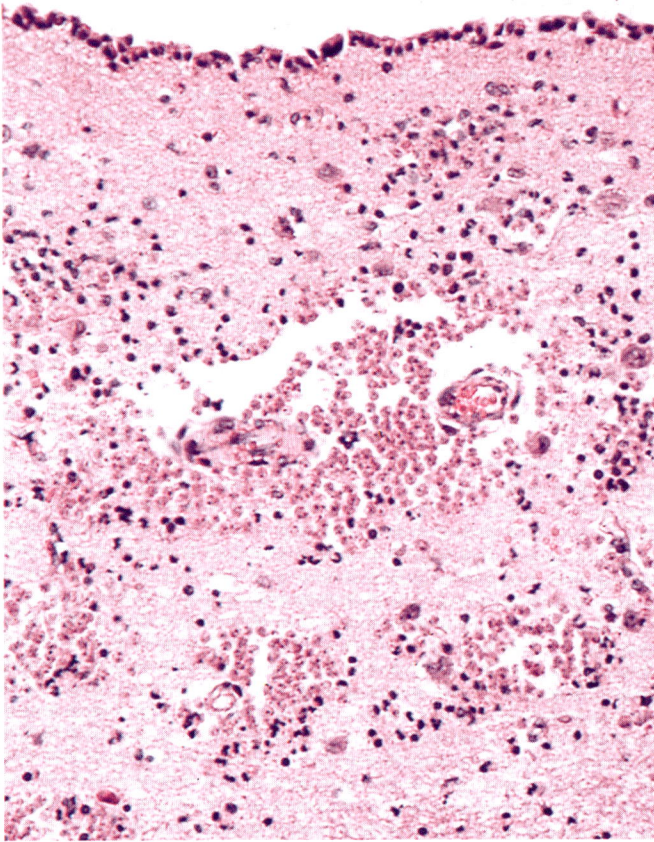

Fig. 9.4 Numerous soil amoebae in brain tissue with inflammation. H&E

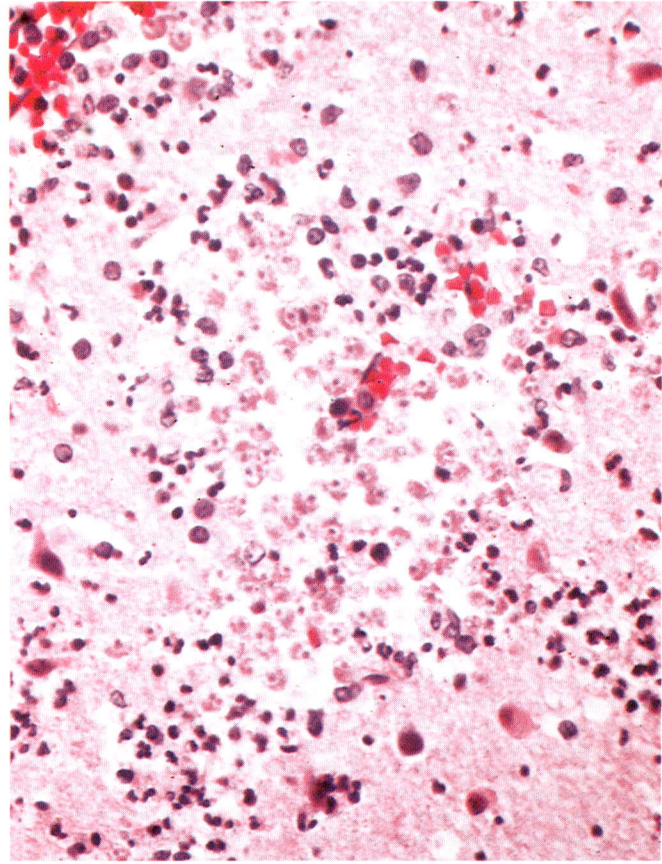

Fig. 9.5 Acanthamoebiasis. In addition to parasites, marked leukocytic inflammation is seen. H&E

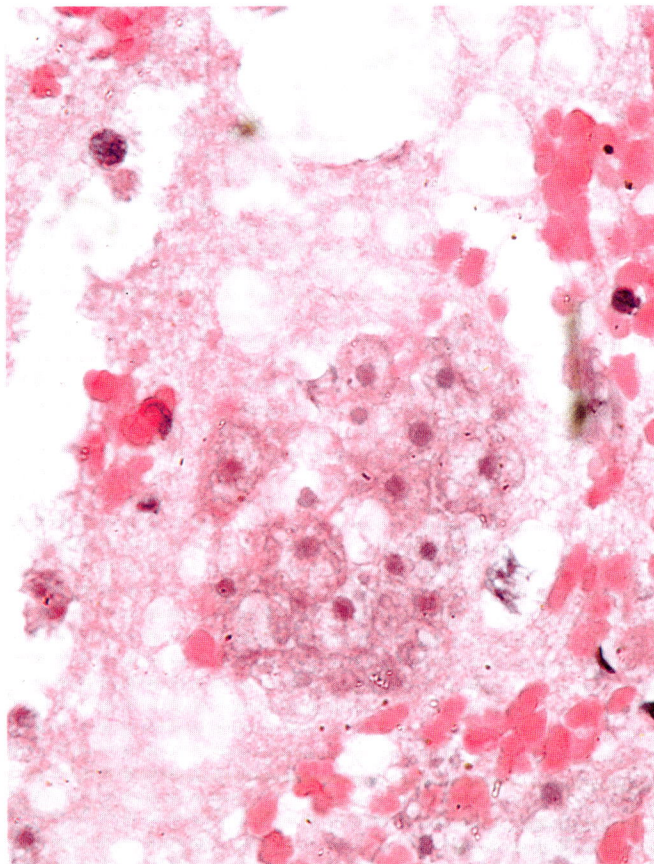

Fig. 9.6 Nest of soil amoebae in necrotic brain tissue. H&E

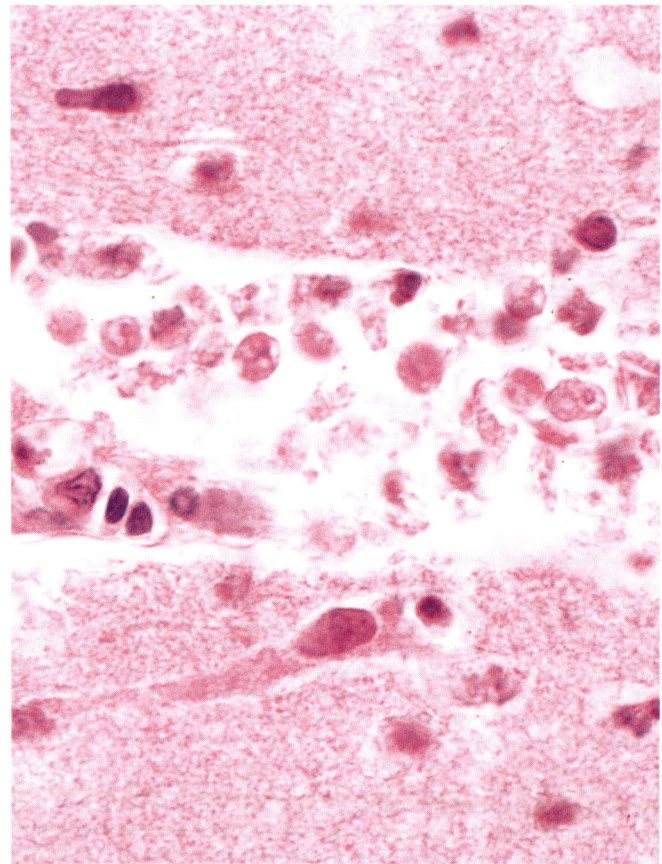

Fig. 9.7 Cluster of soil amoebae in a perivascular space. H&E

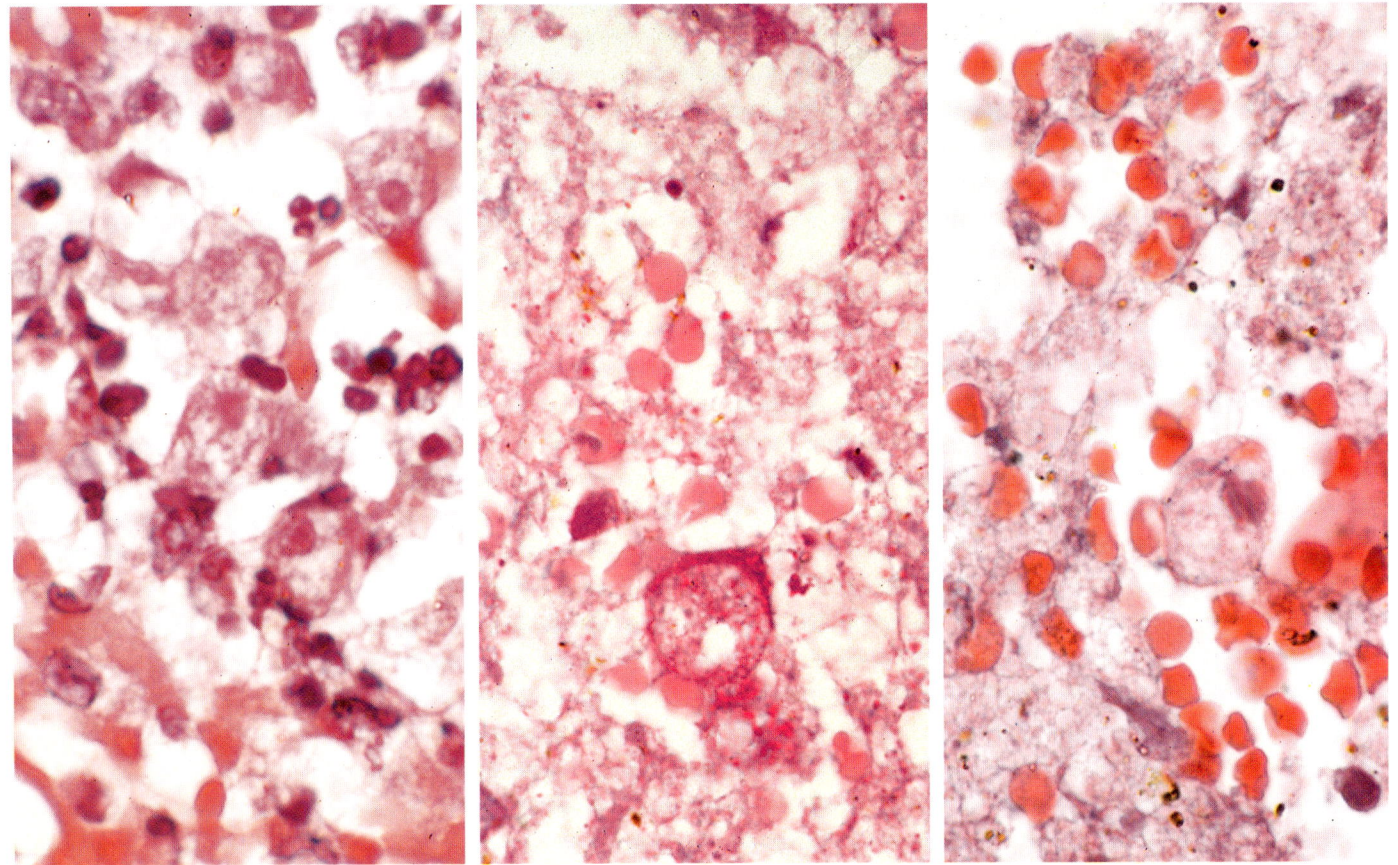

Fig. 9.8   Soil amoebae in brain tissue at high magnification. H&E

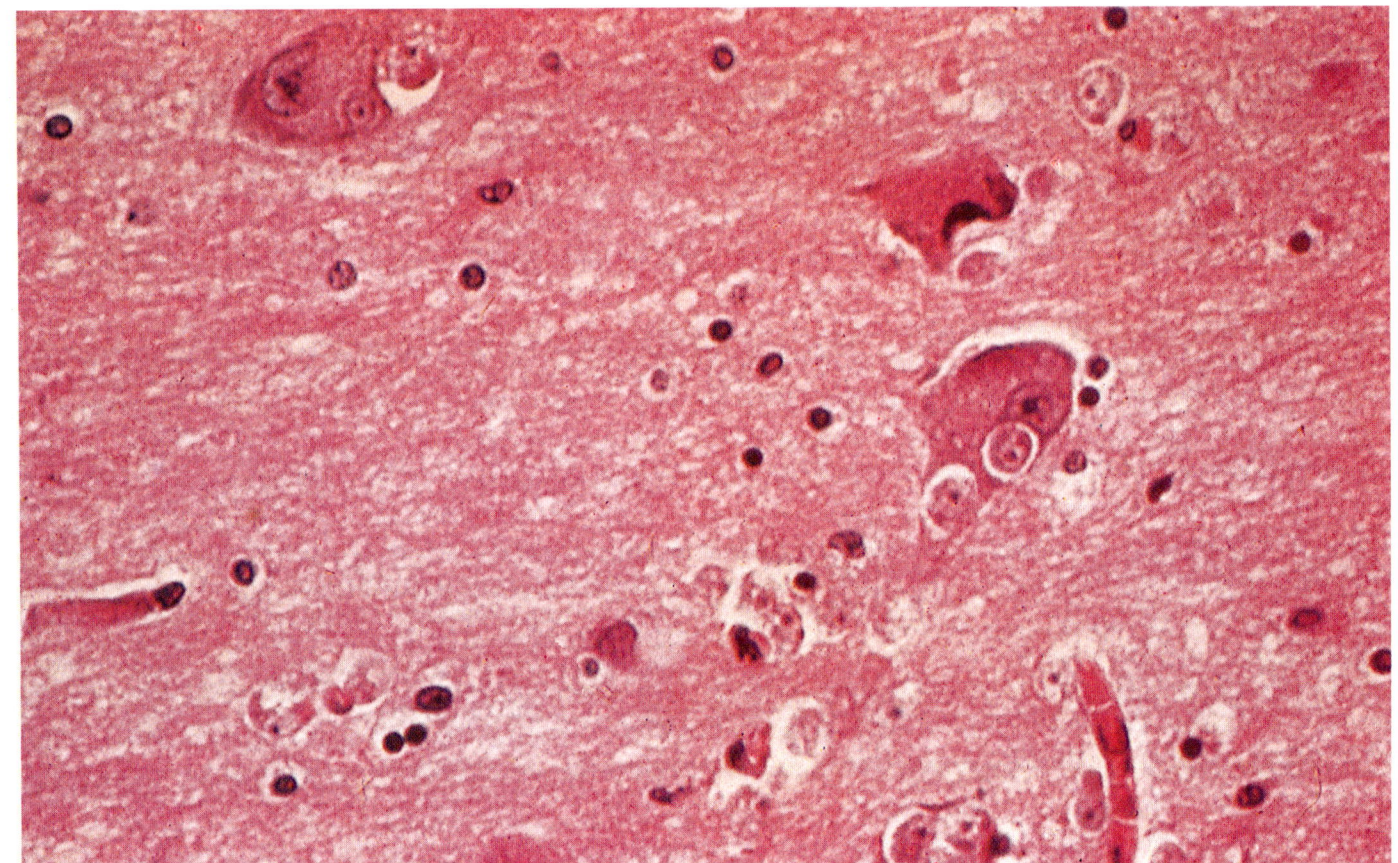

Fig. 9.9   'Soil amoeba' in the brain are phagocytising nerve cells (neurophagy). H&E

histolytica) are pleomorphic, show erythrophagia and stain with PAS and weakly with Grocott. In addition, the purulent tissue reaction in acanthamoebiasis is not found in the lesions produced by *E. histolytica*.

References

1. Witschel, H., Sundmacher, R. and Seitz, H. M. (1984). Amoeben-Keratitis. Ein klinisch-histopatologischer Fallbericht. *Klin. Mbl. Augenheilk.*, **185**, 46
2. Florakis, G. J., Folberg, R., Krachmer, J. H., Tse, D. T., Roussel, T. J. and Vrabec, M. P. (1988). Elevated corneal epithelial lines in Acanthamoeba keratitis. *Arch. Ophthalmol.*, **106**, 1202
3. Wilhelmus, K. R., McCulloch, R. R. and Osato, M. S. (1988). Photomicrography of Acanthamoeba cysts in human cornea. *Am. J. Ophthalmol.*, **106**, 628
4. Karayianis, S. L., Genack, L. J., Lundergan, M. K. and Schumann, G. B. (1988). Cytologic diagnosis of acanthamoebic keratitis. *Acta Cytol.*, **32**, 491
5. Beattie, A. M. *et al.* (1990). Acanthamoeba keratitis with two species of Acanthamoeba. *Can. J. Opathalmol.*, **25**, 260
6. Brass, K. (1973). Meningo-encefalitis amebiásica primaria (por Naegleriasis). *Arch. Venez. Med. Trop.*, **5**, 291
7. García Tamayo, J., González, J. E. and Martinez, A. J. (1980). Meningoencefalitis amibiana primaria y encefalitis granulomatosa amibiana. *Rev. Med. Venez.*, **27**, 84
8. Ayers, K. N., Billups, L. H. and Garner, F. M. (1972). Acanthamebiasis in a dog. *Vet. Pathol.*, **9**, 221
9. Culbertson, C. G., Smith, J. W., Cohen, H. K. and Minner, J. R. (1969). Experimental infection of mice and monkeys by acanthamoeba. *Am. J. Path.*, **35**, 185
10. Martínez, A. J., Duma, R. R., Nelson, E. C. and Moretta, F. L. (1973). Experimental Naegleria meningoencephalitis in mice. *Lab. Invest.*, **29**, 121
11. Willaert, E. and Stevens, A. R. (1980). Experimental pneumonitis induced by Naegleria fowleri in mice. *Trans. R. Soc. Trop. Med.*

Hyg., **74**, 779
12. Harwood, C. R., Rich, G. E., McAleer, R. and Cherian, G. (1988). Isolation of Acanthamoeba from a cerebral abscess. *Med. J. Aust.*, **148**, 47
13. Martinez, A. J. and Janitschke, K. (1985). Acanthamoeba, an opportunistic micro-organism. A review. *Infections*, **35**, 251
14. Anzil, A. P. *et al.* (1991). Amebic meningoencephalitis in a patient with AIDS caused by a newly recognized opportunistic pathogen. Leptomyxid ameba. *Arch. Pathol. Lab. Med.*, **115**, 21
15. Michel, R. and De Jonckheere, J. F. (1983). Isolation and identification of pathogenic Naegleria australiensis (De Jonckheere 1981) from pond water in India. *Trans. R. Soc. Trop. Med. Hyg.*, **77**, 878
16. Kadlec, V., Skvárová, J., Cerva, L. and Nebáznivá, D. (1980). Virulent Naegleria fowleri in indoor swimming pool. *Folia Parasitol. Prag.*, **27**, 11
17. Michel, R. and Just, H. M. (1984). Acanthamoeben, Naeglerien und andere freilebende Amoeben in Kühl- und Spülwasser von Zahnbehandlungseinheiten. *Zbl. Bakt. I. Abt. Orig. B.*, **179**, 56
18. Michel, R., Roehl, R. and Schneider, H. (1982). Isolierung von freilebenden Amoeben durch Gewinnung von Nasenschleimhautabstrichen bei gesunden Probanden. *Zbl. Bakt I Abt. Orig. B.*, **176**, 155
19. Culbertson, C. G. (1971). The pathogenicity of soil amebas. *Ann. Rev. Microbiol.*, **25**, 231
20. Martinez, A. J. (1991). Infection of the central nervous system due to Acanthamoeba. *Rev. Infect. Dis.*, **13**, Suppl. **5**, 399
21. Kwame Ofori-Kwakye *et al.* (1986). Granulomatous brain tumour caused by Acanthamoeba. *J. Neurosurg.*, **64**, 505
22. Patras, D. and Andujar, J. J. (1966). Meningoencephalitis due to Hartmanella (Acanthamoeba). *Am. J. Clin. Path.*, **44**, 226
23. Robert, V. B. and Rorke, L. B. (1973). Primary amebic encephalitis probably from Acanthamoeba. *Ann. Int. Med.*, **79**, 174
24. Matson, D. O., Rouah, E., Lee, R. T., Armstrong, D., Parke, J. T. and Baker, C. J. (1988). Acanthameba meningoencephalitis masquerading as neurocysticercosis. *Pediatr. Infect. Dis. J.*, **7**, 121

10. BLASTOCYSTIS INFECTION

Introduction

Blastocystis hominis was accepted, previously, as an intestinal yeast, harmless for humans[1]. From the sixties on, it was considered a protozoan[2] and, now, its pathogenicity for man is being discussed[3,4]. It has been found worldwide with an average prevalence of 10–15% in people with enteric symptoms; also in Venezuela[5].

Whether *Blastocystis hominis* occurs naturally in lower animals we do not know. Experimentally, diarrhoea may be produced in guinea pigs and non-human primates[6] when these species are infected with *B. hominis*.

Enterocolitic symptoms, flatulence, diarrhoea, abdominal cramps and pain as well as anorexia, are thought to be caused by this parasite. Clinical diagnosis may be made by examining fresh stools prepared with physiological saline and seen with the light or phase-contrast microscope. However, a single examination of a stool is not sufficient. When, in stools with neutrophilic leukocytes, pathogens are not found, *B. hominis* should be looked for.

The parasite

Blastocystis hominis, known since the beginning of this century as a yeast, has been considered a protozoan, belonging to the Sporozoa, since 1967. The vacuolated cell is spherical in shape and, characteristically, shows a large central vacuole which occupies 75% of the cell volume and is surrounded by a narrow rim of cytoplasm containing nuclei and some inclusions. It has a signet ring appearance (Fig. 10.1). Commonly, there is one nucleus situated in the peripherical membranous-like structure but, occasionally, there are 2–4 nuclei. Mitochondria are confined to the thin peripheral band of

cytoplasm between the membrane surrounding the voluminous inner body and the outer membrane[7,8]. There are wide variations in size. *Blastocystis hominis* may measure from 5–120 μm in diameter. This parasite reproduces rapidly in human serum as culture medium.

In cultures, three morphological forms may be observed: vacuolic, amoeba-like with pseudopodes, and granular. In faecal specimens, the vacuolated and amoeba-like forms are found.

Parasites may be stained permanently with iron haematoxylin (Fig. 10.2), Goldner or the Giemsa method; with the last, they stain weakly. The parasites are Ziehl–Nielsen-, Gram- and Grocott-negative. Their vacuoles do not stain with Lugol. At Mérida, we have achieved good results by staining sections of cell blocks (Figs. 10.3 and 10.4). Reproduction of parasites takes place by binary fission or sporulation.

Pathogenesis

The mechanisms of the pathogenic actions of this parasite have not been elucidated. Massive infections with *Blastocystis hominis* may lead to enterocolitic symptoms. Whether this is due to the parasite alone or to the interaction of *Blastocystis hominis* with other organisms has yet to be resolved.

Invasion of tissues by this parasite has not been confirmed convincingly. In one case, a human death due to these organisms was reported because evidence of mucosal invasion of the colon was shown postmortem[9].

Pathology

Parasites are found in the lower ileum and caecum. Descriptions of gross or microscopic lesions do not exist

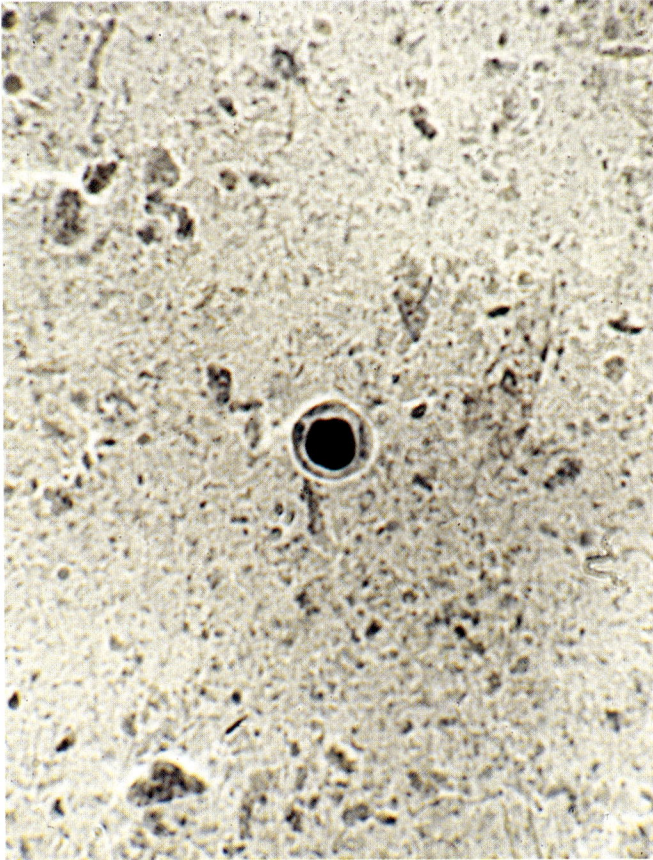

Fig. 10.1 *Blastocystis hominis* cell in smear of faeces. Note the cyst-like appearance with the nucleus in the 'cyst wall'. Iron–haematoxylin

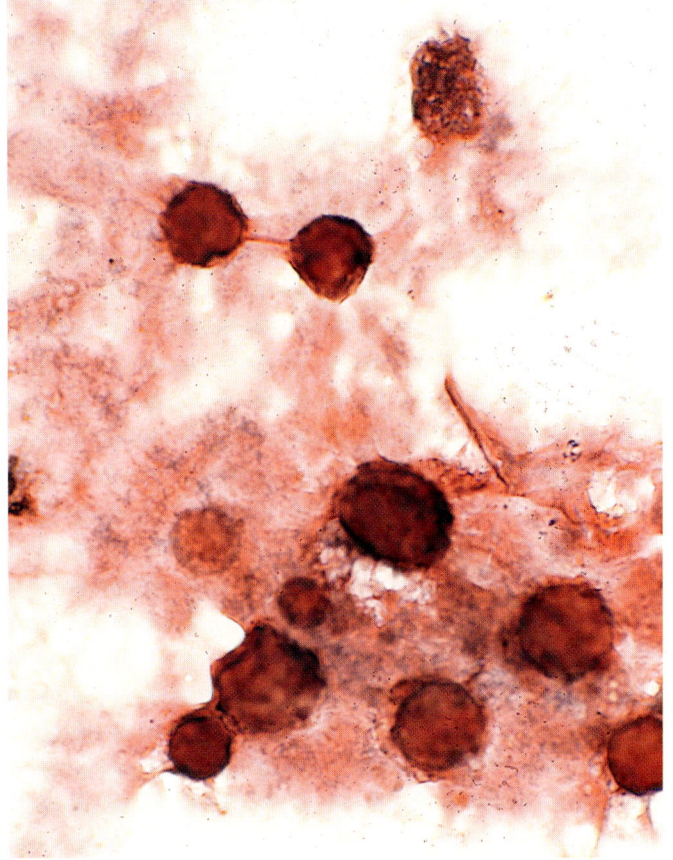

Fig. 10.2 *Blastocystis hominis* cells in smear of faeces. Iron–haematoxylin

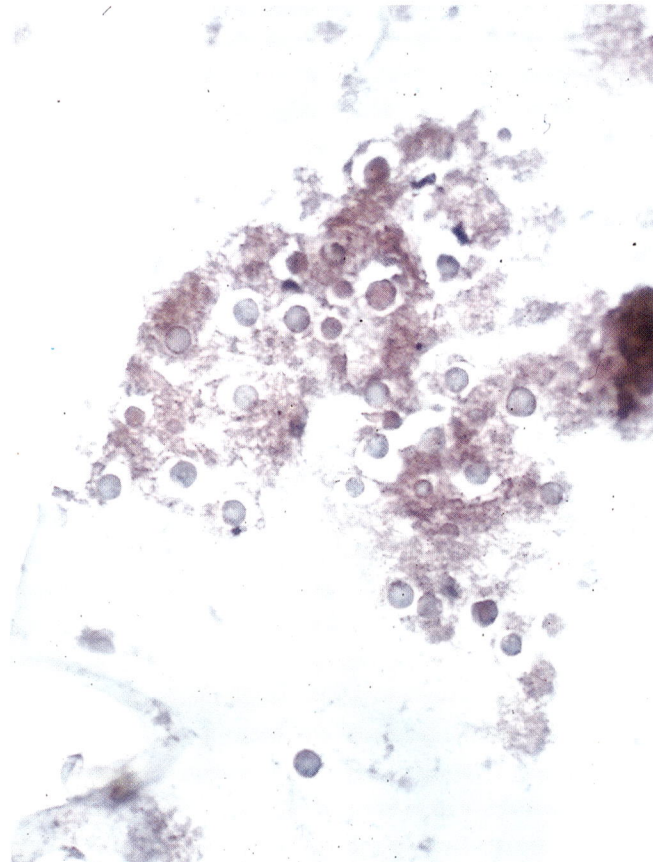

Fig. 10.3 *Blastocystis hominis* cells in section of cell block of faecal material. Iron–haematoxylin

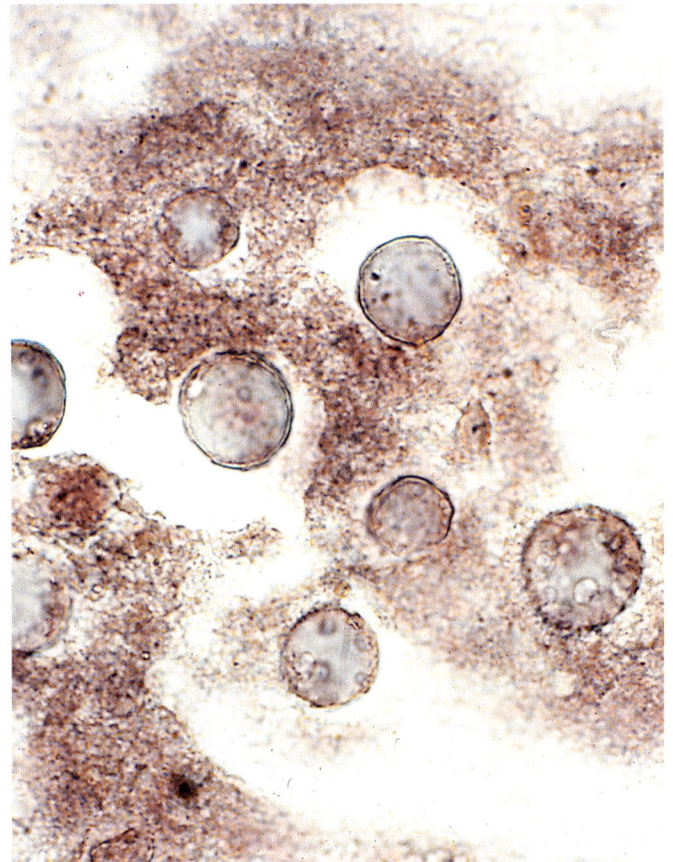

Fig. 10.4 High magnification of Fig. 10.3

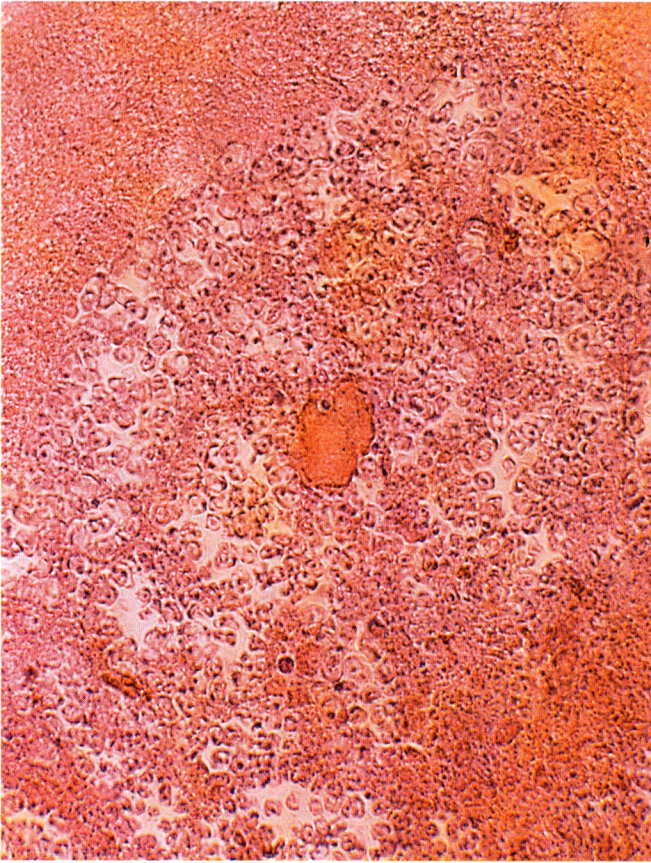

Fig. 10.5 Numerous *Blastocystis hominis* organisms on the surface of the necrotic mucosa of the large bowel. Diffuse pseudomembranous colitis post surgery of carcinoma of the oesophagus. (Case of Dr J. Boehm, München, Germany). Low power. H&E

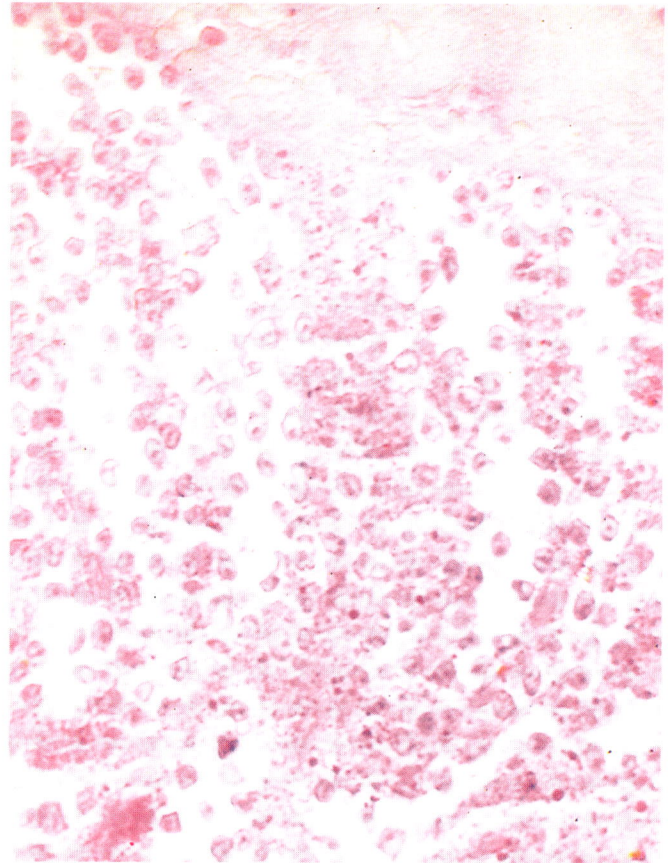

Fig. 10.6 Same case as Fig. 10.5. PAS

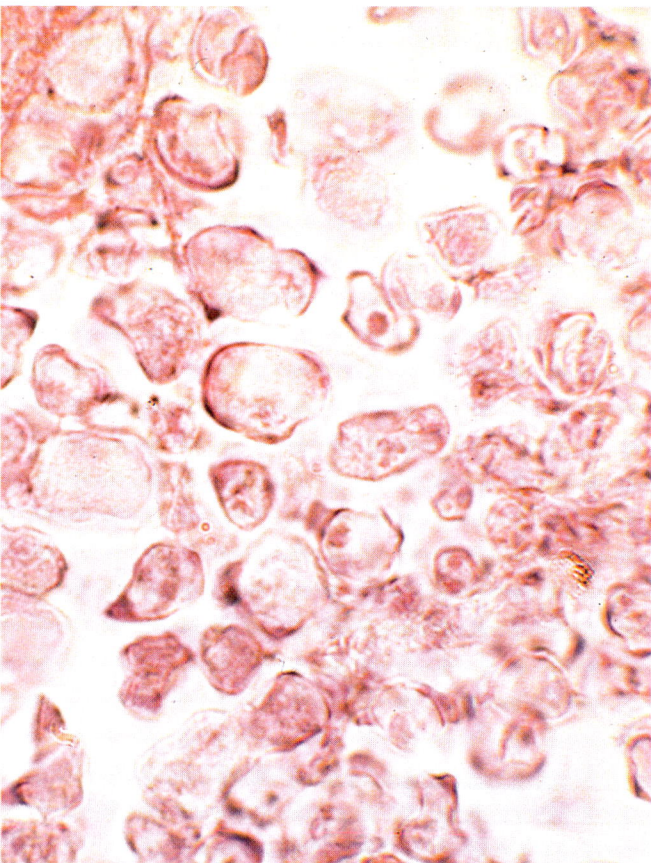

Fig. 10.7 Same case as Figs. 10.5 and 10.6. Nuclei are situated in the peripherical annular-like cytoplasm. This signet-ring appearance cannot be seen. High power. H&E

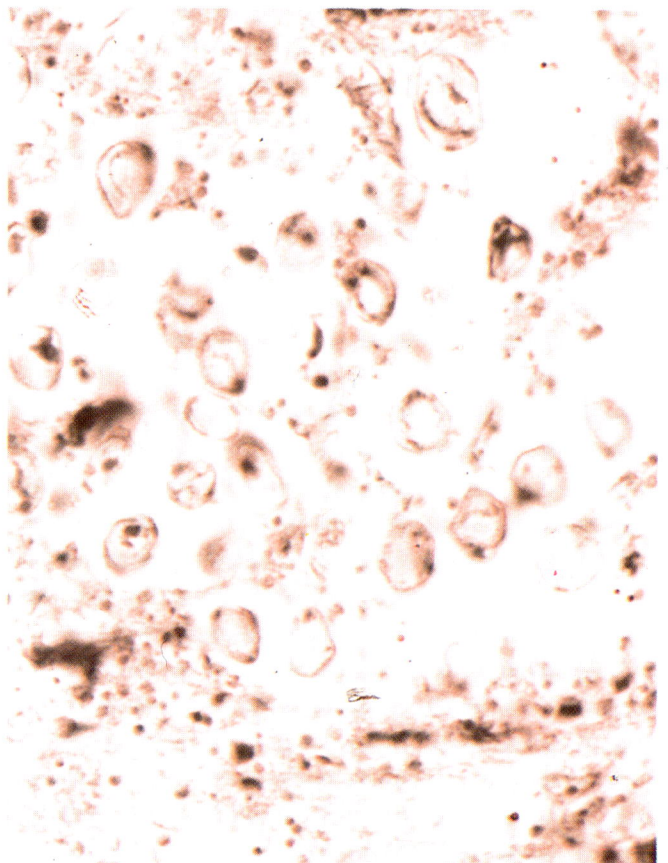

Fig. 10.8 Same case as Figs. 10.5–10.7. High power. Iron–haematoxylin

in the literature. While some reports stress the potential pathogenicity of *Blastocystis hominis*[4,10], there are others who deny that this parasite has a pathogenic role[11]. Recently, an autopsy case was kindly provided from Germany, showing numerous organisms of *Blastocystis hominis*, arranged colony-like and attached to the surface of the large bowel, apparently as secondary non-invasive opportunistic infection in an immunodeficient patient (Figs. 10.5–10.8).

Blastocystis hominis is the most important source of error in stool examinations for protozoa. These parasites may be confused easily with cryptosporidians or intestinal amoebae.

References

1. Brumpt, E. (1912). Blastocystis hominis n. p. et formes voisines. *Bull. Soc. Pathol. Exot.*, **5**, 725
2. Zierdt, C. H. et al. (1967). Protozoan characteristics of Blastocystis hominis. *Am. J. Clin. Pathol.*, **48**, 495
3. Zierdt, C. H. (1983). Blastocystis hominis, a protozoan parasite and intestinal pathogen of human beings. *Clin. Biol. Newslett.*, **5**, 57
4. Zierdt, C. H. (1991). Blastocystis hominis – past and future. *Clin. Microbiol. Rev.*, **4**, 61
5. Tirado Castrillo, de A. et al. (1989). Frecuencia de infección por Blastocystis hominis: un año de estudio. *IV Congreso Panamer. Infect.*, Caracas, Febrero 1989
6. McClure, H. M. et al. (1986). Blastocystis hominis in pig-tailed macaque, a potential enteric pathogen for nonhuman primates. *Lab. Anim. Sci.*, **30**, 890
7. Zierdt, C. H. et al. (1988). Biochemical and ultrastructural study of Blatocystis hominis. *J. Clin. Microbiol.*, **26**, 965
8. Matsumoto, Y. et al. (1987). Light-microscopical appearance and ultrastructure of Blastocystis hominis, an intestinal parasite of man. *Zbl. Bakt. Mikrobiol. Hyg. A.*, **264**, 379
9. Zierdt, C. H. and Tan, H. K. (1976). Ultrastructure and light microscope appearance of Blastocystis hominis in a patient with enteric disease. *Z. Parasitenkd.*, **50**, 277
10. Sheehan, D. J. et al. (1986). Association of Blastocystis hominis and symptoms of human disease. *J. Clin. Microbiol.*, **24**, 548
11. Markell, E. K. and Udkow, M. P. (1986). Blastocystis hominis: Pathogen or fellow traveller. *Am. J. Trop. Med. Hyg.*, **35**, 1028

11. TOXOPLASMOSIS

Introduction

Toxoplasmosis is an important infectious disease. Infection with *Toxoplasma gondii* is, worldwide, of a high prevalence. Latent symptomless infections are far more frequent than disease. Symptomatic disease, on the other hand, is rare but may be severe in man. Today, this is one of the prominent opportunistic infections in immunodeficient persons and typical in AIDS patients[1-5]. The proportion of infected persons is progressively higher in older age groups. More than 80% of the adult rural population in Venezuela[6] was found to have positive serology to *T. gondii*.

The cat (*Felis domestica*) is the specific definitive host for *Toxoplasma gondii*[7-10], although almost all mammals are non-specific intermediate hosts[11,12]. In dogs, lately, toxoplasma-like cyst-forming sporozoans which could not be identified have been reported in nervous tissue[13,14]. Mice and other animal species may be used for experimental purposes[15,16].

There are two principal clinical forms of toxoplasmosis:

1. An extrauterine infection acquired in a natural way. Opportunistic infections with disseminated disease, lymphadenitis and ophthalmitis are of special interest in this group.

2. An intrauterine toxoplasmotic infection in a pregnant woman and the transplacental infection of the fetus.

Clinical diagnosis is only confirmed by the demonstration of the parasite or specific antibodies. Microscopically, the toxoplasmas may be found in the spinal fluid, body and organ fluids as well as organs. Inoculation of specially sensitive *Toxoplasma*-free white mice and special rats may be used for diagnostic purposes.

The parasite

Toxoplasma gondii is the most important of the four coccidian species; the other three are *Sarcocystis bovihominis*, *Sarcocystis suihominis* (Section 13, Sarcosporidiosis) and *Isospora belli* (Section 14, Isosporosis). The Coccidia belong, together with the Plasmodia, to the class of Sporozoa.

It goes through a heteroxenous cycle of evolution, i.e. with several hosts. The final host is solely the cat which becomes contaminated after eating infected mice. In the feline digestive tract, the three phases of the coccidian cycle take place and end with the expulsion of oocysts. After sporulation outside the animals, new infections of mice, domestic animals, e.g. sheep etc., and cats occur. Table 3 shows the cycle of evolution.

The parasite has a half-moon form or is sickle-shaped. It measures $2-5\,\mu m$ when observed in liquid smears and fresh histological preparations, above all as single organism. However, when seen in clusters intracellularly, i.e. in cysts or pseudocysts, they always appear as spherical elements in tissue sections. This is of practical importance because the observer, in order to make a diagnosis, should not look for sickle-shaped structures in tissue sections (Figs. 11.1–11.5). When the parasites reproduce inside tissue cells (muscular, glial or endothelial cells and in macrophages), they form numerous young parasites which fill the cell, pushing cytoplasm and other elements to the periphery, thus forming the already mentioned pseudocysts. Two types of *Toxoplasma* are distinguished by their manner of multiplication: the tachyzoites in pseudocysts, in the acute phase of the disease; and the bradyzoites in cysts with membranes, in the chronic form. However, these two types do not always show visible structural differences. Both types may appear in nests, but the bradyzoites tend to do this more often because they frequently present as cysts which are PAS-positive. This PAS-positivity seems to be related to the storage of glycopolysaccharides.

Artificial culture media which induce growth and multiplication of *Toxoplasma gondii* are not known; however, they may be kept alive in tissue cultures. These parasites can also be preserved in a viable condition for many months by adding glycerol or DMSO and then deep freezing in liquid nitrogen[17].

Pathogenesis

1. The extrauterine and acquired natural infection occurs in two ways:

   a) Raw meat (pigs, sheep or cows) harbouring parasitic cysts may be eaten.
   b) Oocysts or sporocysts of *Toxoplasma gondii* stemming from faeces of a cat may reach the human digestive tract. (Oocysts are highly resistant and may remain viable for longer than a year.)

   From the human gut, haematogenous dissemination takes place. The musculature and the central

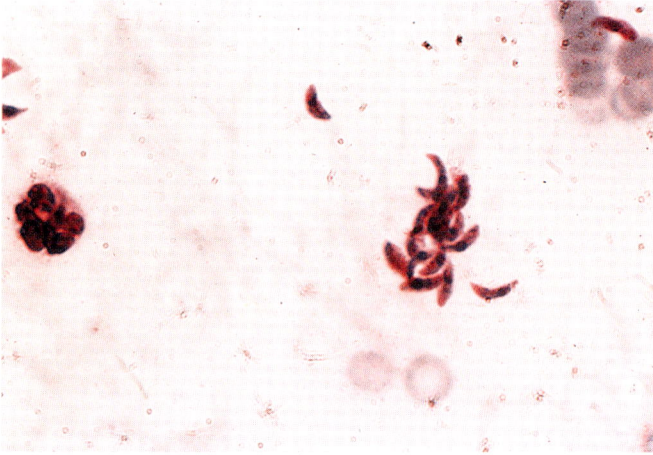

Fig. 11.1 *Toxoplasma gondii* in smear of human bone marrow showing half-moon-shaped parasites. Giemsa

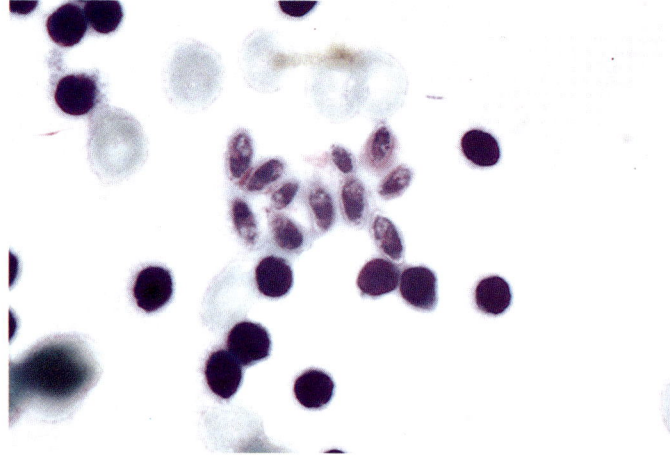

Fig. 11.2 Suspected toxoplasms in smear of pleural exudate, later determined as contaminating fungus cells; here shown as differential diagnostic elements. Giemsa

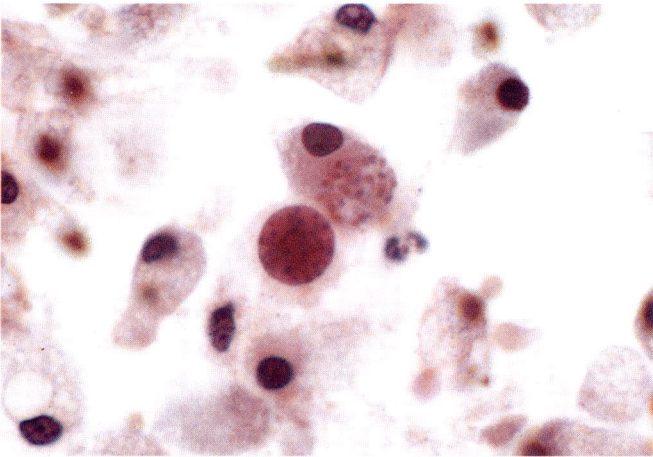

Fig. 11.3 Cyst and pseudocyst with *Toxoplasma gondii* parasites. The densely packed organisms are located in a cyst (dark) and the scarce parasites in a pseudocyst. Section of a toxoplasmic encephalitis. H&E

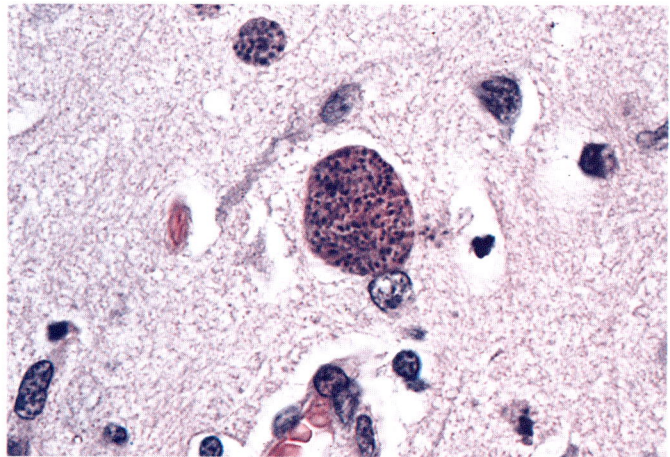

Fig. 11.4 Toxoplasmic cyst without inflammatory reaction at high power in the brain. H&E

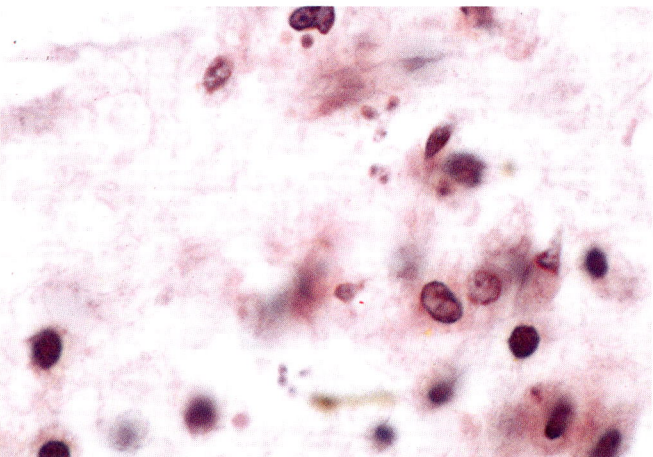

Fig. 11.5 Single, extracystic toxoplasms in tissue section of brain. H&E

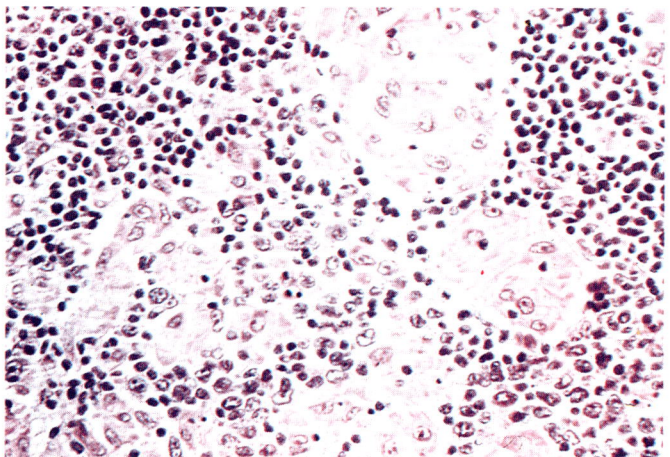

Fig. 11.6 Piringer–Kuchinka lymphadenitis. Cell nodules of variable sizes made up of histiocytes, reticular and epithelioid cells. Parasites of *Toxoplasma gondii* are found only occasionally in this kind of lesion. H&E

Table 3 The evolutionary cycle of *Toxoplasma gondii* (G. Piekarski, *Medical Parasitology*, 1989)

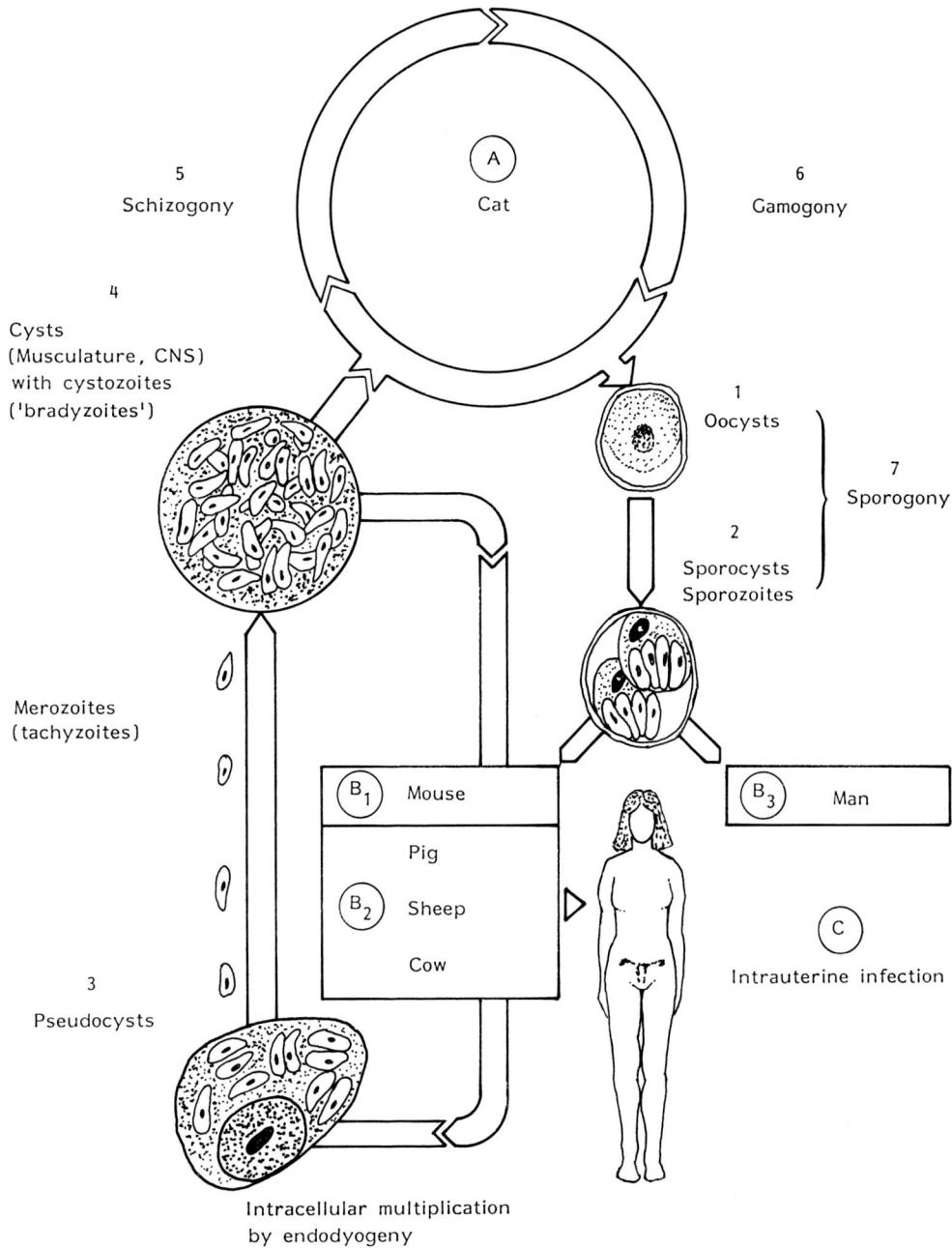

A   Cats, the specific definitive hosts, excrete *Toxoplasma gondii* oocysts in their faeces (*1*). Almost all mammals (non-specific intermediate hosts) can be infected B by the sporocysts (each with four sporozoites, *2*).

B   For example, mouse B_1, pig, sheep, cow B_2, and man B_3.
The parasites multiply intracellularly asexually (*acute phase*) (*3*) and form cysts (*chronic phase*) (*4*). These lead to renewed infection in meat eaters. After a cat is infected, the organisms first multiply asexually in the small intestinal epithelium (schizogony *5*).

Thereafter, they form gamontes and gametes (gamogony, *6*). Development of oocysts and sporocysts, each containing four sporozoites (sporogony, *7*), occurs after fertilization.

C   Intrauterine infection; congenital toxoplasmosis
Infection pathway in man B_3:
a. Through oral ingestion of sporulated oocysts (*2*)
b. Consumption of raw cyst-containing meat from sheep, pig or cow
c. Intrauterine transmission

nervous system are the favoured sites of lesions (tropism). The incubation period is 2–3 weeks. The fact that, all over the world, the prevalence of serologically positive reactions is so high and yet the number of clinical symptomless cases is so low indicates that there must be numerous asymptomatic or subclinical latent infections.

2. If the infected person (see 1) is a woman who is preg-

nant at the time of the first infection with *T. gondii*, she may miscarry or transmit the parasite through the placenta to the fetus with resulting congenital (better described as connatal or prenatal) toxoplasmosis[18–20]. In this situation, the *Toxoplasma gondii* infection seems to be more virulent than when the infection is through the digestive tract. Transplacentally-induced toxoplasmosis has also been detected in fetal pigs[21].

3. Indirect transmission, for example through flies or other insects contaminating food with oocysts, does occur but is in practice of minor importance.

Pathology

The musculature, central nervous system and eyes[22] and lymph nodes[23,24] are the favoured sites of involvement. In cases of disseminated toxoplasmosis, mostly the lungs, liver and adrenal glands are involved. In massive infections, all organs may show lesions.

Natural acquired infection. It is rarely that this infection is followed by an acute or chronic course and fatal cases are even more rare. Gross lesions are of an entirely non-specific nature. It seems appropriate to discuss in this context toxoplasmotic lymphadenitis, toxoplasmotic ophthalmitis and toxoplasmosis due to opportunistic infection.

Lymphadenitis. In adolescents and young adults, toxoplasmotic lymphadenitis appears predominantly in the rear cervical region, or manifests itself as generalized lymphadenopathy. The histological lesions, first described by Piringer-Kuchinka in 1958, have been confirmed by other observers[25]. They are characteristic but not specific for infection with *Toxoplasma gondii*.

Isolated multiple histiocytes or nodules of histiocytic cells, similar to reticular or epithelioid cells, are found. In the cell nodules, neither necrosis nor giant cells are observed (Fig. 11.6), and they do not have the features of true granulomas. Proliferation of this sort of cell and the formation of cell nodules are also seen in Hodgkin disease, infectious mononucleosis and in Whipple disease. The described histological lesions should be confirmed by a positive serological test. Parasites are rarely seen in the lymph node lesions of this aetiology; therefore, definitive aetiological diagnosis should be based on the histological lesions, together with positive results of the serological test.

Ophthalmitis. If toxoplasmotic aetiology has been established, there is a possibility that this is the late consequence of a neonatal infection, or it may be due to haematogenous infection. In toxoplasmotic ophthalmitis, the choroid may present non-specific or necrotizing inflammation, or, less frequently, granulomatous reactions. The nests or cysts of parasites, when present, may show necrobiotic lesions (Figs. 11.7–11.10).

In practice, there is always a problem, in a case of chorioretinitis, in differentiating between toxoplasmotic, histoplasmotic or tuberculous infections or diagnosing an immunological process of undetermined aetiology. It is estimated that a third or a quarter of all cases of chronic ophthalmitis is due to a toxoplasmotic infection (Figs. 11.11–11.13).

Opportunistic infection. Toxoplasmosis, when an infection of this sort, is an acute form of this disease which has, lately, been frequently observed in debilitated patients who have suffered for a long time from various types of chronic diseases. It has been encountered especially in patients treated with cortisone or by irradiation, in individuals with organ transplants, treated with immunosuppression, or in persons with congenital or acquired immunological defects, for instance AIDS. It is thought that this sort of toxoplasmosis did not previously exist but that *Toxoplasma gondii* 'made use of the opportunity' in the above-mentioned conditions to attack without having been present earlier in man as a saprophyte or a facultatively pathogenic micro-organism, as in *Pneumocystis carinii, Candida* sp., etc. This opportunistic infection by *T. gondii* presents neither particular nor specific pathological alterations. Furthermore, this toxoplasmosis is not limited to the central nervous system, as expressed in some books, but, on the contrary, is generalized (Figs. 11.14–11.21). The pathological lesions in the brain are not very extensive, as in neonatal toxoplasmosis (Fig. 11.22). Often, there are other opportunistic infections, for instance cytomegaly, simultaneously present in one patient.

Histologically, when routine tissue sections are reviewed, the parasites are spherical or ovoid in shape. They may be found inside or outside cysts or pseudocysts. We have not always been able to distinguish clearly between these two sorts of intracellular nests of parasites. In cysts, the organisms are densely packed and PAS-positive. The cyst membranes are PAS-positive also. Generally, they do not produce an inflammatory reaction. In pseudocysts, on the contrary, organisms are less numerous and their PAS-positivity is weak. *Toxoplasma* organisms are scarce in tissues because they perish rapidly when outside the nests and when in tissue zones where necrobiosis is occurring. This means that the search for single *Toxoplasma* organisms may be difficult and false negative reports are frequent.

The electron microscope is superior to the light microscope in the identification of *Toxoplasma* organisms: their intracellular localization, type of division, lack of budding and absence of a kinetoplast, are all clearly recognizable ultrastructurally.

Small yeast-like fungus cells of numerous species and *P. carinii* are differentiated from *Toxoplasma* by their Grocott-positivity. Protozoan organisms of other species must be differentiated from *Toxoplasma* on the grounds of their intra- or extracellular localization, presence of kinetoplasts and situation in determined organs or tissues.

Tissue reaction does not show either typical or specific features. Circumscribed necrotic foci, common in toxoplasmotic lesions, may also be observed in other acute infections with massive generalization. In the central nervous system, the parasites are found in necrotic lesions, in cell nodules or situated in areas of undamaged parenchyma. There are numerous coagulative and colliquative necrotic foci. In the periphery of these lesions, proliferation of capillaries and a 'status spongiosus' may be seen. Also, accumulation of foamy cells may be noted.

The glial reaction is characteristic: it consists of the presence of gemistocytic forms of astroglia, some glial nodules and 'naked' astroglial nuclei. The latter mimic Alzheimer nuclei type II, and confusion may also occur with so-called liver-glia seen in the so-called hepatogenic encephalopathy.

Around the small blood vessels are found macrophages (lipophages) and focal infiltrates of scarce lymphocytes and monocytes (Figs. 11.23–11.32). It is not clear whether the necrotic foci are due to damage directly produced by the parasites or whether they are the result of circulatory disorders with hypo- or anoxaemia. The necrotic foci in the brain later become scars and calcification may also occur.

Intrauterine infection. In pregnant women, *Toxoplasma gondii* reaches the uterus after primary infection by haematogenous dissemination and produces placentitis. This does not occur, apparently, in women with latent chronic toxoplasmosis, infected before the beginning of pregnancy. If infection occurs during the first few months of pregnancy, a miscarriage may be the consequence of the placentitis. However, the frequency of miscarriages due to toxoplasmotic infections is lower than was earlier assumed. Only a minimal percentage of all miscarriages can be attributed to infection by *Toxoplasma gondii*. Furthermore, the toxoplasmotic infection has nothing to do with so-called habitual, multiple or repeated miscarriages, as was believed for many years. The inflammatory reaction in the placenta is neither marked nor characteristic, and the parasites are difficult to recognize in the infected placenta (Figs. 11.33–11.35). We, ourselves

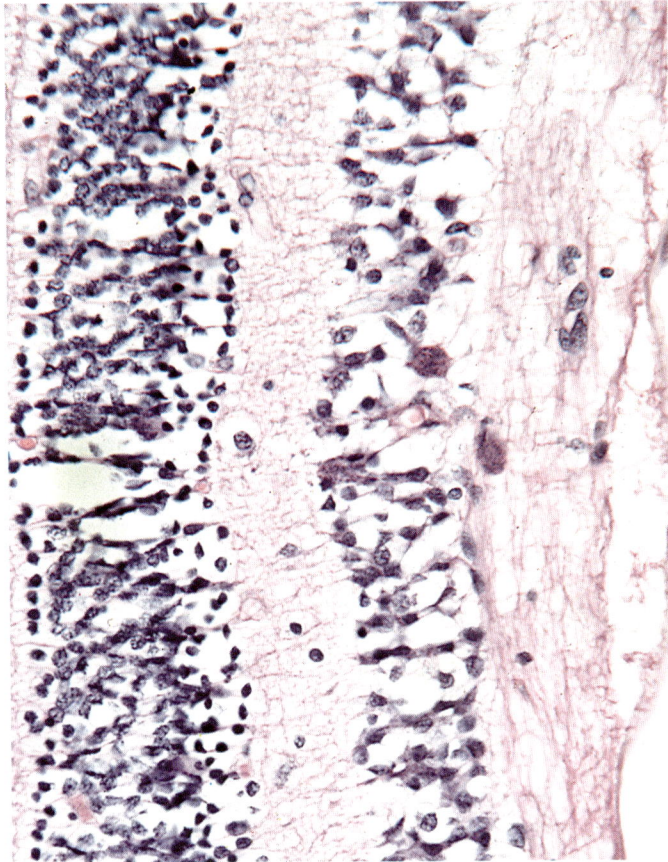

Fig. 11.7 Toxoplasmic chorio-retinitis. Two cysts are seen without inflammatory reaction in this field. H&E

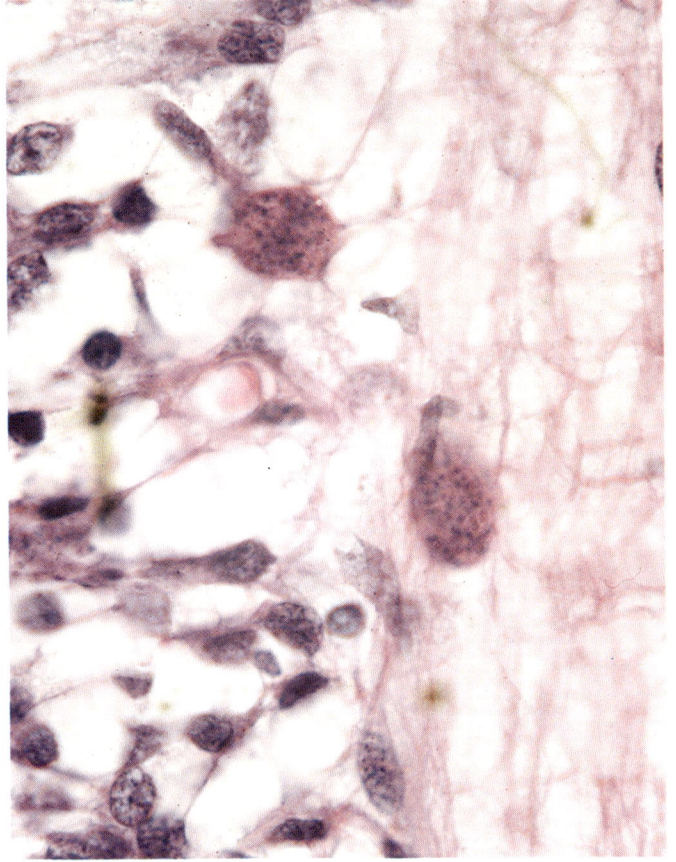

Fig. 11.8 Higher magnification of Fig. 11.7

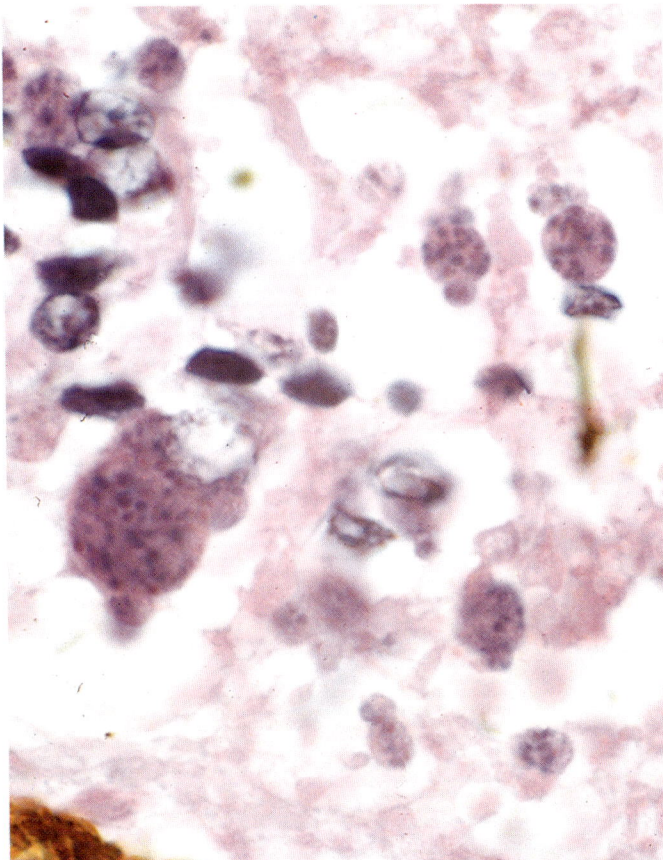

Fig. 11.9 Toxoplasmotic chorio-retinitis with necrobiosis and several parasitic cysts of variable sizes. H&E

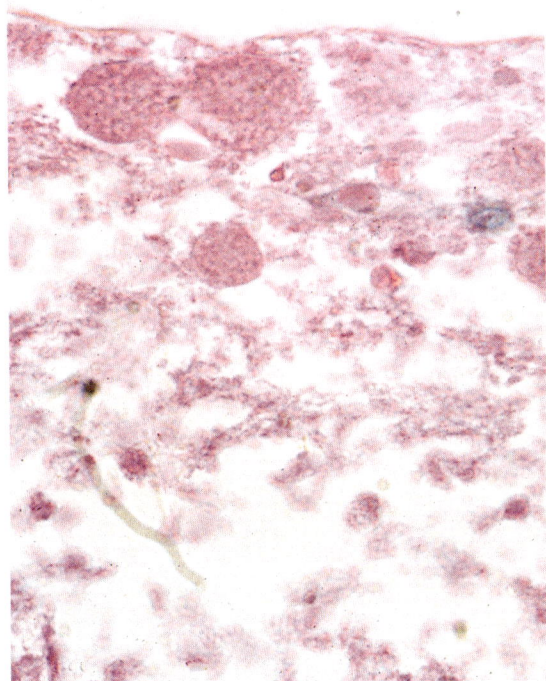

Fig. 11.10 Toxoplasmotic chorio-retinitis with marked necrobiosis of cysts or pseudocysts which are hardly recognizable as such. H&E

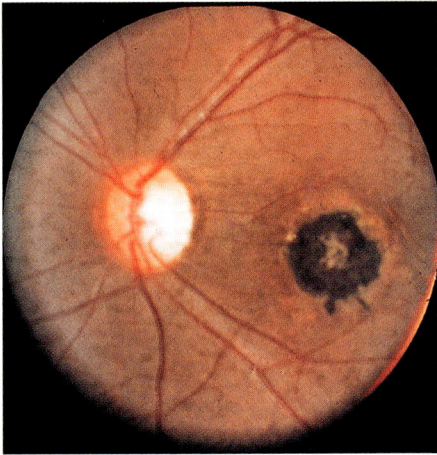

Fig. 11.11 Toxoplasmotic ophthalmitis. Fundus of the eye with an isolated, relatively fresh alteration and a superficial central defect

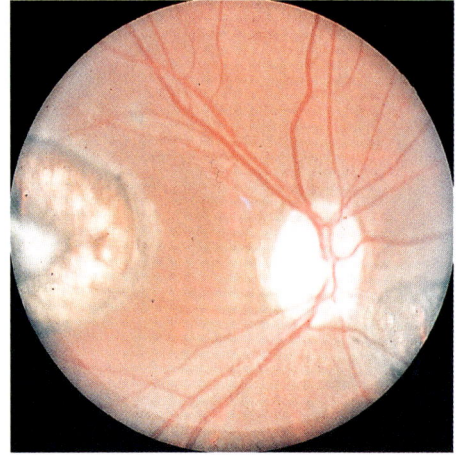

Fig. 11.12 Toxoplasmotic ophthalmitis. Fundus of the eye with an advanced lesion showing a necrosis with a well-defined central ulcer

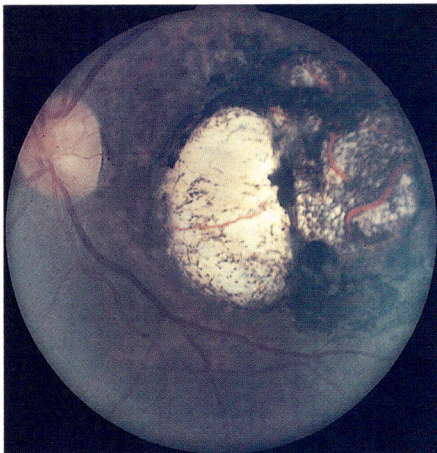

Fig. 11.13 Toxoplasmic ophthalmitis. Fundus of the eye with an extensive chronic lesion. Hyperaemia indicates active inflammation

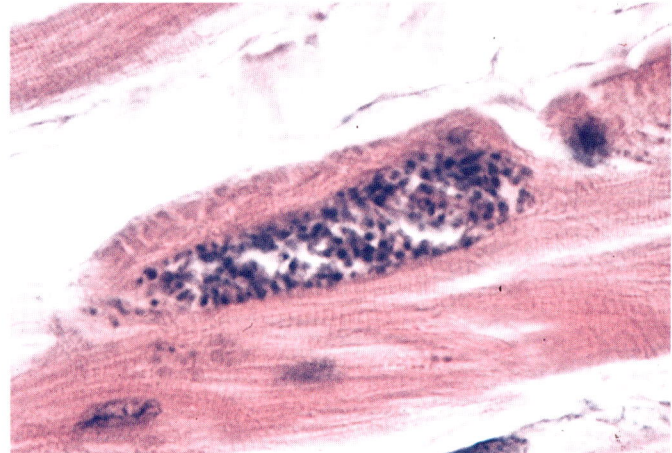

Fig. 11.14 Nest of toxoplasms in a myocardial fibre without inflammation in the vicinity. Originally, this nest was confused with amastigotes of *Trypanosoma cruzi* forming a pseudocyst. H&E

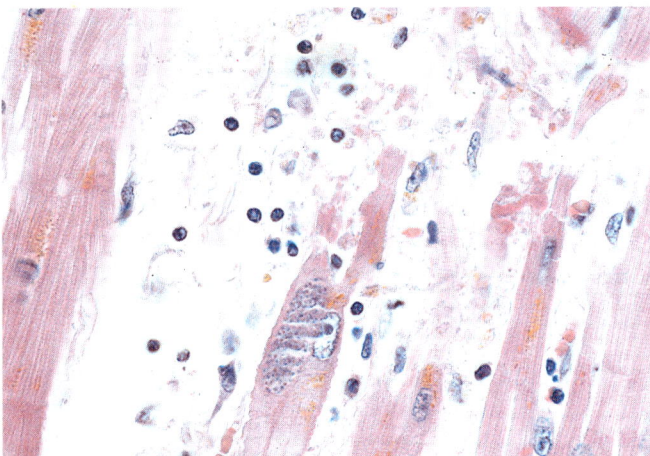

Fig. 11.15 Focal toxoplasmotic myocarditis in a case of generalized toxoplasmosis. The nest of toxoplasms is faintly visible. H&E

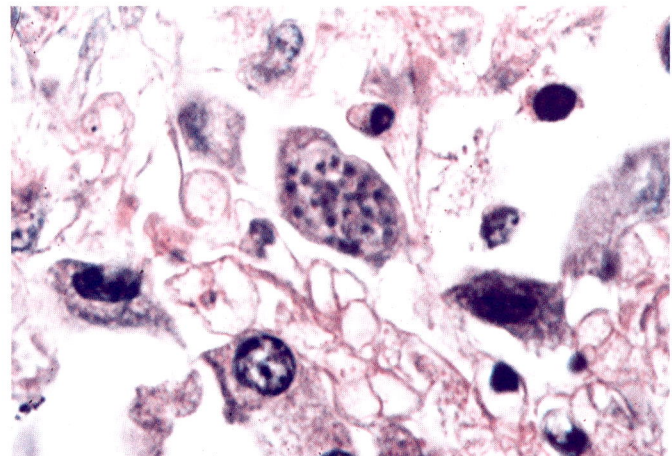

Fig. 11.16 Toxoplasmotic cyst or pseudocyst in lung section. H&E

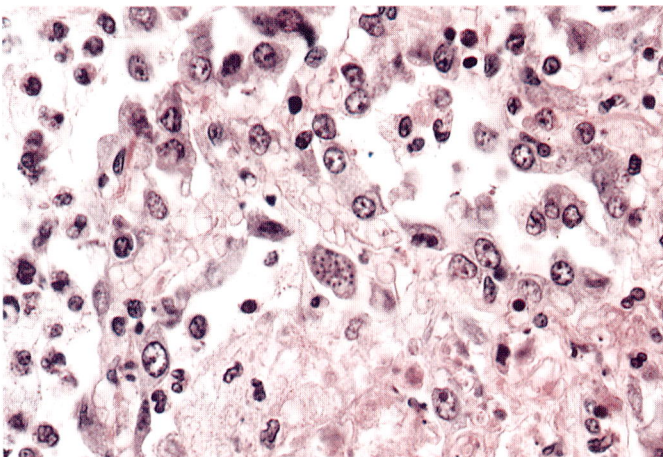

Fig. 11.17 Toxoplasmotic pulmonary lesion. Necrobiosis and acute inflammation are seen together with a small parasitic cyst. H&E

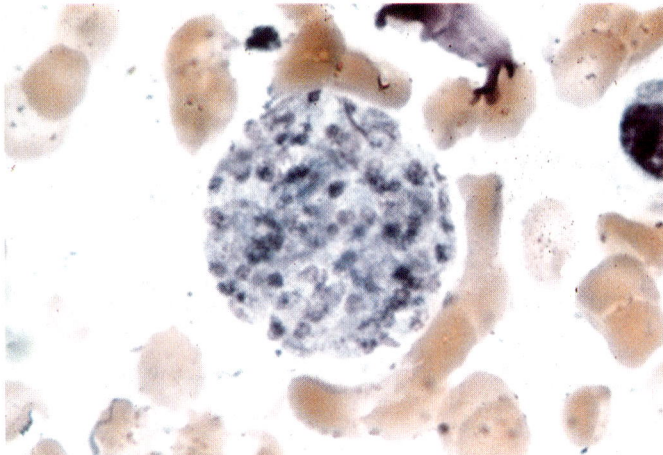

Fig. 11.18 Cyst with *Toxoplasma gondii* organisms in the pleural fluid of a patient with an acquired, disseminated and fatal toxoplasmosis. H&E

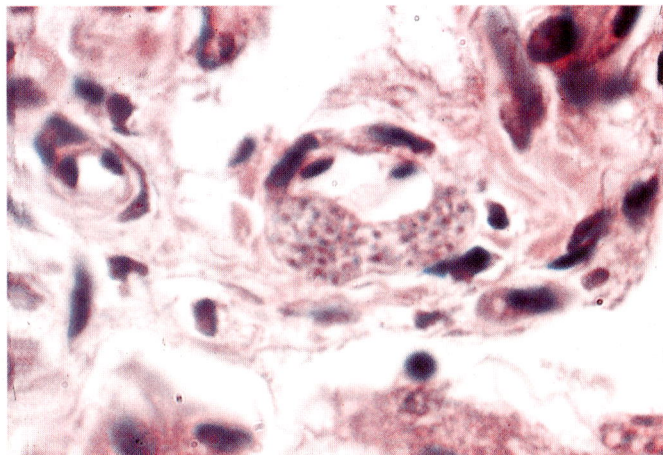

Fig. 11.19 Small toxoplasmotic cyst or pseudocyst in a muscular fibre or endothelial cell of a small blood vessel in the portal space of the liver in a case of generalized toxoplasmosis. H&E

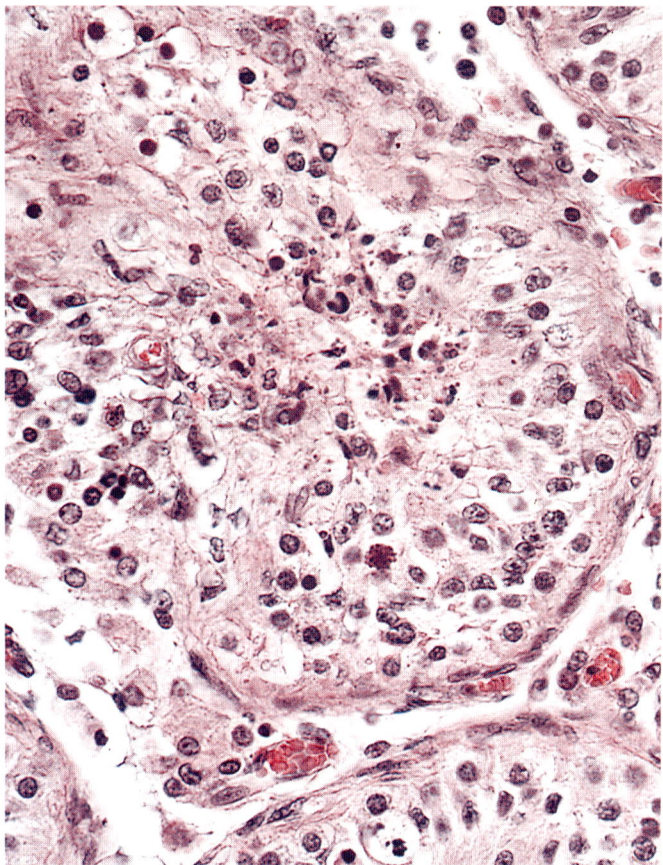

Fig. 11.20 Toxoplasmotic orchitis with necrobiotic changes at a seminiferous tubule and interstitial inflammation. H&E

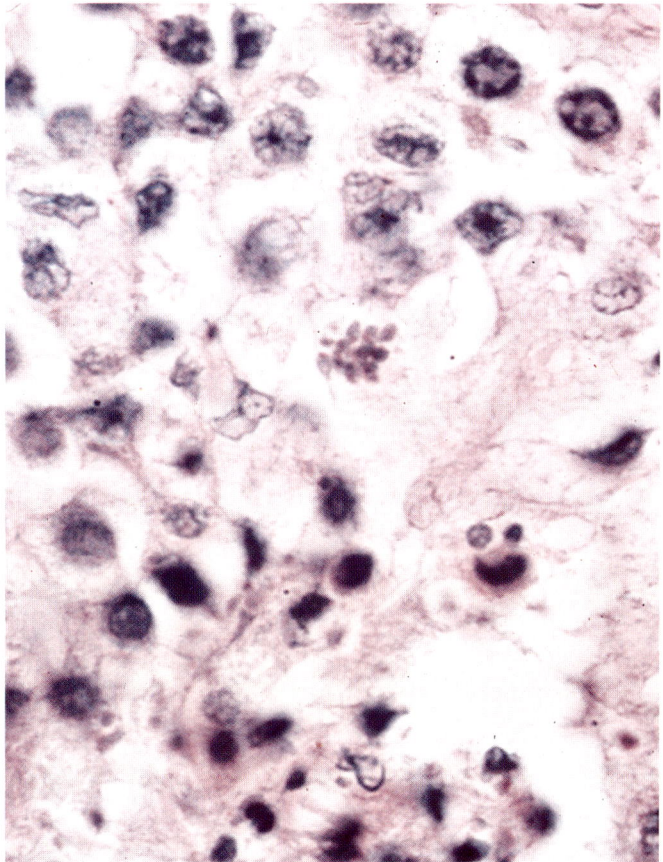

Fig. 11.21 Higher magnification of Fig. 11.20. A cluster of toxoplasms may be discerned. H&E

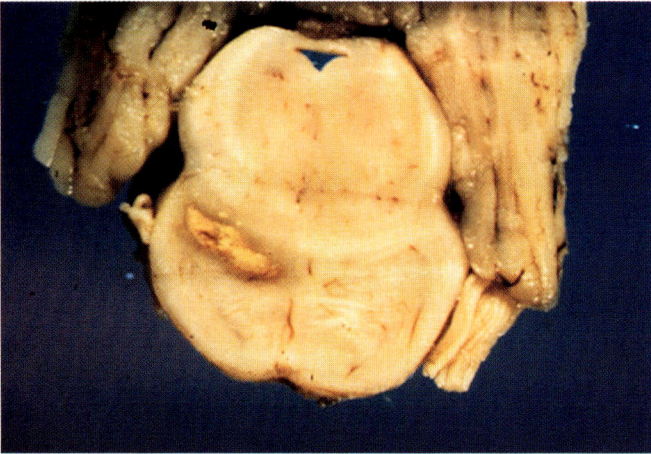

Fig. 11.22 Circumscribed necrotic focus in the medulla oblongata in a case of neonatal toxoplasmosis

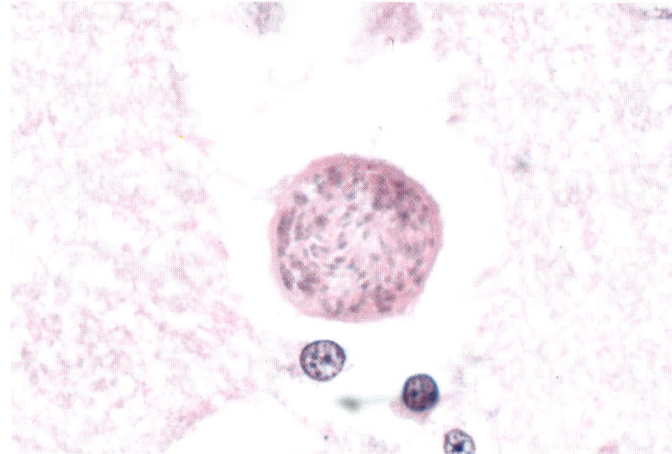

Fig. 11.23 Toxoplasmotic cyst or pseudocyst without inflammatory reaction in the brain. H&E

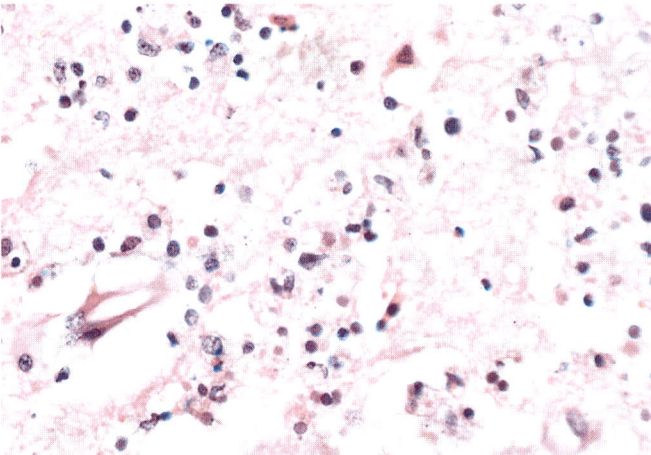

Fig. 11.24 Necrobiotic lesions and inflammation in toxoplasmotic encephalitis. H&E

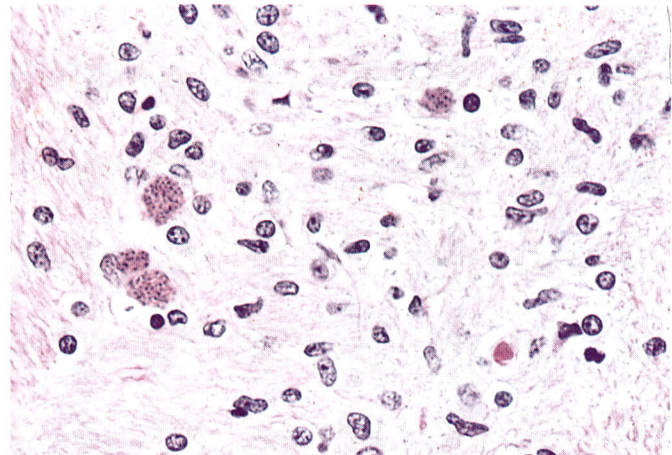

Fig. 11.25 Cell nodule in the brain with several toxoplasmotic cysts or pseudocysts visible in this field. H&E

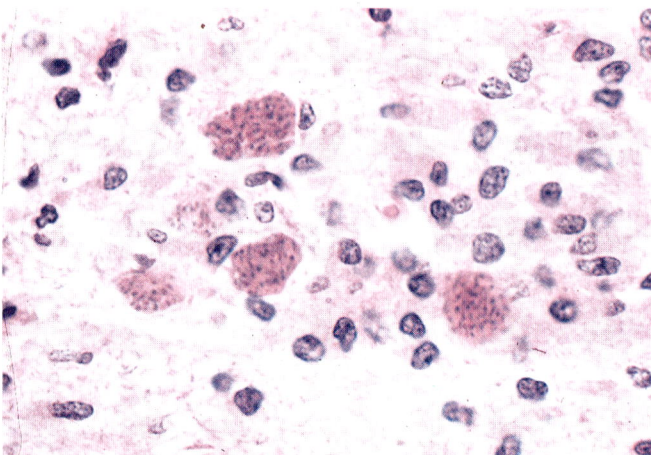

Fig. 11.26 Toxoplasmotic cysts or pseudocysts in cellular infiltrates of the brain with necrobiotic lesions. H&E

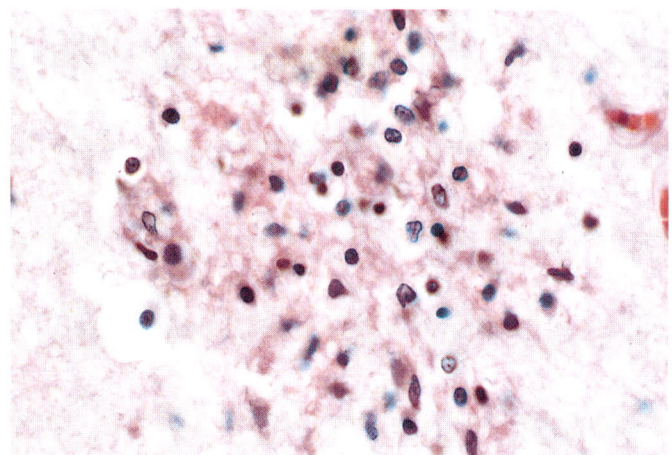

Fig. 11.27 Toxoplasmotic encephalitis with cell nodule not showing parasites. H&E

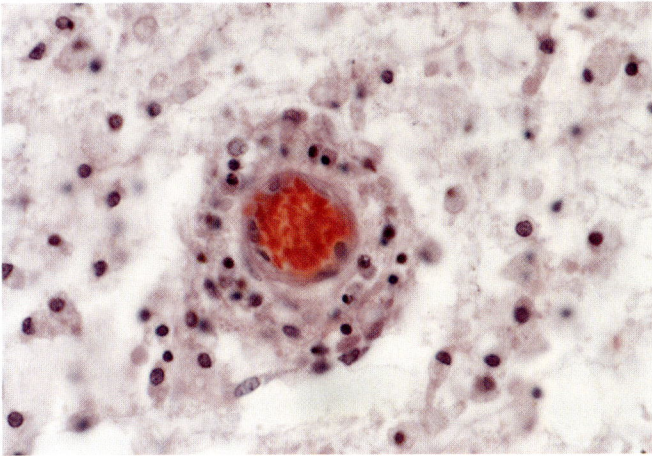

Fig. 11.28 Perivascular infiltrates in toxoplasmotic encephalitis. Parasites are not seen in this field. H&E

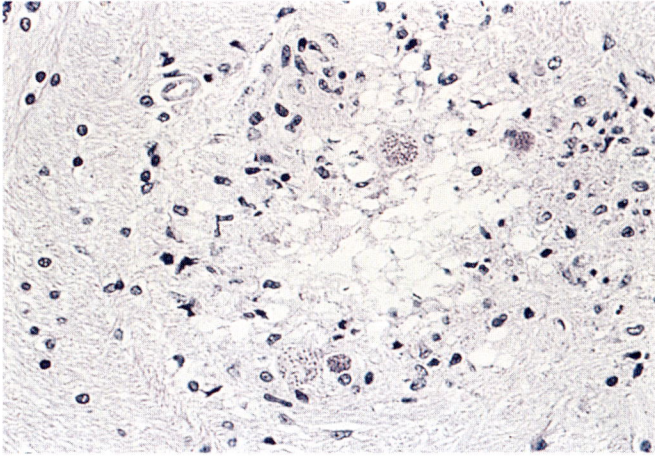

Fig. 11.29 Brain with focal necrobiosis and cell infiltrates. Some toxoplasmotic cysts or pseudocysts faintly visible. H&E

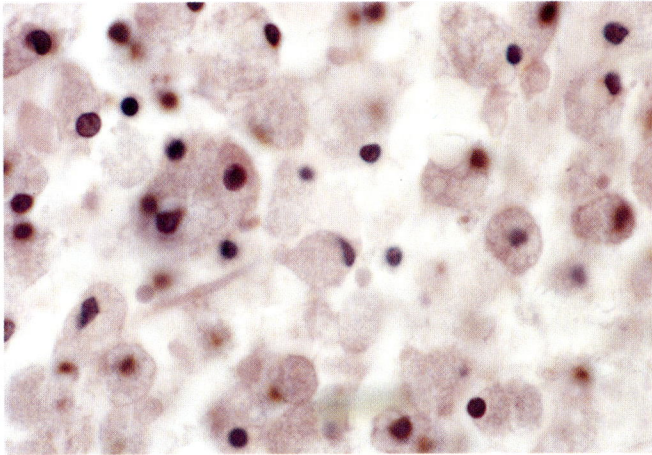

Fig. 11.30 Toxoplasmotic encephalitis with numerous foamy histiocytes in this field. Parasites are not seen in this area. H&E

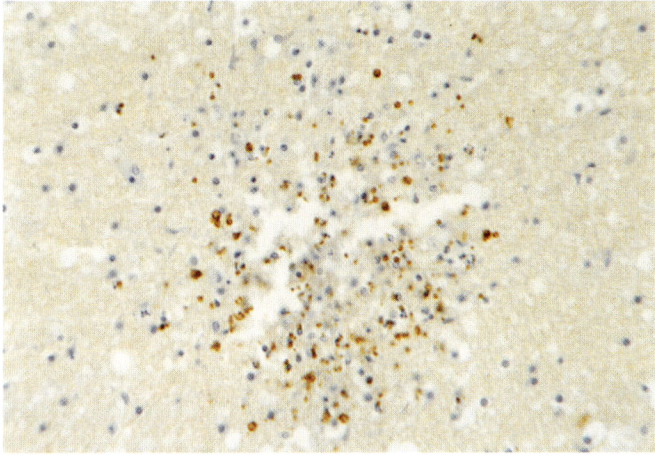

Fig. 11.31 Toxoplasmotic encephalitis. The brownish particles indicate antigen–antibody reaction. Immunoperoxidase

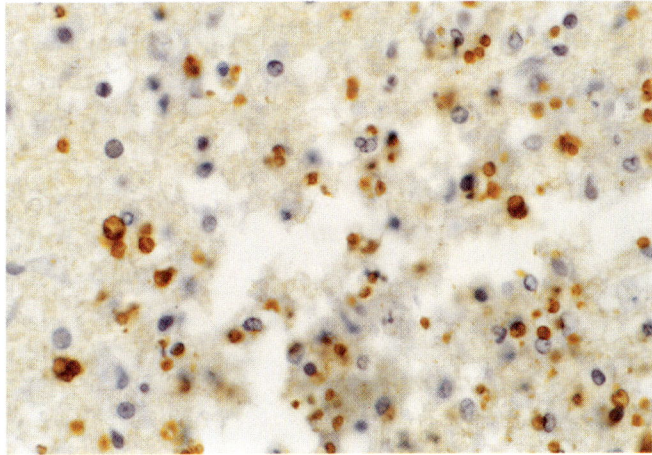

Fig. 11.32 Higher magnification of features in Fig. 11.31

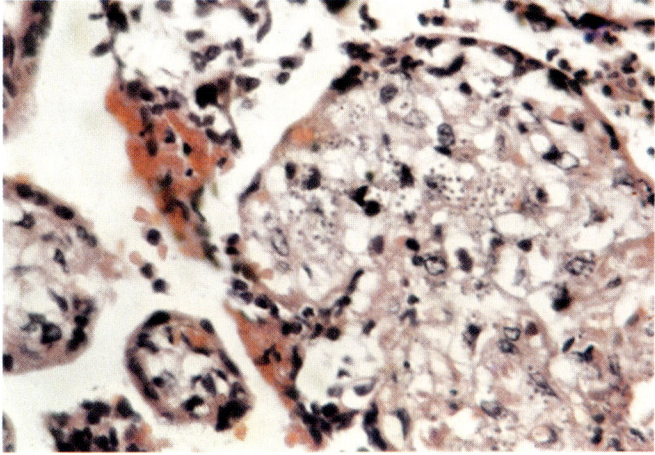

Fig. 11.33 Placenta with several nests of parasites. H&E

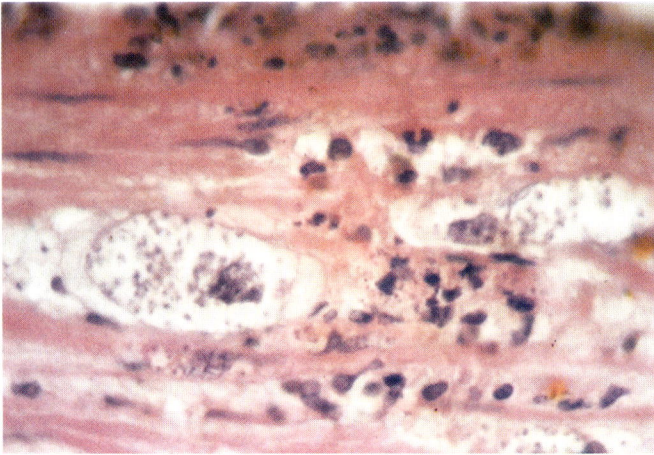

Fig. 11.34 Nest of parasites clearly visible in the placental tissue. H&E

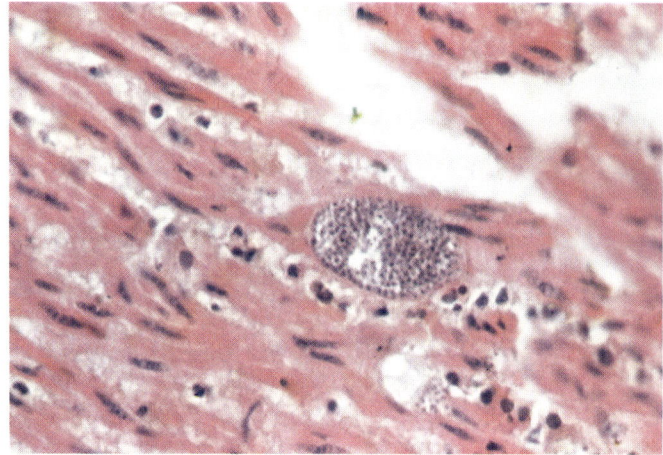

Fig. 11.35 Toxoplasmotic cyst in the umbilical cord. H&E

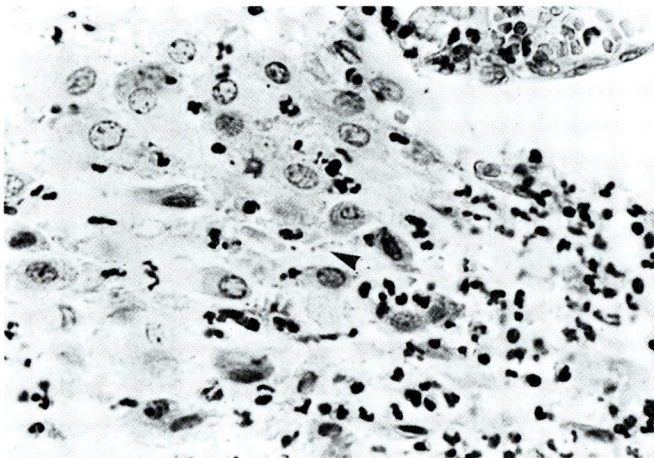

Fig. 11.36 Toxoplasmotic placentitis. The small granular elements in the decidua (arrow) were interpreted by experts as *Toxoplasma gondii* organisms. H&E

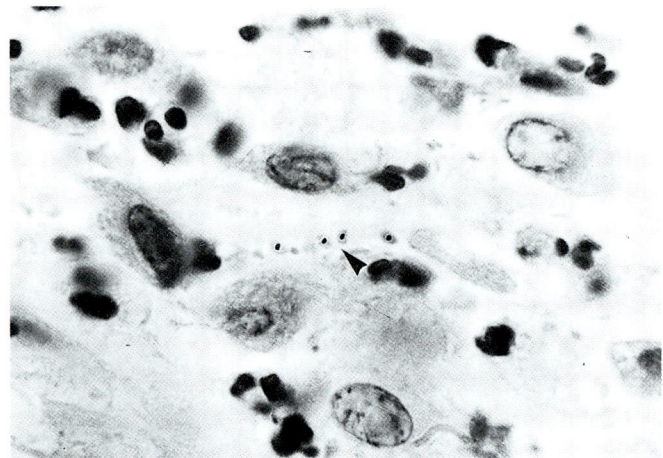

Fig. 11.37 Higher magnification of Fig. 11.36. The toxoplasms are marked with dots. H&E

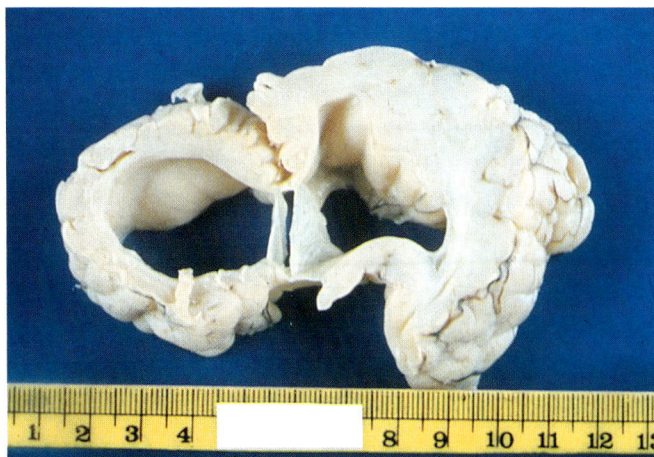

Fig. 11.38 Marked hydrocephalus with cortical atrophy in case of neonatal infection with *Toxoplasma gondii*

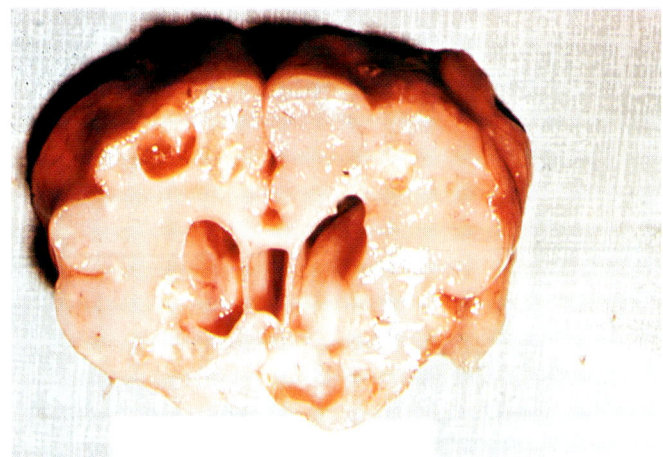

Fig. 11.39 Cut surface of brain with marked oedema, cavities and internal hydrocephalus in case of neonatal toxoplasmosis

were not able to detect parasites in the tissue sections of our cases, although expert parasitologists could demonstrate the micro-organisms in the same cases (Figs. 11.36 and 11.37).

If the toxplasmotic infection occurs during the second three months of pregnancy, premature or still birth may be provoked.

Finally, when infection with *T. gondii* takes place in the last stage of pregnancy, pathological disorders in the pregnancy are almost never seen; birth takes place normally and the fetus also looks normal. However, neonatal toxoplasmosis symptoms may manifest themselves some weeks or months later in a new-born baby, who was born apparently normal and healthy. Cerebral disorders appear, such as fever accompanied by convulsions, states of excitement or lethargy and other signs typical of encephalitis. The majority of the new-born babies with toxoplasmosis die in early infancy. In the autopsies, generalized lesions with parasites are found in the lungs, myocardium, liver and adrenal glands; these have provoked interstitial pneumonia, myocarditis, hepatitis and the formation of necrotic foci in the adrenals. The most significant lesions, however, are always found in the central nervous system. Here, extensive areas of softening, cyst-like lesions and often pronounced internal hydrocephalus are seen. These types of lesions had already been described by Virchow in the last century and were called 'brains resembling Swiss cheese'. Their aetiology, obviously, was unknown at that time (Figs. 11.38 and 11.39).

Under the microscope, areas of softening in different stages of evolution, cellular infiltrates of variable extensions, glial nodules, calcification, vasculitis and thrombotic processes can be found in the brain. Generally, parasites are scarce in this type of lesion. It has not yet been elucidated whether toxoplasmotic chorioretinitis has its origin in this sort of congenital infection or of some other. The percentage of infants with congenital, connatal or neonatal toxoplasmosis who survive is unknown. Also, it would be of interest to know what proportion of all cases of blindness, hydrocephalus, microcephalus, feeblemindedness, imbecility and other cerebral damage is caused by toxoplasmotic infection.

References

1. Enzensberger, W., Helm, E. B., Fischer, P. A. and Stille, W. (1985). Toxoplasmosis of the CNS: an important neurological complication of AIDS. *Trop. Med. Parasit. (Suppl. 11)*, **36**, 19
2. Seitz, H. M. and Kersting, G. (1985). Toxoplasma infection in AIDS patients. *Trop. Med. Parasit. (Suppl. II)*, **36**, 15
3. Tschirhart, D. and Klatt, E. C. (1988). Disseminated toxoplasmosis in the acquired immunodeficiency syndrome. *Arch. Pathol. Lab. Med.*, **112**, 1237
4. Grossniklaus, H. E. *et al.* (1990). Toxoplasma gondii retinochoroiditis and optic neuritis in acquired deficiency syndrome. Report of a case. *Ophthalmology*, **97**, 1342
5. Matturri, L. *et al.* (1990). Cardiac toxoplasmosis in pathology of acquired immunodeficiency syndrome. *Panminerva Med.*, **32**, 194
6. Salfelder, K., Sauerteig, E. and Novoa, M. D. (1987). *Protozoan Infections in Man*. Schwer-Verlag
7. Frenkel, J. K., Dubey, J. P. and Miller, N. L. (1970). Toxoplasma gondii in cats. Fecal stages identified as coccidian oocysts. *Science*, **167**, 893
8. Ruiz, A. and Frenkel, J. K. (1980). Toxoplasma gondii in Costa Rican cats. *Am. J. Trop. Med. Hyg.*, **29**, 1150
9. Dubey, J. P. and Gendron-Fitzpatrick, A. P. (1988). Fatal toxoplasmosis and enteroepithelial stages of Toxoplasma gondii in a Pallas cat (Felis manul). *J. Protozool.*, **35**, 528
10. Dubey, J. P. *et al.* (1990). Acute primary toxoplasmic hepatitis in an adult cat shedding Toxoplasma gondii oocysts. *J. Am. Vet. Med. Assoc.*, **197**, 1616
11. Siim, J. C., Biering-Sorensen, U. and Moller, T. (1963). Toxoplasmosis in domestic animals. *Adv. Vet. Sci.*, **8**, 335
12. Dubey, J. P., Ott-Joslin, J., Torgerson, R. W., Topper, M. J. and Sundberg, J. P. (1988). Toxoplasmosis in black-faced kangaroos (Macropus fuliginosus melanops). *Vet. Parasitol.*, **30**, 97
13. Cummings, J. F., de Lahunta, A., Suter, M. M. and Jacobson, R. H. (1988). Canine protozoan polyradiculoneuritis. *Acta Neuropathol. Berl.*, **76**, 46
14. Bjerkas, I. and Presthus, J. (1989). The neuropathology in toxoplasmosis-like infection caused by a newly recognized cyst forming sporozoon in dogs. *APMIS*, **97**, 459
15. Dubey, J. P. (1988). Lesions in transplacentally induced toxoplasmosis in goats. *Am. J. Vet. Res.*, **49**, 905
16. Dubey, J. P. (1989). Lesions in goats fed Toxoplasma gondii oocysts. *Vet. Parasitol.*, **15**, 133
17. Piekarski, G. (1989). *Medical Parasitology*. Springer-Verlag
18. Werner, H., Schmidtke, L. and Thomaschek, C. (1963). Toxoplasma Infektion und Schwangerschaft. *Klin. Wschr.*, **41**, 96
19. Desmonts, G. and Gonvreur, J. (1974). Congenital toxoplasmosis. A prospective study of 378 pregnancies. *N. Engl. J. Med.*, **290**, 1110
20. Hay, J., Graham, D. I. and Aitken, P. P. (1984). Congenital toxoplasmosis and mental subnormity. *J. R. Soc. Med.*, **77**, 344
21. Dubey, J. P. *et al.* (1990). Lesions in fetal pigs with transplacentally-induced toxoplasmosis. *Vet. Pathol.*, **27**, 411
22. Zimmermann, L. E. (1961). Ocular pathology of toxoplasmosis. *Survey Ophthalmol.*, **6**, 832
23. Piringer-Kuchinka, A. (1952). Eigenartige mikroskopische Befunde an excidierten Lymphknoten. *Verh. Dtsch. Ges. Path.*, **36**, 352
24. Von Arx, D. P. (1988). Cervicofacial toxoplasmosis. *Br. J. Oral. Maxillofac. Surg.*, **26**, 70
25. Soto Urribarri, R. and Soto, Tarazón, S. de (1990). Tratamiento y evolución de la toxoplasmosis ganglionar. *Kasmera*, **18**, 1

12. BABESIOSIS

Introduction

Only isolated cases have been reported in Europe since 1957[1], but, today, human infections of this protozoan disease, which is transmitted by ticks, are increasingly observed and can no longer be considered rare. Cases have been found in Yugoslavia, France, USSR, Ireland, USA and Mexico[2-5], but, to our knowledge, this protozoan infection has, so far, not been found in Venezuela.

Natural *Babesia* infections are well known in cattle and rodents. In the former, *Babesia bovis* and *Babesia divergens* are noted and produce the so-called 'bovine malaria' or piroplasmosis[6-8] in tropical countries. *Theileria* species are similar to *Babesia* spp. and may cause the same disease. In rodents, *Babesia microti* leads to a latent localized infection.

There are two clinical forms in man:

1. The first is mostly observed in Europe, generally takes a fatal course and is produced by *Babesia bovis* or *Babesia divergens*. It has been seen mostly in splenectomized patients.

2. The second form is found, predominantly, in the USA, mostly shows a latent form and is due to *Babesia microti*; the patients often have an intact spleen. Latent *Babesia* infection can lead to a severe, sometimes fatal, disease in the recipients of blood transfusions.

Clinical diagnosis is made by microscopic demonstration of the parasite in Giemsa-stained thin or thick blood films. Also intraperitoneal inoculation of hamsters with the blood of patients allows serological diagnosis of the disease to be made.

Table 4 Developmental cycle of *Babesia microti* (in part from Mehlhorn and Schein, 1984)

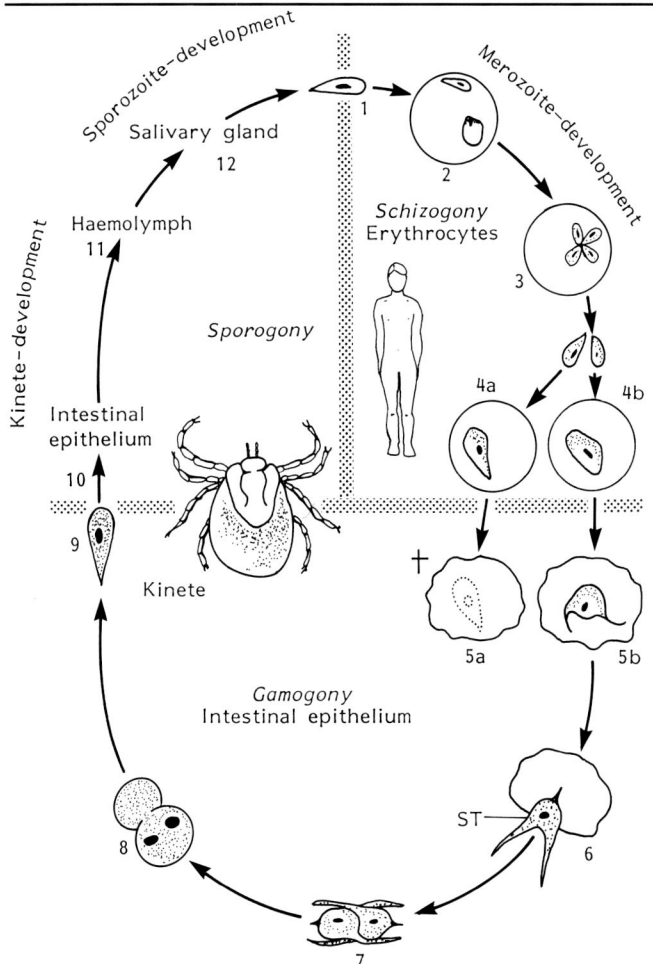

1.   Sporozoite from tick saliva (*Ixodes* species)
2.   Multiplication in erythrocyte by binary schizogony resulting in the formation of merozoites (also in lymphocytes?)
3.   Erythrocyte containing characteristic Maltese cross stage
4a.   Merozoite; disintegrating merozoite in tick intestine (5a)
5b–8. Gamogony with the formation of 'radiating' bodies (6) in the intestinal epithelium of the tick
9.   A kinete develops from the zygote
10–12. Asexual multiplication of the kinetes in the tick; numerous sporozoites develop in the salivary gland

The parasite

Species of the genus *Babesia* belong to the Piroplasmia, a subclass of Sporozoa. Three are pathogenic for man: *Babesia bovis*, *Babesia divergens* and *Babesia microti*. The parasite reservoir hosts are small mammals, e.g. *Microtus* species.

Babesia spp. can easily be confused with the malaria parasite, *Plasmodium falciparum*. There are quite a few morphological similarities, but *Babesia* trophozoites in erythrocytes are more or less pear-shaped. On the other hand, they may also be ring-shaped, about 1 μm in diameter, as are the malaria trophozoites. After division, *Babesia* parasites present themselves inside erythrocytes in pairs or tetrades (also called 'Maltese cross') located marginally (*B. divergens*) or centrally (*B. microti*) within the erythrocyte. Since we do not possess human material we show babesiae in the blood of cattle (Fig. 12.1).

The developmental cycle of *Babesia microti* is seen in Table 4.

Pathogenesis

Vectors of these parasites are hard ticks, for example species of the genus *Ixodidae*, e.g. *Ixodes ricinus* or *Dermacentor reticulatus*. They ingest the intra-erythrocytic stages of *Babesia* when they feed on blood. Sexual development takes place in the tick, and later asexual multiplication and formation of sporozoites in the salivary glands. When the tick next feeds on blood, the parasites are transmitted to a new host[9]. Transmission of the parasites may occur, also, via blood transfusions[10].

The symptoms in the infected human host are similar to those of a recent malaria infection.

Pathology

There are no reports of gross or microscopic tissue lesions due to *Babesia* infections. Parasites of this sort can be found only in blood.

The *Babesia* organisms are similar to trophozoites of *Plasmodium falciparum* inside erythrocytes, as described in Section 16 on Malaria. In contrast to the malaria parasites, however, the *Babesia* organisms may be located in lymphocytes too. The following structural features have to be considered for the differential diagnosis. *Babesia* organisms do **not** have: schizonts, gamontes, the stippling of erythrocytes or pigment. In addition, malaria occurs in tropical or subtropical countries, while babesiosis is found worldwide and infection is acquired in regions where ticks live. Cases with symptoms of malaria resistant to therapy may be due to *Babesia* instead of *Plasmodium* infection. *Babesia* organisms may be confused with haemolysis-induced Pappenheimer bodies[11].

References

1. Skrabalo, Z. and Deanovic, Z. (1957). Piroplasmosis in man. Report of a case. *Docum. Med. Geogr. Trop.*, **9**, 11
2. Fitzpatrick, J. E. P., Kennedy, C. C., McGeown, M. G., Oreopoulos, D. G., Robertson, J. H. and Goyaunwo, M. A. O. (1969). Further details on third recorded case of babesiosis in man. *Br. Med. J.*, **2**, 770
3. Garnham, P. C. C., Donnelly, J., Hoogstrael, H., Kennedy, C. C. and Walton, C. A. (1969). Human babesiosis in Ireland: Further observations and the medical significance of this infection. *Br. Med. J.*, **2**, 768
4. Western, K. A., Benson, G. D., Gleason, N. N. *et al.* (1970). Babesiosis in a Massachusetts resident. *N. Engl. J. Med.*, **283**, 285
5. Anderson, A. E., Cassady, P. B. and Healy, G. R. (1974). Babesiosis in man. *Am. J. Clin. Path.*, **62**, 612
6. Babes, V. (1888). Sur l'hemoglobinurie bactérienne du boeuf. *C. R. Acad. Sci. (Paris)*, **107**, 692
7. Enigk, K., Friedhoff, K. and Wirahadiredja, S. (1963). Die Piroplasmosen der Wiederkäuer in Deutschland. *D. Tierärztl. Wschr.*, **70**, 422
8. McInnes, E. F. *et al.* (1991). An outbreak of babesiosis in imported sable antelope (Hippotragus niger). *J. S. Afr. Vet. Assoc.*, **62**, 30
9. Walter, G. and Weber, G. (1981). Untersuchungern zur Übertragung (transstadial, transovarial) von Babesia microti, Stamm 'Hannover'I, in Ixodes ricinus. *Tropenmed. Parasit.*, **32**, 228
10. Marcus, L. C., Valigorsky, J. M., Fanning, W. L., Joseph, T. and Glick, B. (1982). A case report of transfusion induced babesiosis. *J. Am. Med. Assoc.*, **284**, 465
11. Carr, J. M. *et al.* (1991). Babesiosis. Diagnostic pitfalls. *Am. J. Clin. Pathol.*, **95**, 774

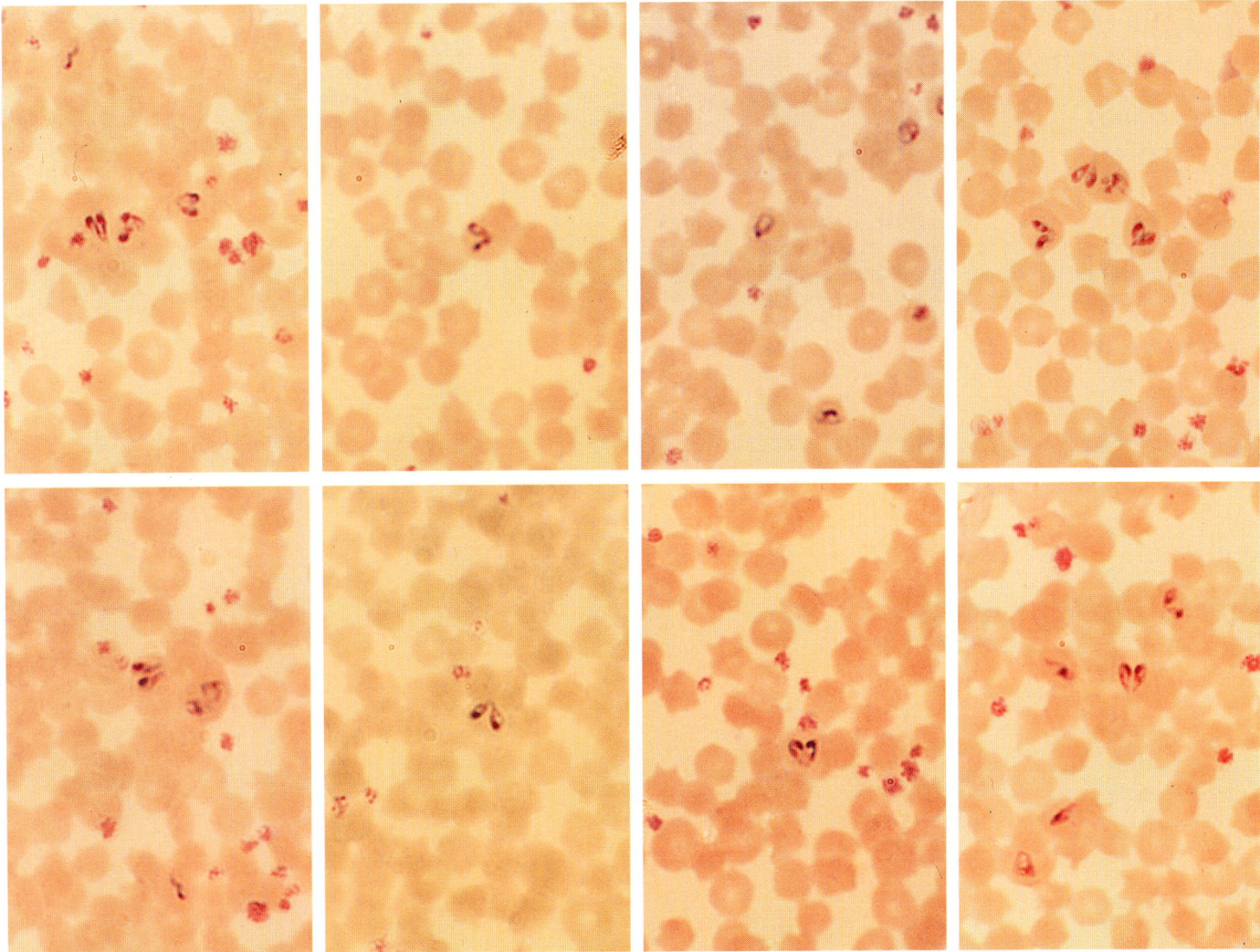

Fig. 12.1 Intraerythrocytic organisms of *Babesia bigemina* in thin blood smear of cattle. Giemsa

13. SARCOSPORIDIOSIS

Introduction

This parasitosis is one of the four important coccidian infections. The others are: **toxoplasmosis** (Section 11), the most significant from the clinical point of view; **isosporosis** (Section 14), today becoming more and more important in AIDS patients; and **coccidiosis**, of interest in veterinary medicine since the causal agents produce disease in poultry, rabbits and other lower animal species[1,2]. Practically, the latter does not cause disease in man and for this reason, it will be omitted here.

Lately, several species have been renamed, the nomenclature of parasites has been modified and details of the evolutionary cycle have been recognized[3,4], thus causing confusion for the non-parasitologists.

Sarcosporidiosis occurs worldwide wherever rare or insufficiently cooked beef or pork is consumed. It is common in North and Central Europe. In Venezuela, to our knowledge, infections of this sort have not been reported in man.

The infection of domestic animals and birds takes place via numerous differentiable species[5-8] (Figs. 13.1 and 13.2). All of these parasites go through an obligatory change of specific hosts. It is easy to infect rodents in the laboratory experimentally by giving them raw meat with cysts of *Sarcocystis* spp.

Clinically, it appears that infection with *Sarcocystis bovihominis* is mild. In contrast, infections with *Sarcocystis suihominis* may produce violent intestinal disorders. In Thailand, fatal intestinal infections have been reported[9].

Clinical diagnosis. The colourless and fragile sporocysts are not easy to detect during routine stool examinations for worms. Concentration procedures must be applied. In biopsies of the small bowel, sarcocysts should be looked for near the epithelium of the mucosa.

The parasite

Sarcocystis species belong to the group Coccidia which form with the *Plasmodia* the class Sporozoa. The species formerly known as *Isospora hominis* has now been named *Sarcocystis bovihominis* and *Sarcocystis suihominis*.

The species *Sarcocystis lindemanni* probably does not exist; it should not be considered a species specific for man. In a critical review by Beaver *et al.*[10], only a few human cases of this sort could be confirmed. The typical Miescher's tubules, known for almost 150 years, are observed frequently in the musculature of domestic animals and do not elicit an inflammatory reaction. *Sarcocystis bovicanis*, *S. suicanis* and *S. bovifelis* are not found in man.

Two *Sarcocystis* species can develop in man: *S. bovihominis* and *S. suihominis*. Their cycle of evolution is shown in Table 5.

Merozoites develop in the lamina propria of the intestinal mucosa into oocysts and sporocysts. Merozoites are banana-shaped intracellular parasites measuring 10–14 μm in length. Oocysts measure about 20 × 10 μm containing 4 sporozoites (about 14 × 8 μm) which later are released from the oocysts (Figs. 13.3–13.6).

Pathogenesis

About 5–10 days after eating parasite-containing raw meat, the first oocysts are excreted with the faeces. After perforation of the walls of the oocysts, sporocysts are released into the intestinal lumen. Oocysts and sporocysts are excreted over more than 6 weeks. The merozoites which derive from sporocysts penetrate into the lamina propria of the small intestine and cause an eosinophilic inflammation. This may be concluded from the reports of cases from Thailand and is inferable from the behaviour of the related species (*S. bovicanis* etc.) which infect only animals. In man, haematogenous dissemination of the parasites into organs other than the small intestine with formation of cysts has not been reported.

Pathology

In man, only involvement of the small intestine has been confirmed, although recently, involvement of skeletal muscles has also been reported in man[11,12]. In the animal host, beside the intestine, lesions have also been found in liver, kidney and brain with formation of whitish elongated foci, visible to the naked eye.

The enteritis found in man is present more often in the ileum than in the jejunum. It is characterized by a marked diffuse oedema of the submucosa and extensive infiltrates of eosinophilic granulocytes in mucosa and submucosa[9]. Oocysts with four sporozoites may be found in tissues. When more or fewer sporozoites are found in oocysts, this is due to cutting.

The cysts of sarcosporidians in lower animals are septate and show the elongated trophozoites of *Sarcocystis* spp.

References

1. Dubey, J. P. (1976). A review of Sarcocystis of domestic animals and of other coccidia of cats and dogs. *J. Am. Vet. Med. Assoc.*, **169**, 1061
2. Lipscomb, T. P. *et al.* (1989). Intrahepatic biliary coccidiosis in a dog. *Vet. Pathol.*, **26**, 343
3. Heydorn, A. O. (1977). Beiträge zum Lebenszyklus der Sarkosporidien. IX. Entwicklungszyklus von Sarcocystis suihominis n. sp. *Berl. Münch. Tieraerztl. Wschr.*, **90**, 218
4. Frenkel, J. K. *et al.* (1979). Sarcocystinae: Nomina dubia and available names. *Z. Parasitenk.*, **58**, 115
5. Dubey, J. P. *et al.* (1991). Acute sarcocystosis-like disease in a dog. *J. Am. Vet. Med. Assoc.*, **198**, 439
6. Gaibova, G. D. and Radchenko, A. I. (1990). An electron microscopic study of the macro- and microcysts of coccidia in the genus Sarcosystis from buffalo. *Tsitologiia*, **31**, 801
7. Borrow-Hagi, A. *et al.* (1989). Sarcocystis in Somali camel. *Parasitologia*, **31**, 133
8. Latimer, K. S. *et al.* (1990). Myocardial sarcocystosis in a grand eclectus parrot (Eclectus roratus) and a Moluccan cockatoo (Cacatua moluccensis). *Avian Dis.*, **34**, 501
9. Bunyaratvey, S., Bunyawongwiroj, P. and Nitiyanant, P. (1982). Human intestinal sarcosporidiosis: report of six cases. *Am. J. Trop. Med. Hyg.*, **31**, 36
10. Beaver, P. C., Gadgil, R. K. and Morera, P. (1979). Sarcocystis in man: a review and report of five cases. *Am. J. Trop. Med. Hyg.*, **28**, 819
11. Pamphlett, R. and O'Donoghue, P. (1990). Sarcocystis infection of human muscle. *Aust. N. Z. J. Med.*, **20**, 705
12. Abdel-Mawla, M. M. (1990). Ultrastructure of the cyst wall of S. lindemanni with pathological correlations. *J. Egypt. Soc. Parasitol.*, **20**, 319

Table 5 Developmental cycle of *Sarcocystis suihominis* (Mehlhorn, 1980)

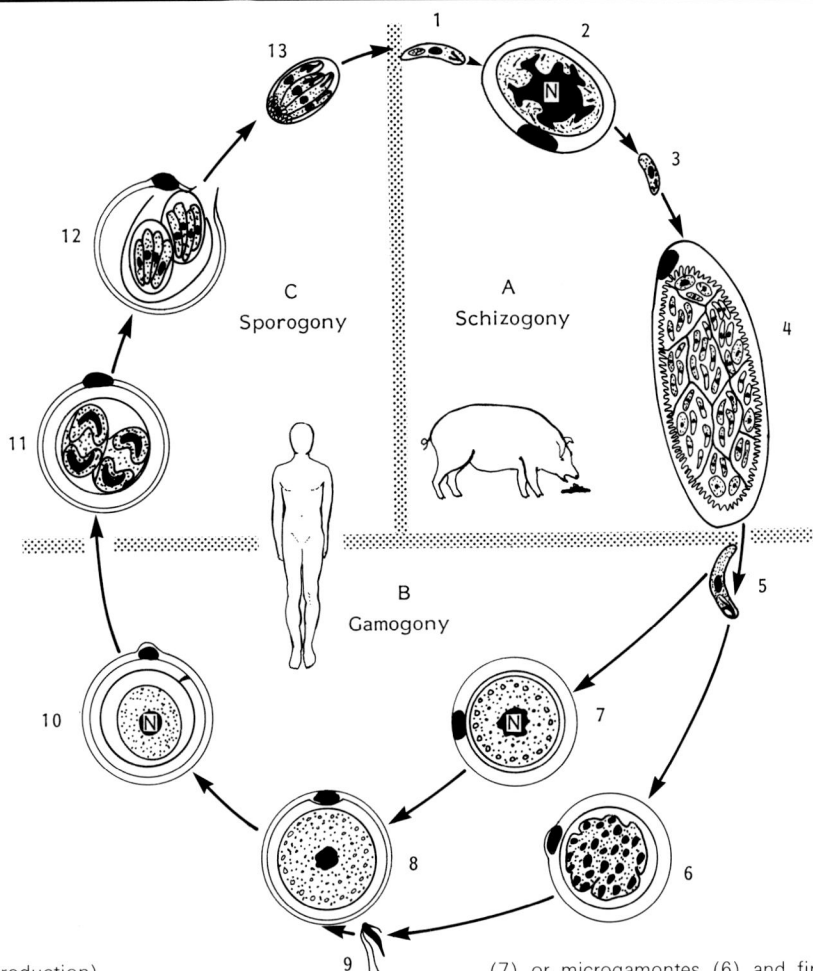

A. Schizogony (asexual reproduction)
Fully developed sporocysts (13) are ingested orally and reach the gastrointestinal canal; from them sporozoites are released (1), which multiply asexually in the endothelial cells of the liver, kidneys, lungs and other internal organs and form merozoites (2–5). This intracellular reproduction can repeat itself many times (5 → 2)
  2. Schizont
  3. Merozoite } Stages of development in pigs
  4. Cysts in the musculature
  5. Merozoites from one cyst after consumption of infected muscle
B. Gamogony (sexual development)
Merozoites (5) develop in the lamina propria to macrogamontes

(7) or microgamontes (6) and finally to macrogametes (8) or microgametes (9)
C. Sporogony
  10. The oocyst develops from the zygote
  11. Beginning of sporulation (still within the host cell)
  12. Oocysts with two sporocysts: the oocyst wall splits open in the intestinal lumen
  13. Free sporocysts containing four sporozoites (capable of infection)

14. ISOSPOROSIS

Introduction

Infection with *Isospora belli* does not generally produce severe disease except in those patients with AIDS. Isosporosis is found mostly in Asia and South America and also in the Mediterranean countries. It is rarely observed in regions with a temperate climate[1]. We do not know of any reports of this disease in Venezuela.

The reservoir hosts of *Isospora belli* are not well known at present. Experimentally, the gibbon may be infected with this parasite.

Frequently, infection with *Isospora belli* is symptomless, i.e. more than half of the infected persons are only carriers of this parasite. Symptoms of enterocolitis may be noted but severe and lasting damage is unlikely[2,3]. However, immunodeficient patients may present severe colitis.

In order to obtain a clinical diagnosis, concentration techniques of stools must be used. The uninucleate oocysts may be distinguished from sporocysts of Sarcosporidia.

The parasite

Isospora belli, today, is considered the sole causal agent of isosporosis. The species, *Isospora hominis*, has now been transferred to the Sarcosporidia, *S. bovihominis* and *S. suihominis*.

Only the oocysts of *Isospora belli* have been recognized until now. They are oval shaped, $20 \times 30\,\mu m$ in size and are pointed at one pole with a 'neck-like' constriction[4]. Soon, two sporocysts, each containing four sporozoites, develop from the oocysts (Figs. 14.1–14.3).

Pathogenesis

Transmission of *Isospora belli* to man occurs via the resistant oocysts or sporocysts without an intermediate host. The sporocysts liberate sporozoites which penetrate the intestinal mucosa. It is quite possible that *Isospora* in man behaves like the *Isospora* species in the dog and in

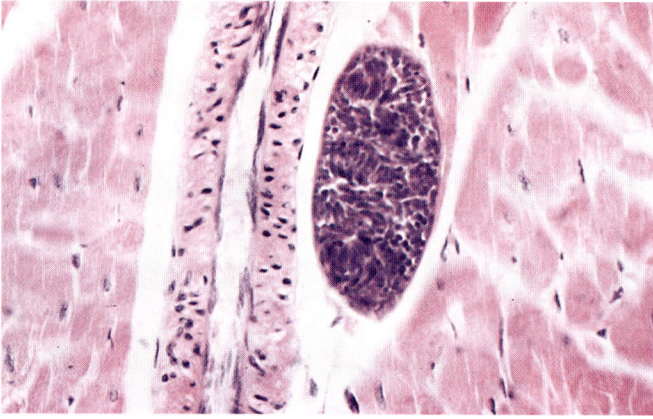

Fig. 13.1 Sarcosporidian cyst in myocardial fibre of cattle. H&E

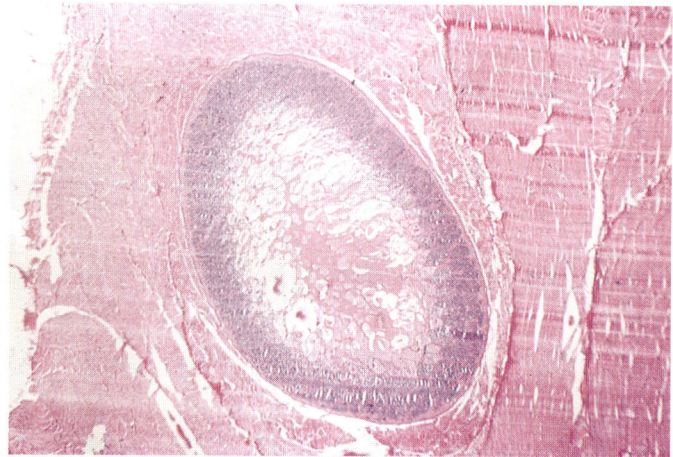

Fig. 13.2 *Sarcocystis* sp. cyst in the oesophageal musculature of buffalo from Thailand. H&E

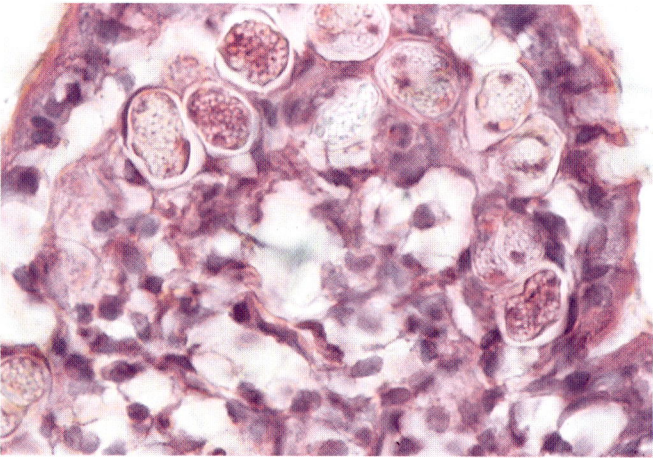

Fig. 13.3 Oocysts of *Sarcocystis* sp. in the small intestine of dog. H&E

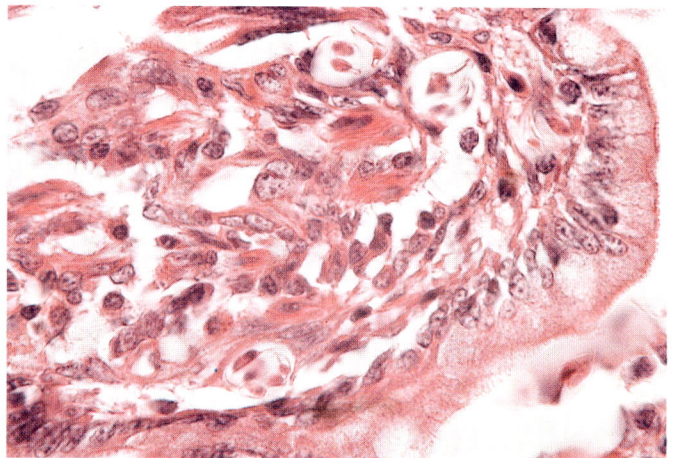

Fig. 13.4 Several oocysts of *Sarcocystis* sp. in the small intestine of a patient from Thailand. There was a marked eosinophilic enteritis in this case. H&E

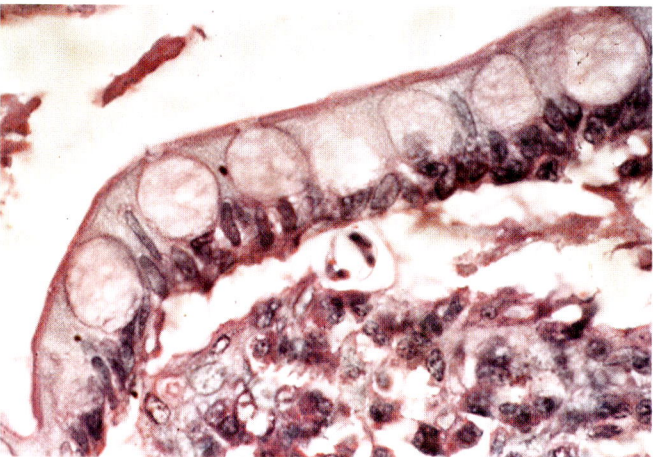

Fig. 13.5 Same case as in Fig. 13.4 with higher magnification. Oocysts contain 4 sporocysts which, however, do not show in every section. H&E

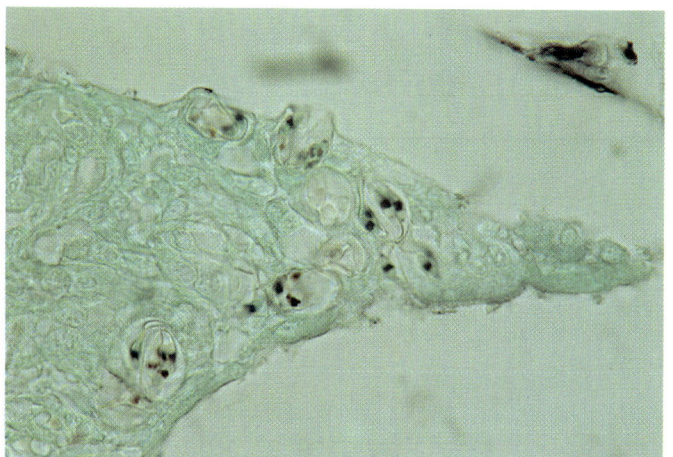

Fig. 13.6 Same case as Figs. 13.4 and 13.5. The oocysts with their sporocysts are marked also with this special staining method. Grocott

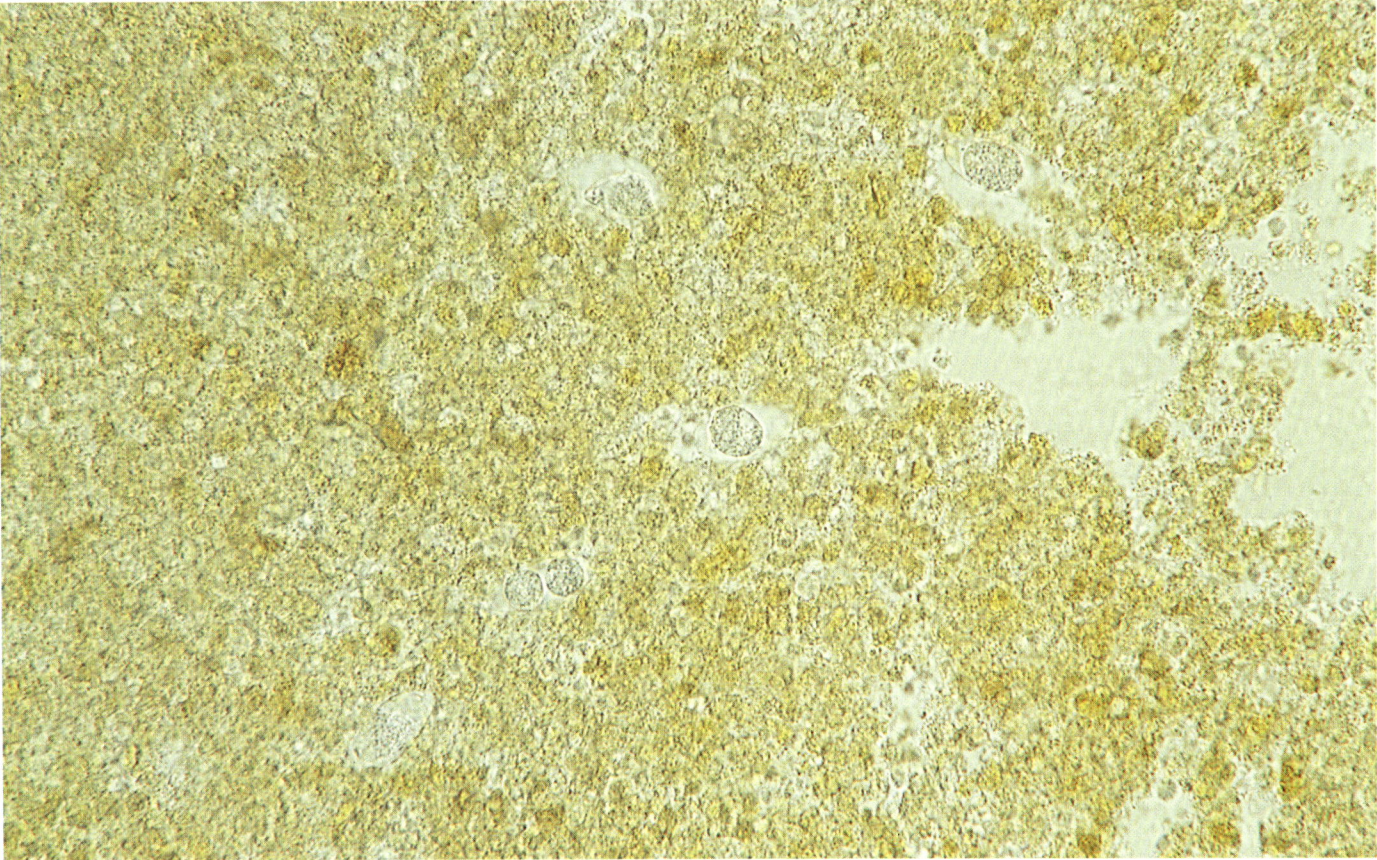

Fig. 14.1 Oocysts of *Isospora belli* in faeces at low power. Unstained fresh smear

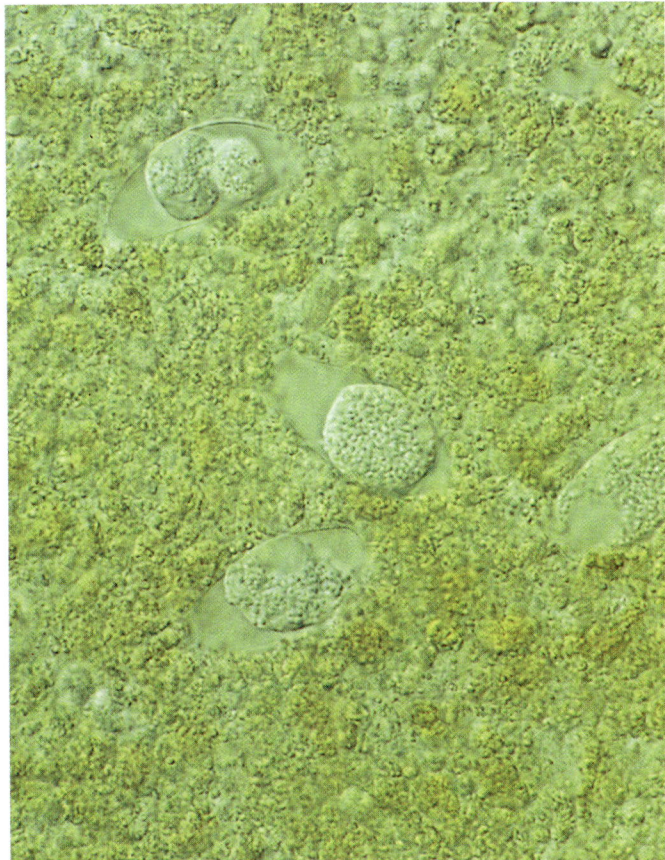

Fig. 14.2 The evolution starts with formation of 2 sporoblasts inside oocysts of *Isospora belli*. Unstained faecal smear

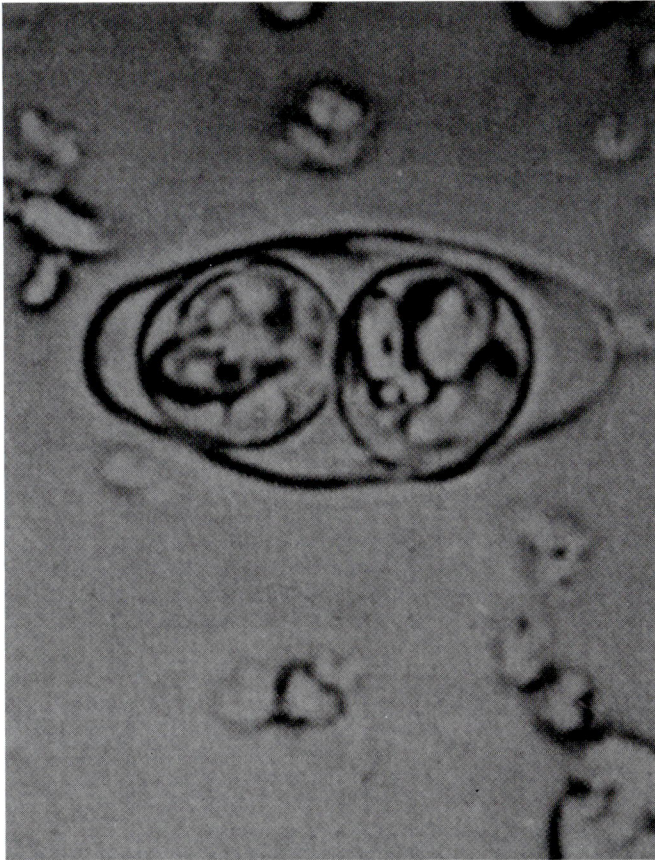

Fig. 14.3 Oocyst of *Isospora belli* with two sporoblasts. Unstained faecal smear

the cat. Minute microscopic superficial lesions in the intestinal mucosa may result[5,6].

Pathology

The ileum and caecum may be involved in infections with *Isospora belli*. Gross lesions and forms of *Isospora belli* in tissues have not yet been studied in man.

References

1. Piekarski, G. (1989). *Medical Parasitology*. Springer-Verlag
2. French, J. M., Whitby, J. L. and Whitfield, A. G. W. (1964). Steatorrhea in man infected with coccidiosis (Isospora belli). *Gastroenterology*, **47**, 642
3. Sanders, A. (1967). Human infection with Isospora belli. *Am. J. Clin. Path.*, **47**, 347
4. Mehlhorn, H. and Peters, W. (1983). *Diagnose der Parasiten des Menschen, einschließlich der Therapie einheimischer und tropischer Parasitosen*. Gustav Fisher-Verlag
5. Webster, B. H. (1957). Human isosoporiasis. A report of three cases with necropsy findings of one case. *Am. J. Trop. Med. Hyg.*, **6**, 86
6. Trier, J. S. *et al.* (1974). Chronic intestinal coccidiosis in man: Intestinal morphology and response to treatment. *Gastroenterology*, **66**, 923

15. CRYPTOSPORIDIOSIS

Table 6 Developmental cycle of *Cryptosporidium* sp. (according to Current, 1985)

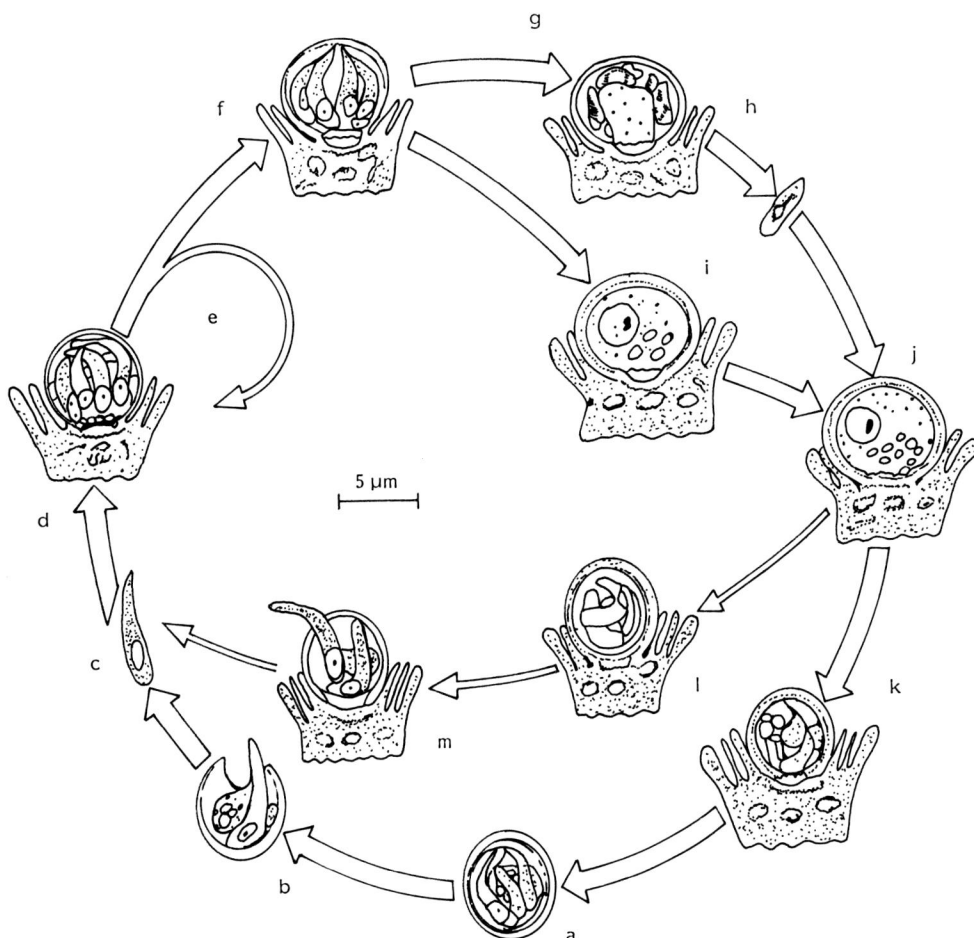

a. Sporozoite-containing oocysts from the faeces; b. excysting sporozoites; c. free sporozoite; d. schizont with 6–8 merozoites; e. new infection of intestinal cells; f. schizogony, which leads to micro- and macrogamontes (g, h, i) and a zygote (j) with a thick-walled oocyst (k). Thin-walled oocysts, which cause auto-infection can also be formed (l, m)

Introduction

Infection by cryptosporidians, a coccidian protozoan parasite, is a relatively 'new' human disease. The parasite was first described in mice at the beginning of this century, and has been reported in man only since 1976. Because of an increased veterinary interest and also the increasing importance of *Cryptosporidium* spp. as an opportunistic parasite, for instance in AIDS patients[1-3], there have been numerous publications on these parasites in the medical literature of recent years[4-6].

The distribution of this organism is worldwide. There is a high risk of infection for people in rural areas. The infection and symptomatic disease is well known in Venezuela[7].

The source of human infections are, in addition to pets, cattle, pigs, sheep and goats, also guinea pigs, mice, rats, as well as birds, snakes and fish, all of which may be carriers of cryptosporidians[8-17]. Several laboratory animal species may be used for experimental work[18-21].

In man, infection may be silent, but the symptomatic disease shows a picture of gastroenteritis with diarrhoea and watery stools which may continue for 3–14 days. The considerable loss of water and cramp-like abdominal pain may be followed by obstipation. Sometimes, weight loss, vomiting and low fever may be associated. After about 3 weeks, the symptoms disappear or the condition becomes chronic. In AIDS patients, the course is more severe and can lead to death.

For clinical diagnosis, oocysts of *Cryptosporidium* sp. may be found in alcohol-fixed stool smears or in sections of cell blocks stained with Giemsa. The small oocysts are not easy to detect with this staining technique. We prefer to stain the oocysts with the Ziehl–Neelsen method.

The parasite

The parasite has been named *Cryptosporidium* sp. and belongs to the class of Sporozoa. It goes through a complicated cycle of evolution which cannot be followed using the light microscope; see Table 6. The thick-walled oocysts which contain four sporozoites are excreted and spread the infection transmitting it to a new host.

The oocysts we see in smears of watery stools are spherical in shape and measure 4–7 or 3–6 μm in diameter. They may remain unstained but, with the Ziehl–Neelsen method, they stain positive. Definite inner structures in these oocysts cannot be recognized in routinely examined material. The small banana-shaped sporozoites measure from 5–6 μm.

Pathogenesis

Infections occur by faecal contamination, i.e. by ingestion of oocysts with food, water etc. Transmission takes place directly from man, or domestic animal, to man without an intermediate host; predominantly, the parasites are passed from domestic animals to man. Incubation time is 3–12 days, the prepatent period about 1 week and excretion of oocysts occurs over 2–3 weeks. The sporozoites coming from the oocysts attach themselves to the surface of the gastrointestinal mucosa. This can be observed only with the electron microscope, and the damage produced cannot be confirmed with the light microscope. The sporozoites do not invade tissues.

Pathology

The stomach and the lower parts of jejunum or ileum are involved. Apparently, lung and biliary infections may occur, but only a few cases of this sort have been described[22]. Gross lesions of cryptosporidiosis are not known. The attachment of sporozoites to the surface of the mucosae and the different evolutionary phases of the parasite on the surface may be studied ultrastructurally only. The microvilli of the intestinal epithelium may be destroyed but penetration of the parasite into tissues does not occur.

The oocysts in the gastrointestinal lumen stain easily with the Giemsa and Ziehl–Neelsen methods (Figs. 15.1– 15.3). They are Grocott-negative and may thus be differentiated from small yeasts. They are said to be PAS-positive. In histological sections, they are not always Ziehl–Neelsen-positive (Figs. 15.4–15.6).

References

1. Colebunders, R., Lusakumuni, K., Nelson, A. M., Gigase, P., Lebughe, I., van Marck, E., Kapita, B., Francis, H., Salaun, J. J., Quinn, T. C. *et al.* (1988). Persistent diarrhoea in Zairian AIDS patients: an endoscopic and histological study. *Gut,* **29**, 1687
2. Rene, E., Marche, C., Regnier, B., Saimot, A. G., Vilde, J. L., Perrone, C., Michon, C., Wolf, M., Chevalier, T., Vallot, T. *et al.* (1989). Intestinal infections in patients with acquired immunodeficiency syndrome. A prospective study in 132 patients. *Dig. Dis. Sci.,* **34**, 773
3. Silverman, J. F. *et al.* (1990). Small-intestinal brushing cytology in the diagnosis of cryptosporidiosis in AIDS. *Diagn. Cytopath.,* **6**, 193
4. Tzipori, S., Smith, M., Birch, C., Barnes, G. and Bishop, R. (1983). Criptosporidiosis in hospital patients with gastroenteritis. *Am. J. Trop. Med. Hyg.,* **32**, 931
5. Burchard, G. D. and Kern, P. (1985). Kryptosporidiose bei Patienten mit und ohne AIDS. *Mit. Oesterr. Ges. Tropenmed. Parasit.,* **7**, 33
6. Casemore, D. P., Sands, R. L. and Curry, A. (1985). Cryptosporidium species a 'new' human pathogen. *J. Clin. Pathol.,* **38**, 1321
7. Tirado, de A. L. C., Hidalgo, C. and Morales, O. (1988). Brote familiar de criptosporidiosis en Venezuela. *Conv. An. ASOVAC,* Maracay
8. Harp, J. A., Wannemuehler, M. W., Woodmansee, D. B. and Moon, H. W. (1988). Susceptibility of germfree or antibiotic treated adult mice to Cryptosporidium parvum. *Infect. Immun.,* **56**, 2006
9. Gibson, S. V. and Wagner, J. E. (1986). Cryptosporidiosis in guinea pigs: a retrospective study. *J. Am. Vet. Med. Assoc.,* **1**, 1033
10. Rehg, J. E., Gigliotti, F. and Stokes, D. C. (1988). Cryptosporidiosis in ferrets. *Lab. Anim. Sci.,* **38**, 155
11. Goodwin, M. A. and Brown, J. (1988). Histologic incidence and distribution of Cryptosporidium sp. infection in chickens: 68 cases in 1986. *Avian Dis.,* **32**, 365
12. Wages, D. P. and Ficken, M. D. (1989). Cryptosporidiosis and turkey viral hepatitis in turkeys. *Avian Dis.,* **33**, 191
13. Boch, J., Goebel, E. *et al.* (1982). Kryptosporidose-Infektion bei Haustieren. *Berl. Münch. Tierärztl. Wschr.,* **95**, 361
14. Hatkin, J. M. *et al.* (1990). Experimental biliary cryptosporidiosis in broiler chickens. *Avian Dis.,* **34**, 454
15. Mair, T. S. *et al.* (1990). Concurrent cryptosporidium and corona-virus infections in an Arabian foal with combined immunodeficiency syndrome. *Vet. Rec.,* **126**, 127
16. Argenzio, R. A. *et al.* (1990). Villous atrophy, crypt hyperplasia, cellular infiltration, and impaired glucose–Na absorption in enteric cryptosporidiosis of pigs. *Gastroenterology,* **98**, 1129
17. Mead, J. R. *et al.* (1991). Chronic Cryptosporidium parvum infections in congenitally immunodeficient SCID and nude mice. *J. Infect. Dis.,* **163**, 1297
18. Kim, C. W., Joel, D., Woodmansee, D. and Luft, B. J. (1988). Experimental cryptosporidiosis in fetal lambs. *J. Parasitol.,* **74**, 1064
19. Bayer, R. *et al.* (1990). Immunotherapeutic efficacy of bovine colostral immunoglobulins from a hyperimmunized cow against cryptosporidiosis in neonatal mice. *Infect. Immun.,* **58**, 2962
20. Levy, M. G., Ley, D. H., Barnes, H. J., Gerig, T. M. and Corbett, W. T. (1988). Experimental cryptosporidiosis and infectious bursal disease virus infection of specific-pathogen-free chickens. *Avian Dis.,* **32**, 803
21. Lindsay, D. S., Hendrix, C. M. and Blagburn, B. L. (1988). Experimental Cryptosporidium parvum infections in opossums (Didelphis virginiana). *J. Wildl. Dis.,* **24**, 157
22. Travis, W. D. *et al.* (1990). Respiratory cryptosporidiosis in a patient with malignant lymphoma. Report of a case and review of the literature. *Arch. Pathol. Lab. Med.,* **114**, 519

16. MALARIA

Introduction

Malaria is called also paludism, swamp or intermittent fever. It is still a very important and uncontrolled disease because the campaigns of eradication have not led to the desired results. It is estimated that still 200 million people are infected.

Circumscribed epidemic zones of malaria, situated between 40° latitude north and 30° latitude south, are found in Central America, South America, Southern Europe, Africa, Asia, the Philippines and many islands of the Pacific Ocean. The endemic zones in the South of the USA have practically disappeared since World War II. Today, malaria infections in the USA and Northern Europe are all 'imported' cases. Imported malaria, actually, is of great importance because symptomatology is often atypical and the diagnosis may not be made at the time. Each one of the four species of *Plasmodium* has, in

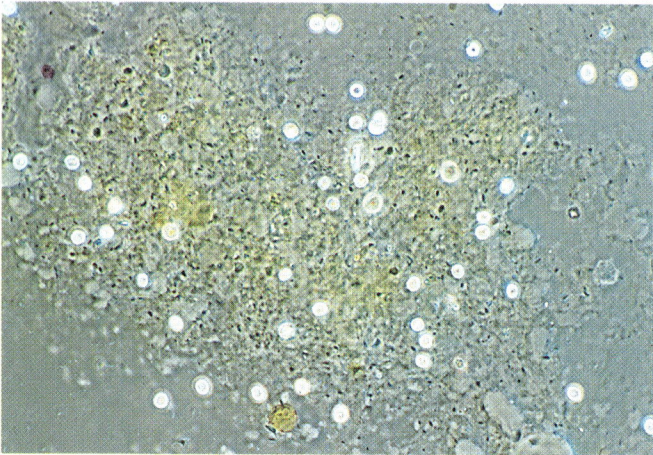

Fig. 15.1   Unstained smear of faecal material with numerous organisms of *Cryptosporidium* sp. Phase-contrast

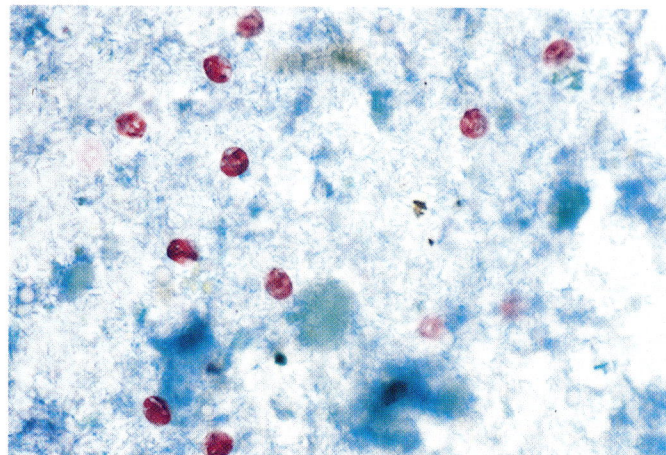

Fig. 15.2   Smear of faecal material with acid-fast organisms of *Cryptosporidium* sp. Ziehl–Neelsen

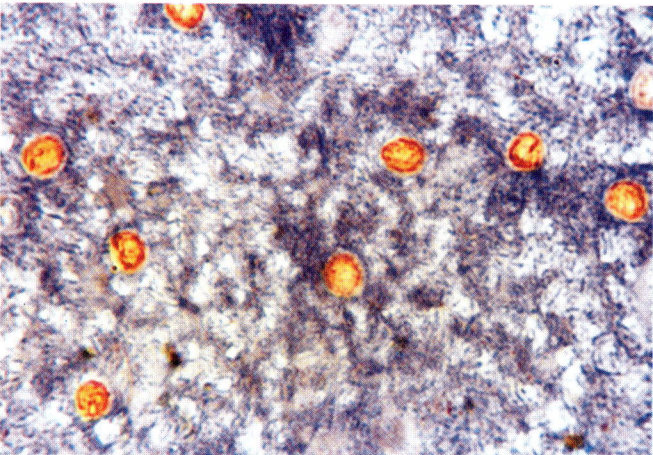

Fig. 15.3   Numerous acid-fast organisms of *Cryptosporidium* sp. in smear of faeces at high power. Ziehl–Neelsen

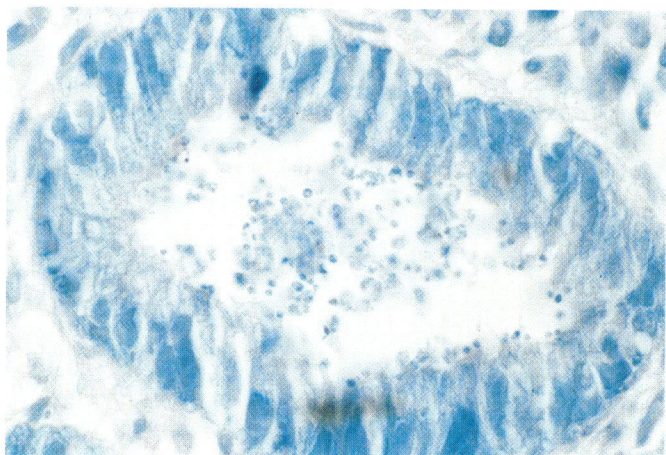

Fig. 15.4   Numerous cryptosporidians in the lumen of the intestine in case of AIDS (tissue section). Giemsa

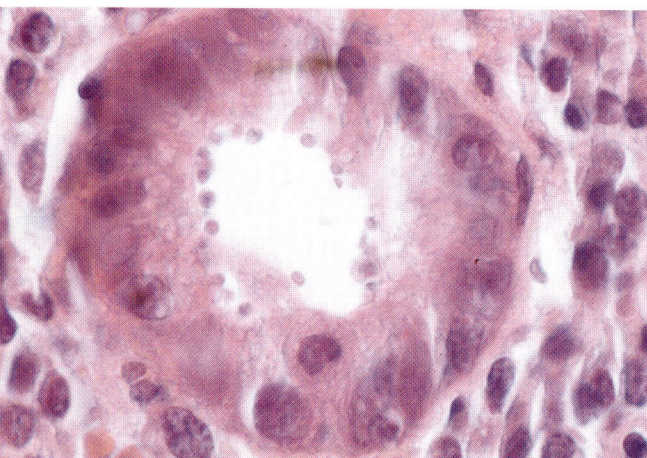

Fig. 15.5   Same case as Fig. 15.4 H&E

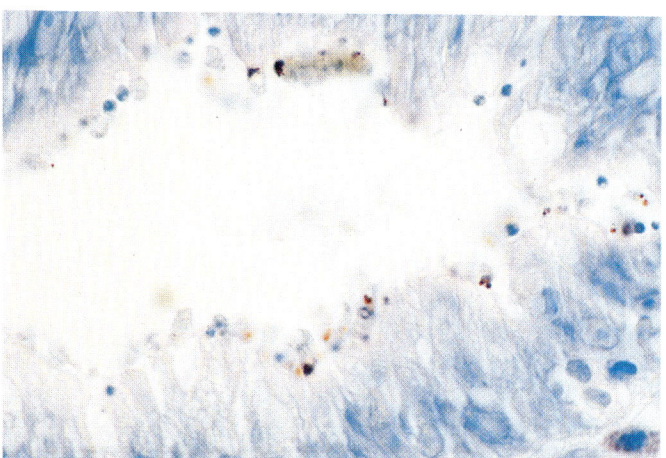

Fig. 15.6   Same case as Figs. 15.4 and 15.5. Cryptosporidians are partly impregnated with faecal material. Giemsa

Table 7 Intraerythrocytic structures of species of *Plasmodium*

P. vivax	P. falciparum	P. malariae	P. ovale
Middle aged trophozoite with Schueffner's punctuation	Young trophozoite with two dots	Young trophozoite	Young trophozoite annular form
Trophozoite with basophilic dots	Multiple trophozoites	Adult trophozoite, band-shaped	Trophozoite, double infection
Segmented schizont	Presegmented schizont	Segmented schizont	Schizont, progressive form
Young gametocyte	Adult macrogametocyte	Young microgametocyte	Mature gametocyte

addition to diverse vectors, a different geographic distribution. Malaria is becoming endemic in Venezuela again, after having been completely eradicated in the fifties and sixties. In 1991 newspapers called it a 'national emergency'.

Hundreds of species of vertebrates and non-vertebrates may be infected by some 50 species of the genus *Plasmodium*. Monkeys may be affected naturally by three species of *Plasmodium* (*P. knowlesi*, *P. cynomolgi* and *P. brazilianum*). All of these may, rarely, infect man. *Plasmodium berghei* and other *Plasmodium* species are used for experimental work in various lower animal species[1-3].

The clinical course, at least in endemic regions, is relatively benign, possibly as a result of a relative immunity. Fatal outcome is observed practically only in infections with *Plasmodium falciparum*, and mainly among tourists. Almost one million deaths are estimated to occur per year.

The denominations of clinical forms of malaria do not depend only on the bouts of fever. Infections with *P. vivax* and *P. ovale* are called the 'tertiana type'; with *P. malariae* the 'quartana type'; and with *P. falciparum*

Table 8 Cycle of *Plasmodium* in man and vector

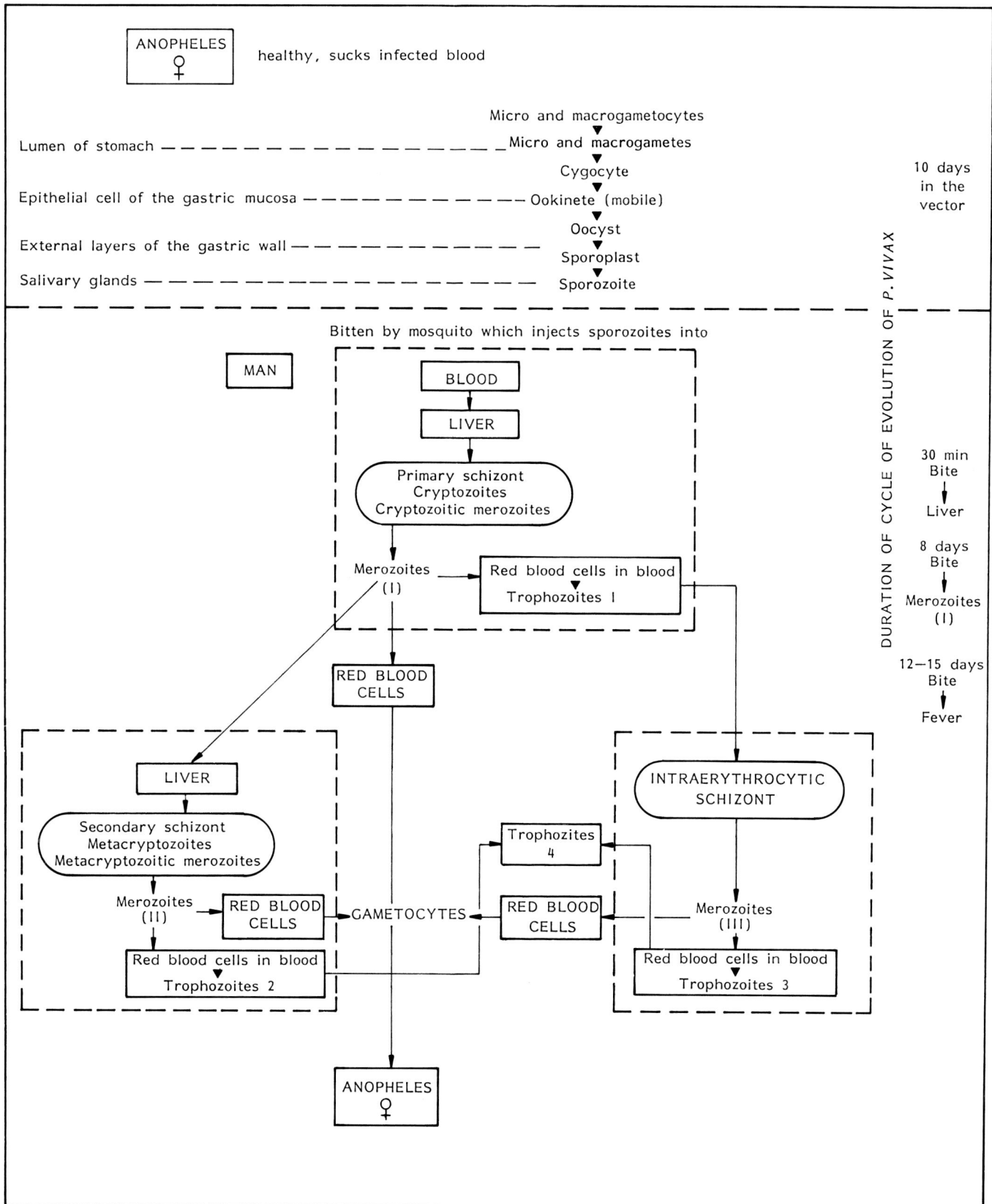

'tropical', 'pernicious' or 'malignant' malaria.

For clinical diagnosis, the plasmodians should be recognized in Giemsa-stained thin or thick blood films. Blood may be drawn at any time between or during the attacks of fever. The trophozoites of *Plasmodium falciparum* are one fifth the size of the diameter of a red blood cell.

The parasite

The four species of *Plasmodium* pathogenic for man (*P. vivax, P. falciparum, P. malariae* and *P. ovale*) belong to the group Haemosporidia of the class Sporozoa. The characteristic structures of the diverse species of *Plasmo-*

dium in red blood cells are shown schematically in Table 7. Trophozoites, schizonts and gametocytes are illustrated in Fig. 16.1. The red dot in the trophozoites represents the nucleus. The Schüffner dots in *Plasmodium vivax*-infected human erythrocytes are important in the identification of this malarial species[4].

Pathogenesis

Man acquires this disease mostly through the bite of an infected female *Anopheles* mosquito, which is haematophagous; the male mosquito does not suck blood. Exceptionally, malaria may be transmitted by blood transfusion. Infections do occur from mosquitos carried via airports from the tropics to countries with a temperate climate[5]. The genus *Anopheles* comprises more than 400 species; 65 of them are able to transmit human malaria. More than 300 species are considered potential vectors. The evolutionary cycle of *Plasmodium* is shown schematically in man and the vector in Table 8.

The three principal stages of evolution are:

1. Sexual reproduction of parasites in the female *Anopheles* mosquito, followed later by asexual development and sporozoites invading the salivary glands, through which humans are infected when bitten.
2. Asexual multiplication in the hepatic cells of the host (pre-erythrocytic stage) with formation of merozoites and subsequent invasion of red blood cells as trophozoites.
3. Asexual repeated multiplication in the erythrocytes, causing the clinical picture of the intermittent fever. The red blood cells may harbour multiple plasmodians[6].

The prepatent period (until the appearance of the parasite in blood) is 8 days for *P. falciparum*; the incubation period (until the first bout of fever) 12–15 days. The parasites destroy erythrocytes with the formation of iron-free malarial pigment, also called haemozoin. Symptomatology and the periodic bouts of fever are classical.

Pathology

The destruction of red blood cells leads to pathological alterations which may be summarized as: terminal circulatory disorders, storage phenomena in the PMS system and consequences of hypoxaemia. Ultrastructural lesions will not be discussed here[7–10]. With the light microscope, it may be possible to detect: thromboses, disseminated intravascular coagulation, micro-infarcts, necroses, haemorrhages and a slight inflammatory reaction.

In fatal cases, characteristics gross lesions are present in the liver and spleen; these organs show a diffuse greyish or black colour, while the other viscera and tissues show a less pronounced blackish colour. Kidneys, liver and spleen are slightly enlarged. In the chronic forms of malaria, the splenomegaly is more notable than in the acute fatal forms. Petechiae and oedema are observed in the brain (Figs. 16.3–16.8).

Regarding histological lesions, plasmodians are said to be seen in sections in red blood cells, situated in capillaries. Personally, we have been able to detect parasitized erythrocytes only in sections of a placenta (Fig. 16.9) and bone marrow in a *P. falciparum* infection. This case was kindly provided by Dr Francis W. Chandler from the CDC, Atlanta/Georgia, USA. Later, after a prolonged search, we could also see plasmodians in erythrocytes situated in cerebral capillaries (Fig. 16.10). However, these intra-erythrocytic structures, which may be trophozoites or schizonts of *Plasmodium*, were only faintly visible. The dark dots in red blood cells represent malaria pigment.

By contrast, malaria pigment is present in numerous organs (Figs. 16.11 and 16.12). It is called haematin or haemozoin and is a derivative of haemoglobin but is iron free and difficult to distinguish from formalin pigment. No histochemical methods are known by which it can be recognized as such. The malarial pigment is encountered as small black dots in erythrocytes and as blackish-brown irregular granules in circulating and fixed macrophages, above all in von Kupffer cells of the liver. The pigment is formed in erythrocytes and tissue cells each time an acute bout of fever, with destruction of red blood cells, occurs. In autopsies of individuals from endemic zones who suffered from acute malaria years ago, malaria pigment was found in viscera only exceptionally, i.e. the pigment disappears slowly from tissues. Double refraction of malarial pigment with polarization, as described in the literature, could not be detected in our material.

Renal lesions are frequent and typical in infections with *Plasmodium* species. Characteristic is blackwater fever or haemoglobinuric nephrosis, an intravasal haemolysis which leads to haemoglobinaemia and haemoglobinuria. In the renal tubules, destroyed red blood cells and haemosiderin are found in the haemoglobin casts. The dark colour of the urine, therefore, is not due to malarial pigment. The latter is not deposited in the spaces of Bowman nor in renal tubules. Renal insufficiency, azotaemia and uraemia are possible consequences of blackwater fever.

The classical malarial lesions in the brain are annular haemorrhages and granulomas of Dürck. Parasites are not found in the red blood cells situated in the annular haemorrhages around necrotic foci. The subcortical granulomas of Dürck consist of proliferated glial cells and appear only in patients who survive more than 12 days. The blockage of capillaries by *P. falciparum*-infected erythrocytes seems to be the principal cause of cerebral malaria[11–14].

The placenta is probably the organ where most parasitized red blood cells and pigment accumulate. *Plasmodium falciparum* matures in the placenta and, consequently, may cause miscarriages, or there may be transmission through the placenta, as described in the USA (congenital malaria)[15,16]. In the heart, thromboses of coronary arteries, infarcts and interstitial inflammatory reactions have been described, but only occasionally.

References

1. Gupta, N., Sehgal, R., Mahajan, R. C., Banerjee, A. K. and Ganguly, N. K. (1988). Role of immune complexes in cerebral malaria. *Pathology*, **20**, 373
2. Stevenson, M. M. and Kraal, G. (1989). Histological changes in the spleen and liver of C57BL/6 and A/J mice during Plasmodium chabaudi AS infection. *Exp. Mol. Pathol.*, **51**, 80
3. Wangoo, A. *et al.* (1990). Immunosuppression in murine malaria: suppressor role of macrophages and their products during acute and chronic Plasmodium berghei infection. *APMIS*, **98**, 407
4. Udagama, P. V., Atkinson, C. T., Peiris, J. S., David, P. H., Mendis, K. N. and Aikawa, M. (1988). Immunoelectron microscopy of Schüffner's dots in plasmodium vivax-infected human erythrocytes. *Am. J. Pathol.*, **131**, 48
5. Majori, G. *et al.* (1990). Two imported malaria cases from Switzerland. *Trop. Med. Parasitol.*, **41**, 439
6. Prasad, R. N. *et al.* (1990). Detection of multiple invasion of erythrocytes by Plasmodium vivax. *Trop. Med. Parasitol.*, **41**, 437
7. Nash, G. B., O'Brien, E., Gordon-Smith, E. C. and Dormandy, J. A. (1989). Abnormalities in the mechanical properties of red blood cells caused by Plasmodium falciparum. *Blood*, **1**, 855
8. Pongponratn, E., Riganti, M., Harinasuta, T. and Bunnag, D. (1989). Electron microscopic study of phagocytosis in human spleen in falciparum malaria. *Southeast. Asian J. Trop. Med. Public Health*, **20**, 31
9. Aikawa, M. (1988). Morphological changes in erythrocytes induced by malarial parasites. *Biol. Cell.*, **64**, 173

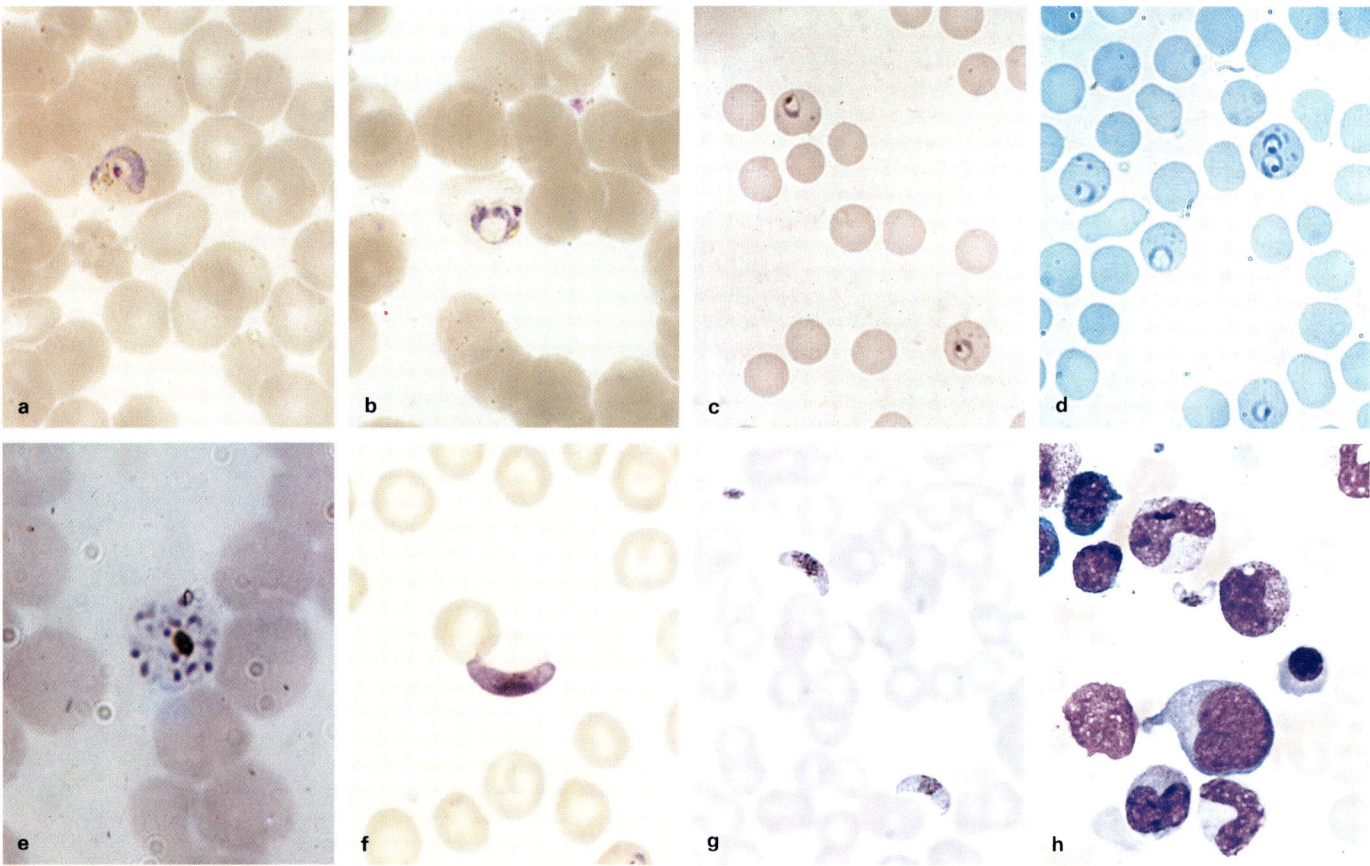

Fig. 16.1 Plasmodians: **a–d**. Trophozoites of *Plasmodium vivax*
e. Schizont of *Plasmodium vivax*
f, g. Gametocytes of *Plasmodium falciparum*
h. Gametocyte in bone marrow. Giemsa + May–Grünwald

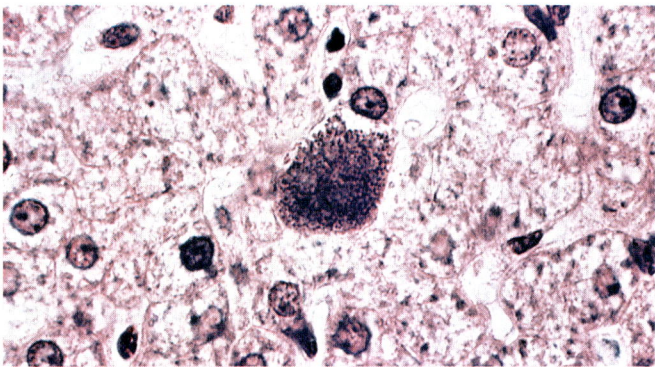

Fig. 16.2 Schizont in hepatocyte containing cryptozoites or metacryptozoites. Fortuitous finding at autopsy. H&E

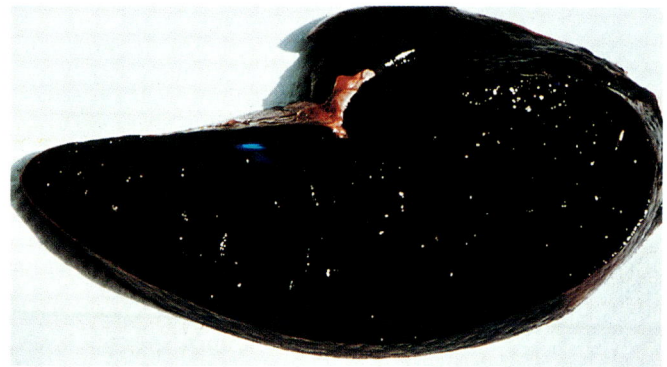

Fig. 16.4 Cut surface of spleen in the same case as Fig. 16.3

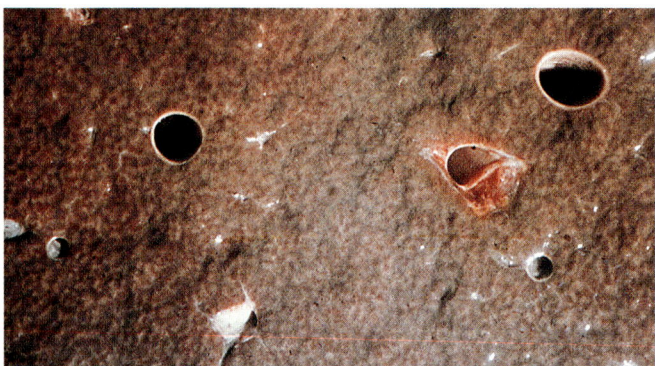

Fig. 16.3 Cut surface of liver in case of fatal tropical malaria (infection with *Plasmodium falciparum*)

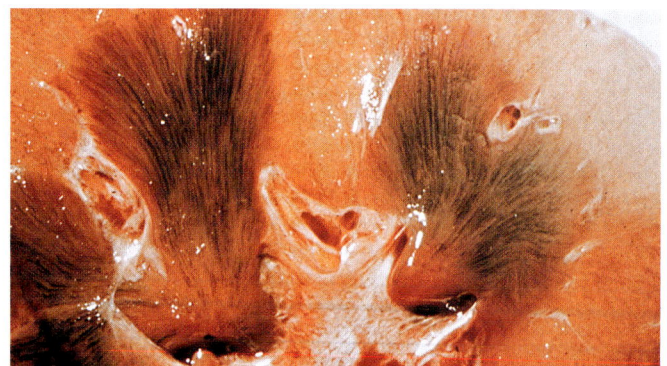

Fig. 16.5 Cut surface of kidney in the same case as Figs. 16.3 and 16.4

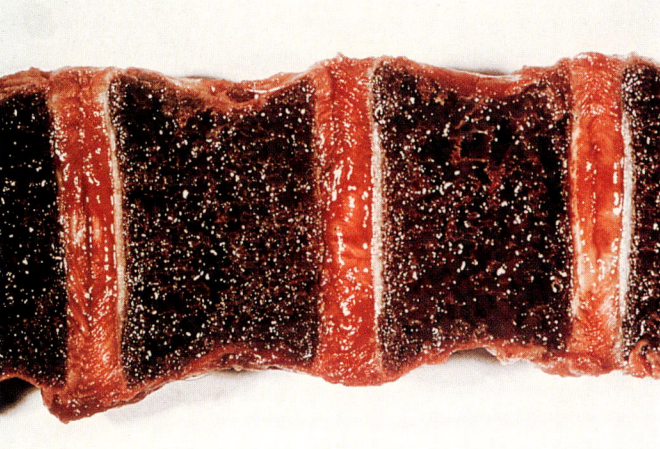

Fig. 16.6 Bone marrow in the same case as Figs. 16.3–16.5

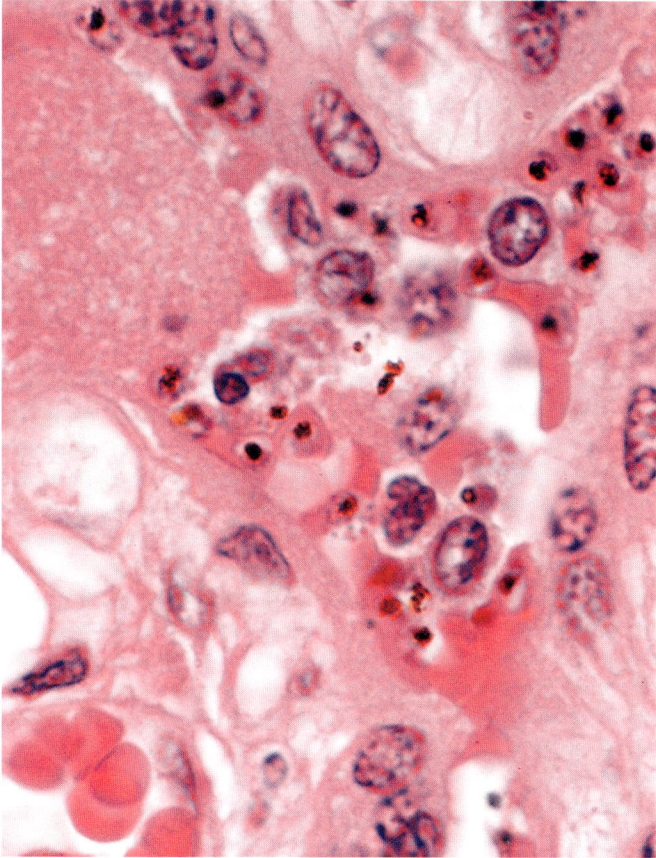

Fig. 16.7 Cut surface of brain with oedema and petechiae in the same infection as Figs. 16.3–16.6

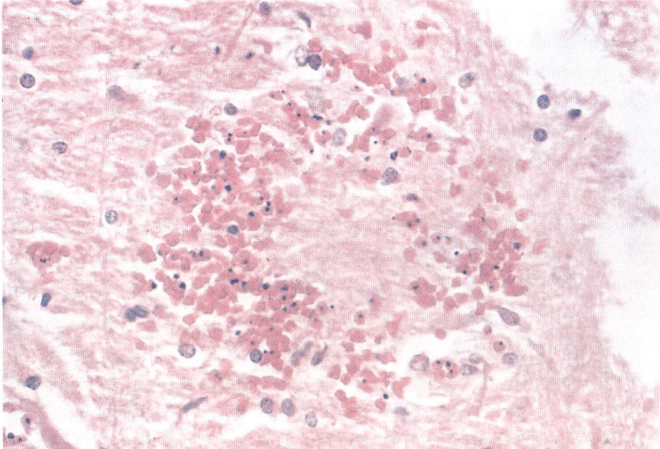

Fig. 16.8 Brain with annular haemorrhage in the same case as Fig. 16.7. The dark dots are granules of malaria pigment inside erythrocytes. H&E

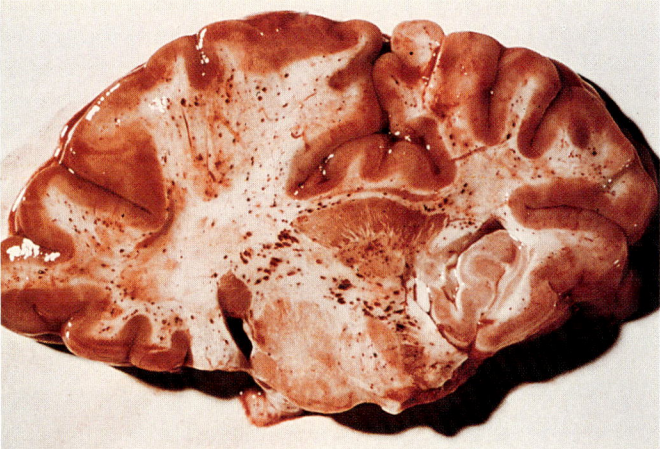

Fig. 16.9 Placenta with plasmodians and abundant deposits of malaria pigment. H&E

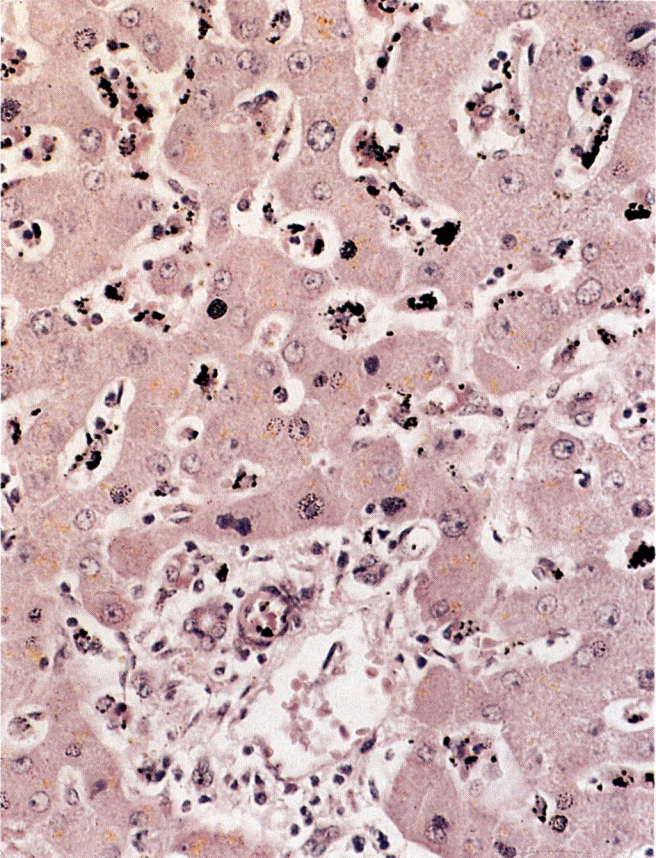

Fig. 16.10 Malaria pigment in Kupffer cells of the liver. H&E

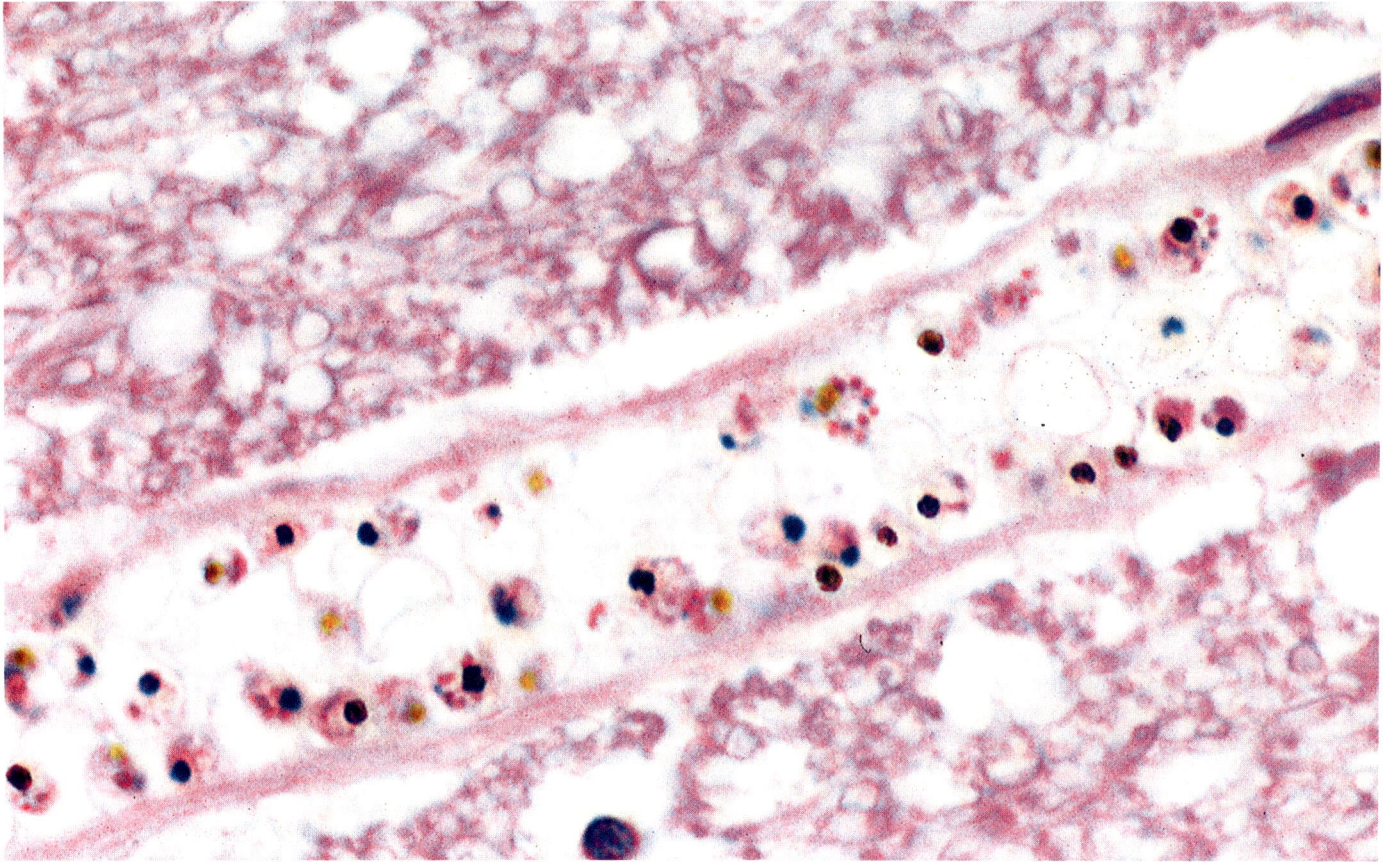

Fig. 16.11 Schizonts of *Plasmodium falciparum* seen faintly in a blood vessel of brain in addition to granules of malaria pigment. Plasmodians, as a rule, are not seen in tissue sections. H&E

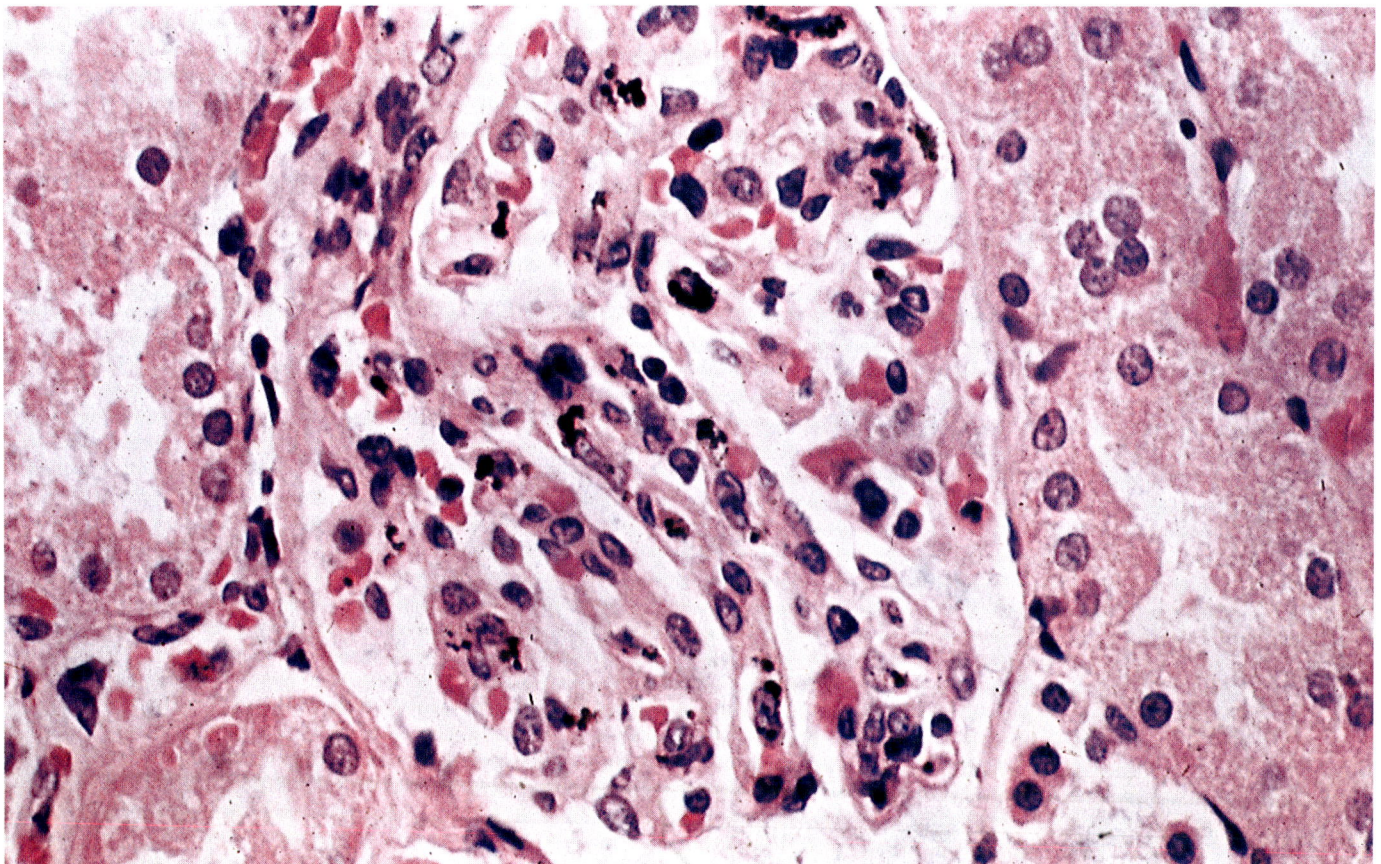

Fig. 16.12 Glomerulus in case of infection with *Plasmodium falciparum* showing malaria pigment. H&E

10. Torii, M., Adams, J. H., Miller, L. H. and Aikawa, M. (1989). Release of merozoite dense granules during erythrocyte invasion by Plasmodium knowlesi. *Infect. Immun.*, **57**, 3230
11. Aikawa, M. (1988). Human cerebral malaria. *Am. J. Trop. Med. Hyg.*, **39**, 3
12. Riganti, M. *et al.* (1990). Human cerebral malaria in Thailand: a clinico-pathological correlation. *Immunol. Lett.*, **25**, 199
13. Boonpucknavig, V. *et al.* (1990). An immunofluorescence study of cerebral malaria. A correlation with histopathology. *Arch. Pathol. Lab. Med.*, **114**, 1028
14. Pongponratn, E. *et al.* (1991). Microvascular sequestration of parasitized erythrocytes in human falciparum malaria: a pathological study. *Am. J. Trop. Med. Hyg.*, **44**, 168
15. Yamada, M., Steketee, R., Abramowsky, C., Kida, M., Wirima, J., Heymann, D., Rabbege, J., Breman, J. and Aikawa, M. (1989). Plasmodium falciparum associated placental pathology: a light and electron microscopic and immunohistologic study. *Am. J. Trop. Med. Hyg.*, **41**, 161
16. McGregor, I. A., Wilson, M. E. and Billewicz, W. Z. (1983). Malaria infection of the placenta in the Gambia, West Africa; its incidence and relationship to stillbirth, birthweight and placental weight. *Trans. R. Soc. Trop. Med. Hyg.*, **77**, 232

17. PNEUMOCYSTOSIS

Introduction

This disease is also called Pneumocystis pneumonia or interstitial plasma cell pneumonia due to *Pneumocystis carinii* infection. It is an important and worldwide, mostly opportunistic, infection manifesting itself as a consequence of immunosuppressive treatment, primary immunodeficiency in premature newborns and AIDS. Here, often, disseminated forms and/or tumour-like manifestations with granulomatous tissue reaction are observed[1-8]. The number of individuals who become ill with Pneumocystis pneumonia is increasing constantly. In Venezuela, a tropical country, infections have been confirmed too[9,10].

Spontaneous infections have been found in numerous animal species: rats, mice, rabbits, dogs, cats, cattle and sheep. Experimentally, pneumocystosis may be produced easily by injecting rats for 10–14 days with corticosteroids.

The massive, epidemic and often fatal form of the disease, due to nosocomial infections in premature newborns and undernourished infants[11,12], hardly occurs any longer. This was a typical infection, with a high prevalence and a high mortality rate, in the years after World War II in Europe. Opportunistic infection in adults, is a consequence of immunodeficiencies of all sorts, is the most common form of this disease nowadays[13]. A latent, asymptomatic, pauci-parasitic and pauci-reactive form exists in immunocompromised and immunocompetent persons, above all infants. Connatal[14] and familial forms of the disease and cases with involvement of extrapulmonary sites are all rare. In pneumocystosis, commonly, the characteristic radiological picture of an interstitial pneumonia exists. Fever is generally present. The patients become cyanotic and death occurs due to pulmonary insufficiency and/or associated bacterial bronchopneumonia. The prognosis is bad, at least in untreated patients.

Clinical diagnosis is made by observing *Pneumocystis carinii* organisms. They are demonstrated, rarely, in smears of sputum or bronchial secretions. A special cytocentrifuge is recommended for processing sputa and fluids from broncho-alveolar lavage[15]. Examination of BAL sediments is the method of choice today.

In the books, the Giemsa method is recommended to stain the parasites. However, in our experience of examining routine material, the parasites are found only when stained by the Grocott or toluidine blue method. Immunobiological methods for diagnosis exist, as indirect fluorescent staining techniques. Not all are reliable.

The parasite

Pneumocystis carinii is the causal agent of the disease. It has not been encountered living free in nature, nor has it been cultured in artificial media. It seems to belong, on the basis of its appearance, to the Protozoa. The majority of scientists believe it belongs to the class Sporozoa and subclass Haplosporidia. Others assume it is probably related to the microsporidia. However, in all the classifications of Protozoa we know, it is not mentioned and some people consider it a fungus. This was stressed at the ISHAM Congress, June 1991, in Montreal, Canada.

Some scientists believe that the species of *Pneumocystis carinii* in man is different from that which is found in the rat, in spite of both being structurally the same.

The *Pneumocystis carinii* organisms in sections and smears are spherical, relatively thick-walled, cyst-like structures. Also, thin-walled parasites are said to be found. They measure about 3–8 μm in diameter and sometimes appear to be crescent-shaped or coffee bean-like when the cysts collapse. However, this happens too with the large yeast-like fungus cells in tissue sections. The Grocott and toluidine blue methods are the best techniques for bringing out these parasites. It must be emphasized, especially, that *P. carinii* does not stain with H&E. With the Giemsa method, the organisms are mostly difficult to recognize. We have seen them with this technique but only occasionally, in special cases and after a prolonged search. With the Giemsa and the Rhodamine stains, 'intracystic bodies' which measure about 1–2 μm, can be demonstrated. There may be up to 8 bodies (sporozoites?) in each parasite. Some investigators have observed PAS-positive membranes of the *P. carinii* organisms (Figs. 17.1–17.3). The cycle of evolution of *Pneumocystis carinii* in man and lower animals is not well understood (like its taxonomic position), and there are too many controversial concepts in this subject to venture a personal opinion.

Pathogenesis

Apparently, a latent infection occurs in humans, rodents and some domestic lower animals. The portal of entry of the parasites is the respiratory tract. Then, suddenly, the saprophyte-like inactive parasites multiply copiously, transforming into aggressive organisms, and produce pulmonary disease. They colonize the inferior airways and become attached to the surface of the bronchiolar mucosa and alveoli, obstructing the lumens of the cavities mechanically. The parasites reproduce rapidly, covering the remaining respiratory surface, and the patient practically suffocates. When, in addition, interstitial cell infiltrates form, the lung function is still more compromised. Extrapulmonary sites used to be involved only exceptionally, but such localizations are now seen with increasing frequency.

Pathology

The lungs are always involved in infections with *Pneumocystis carinii*. Additionally extrapulmonary lesions are found in lymph nodes, bone marrow, liver (Fig. 17.4) and spleen[16,17]. Recently, involvement of the small intestine, choroid and adrenal glands has been reported in AIDS patients[18-20]. Here, the granular and foamy masses are

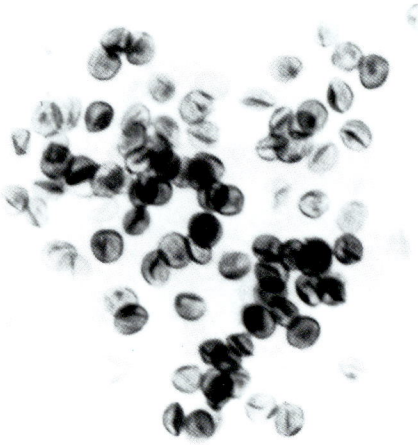

Fig. 17.1 Cluster of *Pneumocystis carinii* organisms in smear of a cut lung surface in a case of massive pneumocystosis. Folds, 'sickle' and 'hat' forms as well as other deformations of the parasites, known in large yeast-like cells, are seen. *Pneumocystis carinii* does not stain with H&E. Grocott

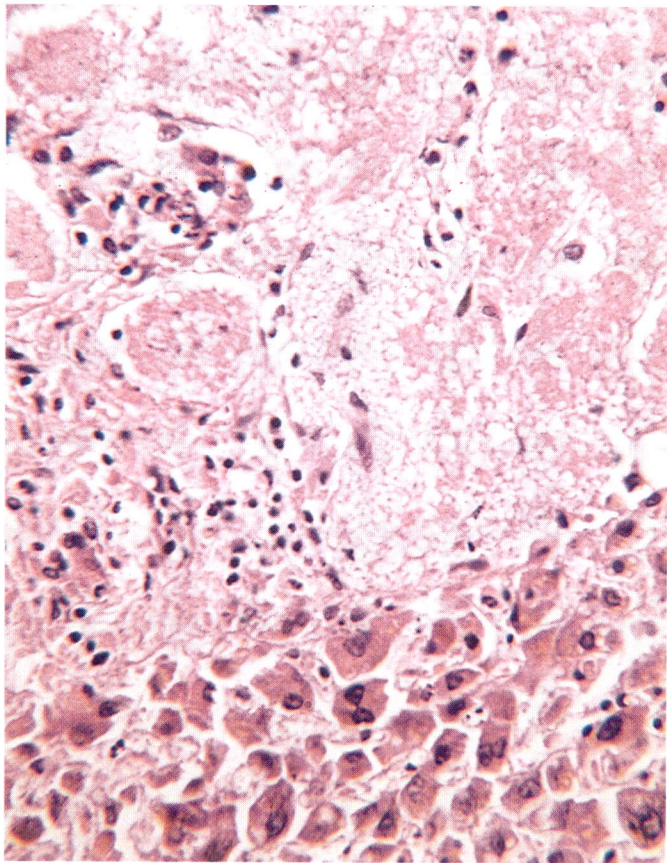

Fig. 17.2 Cystic parasites of *Pneumocystis carinii* showing internal corpuscles. This is from a smear of the cut surface of a rat lung. Giemsa

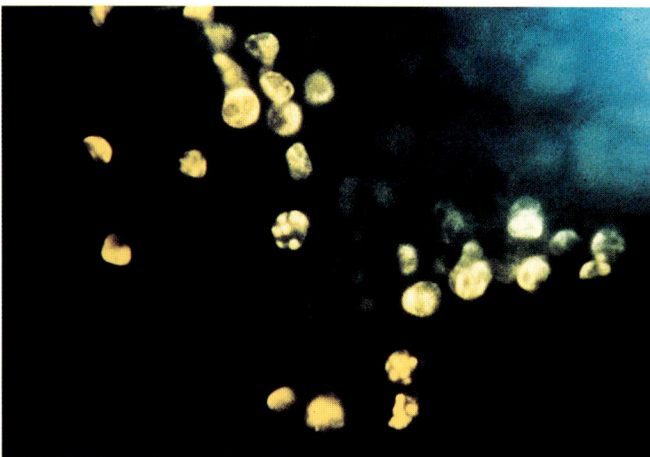

Fig. 17.3 Smear of the same case as Fig. 17.2 with the same internal corpuscles. Rhodamine; UV light

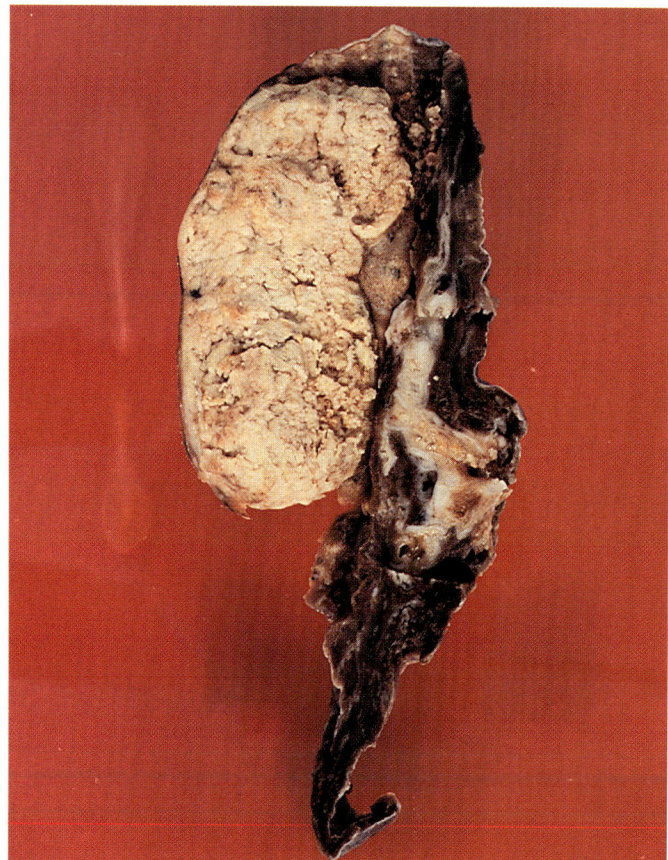

Fig. 17.4 In this human liver the parenchyma is replaced by the typical granular and foamy eosinophilic masses found inside pulmonary alveoli in cases of pneumocystosis. H&E

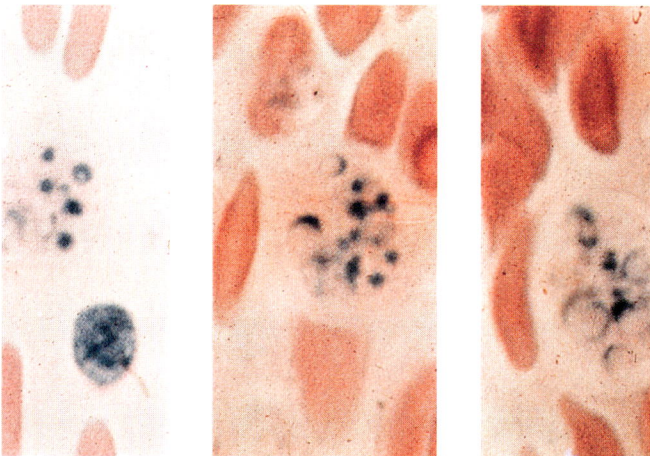

Fig. 17.5 Unfixed, resected pulmonary specimen with a tumorous mass (pneumocystoma) in an AIDS patient. (Case of Dr P. Deicke, Berlin)

the same as those present in the pulmonary alveoli. Additionally, necrobiotic lesions are found with replacement of the organic structure, together with parasites in these focal lesions.

Grossly, the pulmonary lesions resemble foci of bacterial bronchopneumonia. Irregularly delimited areas show increased consistency. Furthermore, large tumour-like nodules may be found in lungs and other organs[2,3,7] (Figs. 17.5 and 17.6).

Histologically, the organisms of *P. carinii* are found almost exclusively extracellularly and only inside the pulmonary alveoli. They cannot be detected in sections stained routinely with H&E. Often, they are arranged in clusters and attached to the alveolar or bronchiolar walls (Figs. 17.7–17.9). With the Giemsa method, it is very difficult and time-consuming to look for this species of parasites. Sometimes the internal bodies of the organisms can be seen with the Giemsa method (Fig. 17.2) or with Rhodamine stain (Fig. 17.3). The best method for staining pneumocysts is the Grocott technique, both in smears and in tissue sections. Stained in this way, they look like small yeast-like fungus cells, occasionally showing single internal dots (Fig. 17.9). Collapsed or squeezed protozoan cells may be seen, showing hat-, sickle- and pot-like forms. Another good stain for *P. carinii* organisms is toluidine blue.

In the lumens of the alveoli, it is possible to see single pneumocysts detached from the walls, together with typical inhomogeneous, granular and foamy substances. These are eosinophilic with H&E and stain faintly with the PAS method (Figs. 17.10–17.13). With the Grocott method, these intra-alveolar substances often stain blackish and may represent debris of destroyed *P. carinii* parasites. This foamy alveolar content is found mostly in infants who also show an interstitial pneumonia. The latter is said to be missing in immunocompromised patients. However, we found it recently in an AIDS patient in Mérida. In this case, additional bronchopneumonic foci were found, apparently due to an associated bacterial infection (Figs. 17.14 and 17.15). This type of alveolar content in cases of pneumocystosis can be distinguished from ordinary oedema or the lipoproteinaceous content of alveoli observed in histoplasmosis capsulati and other infections (see the *Atlas of Fungal Pathology* in this series). This was previously considered as typical in so-called lipoproteinosis. In cases of marked PAS-positivity of the alveolar content, an additional lipoproteinaceous reaction may be present.

In the interstitium, a cellular infiltrate consisting of mononuclear elements, lymphocytes and sometimes numerous plasma cells is found. These interstitial infiltrates are present mostly in cases of immunocompetent patients, while they are said to be absent in immunocompromised patients, as mentioned above.

Exceptionally, a granulomatous reaction has been noted in cases of pneumocystosis with formation of granulomas and giant cells[21] (Figs. 17.16–17.20). In the latter, parasites may be located. Granulomas of this sort cannot be distinguished from granulomas due to *Mycobacterium tuberculosis*. Granulomatous reaction is reported with increasing frequency in AIDS cases[2,4,7]. In the necrotic masses of the nodular (tumour-like) lesions, calcifications are often found (Fig. 17.21).

Frequently, in cases of infection with *Pneumocystis carinii*, another associated opportunistic infection may be present, e.g. cytomegaly or fungal infections.

The organisms of *P. carinii* must be differentiated from small yeast-like fungus cells, which are also Grocott-positive.

References

1. Ognibene, F. P., Masur, H. *et al.* (1988). Nonspecific interstitial pneumonitis without evidence of Pneumocystis carinii in asymptomatic patients infected with human immunodeficiency virus (HIV). *Ann. Intern. Med.*, **109**, 874

2. Hartz, J. W. *et al.* (1985). Granulomatous pneumocystosis as a solitary pulmonary nodule. *Arch. Pathol. Lab. Med.*, **109**, 466

3. Barrio, J. *et al.* (1986). Pneumocystis carinii pneumonia presenting as cavitating and noncavitating solitary pulmonary nodules in patients with acquired immunodeficiency syndrome. *Am. Rev. Respir. Dis.*, **134**, 1094

4. Bleiweiss, I. *et al.* (1988). Granulomatous Pneumocystis carinii pneumonia in three patients with the acquired immune deficiency syndrome. *Chest*, **94**, 580

5. Pilon, V. A. *et al.* (1987). Disseminated Pneumocystis carinii infection in AIDS. *N. Engl. J. Med.*, **316**, 1410

6. Leoung, G. (1989). Pneumocystis carinii pneumonia. *AIDS Clinical Care*, **1**, 9

7. Baumgarten, R. *et al.* (1990). Pulmonales 'Pneumozystom'-granulomatoes-nekrotisierende Pneumozystose bei einem AIDS-Patienten. *AIFO*, **6**, 297

8. Comite du Consensus de la premiere conference de consensus en therapeutique anti-infectieuse de langue francaise. La pneumocystose au cours de l'infection par le VIH. *Rev. Pneumol. Clin.*, **46**, 141

9. Salfelder, K., Schwarz, J., Sethi, K. K., González, R., Liscano, T. R. de and Carlesso, J. (1965). *Neumocistosis*, p. 141. Universidad de Los Andes, Mérida/Venezuela

10. Salfelder, K., Liscano, T. R. de, González, R. and Carlesso, J. (1967). Pauciparasitic pneumocystosis. *Mykosen*, **10**, 589

11. Vanek, J. and Jirovec, O. (1952). Parasitaere Pneumonie: 'Interstitielle' Plasmazellenpneumonie der Frühgeborenen, verursacht durch Pneumocystis carinii. *Zbl. Bakt. I. Abt. Orig.*, **158**, 120

12. Giese, W. (1953). Pathogenese und Ätiologie der interstitiellen plasmazellulären Säuglingspneumonie. *Verh. Dtsch. Ges. Path.*, **36**, 284

13. Gryzan, S., Paradis, I. L. *et al.* (1988). Unexpectedly high incidence of Pneumocystis carinii infection after lung-heart transplantation. Implications for lung defense and allograft survival. *Am. Rev. Respir. Dis.*, **137**, 1268

14. Pavlica, F. (1966). The first observation of congenital pneumocystis pneumonia in a fully developed still-born child. *Ann. Paediatr.*, **198**, 177

15. Gill, V. J., Nelson, N. A., Stock, F. and Evans, G. (1988). Optimal use of the cytocentrifuge for recovery and diagnosis of Pneumocystis carinii in bronchoalveolar lavage and sputum specimens. *J. Clin. Microbiol.*, **26**, 1641

16. Jarnum, S., Rasmussen, E. F., Ohlsen, A. S. and Sorensen, A. W. S. (1968). Generalized pneumocystis carinii infection with severe idiopathic hypoproteinemia. *Ann. Int. Med.*, **68**, 138

17. Barnett, R. N., Hull, J. G., Vortel, V., Kralove, H. and Schwarz, J. (1969). Pneumocystis carinii in lymph nodes and spleen. *Arch. Path.*, **88**, 175

18. Carter, T. R., Cooper, P. H., Petri, W. A. Jr., Kim, C. K., Walzer, P. D. and Guerrant, R. L. (1988). Pneumocystis carinii infection of the small intestine in a patient with acquired immune deficiency syndrome. *Am. J. Clin. Pathol.*, **89**, 679

19. Freeman, W. R., Gross, J. G., Labelle, J., Oteken, K., Katz, B. and Wiley, C. A. (1989). Pneumocystis carinii choroidopathy. A new clinical entity. *Arch. Ophthalmol.*, **107**, 863

20. Unger, P. D., Rosenblum, M. and Krown, S. E. (1988). Disseminated Pneumocystis carinii infection in a patient with acquired immunodeficiency syndrome. *Hum. Pathol.*, **19**, 113

21. Schmid, O. (1964). Studien zur Pneumocystis-Erkrankung des Menschen. I. Mitt. Das wechselnde Erscheinungsbild der Pneumocystis Pneumonie beim Säugling. Konkordante und diskordante Form. Pneumocystis granulomatosa. *Frankf. Z. Path.*, **74**, 121

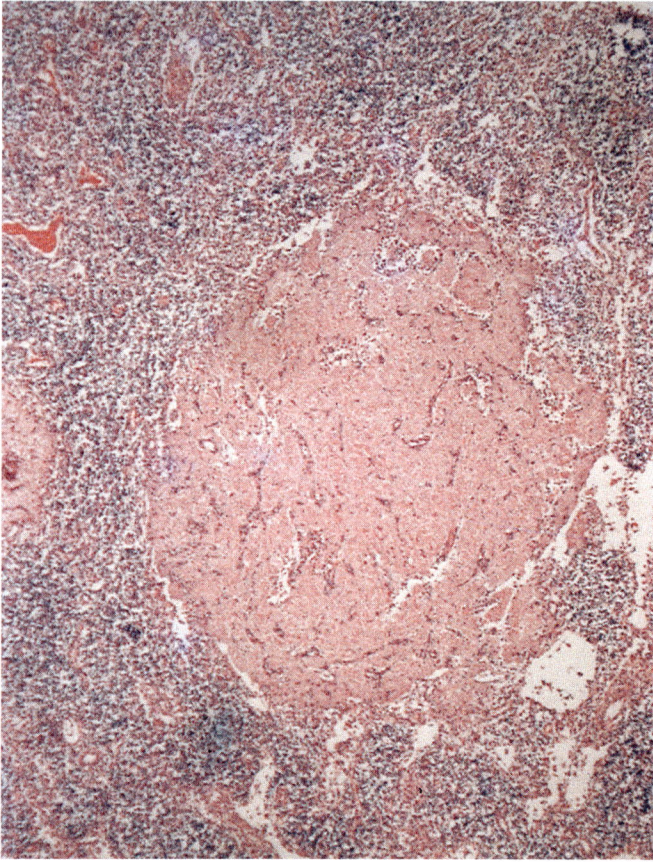

Fig. 17.6 Tumour-like focus of pneumocystosis in lymph node. H&E

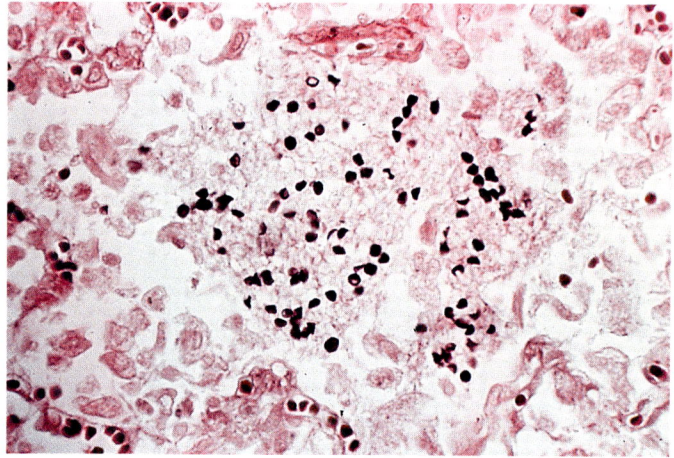

Fig. 17.8 Cluster of pneumocysts inside pulmonary alveoli in man. Grocott.

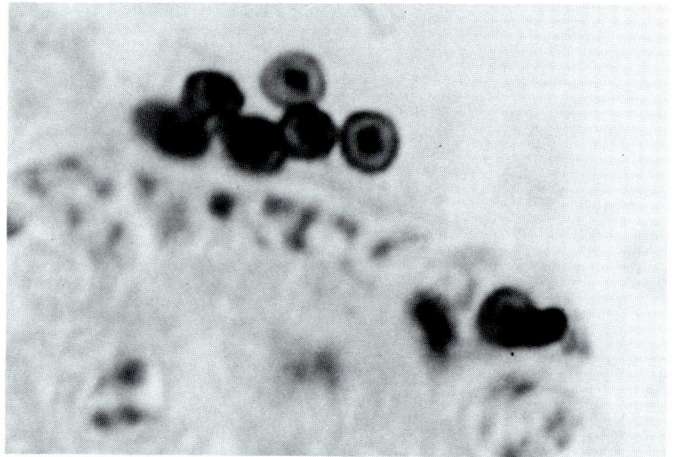

Fig. 17.9 Small cluster of organisms of *Pneumocystis carinii* attached to an alveolar wall in a case of pauciparasitic and paucireactive pneumocystosis in an infant from Mérida, observed many years ago. These organisms were first considered to be yeast-like fungus cells. Grocott

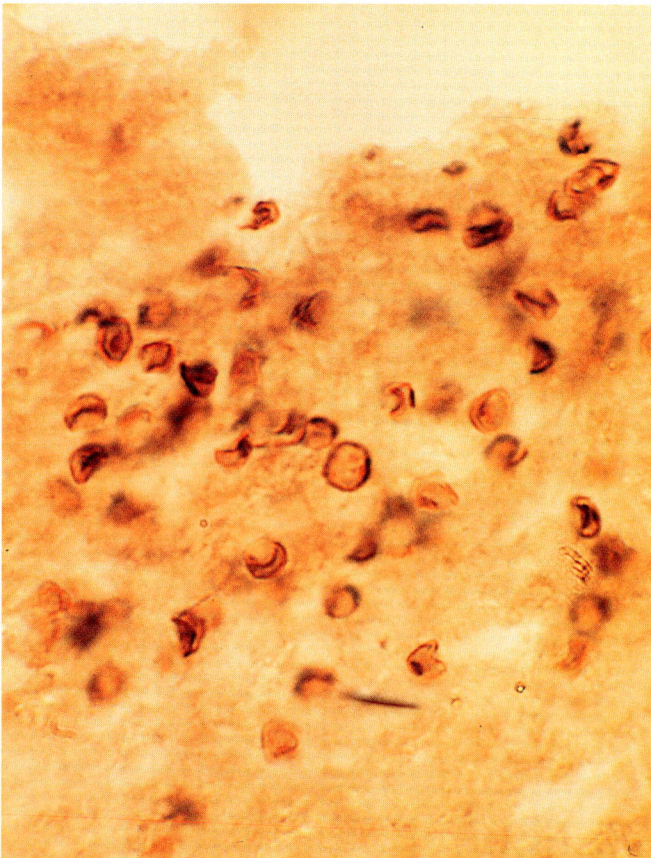

Fig. 17.7 Organisms of *Pneumocystis carinii* in lung tissue with deformation of parasites. A case of AIDS from Mérida. Grocott

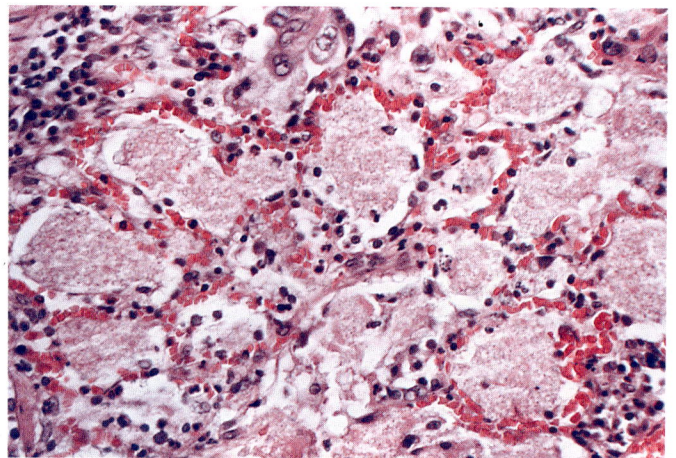

Fig. 17.10 The typical alveolar content in a human case of massive pneumocystosis. It is constituted, apparently, by necrotic parasites mixed with exudate. H&E

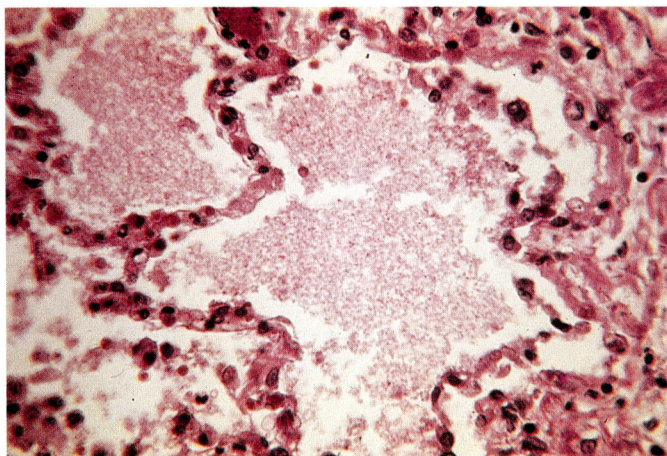

Fig. 17.11 The typical foamy alveolar content of pneumocystosis at higher power. H&E

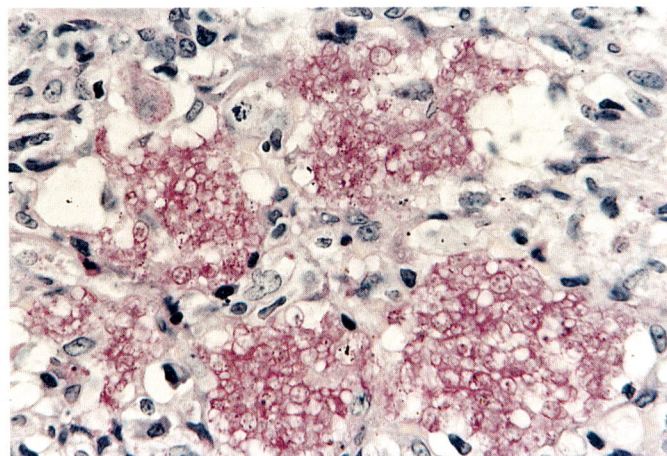

Fig. 17.12 The foamy structure of the alveolar content is clearly seen. Numerous unstained cyst-like forms may be discerned. Material from an AIDS patient. PAS

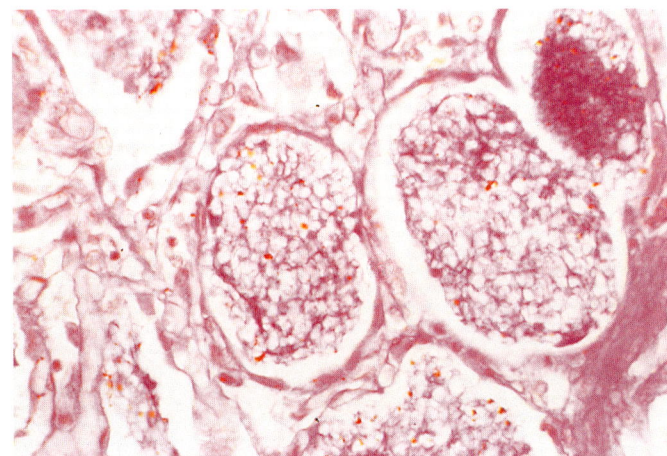

Fig. 17.13 The typical foamy alveolar content at higher magnification. An AIDS case from Mérida. PAS

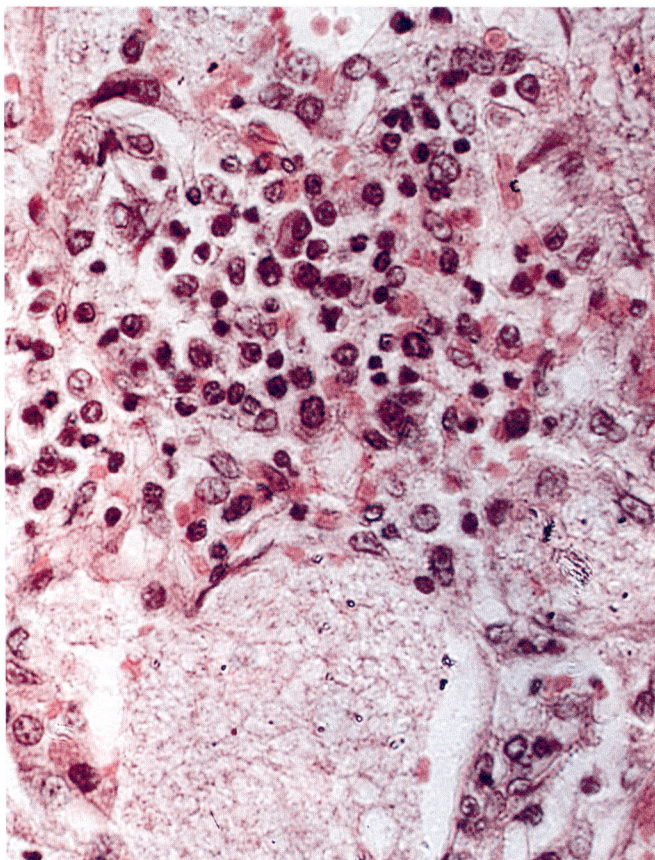

Fig. 17.14 Interstitial pneumonia with plasma cells in the AIDS case from Mérida. H&E

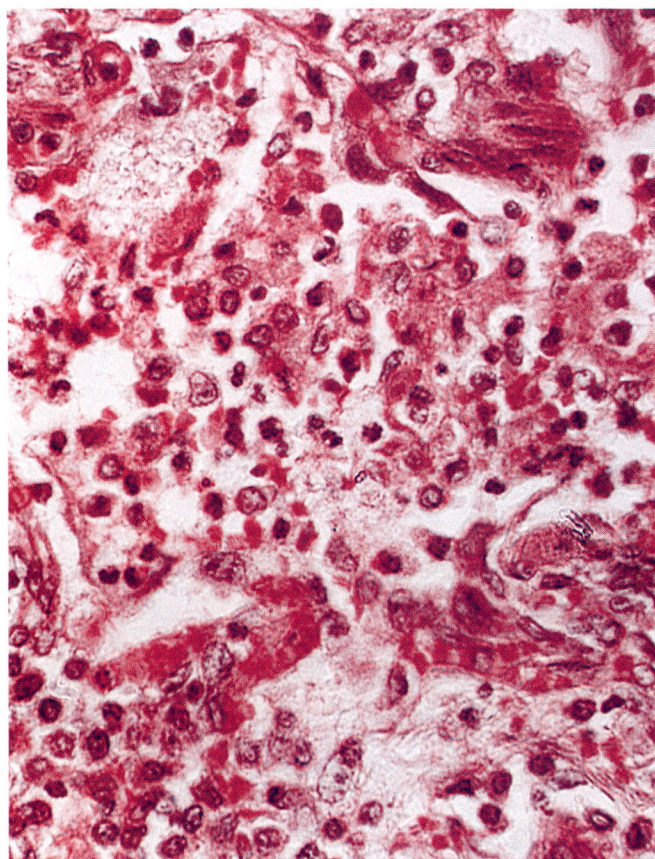

Fig. 17.15 Intra-alveolar exudate with granulocytes in the AIDS case from Mérida. H&E

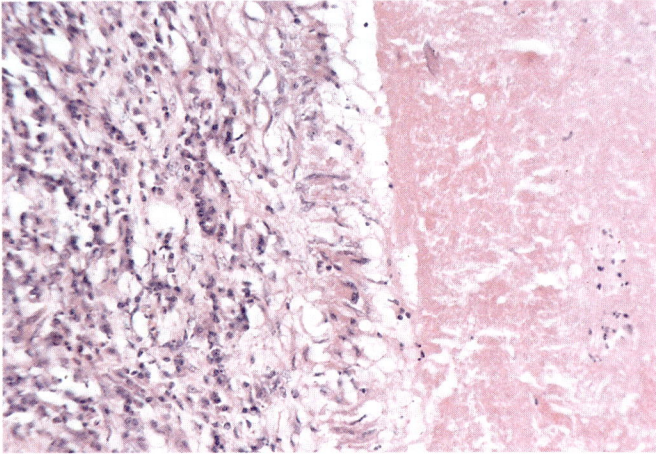

Fig. 17.16 Granulomatous reaction, i.e. epithelioid cells in a palisade-like fashion in the periphery of a pneumocystoma (AIDS patient). H&E

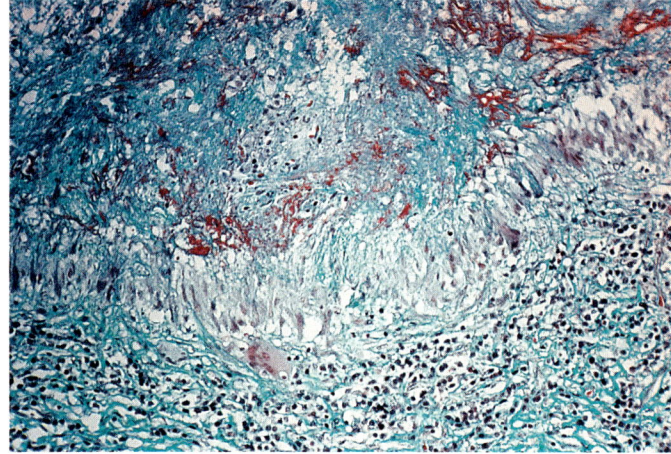

Fig. 17.17 The same pattern as in the case of Fig. 17.16. Trichrome (Goldner)

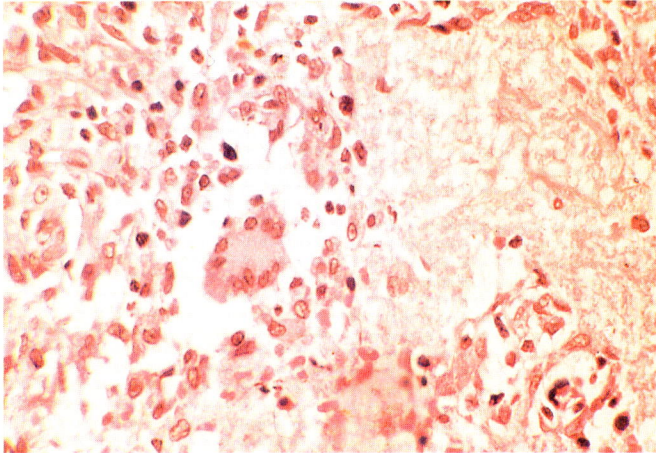

Fig. 17.18 Giant cell in the case of Figs. 17.16 and 17.17. H&E

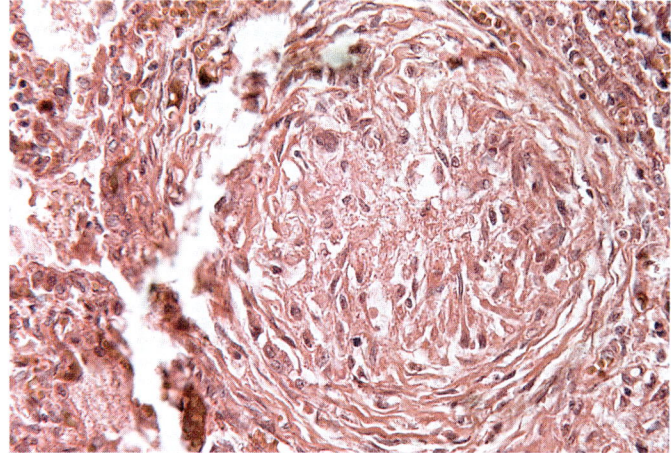

Fig. 17.19 Pulmonary granuloma in case of infection with *Pneumocystis carinii*. H&E

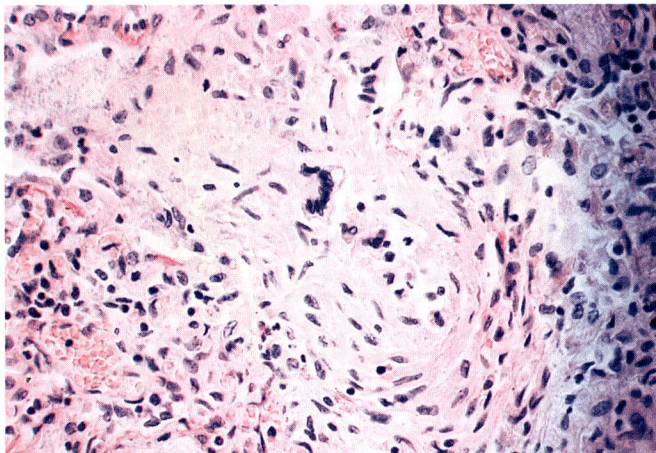

Fig. 17.20 Another case of pulmonary granuloma in a case of pneumocystosis. Organisms of *Pneumocystis carinii* may be found inside giant cells but are not seen in this field. H&E

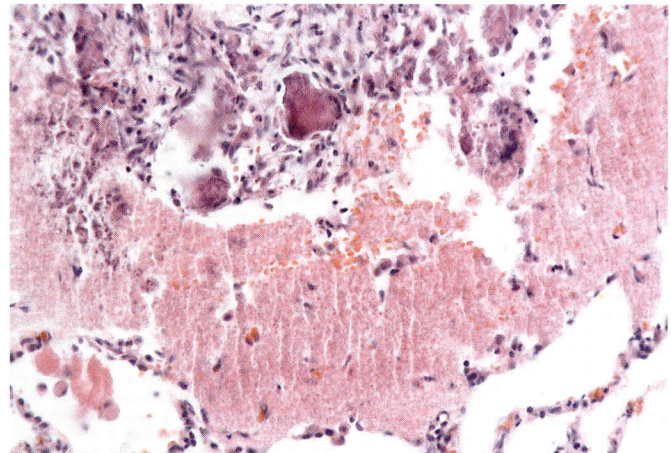

Fig. 17.21 Pulmonary pneumocystosis with granulomatous reaction and calcifications. H&E

18. BALANTIDIASIS

Introduction

This disease is also called balantidial dysentery or balantidial colitis. It is relatively rare in man because he is not the principal, but only the secondary or occasional host. The disease occurs worldwide, mostly in people dealing with pigs, such as pig breeders, veterinarians and butchers.

This infection is mostly observed in Eastern Europe, the former USSR, Asia and the Americas[1-3]. It is well known in Venezuela where its frequency has not increased over the last few years[4,5]. Fatal cases no longer exist (as they did some 30 years ago). There have been no reports on this protozoan infection in the medical literature for the past two years.

Almost all pigs are infected, but they rarely develop any disease. In addition, monkeys constitute a parasite reservoir, but, by contrast with pigs, they are sometimes severely ill. Cats, rabbits, rats and guinea pigs may be used for experimental infection[6].

In man, asymptomatic carriers are more common than cases of disease. Balantidiasis does not have characteristic symptoms, often takes a chronic course and may remain undiagnosed. Bloody stools and numerous leukocytes in faeces are typical of this infection. A fatal outcome may occur in cases with symptomatology for years, in cases with perforated ulcers and peritonitis and in cases not treated adequately[7].

Clinical diagnosis is made by examining fresh faeces. The trophozoites of *Balantidium coli* are easily recognized by their size and typical movement. Their cilia are not seen in permanent preparations and tissue sections. For diagnostic purposes, balantidians may also be cultured in artificial media, similar to amoebae.

The parasite

Balantidium coli is the largest protozoan pathogenic to man. It is ciliated and belongs to the class Ciliophora. Reproduction takes place asexually by transverse division. The parasite shows two forms:

1. The trophozoites (or vegetative forms) of *Balantidium coli* are spherical or oval shaped. Their maximum size is 70–150 μm. Cilia cover the entire surface of the trophozoites and make them mobile (Figs. 18.1 and 18.2).

2. The cysts are more roundish and a little bit smaller. The membrane is thicker than that of the trophozoites and there are no cilia. They do not develop in man.

At one pole of the balantidia, there is a funnel-shaped invagination (mouth) and, at the other pole, an anal orifice which is difficult to detect. Bacteria and other faecal material are the food for the balantidia. Typically, there are two nuclei, a kidney-shaped macronucleus and a smaller spherical micronucleus. Vacuoles are present in the cytoplasm. *Balantidium coli* may be cultured and grows like amoeba.

Pathogenesis

Balantidium coli is mostly an inoffensive commensal in the lumen of the large bowel of pigs. Seldom does the pig become ill. In nature, cysts derive from trophozoites of *B. coli* in faeces of pigs. They hardly ever form in man. Therefore, infection from man to man is rare. The resistant cysts are ingested with contaminated food or water and reach the large bowel of man. There they remain in the intestinal lumen; asymptomatic infection is more frequent than disease, as in pigs. In certain circumstances, however, the balantidia become virulent and aggressive and invade the intestinal wall, causing colitis. Balantidial dysentery is similar to amoebic dysentery in many respects.

Theories about the action of balantidia, i.e. how and why the parasites penetrate the intestinal wall, perhaps by production of proteolytic enzymes, and the following action of pathogenic bacteria, are still theories and need confirmation. Haematogenous and lymphogenous dissemination of parasites to extraintestinal sites occurs very rarely.

Pathology

The organ involved is almost exclusively the large bowel in its entire length (Fig. 18.3). Occasionally, the appendix is affected[4] and, exceptionally, the terminal ileum. Extraintestinal organs are involved very seldom: in single cases, involvement of mesenteric lymph nodes (Fig. 18.4), liver[5], lungs, ureter and bladder, vagina[8] and exocervix (Fig. 18.5) has been reported.

Grossly, intestinal lesions are very similar to those caused by amoebae. Also, ulcers of the mucosa with undermined borders may be found in the large bowel.

Microscopically, the balantidia in smears and tissue sections cannot be overlooked because they are so large and show characteristic structures. In fresh preparations, they are very mobile. With routine staining methods, like H&E (Figs. 18.6 and 18.7), iron haematoxylin and also the PAS method (Fig. 18.8), they come out well. Special staining techniques are not necessary for the detection of these large protozoans. Small balantidia may be confused with amoebae.

The tissue reaction consists of non-specific inflammation with exudation of leukocytes and abscess formation. Almost always, bacterial infection is associated.

References

1. De Carneri, I. (1958). The frequency of balantidiasis in Milan pigs. *Trans. R. Soc. Trop. Med. Hyg.*, **52**, 475
2. Arean, V. M. and Koppisch, E. (1956). Balantidiasis. A review and report of cases. *Am. J. Path.*, **32**, 1089
3. Walter, P. D., Judson, F. N., Murphy, K. D. *et al.* (1973). Balantidiasis outbreaks in Truk. *Am. J. Trop. Med. Hyg.*, **22**, 33
4. Jaffé, R. and Kann, C. (1943). Sobre el Balantidium coli en el apéndice y la apendicitis balantidiana. *Rev. Sudam. Morfol.*, **1**, 74
5. Wenger, F. (1943). Absceso hepático producido por el Balantidium coli. *Kasmera (Univ. Zulia)*, **2**, 433
6. Westphal, A. (1957). Experimentelle Infektionen des Meerschweinchens mit Balantidium coli. *Z. Tropenmed. Parasit.*, **8**, 288
7. Garcia-Pont, P. H. and Ramirez, de Arellano, G. (1966). Fatal balantidial colitis. *Bol. Assoc. Med. Puerto Rico*, **58**, 195
8. Isasa Mejia, G. (1955). Balantidiasis vaginal. *Antioquia Med.*, **5**, 488

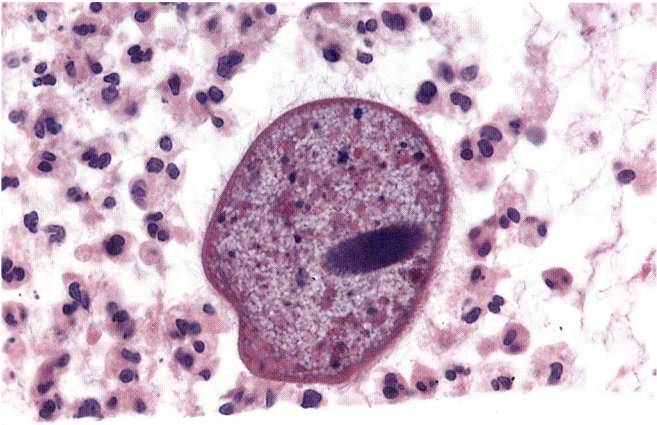

Fig. 18.1 Trophozoite of *Balantidium coli* in a faecal smear. H&E

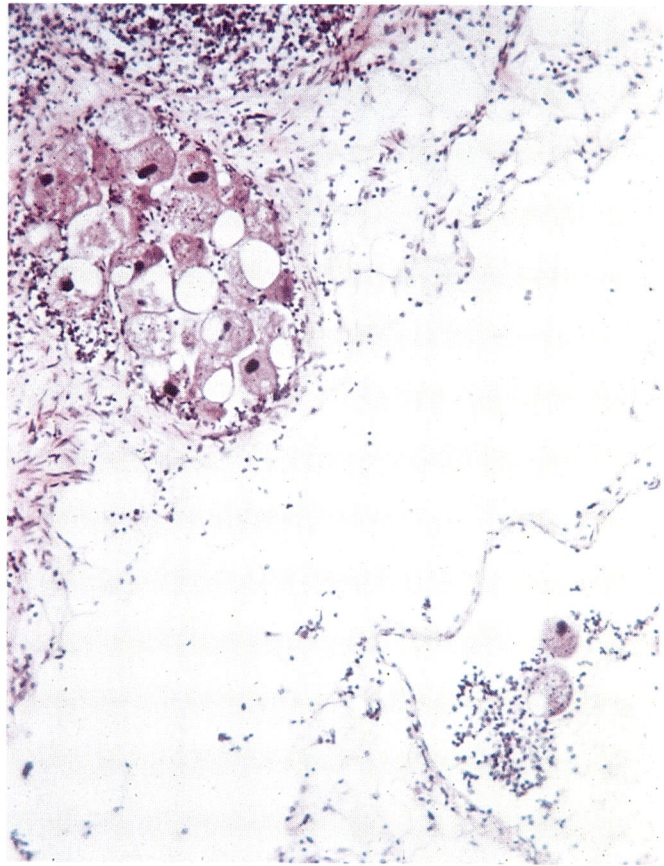

Fig. 18.2 Cysts of *Balantidium coli* in a faecal smear. H&E

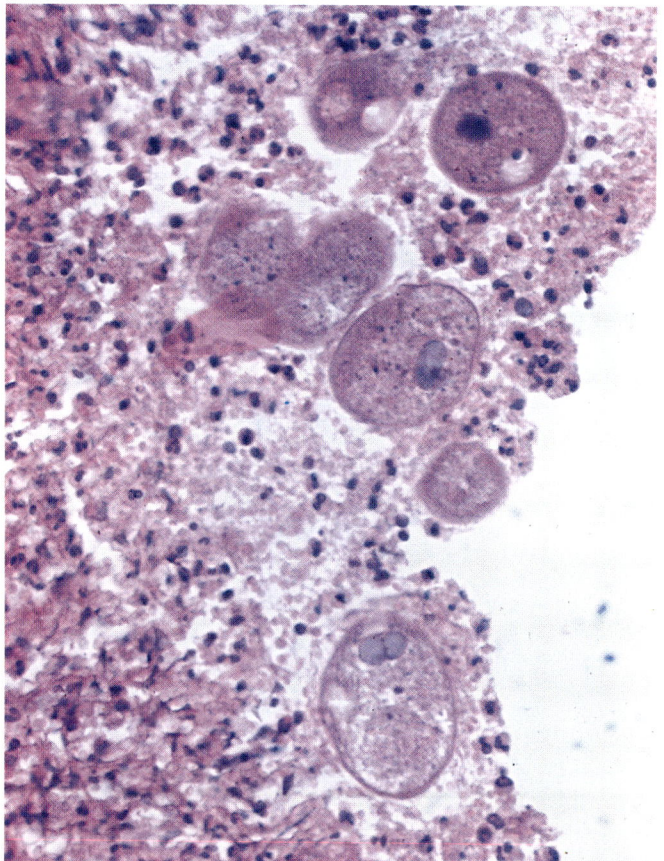

Fig. 18.3 Perforated ulcers in the ileum and colon due to balantidiasis. Autopsy material

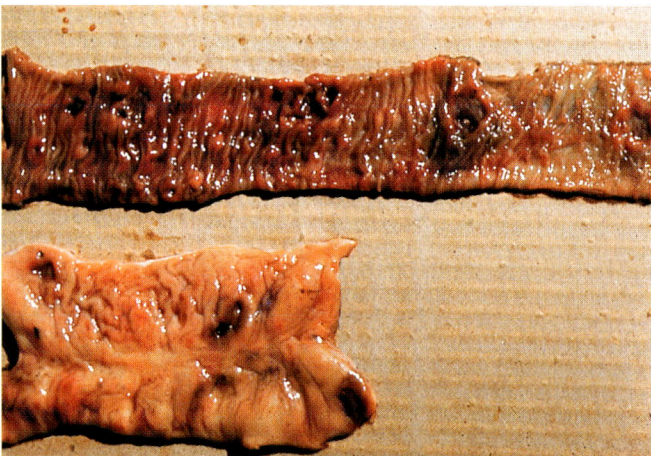

Fig. 18.4 Numerous balantidia inside a lymph vessel near a mesenteric lymph node and several parasites in a lymph vessel of the mesocolon. H&E

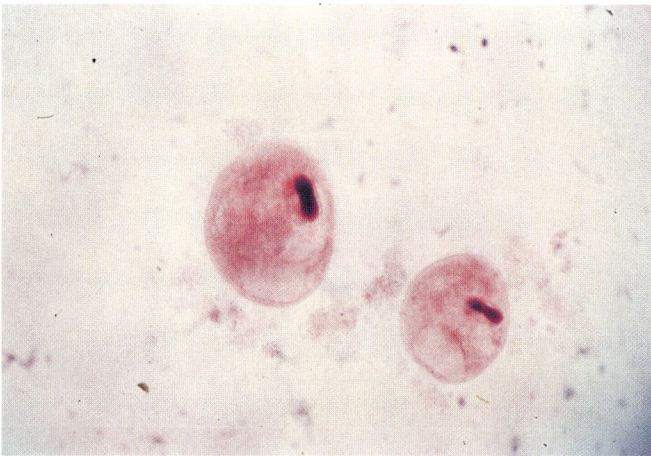

Fig. 18.5 Marked necrotizing inflammation at the exocervix with several balantidia. H&E

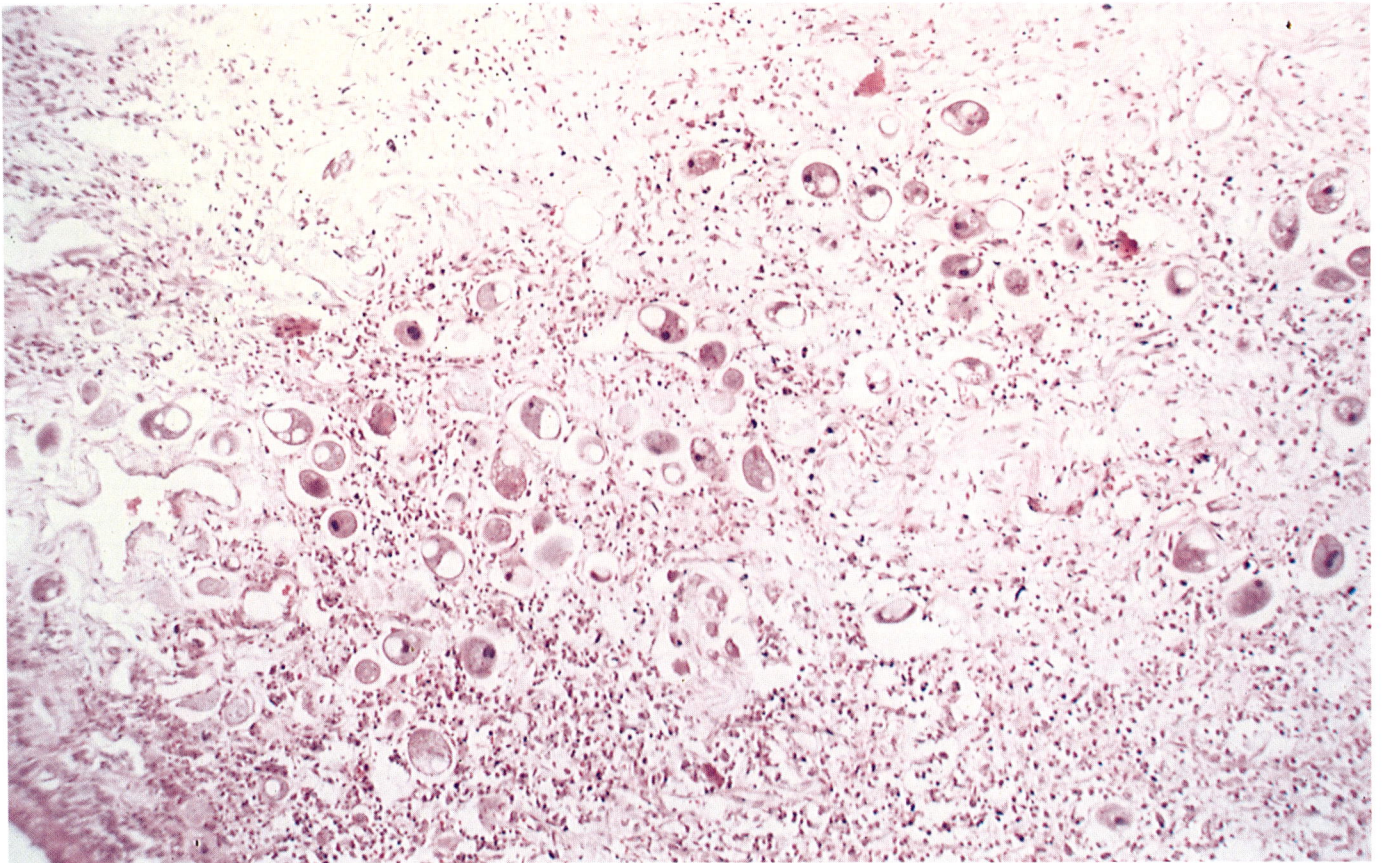

Fig. 18.6 Numerous balantidia in the wall of the large bowel (balantidial colitis) at low power. H&E

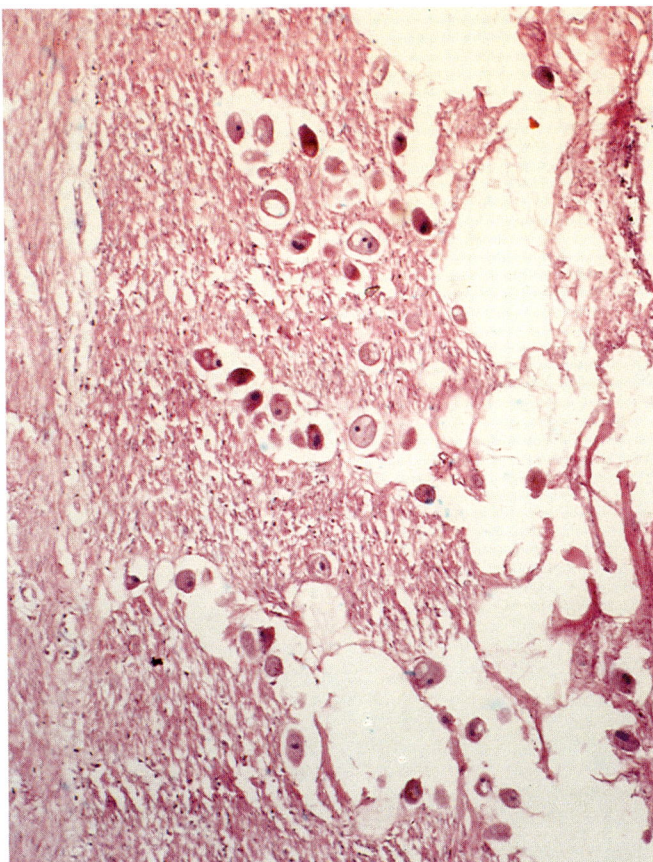

Fig. 18.7 Necrotizing colitis with groups of balantidia in the mucosa. H&E

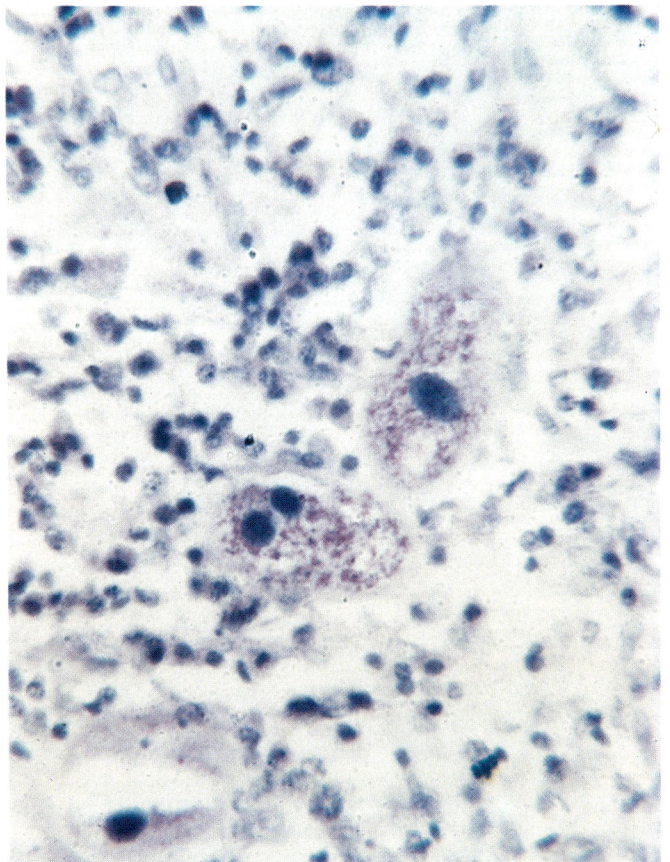

Fig. 18.8 Balantidia with red granulae in tissue section. PAS

19. MICROSPORIDIOSIS

Introduction

This protozoan disease is also named microsporidosis or nosematosis, and, lately, other names have been proposed since other microsporidians have been described. Microsporidiosis, to our knowledge, is not mentioned in European medial literature. The first case of human infection was reported in 1959[1].

Only a few cases of infection in humans have been reported, but, in recent years, their number has increased, although named differently. A few cases seem to have been opportunistic infections. The majority of cases have occurred in Asia and in children. This disease has not been reported in Venezuela.

The first natural infection in a lower animal species was described by Pasteur in 1870 in the silk worm (*Bombyx mori*). Later, microsporidians were found in numerous animal species (dogs, insects, fish and laboratory animals[2-7]). Vervet monkeys and rabbits may be infected experimentally[2,8].

Little is known about the clinical course or form. Only a few of the human cases have survived. Infections are known in immunocompromised persons and AIDS patients, with increasing frequency lately[6-17].

Clinical diagnosis is based on the observation of microsporidians in tissue sections of biopsies or in smears of fluids. Inoculation of laboratory animals cannot be used as a diagnostic tool because natural infection with microsporidians in these animals is normal.

The parasite

Microsporidia belong to the class Cnidosporidia and phylum Microspora. The species of the genera *Nosema*, *Encephalitozoon*, *Enterocytozoon* and *Thelohania* are the agents which produce the infection in mammals and, occasionally, man. The spores of *Nosema connori* are oval in shape and measure 2–4 μm. They stain weakly with H&E, are sometimes birefractive with polarized light[18] and their membranes stain weakly with the Grocott method. A characteristic element of the spores is a PAS-positive corpuscle. With a phase contrast microscope or an electron microscope, typical filaments arranged in a spiral form may be discerned.

Pathogenesis

Very little is known about transmission or infection. The portal of entry seems to be the digestive tract. The cycle of evolution of the microsporidians is not completely known at present.

Pathology

Mostly, musculature (Fig. 19.1) is involved, although several other tissues may be affected too. In some reported cases[17,19,20], the ocular cornea was invaded by this parasite, and, in another[21], tumour cells of a pancreatic carcinoma harboured microsporidians. Intestinal involvement has been reported mostly in AIDS patients[12-15]. Details of gross lesions are not known.

Microscopically, the spores of microsporidians are arranged in clusters, mostly intracellularly. Some microsporidians show a halo (Fig. 19.2), others a PAS-positive dot (Fig. 19.3) and others are slightly Gram-positive. The Grocott-positive membranes indicate fungal cells (Fig. 19.4).

Regarding differential diagnosis of the microsporidians, all small micro-organisms and inclusion bodies must be mentioned (Figs. 19.5 and 19.6). Muscle fibres may be invaded by the following protozoa: *Trypanosoma cruzi*, *Toxoplasma gondii*, *Sarcocystis* sp. and *Nosema connori*.

References

1. Matsubayashi, H. *et al.* (1959). A case of Encephalitozoon-like body infection in man. *Pathology*, **67**, 181
2. van Dellen, A. F., Stewart, C. G. and Botha, W. S. (1989). Studies of encephalitozoonosis in vervet monkeys (Cercopithecus pygerythrus) orally inoculated with spores of Encephalitozoon cuniculi isolated from dogs (Canis familiaris). *Onderstepoort. J. Vet. Res.*, **56**, 1
3. Van Heerden, J., Bainbridge, N., Burroughs, R. E. and Kriek, N. P. (1989). Distemper-like disease and encephalitozoonosis in wild dogs (Lycaon pictus). *J. Wildl. Dis.*, **25**, 70
4. Cutlip, R. C. and Beall, C. W. (1989). Encephalitozoonosis in arctic lemmings. *Lab. Anim. Sci.*, **39**, 331
5. Ansbacher, L., Nichols, M. F. and Hahn, A. W. (1988). The influence of Encephalitozoon cuniculi on neural tissue responses to implanted biomaterials in the rabbit. *Lab. Anim. Sci.*, **38**, 689
6. Powell, S. *et al.* (1989). Microsporidiosis in a lovebird. *J. Vet. Diagn. Invest.*, **1**, 69
7. Bjerkas, I. (1990). Brain and spinal cord lesions in encephalitozoonosis in mink. *Acta Vet. Scand.*, **31**, 423
8. Wicher, V. *et al.* (1991). Enteric infection with an obligate intracellular parasite, Encephalitozoon cuniculi, in an experimental model. *Infect. Immun.*, **59**, 2225
9. Margileth, A. M., Strano, A. J., Chandra, R. *et al.* (1973). Disseminated nosematosis in an immunologically compromised infant. *Arch. Path.*, **95**, 145
10. Zender, H. O., Arrigoni, E., Eckert, J. and Kapanci, Y. (1989). A case of Encephalitozoon cuniculi peritonitis in a patient with AIDS. *Am. J. Clin. Pathol.*, **92**, 352
11. Rijpstra, A. C., Canning, E. U. *et al.* (1988). Use of light microscopy to diagnose small-intestinal microsporidiosis in patients with AIDS. *J. Infect. Dis.*, **157**, 827
12. Greenson, J. K. *et al.* (1991). AIDS enteropathy: occult enteric infections and duodenal mucosal alterations in chronic diarrhea. *Ann. Intern. Med.*, **114**, 366
13. Orenstein, J. M. *et al.* (1990). Intestinal microsporidiosis as a cause of diarrhea in human immunodeficiency virus-infected patients: a report of 20 cases. *Hum. Pathol.*, **21**, 475
14. Kotler, D. P. *et al.* (1990). Small intestinal injury and parasitic diseases in AIDS. *Ann. Intern. Med.*, **113**, 444
15. Peacock, C. S. *et al.* (1991). Histological diagnosis of intestinal microsporidiosis in patients with AIDS. *J. Clin. Pathol.*, **44**, 558
16. Shadduk, J. A. *et al.* (1990). Isolation of a microsporidian from a human patient. *J. Infect. Dis.*, **162**, 773
17. Friedberg, D. N. *et al.* (1990). Microsporidial keratoconjunctivitis in acquired immunodeficiency syndrome. *Arch. Ophthalmol.*, **108**, 504
18. Tiner, J. D. (1988). Birefringent spores differentiate Encephalitozoon and other microsporidia from coccidia. *Vet. Pathol.*, **25**, 227
19. Ashton, N. and Wiransnha, P. A. (1973). Encephalitozoonosis (nosematosis) of the cornea. *Br. J. Ophthalmol.*, **57**, 669
20. Davis, R. M. *et al.* (1990). Corneal microsporidiosis. A case report including ultrastructural observations. *Ophthalmology*, **97**, 953
21. Marcus, P. P., Van der Walt, J. J. and Burger, P. J. (1973). Human tumour microsporidiosis. *Arch. Path.*, **95**, 341

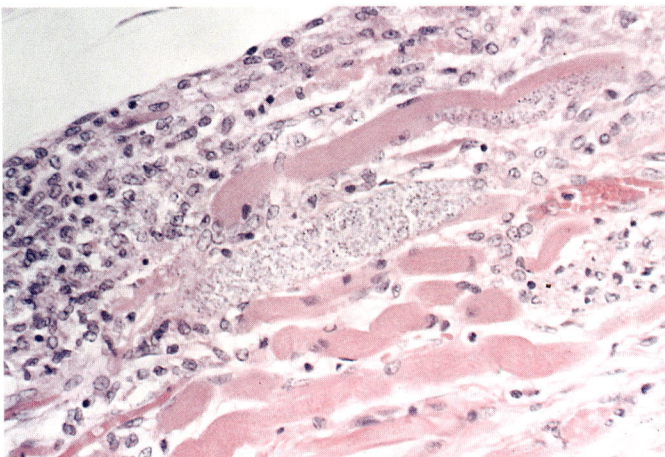

Fig. 19.1 Cluster of microsporidians in a muscle fibre of the diaphragm with inflammation in the vicinity. H&E

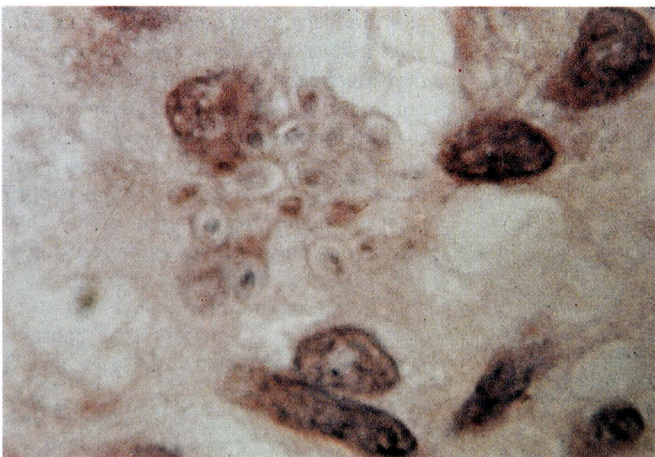

Fig. 19.2 Spores with a halo in a lesion caused by microsporidians. H&E

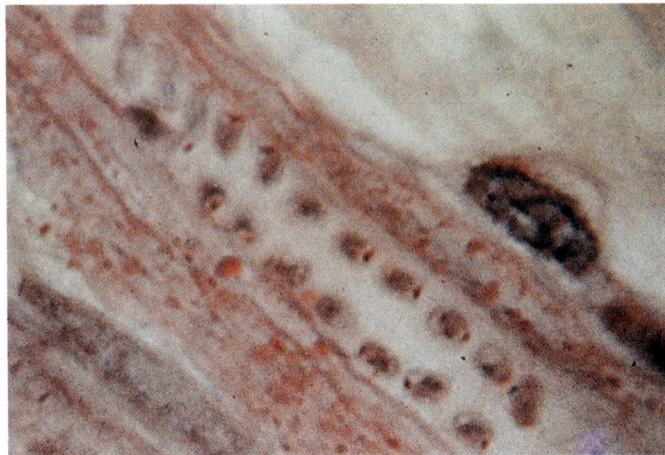

Fig. 19.3 Spores with PAS-positive dots inside a muscle fibre. PAS

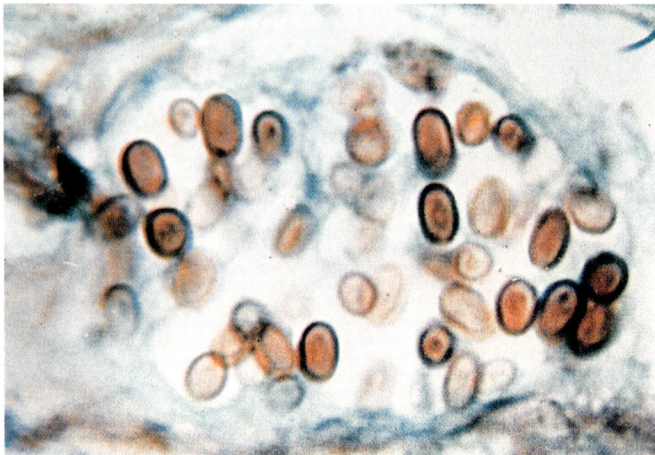

Fig. 19.4 These microsporidians at high power are partly Grocott-positive. Grocott

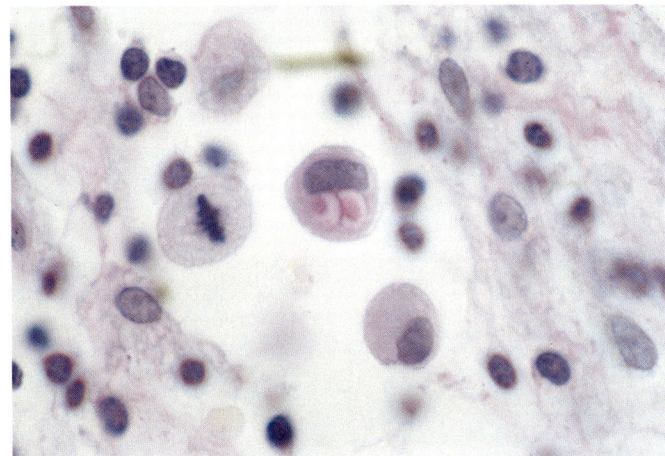

Fig. 19.5 Cytoplasmic inclusion bodies in carcinoma cells (metastasis of gastric carcinoma) are similar to microsporidians. PAS

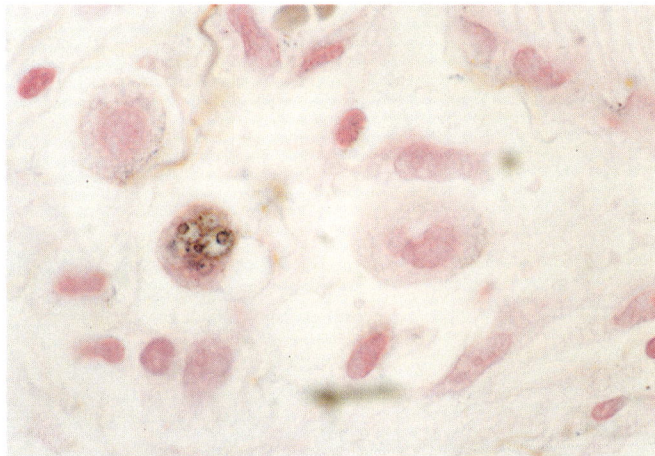

Fig. 19.6 Same case as Fig. 19.5. The inclusion bodies, variable in size, are positive with this special staining method. Grocott

Helminthic diseases

The parasitic helminths belong to multicellular living organisms (Metazoa of the fifth kingdom), are male, female or hermaphrodite and do not usually multiply in man. They may live in the human digestive tract or in determined tissues, and they may produce up to 100 000 eggs per day. Many species have teeth or hooks for adherence to the wall of hollow organs.

Sources of infection and portals of entry are listed in Table 9.

Frequently, the presence of worms in an individual is not noticed. Signs of worm infection may be:

1. Loss of weight because the worms consume too much food destined for the host;

2. Anaemia, because worms suck blood from the host; and

3. Obstruction and/or perforation of hollow organs.

Consequences of their toxic action may be allergies or inflammation with eosinophilic leukocytes in the blood and/or in tissues. Often, the number of parasites determines symptoms and severity of disease. For the prepatent period and the lifespan of helminths in man, see Table 10.

The diseases produced by the three large groups of helminths are: A. nematodiasis, B. cestodiasis, and C. Trematodiasis (flukes).

Table 9 Principal sources of infection in helminthic diseases

Source of infection	Species of parasite
Oral infection	
1. Drinking water	
Ingestion of cyclops and larvae	*Dracunculus*
	Sparganum
Salad and vegetables contaminated by human faeces	*Ascaris, Trichuris*
Lettuce, radish, all kinds of fruit	*Cysticercus cellulosae*
Cress	*Fasciola*
Water nuts	*Fasciolopsis*
2. Uncooked food	
Meat	
Pork	*Taenia solium, Trichinella spiralis*
Cattle	*Taenia saginata*
Fish	*Diphyllobothrium latum*
Several species	*Opisthorchis*
Crabs and crayfish	*Paragonimus*
3. Dirt	
Earth	*Ascaris, Trichuris, Cysticercus cellulosae, Echinococcus*
Anus–finger–mouth	*Enterobius, Hymenolepis nana*
	Cysticercus cellulosae
House dust	*Enterobius*
Contact with dogs	*Echinococcus*
Percutaneous infection	
1. Soil	*Ancylostoma, Necator Strongyloides*
2. Water	*Schistosoma*
	Various species causing Cercaria dermatitis
3. Insect bite	Species of Filaria

A. NEMATODIASIS

The nematodes, threadworms or roundworms belong to the phylum of Nemathelminthes; they are non-segmented parasites and have separate sexes. They measure from a few mm (*Strongyloides stercoralis*, almost invisible to the naked eye) up to 60 cm (*Dracunculus medinensis*) and all have pointed ends. Tables 11 and 12 show structural details of the digestive tract, the separate genital organs and the cuticle on the surface with collagen fibres which produce contractions. There are several developmental stages from the egg, through 4 moults of larvae, to the mature worm. Details of larvae, whether rhabditiform or filariform, will not be discussed here.

Four different types of cycles of evolution in man may be distinguished:

1. The *Enterobius* type
   The ova are ingested → mature in the intestinal tract
2. The *Ascaris* type
   Ova are ingested → larvae in the digestive tract → transenteral passage → blood → heart → lungs → pharynx → digestive tract (maturing)
3. The hookworm type
   Ova in nature become larvae → transcutaneous passage

age → blood heart → lung → pharynx → digestive tract (maturing)

4. The *Trichinella* type
Encysted larvae are ingested with meat → larvae are set free in digestive tract → transenteral passage →

blood → heart → musculature (larvae become again encysted)

Recently, strongyloidiasis as an opportunistic infection has become important because latent infections of this kind are exacerbated in immunocompromised individuals.

20. ENTEROBIASIS

Introduction

This disease is also named oxyuriasis or pinworm infection. It occurs worldwide and is perhaps one of the most frequent worm infections. It is found mainly in regions with temperate or colder climates and in middle and upper class people, i.e. contrary to most other worm infections,

it is observed in wealthy individuals. Furthermore, it is seen predominantly in children. The infection is unusual in Venezuela. This parasite does occur in lower animals but only occasionally[1]; it develops in man without intermediate hosts.

Table 10 Prepatent period of various helminths (eggs in the faeces or microfilariae in the blood). From Piekarski, G. (1989) *Medical Parasitology*

	Developmental stage		Prepatent period	Lifespan in man (extreme values)
Nematodes				
Trichuris trichiura	Egg		60–90 days	Several years
Enterobius vermicularis	Egg		37–101 days	ca. 100 days
Ascaris lumbricoides	Egg		50–80 days	1–1.5 years
Ancylostoma duodenale	Egg		35–42 days	5–12 years
Necator americanus	Egg		35–42 days	5–8 years
Strongyloides stercoralis	Larva		17–28 days	20 years
Trichostrongylus orientalis	Egg		25–30 days	
Wuchereria bancrofti		Blood	ca. 1 year	17 years
Brugia malayi		Blood	50–60 days	8–10 years
B. timori		Blood	90 days	
Loa loa	Microfilariae	Blood	ca. 1 year	17 years
Onchocerca volvulus		Skin	12–15 months	15–18 years
Mansonella ozzardi		Blood	?	
Dipetalonema perstans		Blood	8–12 months	
D. streptocerca		Skin	3–4 months?	
Cestodes				
Taenia saginata	Proglottid		77–84 days	up to 20 years
Taenia solium	Proglottid		35–74 days	up to 25 years
Hymenolepis nana	Egg		14–28 days	2 weeks to months
Diphyllobothrium latum	Egg		18–21 days	15–20 years
Dipylidium caninum	Proglottid		20 days	
Trematodes				
Fasciolopsis buski	Egg		ca. 30–90 days	6 months
Echinostoma ilocanum	Egg			
Metagonimus yokogawai	Egg		10–14 days	2 years
Heterophyes heterophyes	Egg		7–8 days	2–4 months (?)
Schistosoma mansoni	Egg (lateral spine)		49 days	up to 30 years
Schistosoma intercalatum	Egg (terminal spine)		50–55 days	up to 25 years
Schistosoma japonicum	Egg Small lateral		20–26 days	
Schistosoma mekongi	Egg knob		35 days	

Table 11 Typical features of nematodes. *Enterobius*, about 10 mm (female, above) and 4 mm (male, below) in length

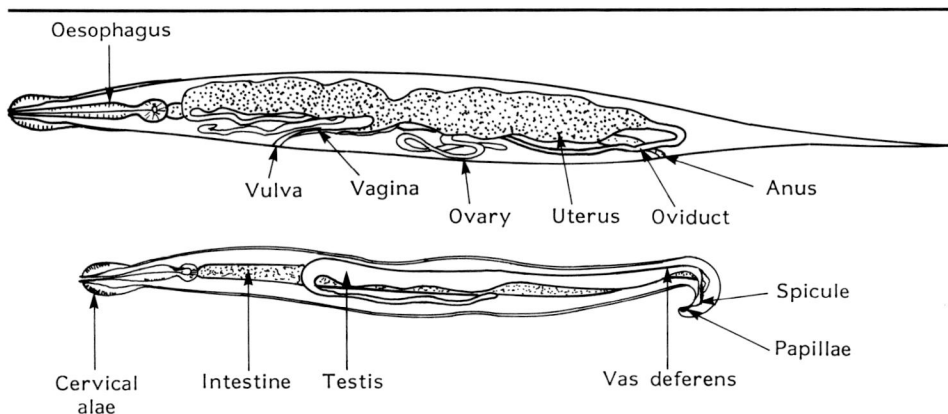

Table 12   Schematic cross-section from various groups of female nematodes

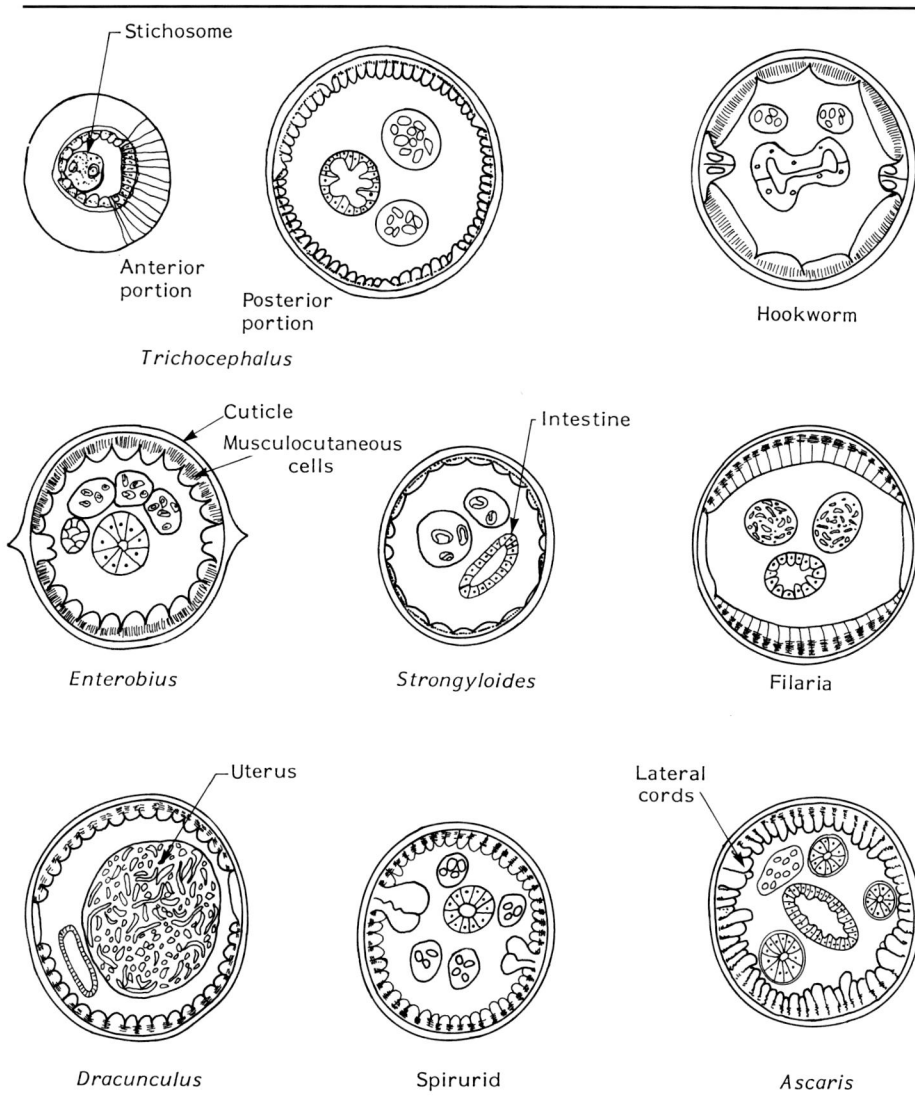

Trichocephalus

Hookworm

Enterobius

Strongyloides

Filaria

Dracunculus

Spirurid

Ascaris

The clinical picture is typical. The children become sleepless, restless and inattentive. The bad feeling, and sometimes diarrhoea, may mimick appendicitis. In the genito-anal region, the parasites may lead to marked scratching with cutaneous irritation. Clinical diagnosis is made by looking for pinworm eggs in anal swabs or on strips of clear adhesive tape from the genito-anal region. Adult worms may be found in smears from stools. Eggs or worms may be stained with toluene blue.

The parasite

This roundworm is called *Enterobius vermicularis* or *Oxyuris vermicularis*. It measures from 2–13 mm, the females being larger (Figs. 20.1 and 20.2). Tables 11 and 12 show the structure of male and female pinworms schematically. These worms may be vectors of micro-organisms[2,3]. Characteristically, the ova of *E. vermicularis* are oval and flattened on one side; they measure 55 × 25 μm (Fig. 20.3).

Pathogenesis

The ova are ingested. Autoinfection may take place, mainly in children. Larvae and eggs in the anal and genital region lead to scratching, and reach the mouth via the fingers. Infections may also occur by direct contact of the

hands with clothes, dust or food where worm eggs may be present. Retrograde migration of larvae from the anal region to the gut may occur[4], usually in adults. The larvae reach the appendix; here, male pinworms are seen more frequently than female[5].

After oral ingestion, larvae enter the small intestine where they mature. The male worms die soon after mating. During the night, the females migrate to the anal region where they lay their eggs. Within a few minutes they can lay up to 10 000 eggs. Adult worms, larvae and eggs do not penetrate into tissues.

Pathology

The adult worms are found in the terminal small intestine, the region of the ileocaecal valve, the appendix and the caecum (Fig. 20.4). The parasites, larvae and eggs may produce superficial irritation but, as a rule, do not invade mucosa or skin (Fig. 20.5). They do not cause appendicitis[5,6].

References

1. Zhang, G. W. *et al.* (1990). The presence of pinworms (Enterobius sp.) in the mesenteric lymph nodes, liver and lungs of a chimpanzee, Pantroglodytes. *J. Helminthol.*, **64**, 29
2. Burows, R. B. and Swerdlow, M. A. (1956). Enterobius vermicularis

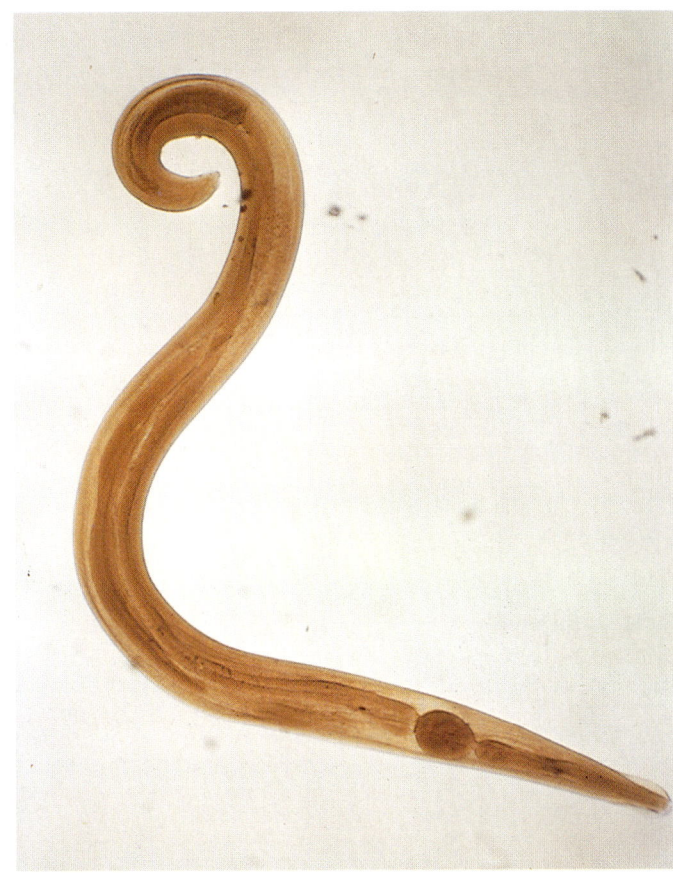

Fig. 20.1 Mature male *Enterobius vermicularis* (pinworm)

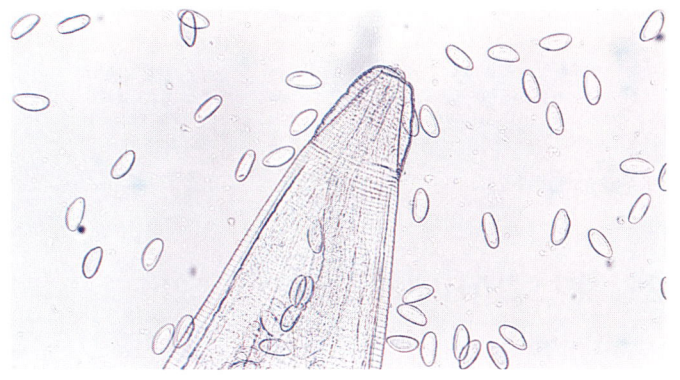

Fig. 20.2 Fore-end of female *Enterobius vermicularis* and numerous eggs of this nematode

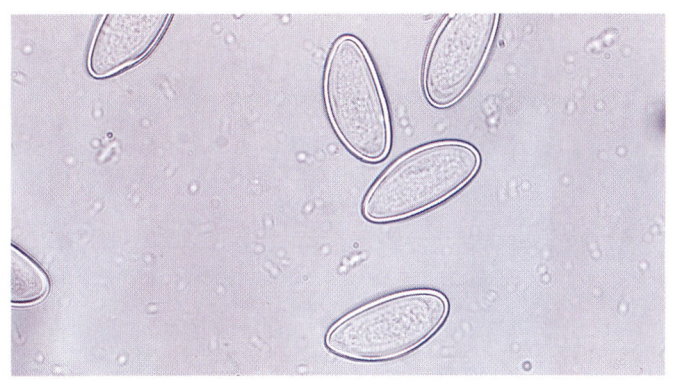

Fig. 20.3 Eggs of pinworm, almost colourless, ovoid and flattened on one side, i.e. with characteristic structural features

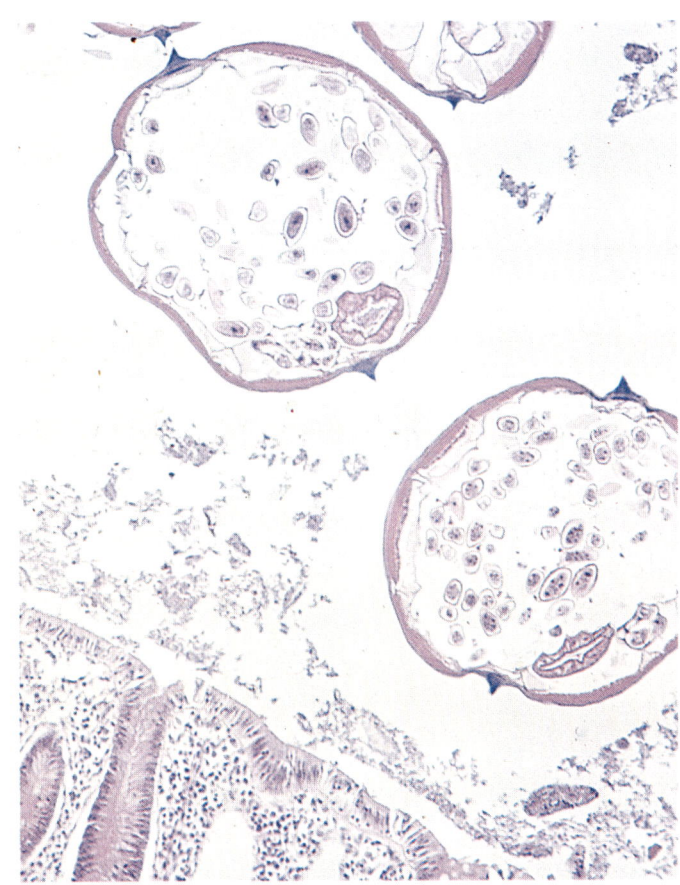

Fig. 20.4 Pinworms in the lumen of the appendix. H&E

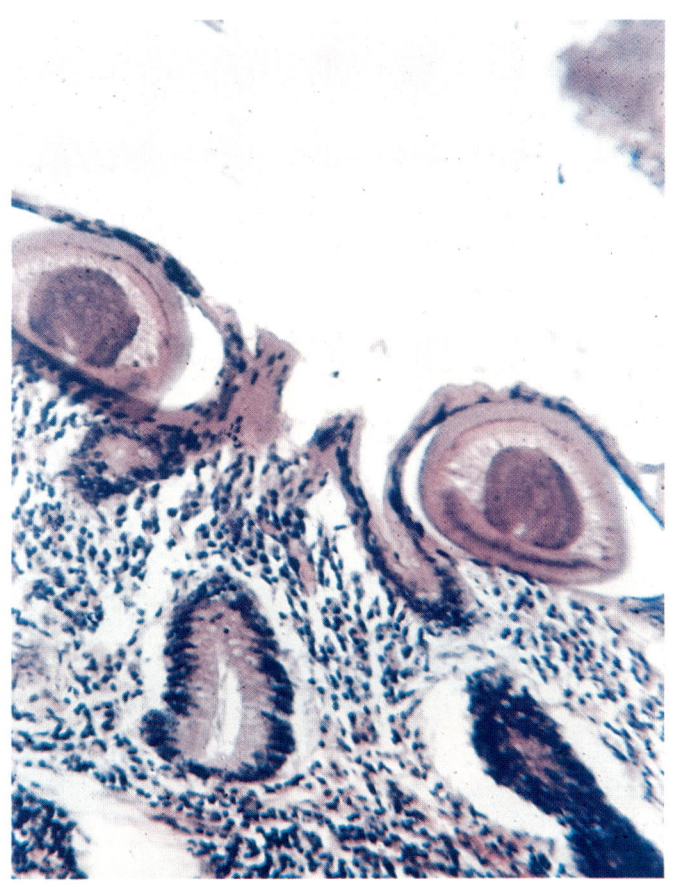

Fig. 20.5 Superficial tissue invasion of pinworms into the intestinal mucosa. H&E

as a probable vector of Dientamoeba fragilis. *Am. J. Trop. Med. Hyg.*, **5**, 258

3. Ockert, G. (1972). Zur Epidemiologie von Dientamoeba fragilis. II. Versuch der Übertragung der Art mit Enterobius-Eiern. *J. Hyg. Epidemiol. Microbiol. Immunobiol.*, **16**, 222

4. Schüffner, W. and Swellengrebel, N. H. (1949). Retrofection in

oxyuriasis. A newly discovered mode of infection with Enterobius vermicularis. *J. Parasit.*, **35**, 138

5. Williams, D. J. and Dixon, M. F. (1988). Sex, Enterobius vermicularis and the appendix. *Br. J. Surg.*, **75**, 1225

6. Symmers, W. S. C. (1950). Pathology of oxyuriasis. *Arch. Path.*, **50**, 475

21. ASCARIASIS

Introduction

This worm infection was described more than 2000 years ago[1]. *Ascaris lumbricoides* is cosmopolitan. It is found more frequently in children than in adults. It has been estimated that about a quarter of the world population is a carrier of this worm[2]. The prevalence of ascariasis is especially high in tropical countries. In Venezuela, we find it often in combination with whipworms and hookworms in the intestinal tract of members of the rural population where it occasionally causes severe complications.

Man is the only host. Ascariasis is not seen in lower animals. Piglets and pigs may be infected experimentally with *A. suum* and *A. lumbricoides*[3-5].

Clinically, this intestinal parasitosis is often asymptomatic. Symptoms may consist of allergic reactions, abdominal pain, anaemia and numerous other symptoms due to diverse complications (see *Pathology* below). Complications may be fatal. The death rate is estimated at 6 per 100 000 carriers. Weakness and lowered resistance, as well as immunological defects, may be due to a massive deprivation of food and vitamins by the worms.

Clinical diagnosis is made by finding the parasites or their eggs in stools or vomited masses. Transient pulmonary infiltrates or worms in hollow organs may be detected by X-ray. Eosinophilia of the blood may indicate worm infection.

The parasite

Ascaris lumbricoides is called the ascarid roundworm and is one of the largest and most common intestinal parasites in man. The mature worms measure up to 40 cm in length and may survive 1-2 years in the human body. They look like earthworms, hence their denomination. The female worms are a little larger than the males. They may lay up to 240 000 eggs per day. Fertilized and non-fertilized eggs may be distinguished morphologically; they measure 60-70 × 50 μm and, typically, are surrounded by three coverings.

Pathogenesis

The ova excreted in the faeces may remain infectious for many months or even years in appropriate humid conditions. They are ingested and go through a special developmental cycle, called the *Ascaris* type, which was mentioned in the introductory remarks about nematodiasis and is shown schematically in Table 13. There is no intermediate host.

The larvae go through consecutive moults while passing through the small bowel wall. They may cause the Löffler syndrome in the lungs, and the so-called larva migrans condition which will be discussed separately (Section 37). Migrating *Ascaris* larvae may carry bacteria[3].

Pathology

The adults of *Ascaris lumbricoides* normally inhabit the small intestine, but may be found in all body cavities, and leave through all body orifices. Sometimes, they are present in large numbers in the lumen of the small bowel

Table 13 *Ascaris lumbricoides*. Schematic representation of the life cycle

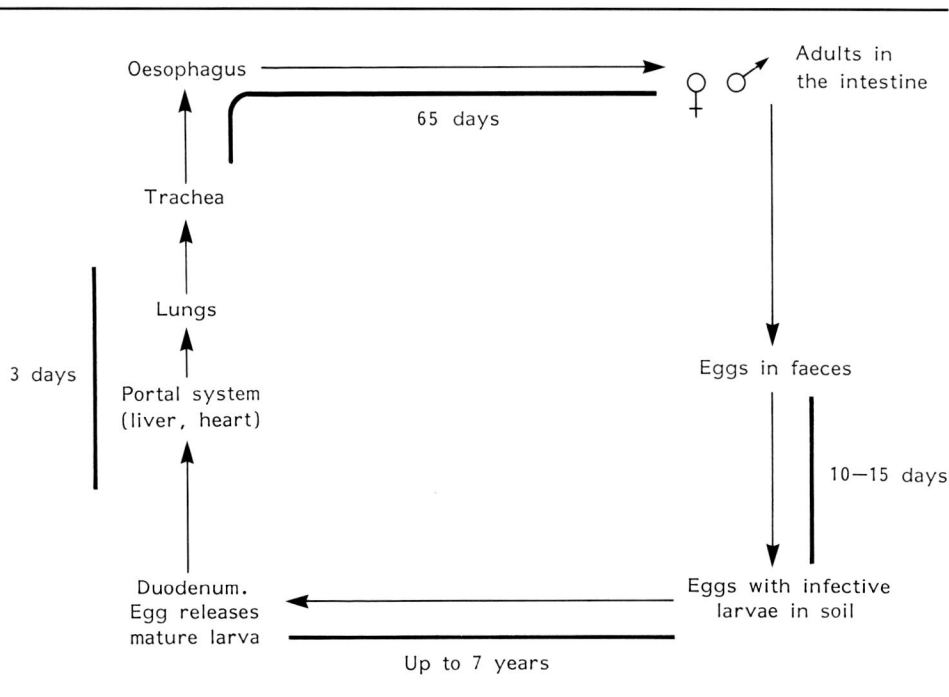

and may produce mechanical ileus, volvulus or intestinal perforation, followed by purulent peritonitis[6] (Figs. 21.1–21.4). Also, a granulomatous peritonitis may be seen due to worm eggs[7] (Figs. 21.5–21.7). Occasionally, perforation of the intestinal wall takes place postmortem.

Coming to, and remaining in, the appendix, they may cause appendicitis. When the worms invade pancreatic ducts, acute obstructive pancreatitis may be the consequence. More often, they obstruct bile ducts and provoke purulent cholangitis and liver abscesses[8–11] (Figs. 21.8–21.10). Also, formation of tumour-like nodules or necrotic foci, sometimes called ascaridiomas, may take place in the liver. In the abscesses and ascaridiomas (Figs. 21.11 and 21.12), numerous *Ascaris* eggs may be encountered (Fig. 21.13). Obstruction of the nasolacrimal duct by this nematode is exceptional[12].

The passage of the larvae of *A. lumbricoides* (and of other worms) through the lungs leads to focal and transient eosinophilic infiltrates (Löffler syndrome). In these organs, the lesions are usually found fortuitously when the organs are examined histologically at autopsy since these foci may not be detected with the naked eye. Microscopic lesions caused by these larvae in other organs will be described later (Section 37).

References

1. Ferreira, L. A. *et al*. (1980). The finding of eggs and larvae of parasitic helminths in archaeological material from Unai, Minas Gerais, Brazil. *Trans. R. Soc. Trop. Med. Hyg.,* **74**, 798
2. Crompton, D. W. T. (1988). The prevalence of ascariasis. *Parasitol. Today,* **4**, 162
3. Adedeji, S. O. *et al*. (1989). Synergistic effect of migrating Ascaris larvae and Escherichia coli in piglets. *J. Helminthol.,* **63**, 19
4. Bernardo, T. M. *et al*. (1990). A critical assessment of abattoir surveillance as a screening test for swine ascariasis. *Can. J. Vet. Res.,* **54**, 274
5. Bernardo, T. M. *et al*. (1990). Ascariasis, respiratory diseases and production indices in selected Prince Edward Island swine herds. *Can. J. Vet. Res.,* **54**, 267
6. Tie-Hsiung, T. and Pin-Liang, C. A. (1963). A case report of panperitonitis due to perforation of Meckel's diverticulum caused by ascariasis. *J. Formosa Med. Assoc.,* **62**, 89
7. Walter, N. and Krishnaswami, H. (1989). Granulomatous peritonitis caused by Ascaris eggs: a report of three cases. *J. Trop. Med. Hyg.,* **92**, 17
8. Teoh, T. B. (1963). A study of gallstones and included worms in recurrent pyogenic cholangitis. *J. Path. Bact.,* **86**, 123
9. Strauszer, T. and Candido, J. (1965). Ascaridiasis intracoledociana diagnosticada por colangiografía postoperatoria (communicación de seis casos, uno de ellos fatal). *Bol. Chil. Parasit.,* **20**, 7
10. Schmid, K. O. (1965). Intrahepatische cholangio-ascaridiasis. *Langenbecks Arch. Klin. Chir.,* **310**, 64
11. Gayotto, L. C. *et al*. (1990). Hepatobiliary alterations in massive biliary ascariasis. Histopathological aspects of an autopsy case. *Rev. Inst. Med. Trop. Sao Paulo,* **32**, 91
12. Cunha, M. C. *et al*. (1989). Obstruction of the nasolacrimal duct by Ascaris lumbricoides. *Ophthal. Plast. Reconstr. Surg.,* **5**, 141

22. TRICHURIASIS

Introduction

This helminthic disease, also called whipworm infection, occurs worldwide but is more common in tropical countries than in temperate zones. Here, 90% of the population may be carriers and, in Venezuela, whipworms are very common. Children are affected most often; hundreds of these worms may be encountered in the intestinal tract.

The whipworms found in dogs and monkeys do not appear to be identical to those found in man. However, *Trichuris* ova may be transmitted, experimentally, from monkeys to man[1].

Clinically, this intestinal parasitosis is usually of minor importance, but heavy infections can cause severe damage to man, especially young children, occasionally resulting in death[2–4]. Most infections are asymptomatic, although numerous parasites may impair the nutrition of the host. Since trichuriasis frequently occurs together with uncinariasis and ascariasis, it cannot be determined which parasites cause the damage. Abdominal pain and all kinds of intestinal symptoms may be due to infection with *Trichuris trichiura*.

For a clinical diagnosis, infection with whipworms may be detected by examination of the stools where the typical eggs of *T. trichiura* can be found. Blood eosinophilia is present, as in other worm infections.

The parasite

Trichocephalus trichiuris is a synonym of *Trichuris trichiura* and, commonly, this worm is named whipworm. Without the long whip, the mature whipworm measures 3–6 mm. The whip is a thin thread-like anterior part, previously thought to be a tail (Fig. 22.1). The worm adheres to the intestinal mucosa with the whip and may live for more than a year in the intestinal tract of man.

Eggs of *T. trichiura* have a typical appearance, showing two polar prominences, and cannot be confused with eggs of other worms. They measure 50 × 25 μm (Fig. 22.2).

Pathogenesis

The infection and developmental stages are of the *Enterobius* type. The ingestion of eggs into the gut leads directly to the release of larvae from the eggs which end up and mature in the large bowel. Complicated cycles of evolution, migration to other organs and intermediate hosts do not exist. The prepatent period is about 90 days. The superficial penetration into the intestinal mucosa by the adult worm is the only damage and leads to a mild inflammatory reaction.

Pathology

Mature whipworms are found in the caecum, around the ileocaecal valve and in the large bowel. Since they do not suck blood – like the hookworms, for instance – they always appear white or pale and are easy to detect (Fig. 22.3).

The penetration of their slender anterior part into the intestinal mucosa does not reach the submucosa (Fig. 22.4). Mononuclear cell infiltrates in the stroma of the mucosa are the consequence of an occasional mucosal invasion and are minimal.

References

1. Horii, Y. and Usui, M. (1985). Experimental transmission of Trichuris ova from monkeys to man. *Trans. R. Soc. Trop. Med. Hyg.,* **79**, 423
2. Gilman, R. H. *et al*. (1983). The adverse consequences of heavy Trichuris infection. *Trans. R. Soc. Trop. Med. Hyg.,* **77**, 432
3. Cooper, E. S. and Bundy, D. A. P. (1988). Trichuris is not trivial. *Parasitol. Today,* **4**, 301
4. Arenas, J. V., Brass, K. and Romero Toanyo, H. (1965). Tricocefalosis. Estudio clínico-patológico. *GEN Caracas,* **20**, 177

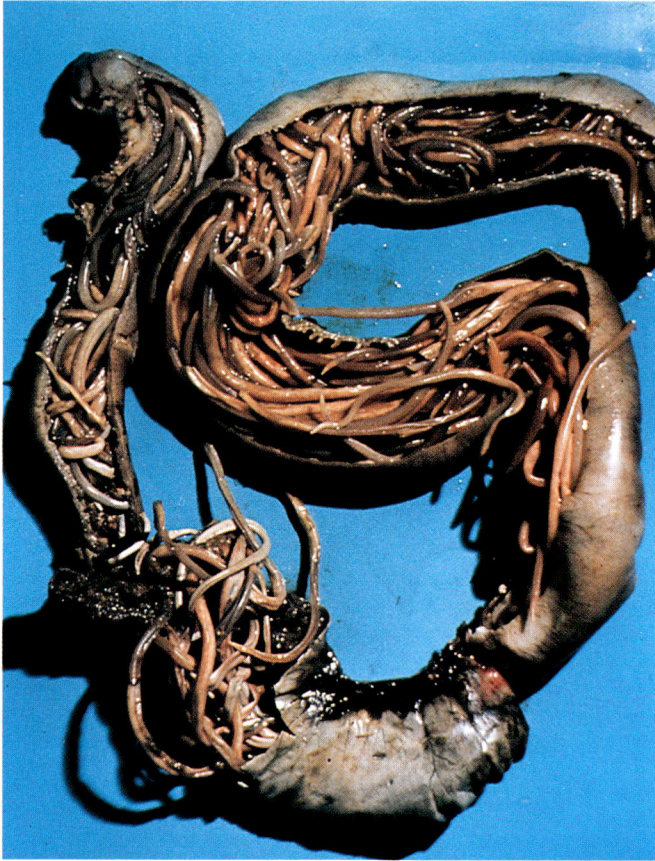

Fig. 21.1   Numerous roundworms (*Ascaris lumbricoides*) filling up the small intestine

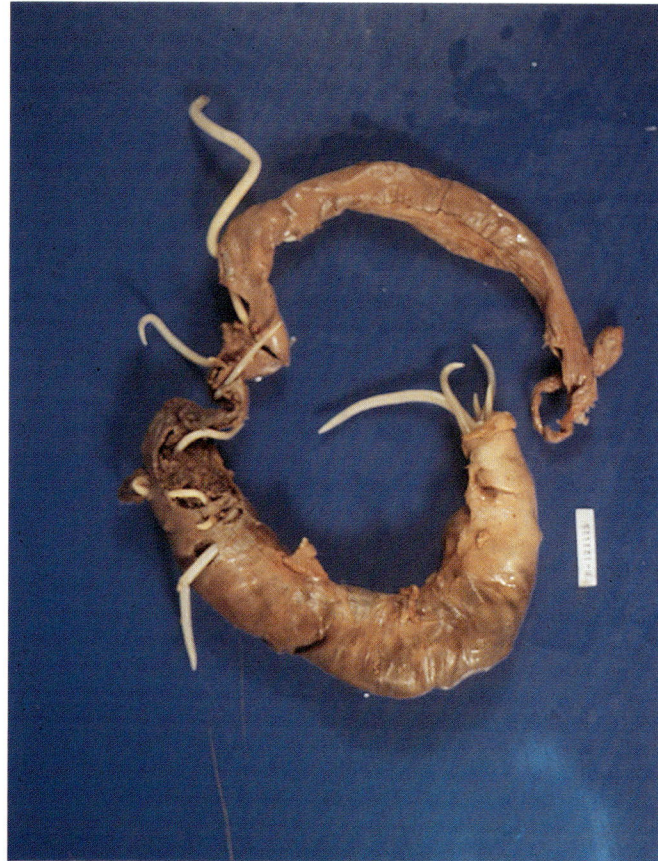

Fig. 21.2   Numerous roundworms perforating the intestinal wall

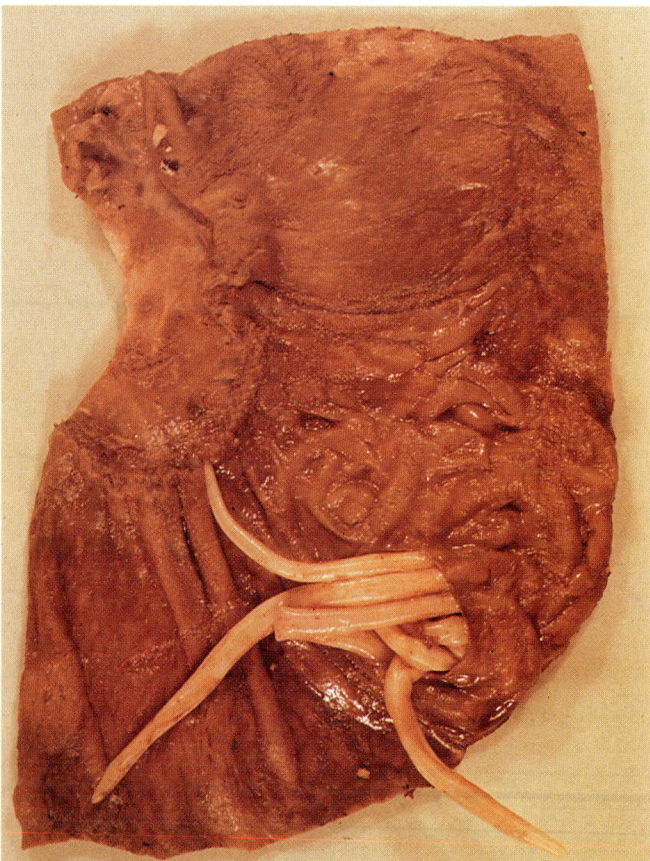

Fig. 21.3   Intestinal perforation by several roundworms, in close-up

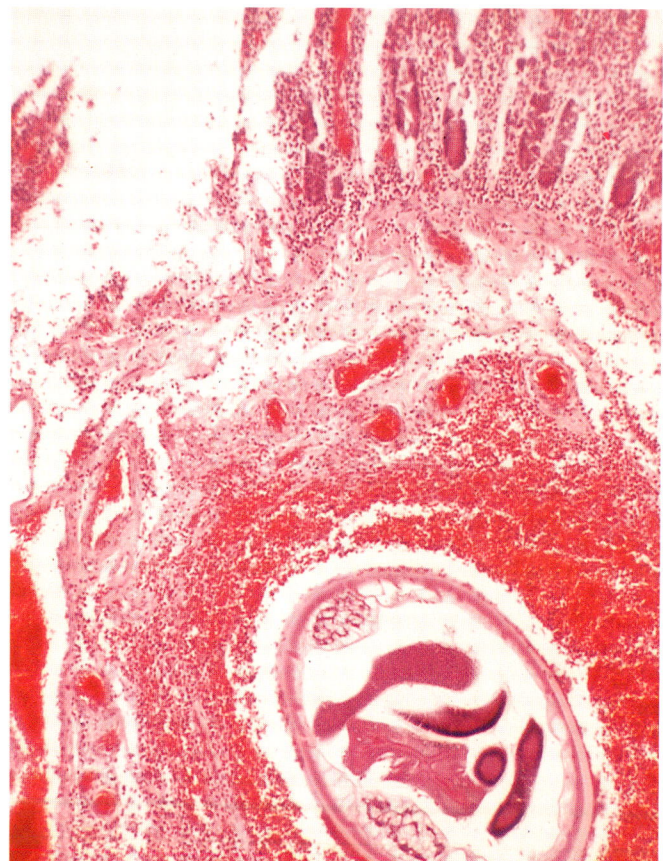

Fig. 21.4   Roundworm, cut transversally, in the intestinal submucosa with massive haemorrhages. H&E

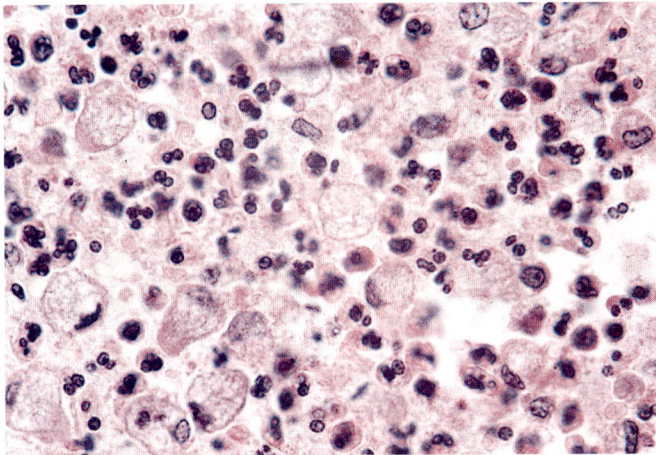

Fig. 21.5 Eggs of *Ascaris lumbricoides* partly necrotized in the granulation tissue of the abdominal wall (after intestinal perforation of worms). The ova are not easily recognizable as deriving from this sort of worm. H&E

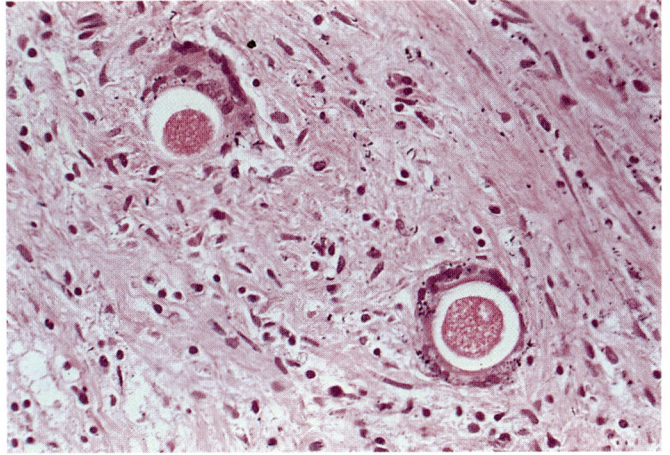

Fig. 21.6 Two eggs of *Ascaris lumbricoides* with foreign body giant cells in an ascaridioma of the liver. H&E

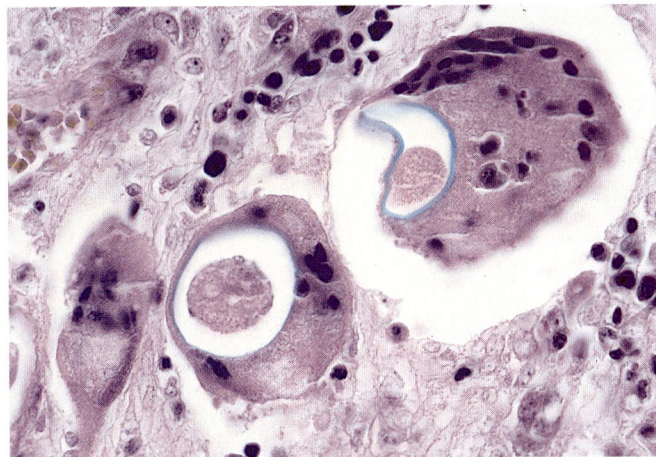

Fig. 21.7 Close-up of a foreign body reaction. Ascaris eggs surrounded by giant cells. The eggs of *Ascaris lumbricoides* in tissues are not easily and surely recognizable as such. H&E

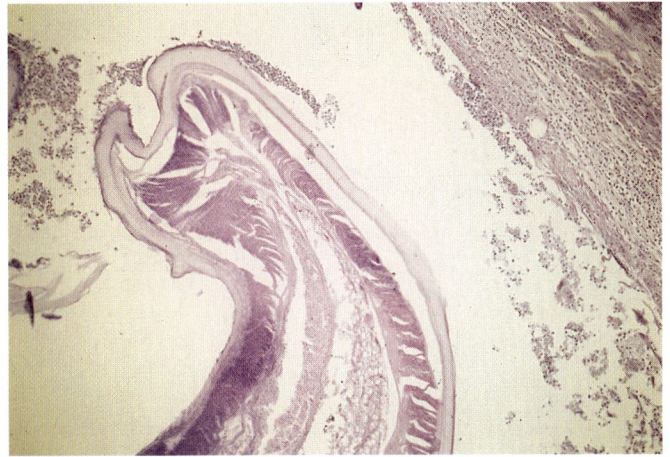

Fig. 21.8 Adult roundworm (*Ascaris lumbricoides*) in a bile duct. H&E

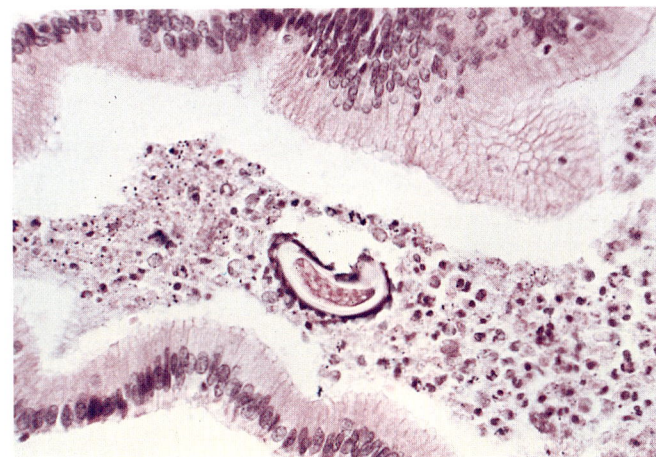

Fig. 21.9 Ascaris egg in the lumen of a bile duct together with leukocytic exudate. H&E

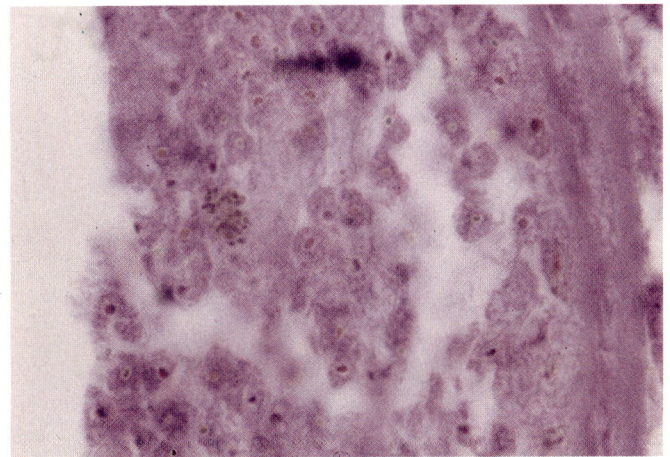

Fig. 21.10 Testicle with spermatozoa of the roundworm in Fig. 21.8 at high power. Male bachelors of *Ascaris lumbricoides* often migrate into the bile and pancreatic ducts in search of female worms. H&E

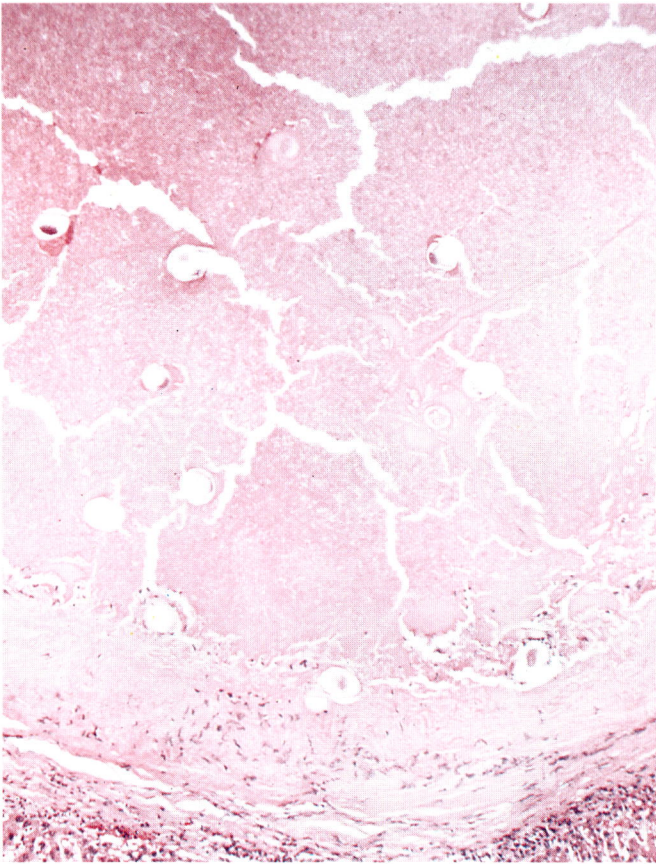

Fig. 21.11 Ascaridioma in the liver at low power. Numerous Ascaris eggs may be seen in the necrotic ('tumour') masses. H&E

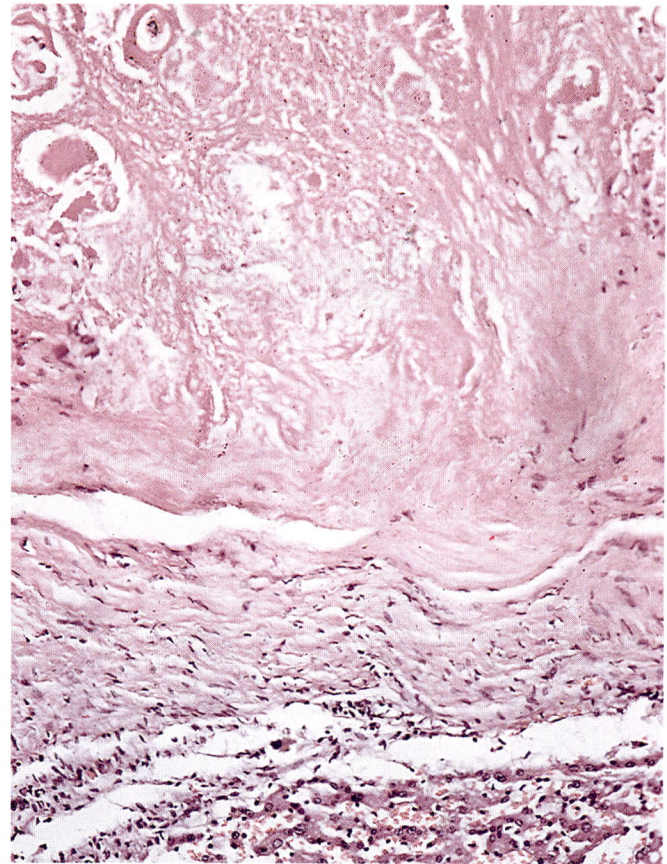

Fig. 21.12 Another field of an 'ascaridioma' of the liver with a fibrous capsule. Worm eggs are also seen. H&E

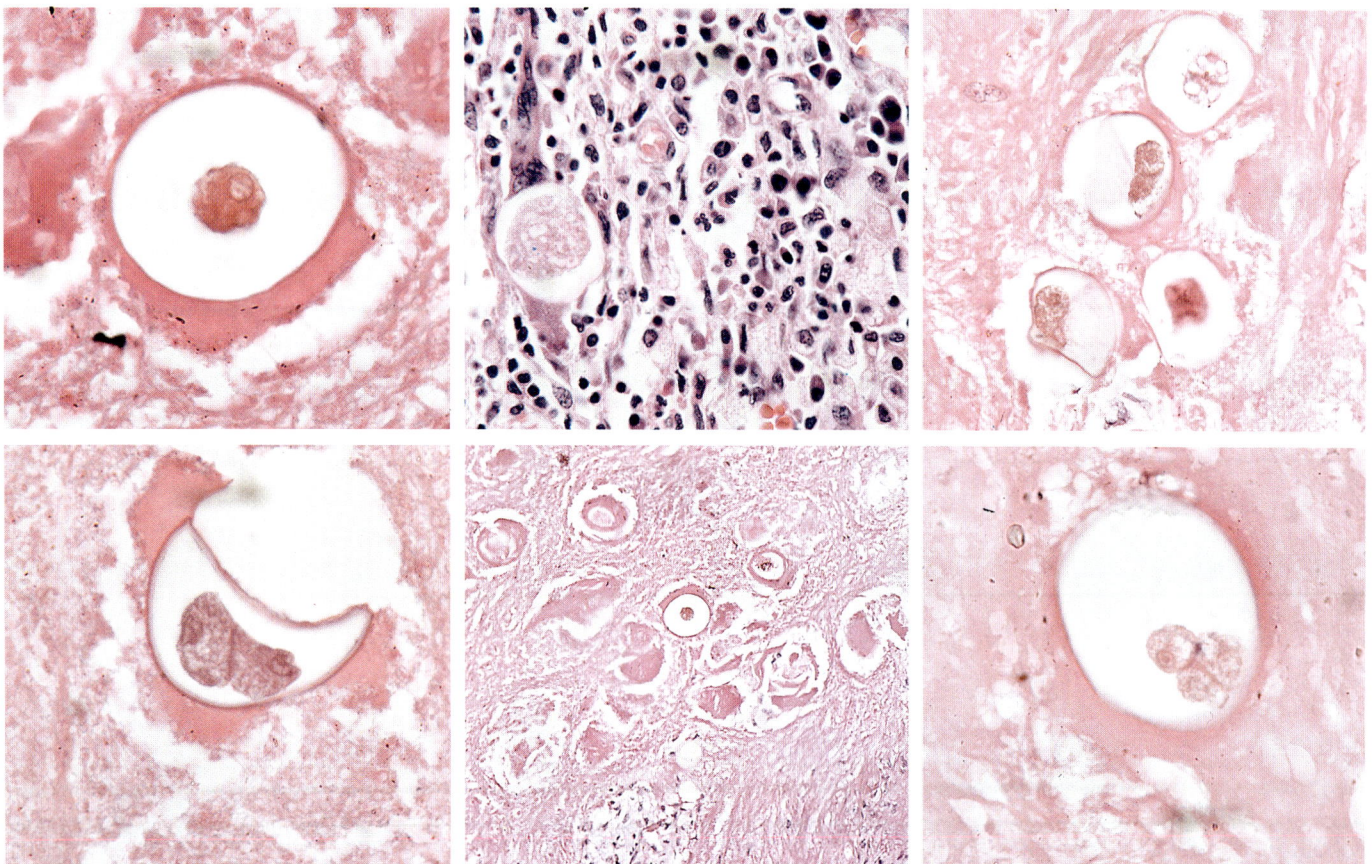

Fig. 21.13 Ova of *Ascaris lumbricoides* from hepatic ascaridiomas and abdominal wall granulomas due to worm eggs. Mostly, they are deformed and not recognizable as Ascaris eggs. H&E

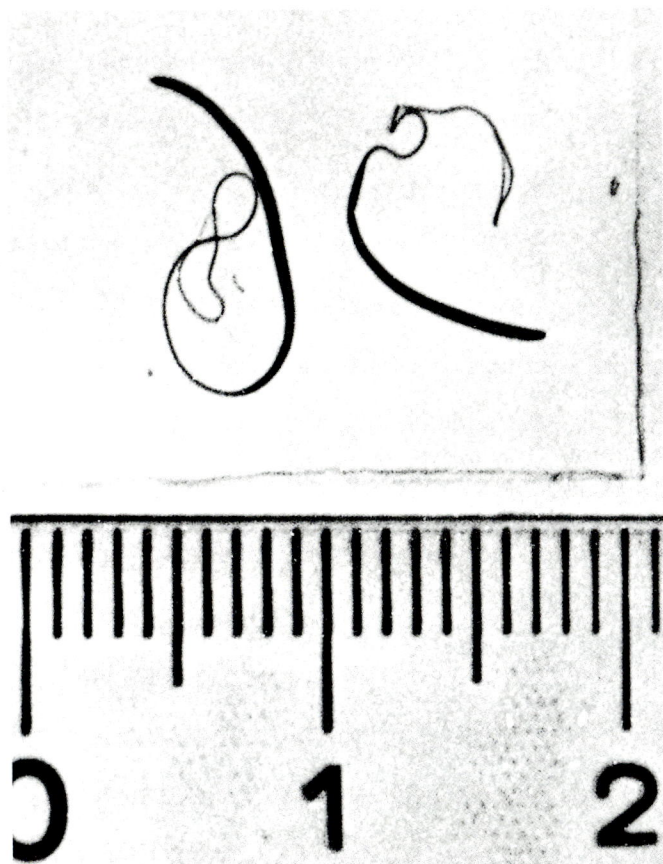

Fig. 22.1 Two whipworms (*Trichuris trichiura*) with the thread-like thin anterior part which mimicks a tail

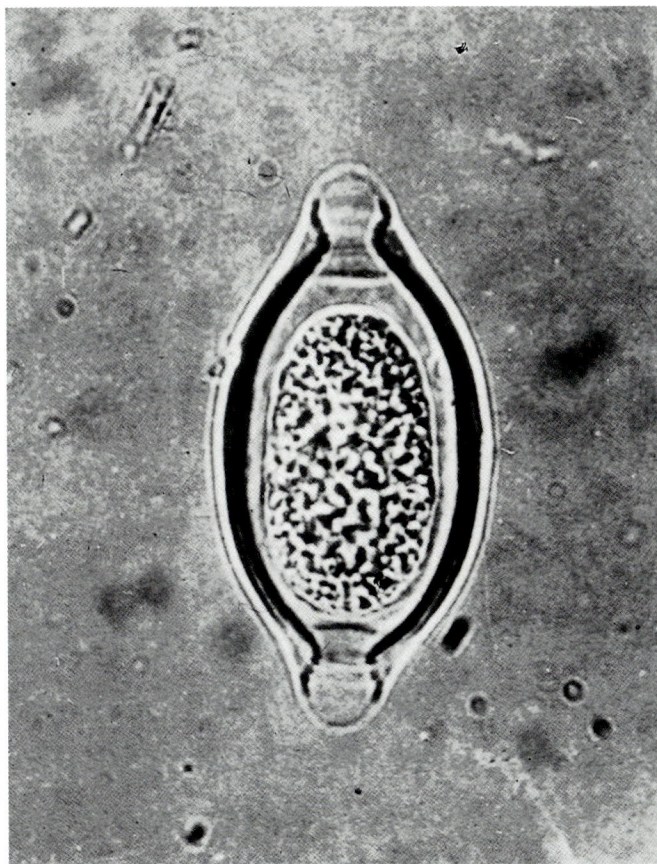

Fig. 22.2 *Trichuris trichiura* egg with the typical two polar prominences

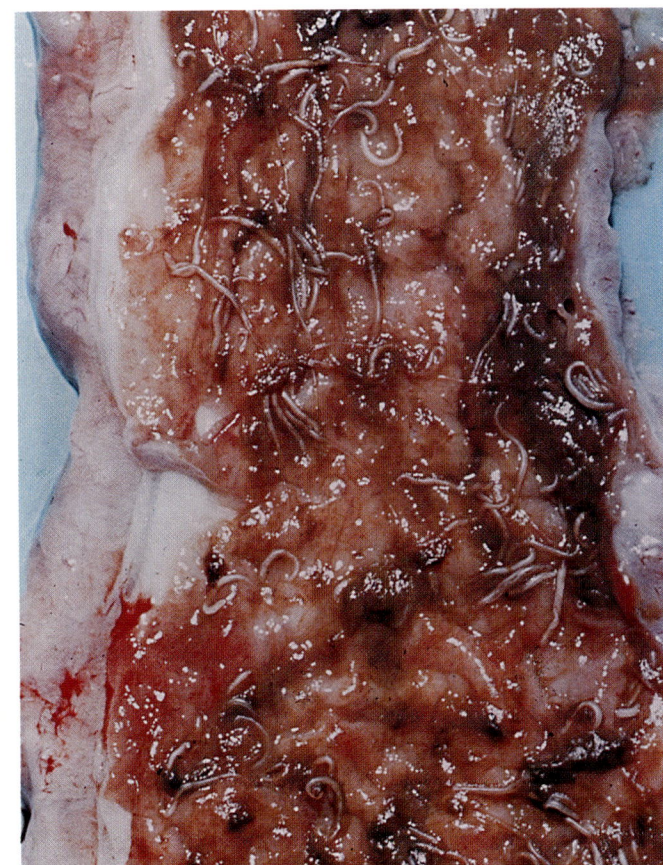

Fig. 22.3 Numerous whitish whipworms in the caecum. Compare with Fig. 23.6

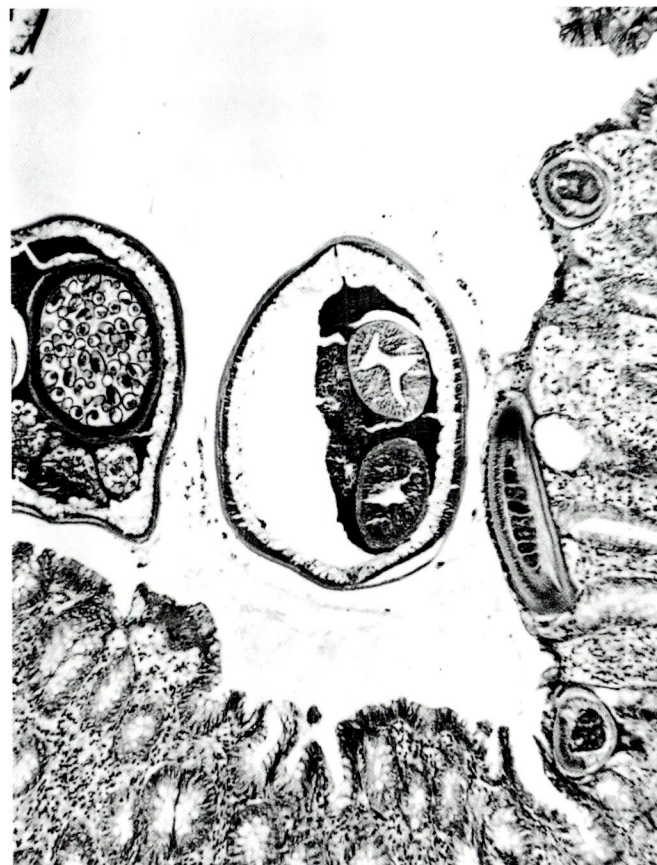

Fig. 22.4 Two whipworms in the lumen of the appendix, one containing numerous eggs. Several worms with superficial penetration into the mucosa. H&E

Table 14 Schematic life cycle of a hookworm

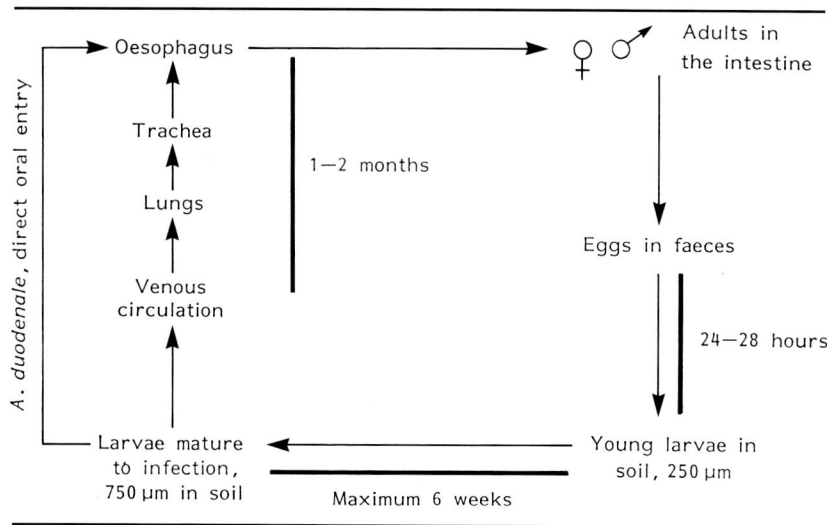

23. UNCINARIASIS

Introduction

Hookworm infections are also called ancylostomiasis, tunnel or miner's disease or necatoriasis. Uncinariasis is a really important worm disease. Twenty to twenty-five per cent of the world population, i.e. more than one billion people, are carriers of hookworms. In addition, it is a dangerous worm disease, unlike many other helminthic infections. In many countries, uncinariasis is a major health problem; about 60 000 individuals die each year from this helminthiasis. Mostly, children are affected.

Hookworm infections are found mainly in tropical countries; *Ancylostoma duodenale* infection is also found in countries with temperate climates. Necatoriasis is well known in Venezuela, particularly in the rural population.

A different hookworm species affects cats and dogs naturally, but it is not pathogenic for man, since, when their larvae enter the human body, they do not mature or migrate. Mice may be used for experimental studies[1].

Clinically, at the site of entering the human body, dermatitis (ground itch) may develop, sometimes persisting for 2 weeks. A few hookworms do not cause disease; however, a massive infection leads to continuous loss of blood, severe anaemia and hypoproteinaemia, weakness and retarded development in children. In the tropics, uncinariasis is one of the important causes of immunodeficiencies and consequent opportunistic infections.

For a clinical diagnosis; numerous eggs of the hookworms can often be found in stools, or the stools may be cultured. Fresh stool specimens should be handled with care, because of the danger of infection for laboratory personnel. Haematologically, a high eosinophilia may be present.

The parasite

Several species of nematodes belong to the hookworms and may produce uncinariasis. The two important hookworms are *Ancylostoma duodenale* which may be found also in the Old World, and *Necator americanus*, observed only in the tropics. In addition, species of the genera *Trichostrongylus* and *Oesophagostomum* may cause uncinariasis. These worms are characterized by microscopic structures similar to teeth or hooks at the oral orifice. Structurally, there are no gross, but only minimal, differences between *Ancylomstoma duodenale* and *Nec-*

ator americanus. Both are 1 cm long on average. Microscopically, *A. duodenale* shows two pairs of fused curved teeth at the mouth, and *N. americanus* has two crescent-shaped cutting plates (Figs. 23.1–23.5). The lifespan of hookworms in the human intestinal tract may be many years (without antihelminthic treatment). Eggs show typical features, are colourless and have a thin shell. They require a minimum temperature of about 18°C with adequate humidity in order to stay alive. The eggs of both species measure 60 × 40 μm.

Pathogenesis

Larvae are released from the eggs of hookworms in a few days and penetrate man, after two moults, transcutaneously. Then, they begin to migrate; see the hookworm type cycle in the general remarks on nematodiasis and the schematic Table 14. *A. duodenale* may also enter man orally. Mature worms, with their hook-like structures at the mouth, actively destroy the mucosa of the small intestine and suck blood. Occasionally, they may penetrate into the submucosa and suck blood at these sites, i.e. from the haemorrhages they themselves have caused. With numerous worms in the intestinal tract, the continuous loss of blood may be considerable.

Pathology

Dog or cat hookworms, penetrating transcutaneously, may produce creeping eruption (cutaneous larva migrans) in man; see Section 37.

During the migration of hookworm larvae (*A. duodenale* or *N. americanus*) in man, foci of eosinophilic infiltrates may be found in the lungs. Often it is difficult to detect larvae in these foci.

Mature hookworms in man are found in the jejunum or ileum. They measure 1 cm on average, and are mostly dark red or black because of the sucked blood (Fig. 23.6). Other short intestinal nematodes, e.g. *Strongyloides stercoralis*, *Enterobius vermicularis* and *Trichuris trichiura*, may be easily distinguished by their size, localization and colour. Grossly, focal haemorrhages of variable extent may be seen in the mucosa. As described above, hookworms produce microscopic destructive lesions of the mucosa of the small bowel when biting with their hooks, and may penetrate into the submucosa (Figs. 23.7 and 23.8).

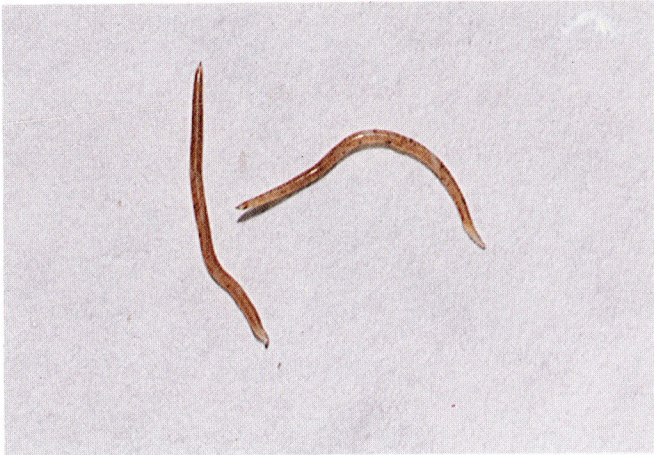

Fig. 23.1   Two *Necator americanus* (mature worms)

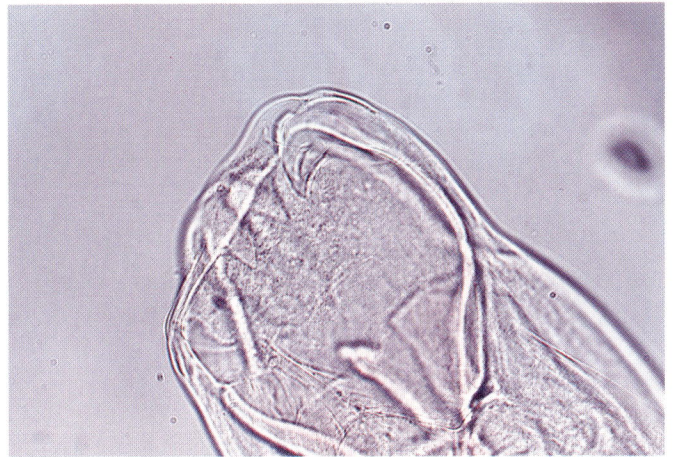

Fig. 23.2   Head of *Ancylostoma duodenale*

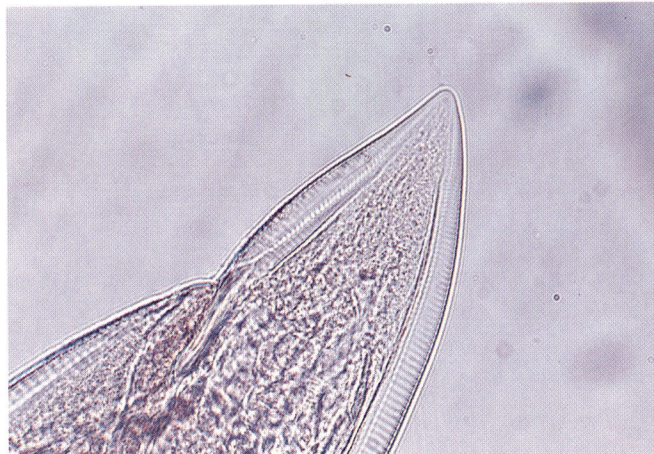

Fig. 23.3   Posterior part of an *Ancylostoma duodenale* female

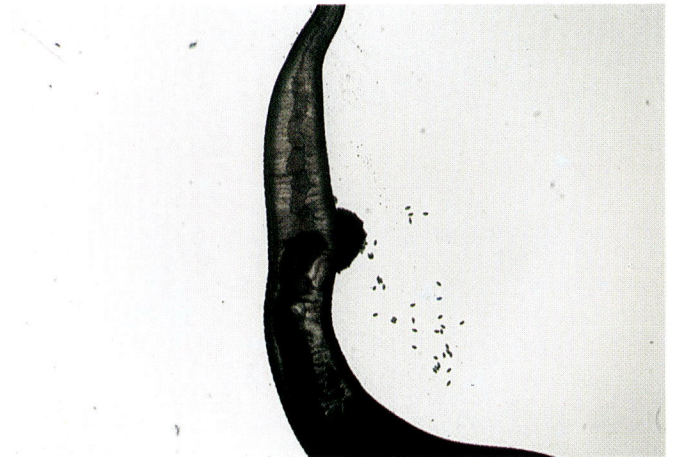

Fig. 23.4   *Necator americanus* expelling eggs

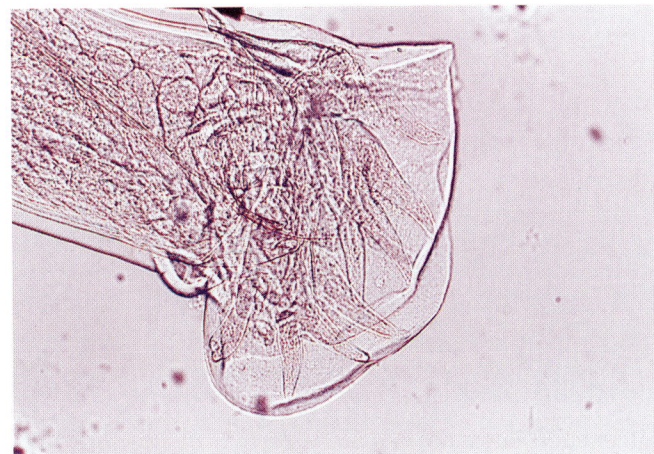

Fig. 23.5   Bolsa copulatrix of a male *Ancylostoma duodenale*

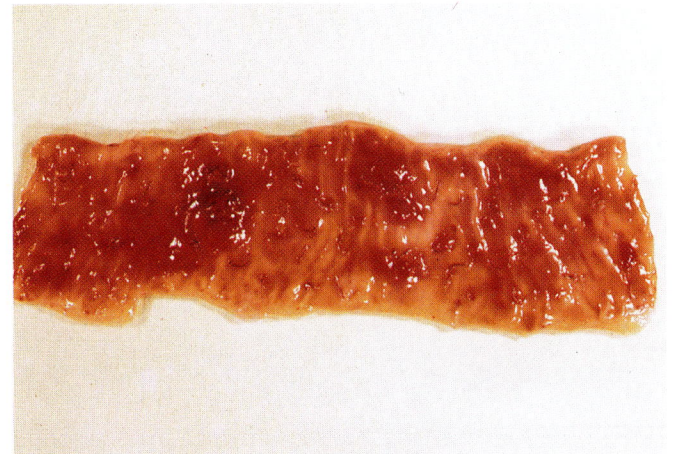

Fig. 23.6   Small intestine with numerous dark hookworms and some haemorrhages in the mucosa. Compare with Fig. 22.3

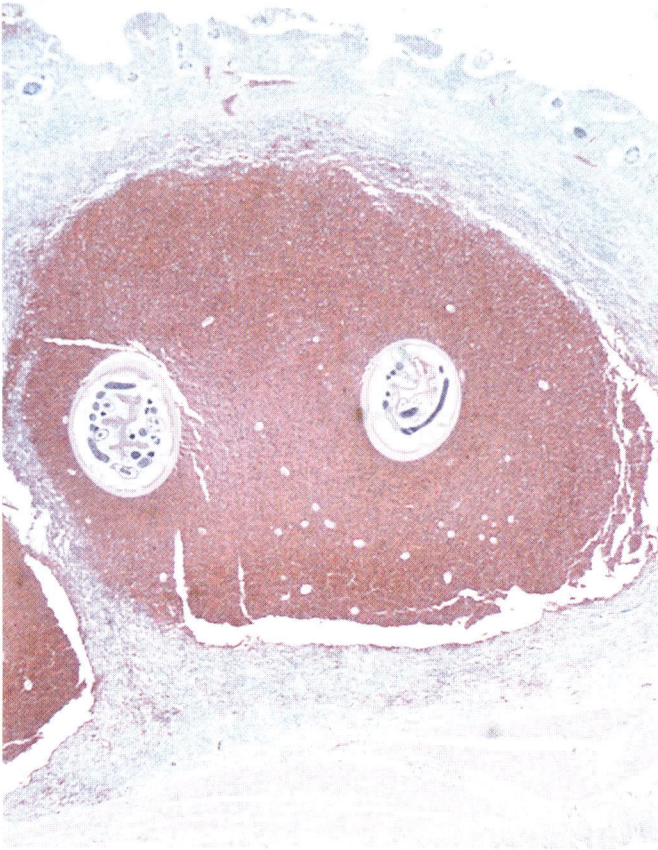

Fig. 23.7 Two horizontally cut hookworms in the haemorrhage of the duodenal submucosa. H&E

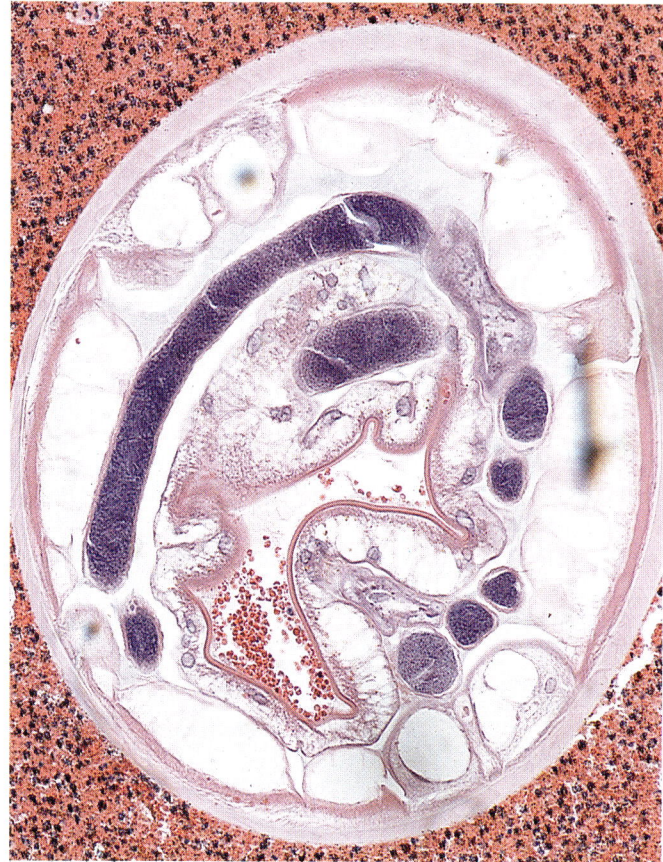

Fig. 23.8 High power view of a horizontally cut hookworm encountered fortuitously in the wall of the duodenum. Same case as Fig. 23.7. The sucked blood (erythrocytes) is seen clearly in the gut of the worm. H&E

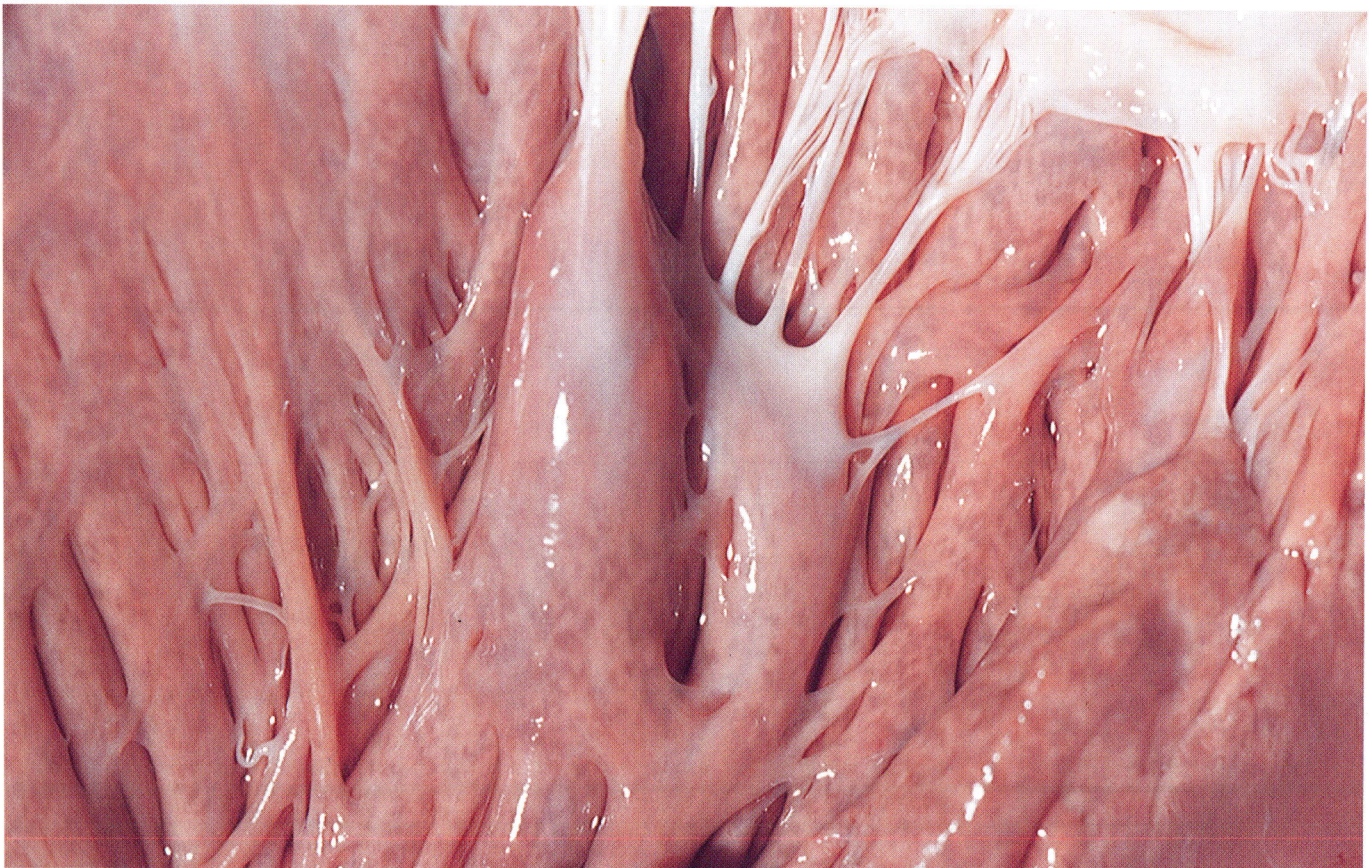

Fig. 23.9 'Tiger heart', i.e. fatty degeneration of the myocardium, in a case of marked chronic anaemia in an infant in Venezuela, due to hookworm parasitosis

The consequences of these intestinal injuries, with the continuous loss of blood, may be severe. The resulting chronic anaemia is of an hypochromic, microcytic and iron-deficiency type[2-4]. Previously, it was called chlorosis or 'green sickness', particularly in adolescent females. Fatty myocardial degeneration, due to chronic hypoxaemia, often leads to cardiac insufficiency and a fatal outcome (Fig. 23.9).

Histologically, eosinophilic enteritis may be observed[5]. Small intestinal mucosal biopsies do not reveal either histological or enzymatic pathological changes[6].

References

1. Wilkinson, M. J. et al. (1990). Necator americanus in the mouse: histopathological changes associated with the passage of larvae through the lungs of mice exposed to primary and secondary infection. Parasitol. Res., **76**, 386

2. Layrisse, M. and Roche, M. (1964). The relationship between anemia and hookworm infection. Results of surveys of rural Venezuela population. Am. J. Hyg., **79**, 279

3. Roche, M. and Layrisse, M. (1966). The nature and causes of hookworm anemia. Am. J. Trop. Med. Hyg., **16**, 1044

4. Martinez-Torres, C. et al. (1967). Hookworm and intestinal blood loss. Trans. R. Soc. Trop. Med. Hyg., **61**, 373

5. Croese, T. J. (1988). Eosinophilic enteritis – a recent North Queensland experience. Aust. N.Z. J. Med., **18**, 848

6. Youssef, M. E. and Abou-Zakham, A. A. (1991). Some histopathological and histochemical aspects of human ancylostomiasis. J. Egypt. Soc. Parasitol., **21**, 219

24. STRONGYLOIDIASIS

Introduction

Typical and special features of this worm infection are the marked tissue lesions in the small, and sometimes in the large, bowel which are often fatal. Strongyloidiasis is a frequent intestinal parasitosis in the tropics. The worms and their larvae require a mean temperature of at least 15°C for their development; this explains partly their geographic distribution which is similar to that of hookworms. In some countries, 30–60% of people are infected, and this worm infection has also been observed in miners. In Japan and South Europe, cases of this infection are only reported occasionally. In Venezuela, this worm disease is common.

Larvae of Strongyloides stercoralis from animal hosts (dogs) enter man and cause creeping eruption, but maturation and migration does not occur in man (as in hookworms for animals). Other species of Strongyloides are found in primates, rats and other mammals[1].

Clinically, the infection may vary from being latent and asymptomatic to massive infection with generalization. A fatal outcome is not exceptional because of the picture of malabsorption syndrome.

In immunocompromised patients, cases of AIDS and cortisone-treated patients, exacerbation of latent worm infections is becoming increasingly important[2-5]. Symptomatology depends on the localization of the parasites; symptoms are mostly those of enterocolitis.

Clinical diagnosis depends on the confirmation of free-moving larvae in stools. Eggs are not always found in stools. Larvae may also be looked for in aspirated material from duodenum, in sputum and in urine. Also, small-bowel biopsies should be considered as a diagnostic tool[6]. Surprisingly, parasites can be detected in gastric or duodenal biopsies when malignant tumours are suspected. Blood eosinophilia might be absent in immunosuppressed patients. Stool cultures may also be used for diagnostic purposes. For handling fresh stool specimens, see Uncinariasis.

The parasite

Strongyloides stercoralis is also named Dwarf threadworm. The important parthenogenetic females of this worm species reach only 2 mm in length in the intestinal tract and are almost impossible to see with the naked eye. The adult worms have a long life-span[7]. When they live for many years in man, this may be due to the long life-span or to continued auto-infection. Eggs are similar to those of hookworms; they measure 55 × 30 μm.

Pathogenesis

Man is the sole host. The possibilities for development and infection are rather complicated:

1. Parthogenetic females lay eggs which hatch out as larvae in the intestinal lumen of the host and pass out in the faeces. In soil, the larvae become infectious (Fig. 24.1) and may penetrate man transcutaneously (*direct development*) going on to migrate through the hookworm type of cycle

2. In addition to direct development (above), there may also be *indirect development*, i.e. free-living female and male worms may mate and produce eggs which become fertilized. Later, larvae may penetrate man (see above).

   In summary, direct and indirect development lead to percutaneous larval invasion. The larvae of S. sterocoralis may move through tissues at speeds up to 10 cm per hour[8].

3. It is also possible to have endo- and exo-auto-(hyper)-infection by endogenous Strongyloides larvae. *Endo-auto-(hyper)-infection* takes place by penetration of the mucosa by larvae which become infectious in the intestinal lumen without reaching the exterior. This occurs mostly in the colon. *Exo-auto-hyper-infection* is the transcutaneous penetration of larvae which derive, not from soil, but directly from the intestinal tract of the host, on the perianal skin, i.e. as in 1 and 2, but with a determined location of transcutaneous penetration.

In addition to transcutaneous infection, oral infection by food or water is possible but very rare. Transmission to newborns via the mother's milk is said to be possible.

Worms and larvae invade the intestinal mucosa. The larvae reach all layers of the intestinal wall, causing inflammation, and become haematogenously generalized.

Pathology

The adult worms, 2 mm long, are almost invisible to the naked eye. They are situated in the upper small bowel.

Grossly, in the small and large intestine, a marked enterocolitis may be present with haemorrhages, necrotic areas and ulcerations in the mucosa. Involvement of the colon usually indicates a hyper or internal auto-infection. Also, linitis plastica has been reported as due to strongyloidiasis[9], as well as gastric strongyloidiasis imitating peptic ulcer[10] (Fig. 24.2).

Microscopically, adult worms and larvae may be found

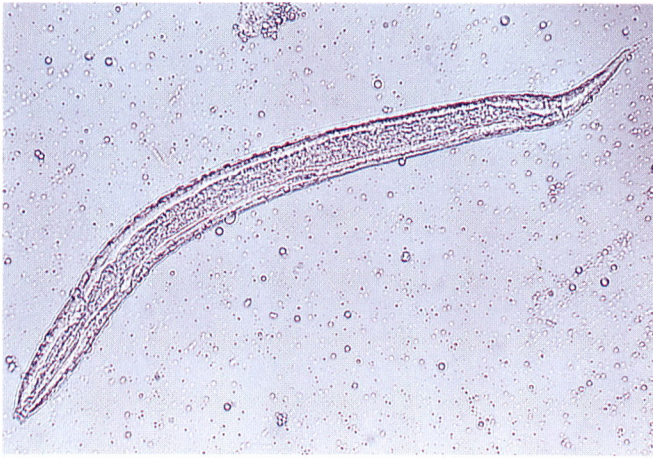

Fig. 24.1   Rhabditiform larva of *Strongyloides stercoralis* in a copro-culture

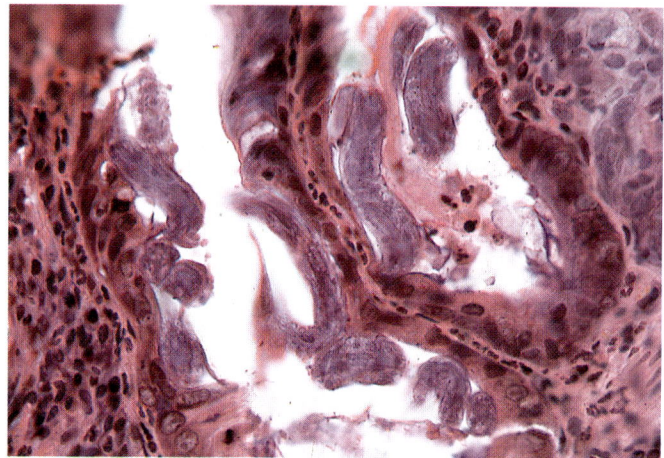

Fig. 24.2   Larvae and adults of *Strongyloides stercoralis* in a gastric biopsy. H&E (Case of Dr Marcelo Mendoza, Mérida)

Fig. 24.3   Numerous adult worms and larvae in the intestinal wall in a case of a marked strongyloidiasis, low power. H&E

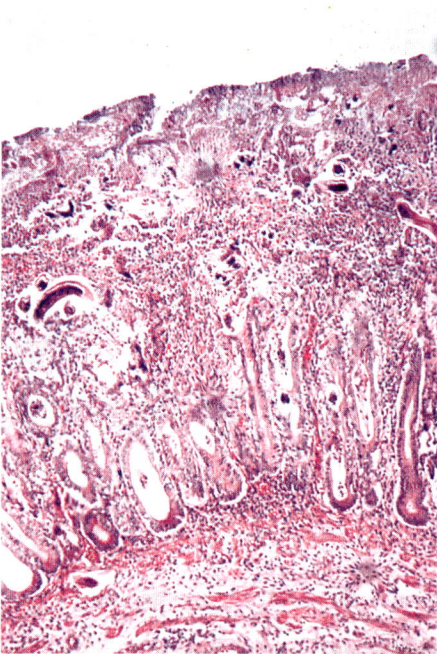

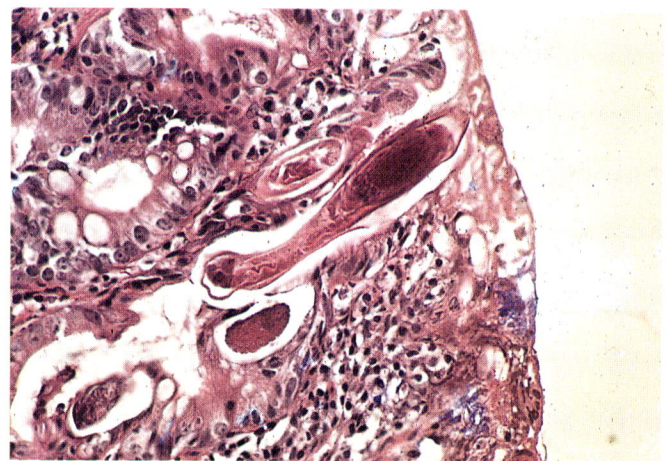

Fig. 24.4   Larvae of *Strongyloides stercoralis* in the intestinal mucosa. H&E

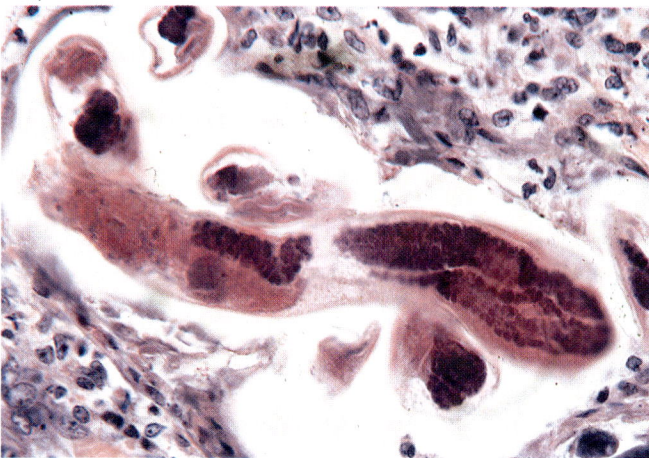

Fig. 24.5   Larvae of *Strongyloides stercoralis* in the intestinal mucosa cut in several directions at high power. H&E

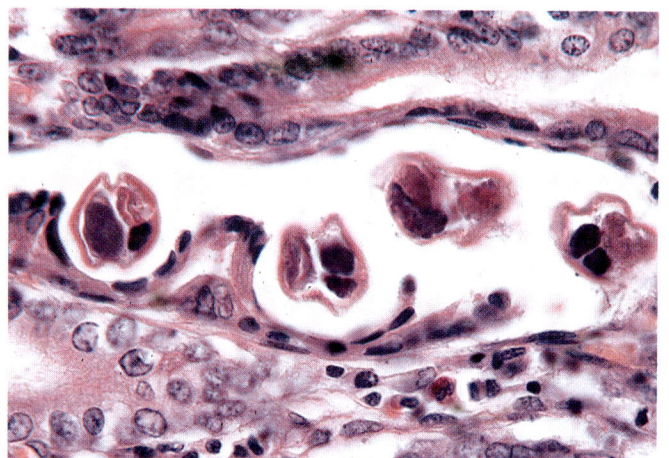

Fig. 24.6   Larvae of *Strongyloides stercoralis* in the intestinal mucosa cut transversally. H&E

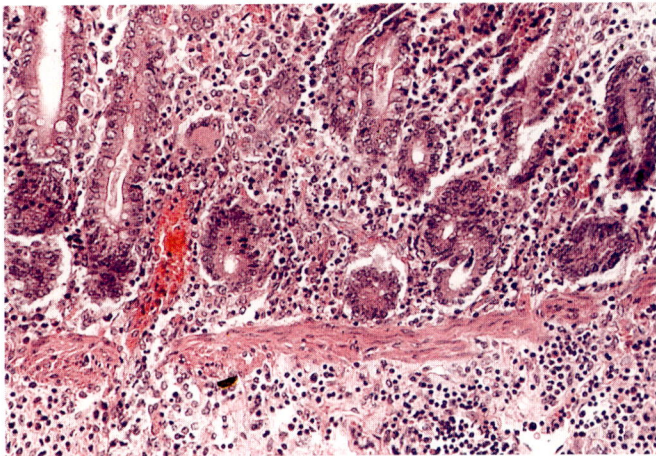

Fig. 24.7 Marked colitis in a case of autoinfection with *Strongyloides stercoralis*. H&E

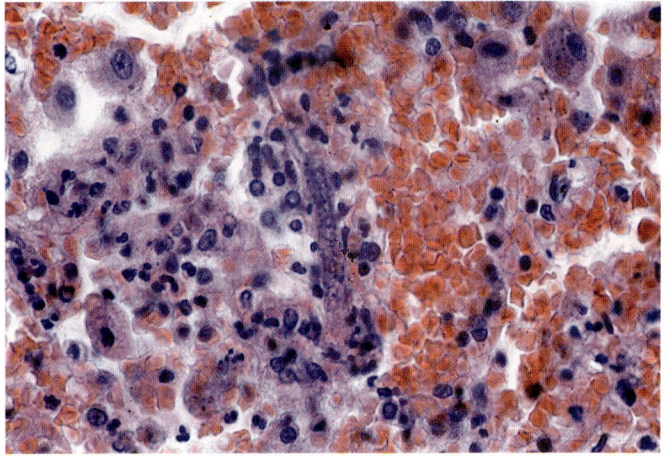

Fig. 24.8 Larva of *Strongyloides stercoralis* in the lung with marked haemorrhagic inflammation. The larva is not easy to detect. H&E

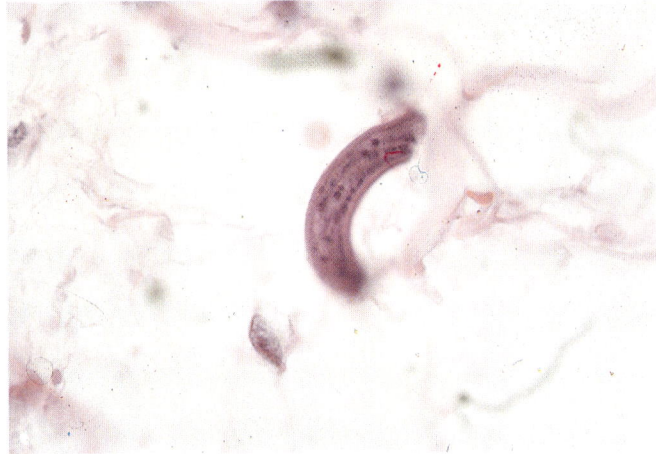

Fig. 24.9 Larva of *Strongyloides stercoralis* in the lung, easy to recognize without inflammatory reaction by the dark dots. H&E

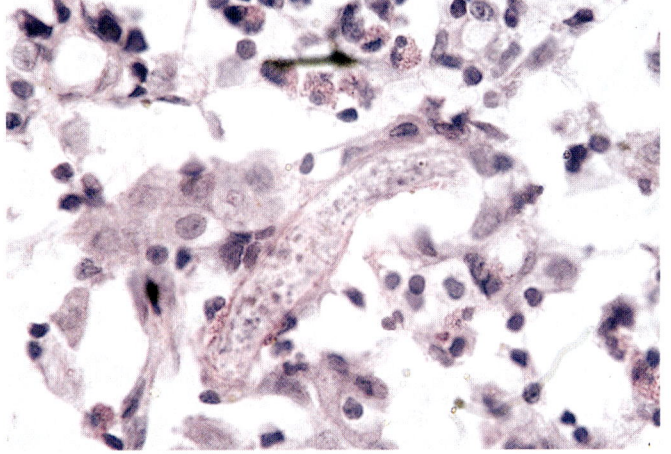

Fig. 24.10 Larva of *Strongyloides* in lymph node with marked eosinophilic lymphadenitis. The microfilaria-like larva is easily recognized by the dark dots. H&E

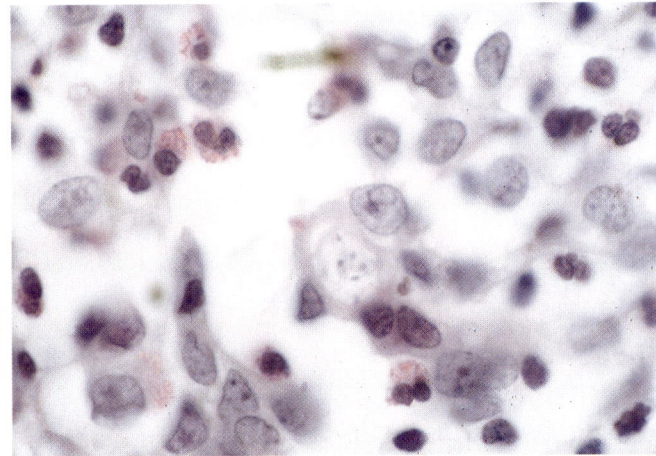

Fig. 24.11 Same lymph node as in Fig. 24.10. At high power eosinophilic lymphadenitis and, in the centre, a transversally cut larva of *Strongyloides stercoralis* may be seen. H&E

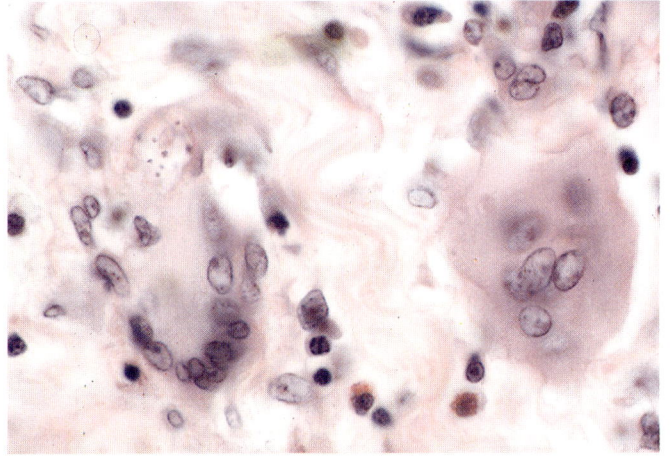

Fig. 24.12 Same lymph node as Figs. 24.10 and 24.11. A transversally cut larva of *Stronglyoides stercoralis* may be detected in the giant cell on the left side. H&E

in the Lieberkühn crypts and deeper, up to the submucosa. Occasionally, it is difficult to differentiate between them (Figs. 24.3–24.7). The larvae are recognized because they show small dots and may be present in all layers of the intestinal wall. Eggs are scarce and difficult to detect in tissues. The tissue reaction consists mostly of non-specific inflammation with lymphocytes, plasma cells and leukocytes. Eosinophilic leukocytes are normally scarce. When numerous eosinophilic leukocytes, giant cells and granulomas are present, it appears that this hypersensibility is due to endo-auto-hyper-infection. Larvae may also be found in skin[11], lungs (Figs. 24.8 and 24.9), liver[12], lymph nodes (Figs. 24.10–24.12) and other extra-intestinal sites; see Section 37.

References

1. Elangbam, C. S. et al. (1990). Strongyloidiasis in cotton rats (Sigmodon hispidus) from central Oklahoma. J. Wildl. Dis., **26**, 398
2. Rogers, W. A. and Nelson, B. (1966). Strongyloidiasis and malignant lymphoma, 'opportunistic infection by a nematode'. J. Am. Med. Assoc., **195**, 685
3. Cruz, T. et al. (1966). Fatal strongyloidiasis in patients receiving corticosteroids. N. Engl. J. Med., **275**, 1093
4. Genta, R. M., Miles, P. and Fields, K. (1989). Opportunistic Strongyloides stercoralis infection in lymphoma patients. Cancer, **63**, 1407
5. Gompels, M. M. et al. (1991). Disseminated strongyloidiasis in AIDS: uncommon but important. AIDS, **5**, 329
6. La Salle, R. et al. (1988). Strongiloidiasis duodenal. V. Congr. Ven. Med. Int. Barquisimeto
7. Grove, D. I. (1982). Treatment of strongyloidiasis with Thiabendazole, an analysis of toxicity and effectiveness. Trans. R. Soc. Trop. Med. Hyg., **76**, 114
8. McKerrow, J. H. et al. (1990). Strongyloides stercoralis: identification of a protease that facilitates penetration of skin by the infective larvae. Exp. Parasitol., **70**, 134
9. Lopez, J. E. (1988). Linitis plástica como manifestación de Strongiloidiasis gástrica. V. Congr. Ven. Med. Int. Barquisimeto
10. Pruglo, I. V. et al. (1990). Gastric strongyloidiasis imitating peptic ulcer. Arkh. Patol., **52**, 53
11. von Kuster, L. C. and Genta, R. M. (1988). Cutaneous manifestations of strongyloidiasis. Arch. Dermatol., **124**, 1826
12. Lopez, J. E. et al. (1988). Strongiloidiasis hepática. Presentación de un caso con confirmación histopatológica. V. Congr. Ven. Med. Int. Barquisimeto

25. TRICHINOSIS

Introduction

This disease is also called trichinellosis. Lesions caused by the larvae of Trichinella spiralis are more important than those caused by the mature worms. It is one of the few parasitoses with high fever. Trichinosis has a worldwide distribution in man and lower animals. It is relatively common in the USA, Canada and Eastern Europe. In Germany, trichinosis has been practically eradicated by obligatory official meat inspection. However, in the eighties, an epidemic was reported in Germany with more than 100 infected people[1]. In the tropics, the prevalence appears to be low. Autochthonous infections have not been reported in Venezuela.

This worm infection is known in almost all mammal species, above all in rodents and wild animals. Domestic[2] and wild pigs are the main sources of human infection. Mice and monkeys are used for experimental work[3–6].

Previously, epidemic outbreaks often occurred and a fatal outcome was not exceptional. Lately, epidemics have also been reported in Central Europe[7].

Worm infection often is asymptomatic. There is a gut trichinosis (caused by adult worms) and a muscle trichinosis (caused by larvae). The first may show gastroenteritic symptoms with fever; the latter occurs with muscle pain and swelling, signs of toxicity and allergy, fever and oedema (eyelid). The fatal outcome is due to pneumonia or cardiac failure.

For clinical diagnosis, mature worms and larvae may be present in stools and larvae may be found in blood or in muscle biopsies. Eosinophilia is not always present. During official meat inspections, larvae are found in muscle samples microscopically, without staining and at low magnification.

The parasite

Trichinella spiralis is the main causal agent. Another species, T. pseudospiralis is of minor importance and shows only minimal differences.

In the intestinal tract, the mature female worm measures 3–4 mm and the male 1.5 mm (Figs. 25.1 and 25.3). They are difficult to see with the naked eye. The female is viviparous and produces up to 1000–2000 larvae. The latter measure from $100\,\mu m$ to 1 mm.

Pathogenesis

Trichinella spiralis goes through the Trichinella type of life cycle (see the general remarks under Nematodiasis). The larvae are ingested by the host, mostly in raw meat. They invade the mucosa of the small bowel (Figs. 25.3 and 25.4) where they develop[8,9]. The mature worms have a short lifespan. The larvae may be disseminated lymphogenously or haematogenously. In the skeletal muscle, they invade muscle fibres where they remain viable for a long time. Inflammatory reaction is scarce. Later, a fibrotic capsule develops and calcification takes place.

Pathology

Mature worms are found in the mucosa of the ileum. The larvae are observed mostly in the muscle fibres of the diaphragm, intercostal muscles, larynx, tongue and extra-ocular muscles (Figs. 25.5–25.8). Muscles of the extremities are seldom involved. Exceptionally, the lungs and central nervous system are affected. Trichinae are never seen in the myocardium.

Non-specific inflammation around the larvae, arranged in a spiral, is minimal. Later, calcified nodules with a fibrotic capsule may develop; these are grossly visible.

References

1. Feldmeier, H. et al. (1984). Untersuchungen über die Epidemiologie der Trichinella-spiralis-Infektion in der Eifel 1982. Dtsch. Med. Wschr., **109**, 205
2. Cowen, P. et al. (1990). Survey of trichinosis in breeding and cull swine, using an enzyme-linked immunoabsorbent assay. Am. J. Vet. Res., **51**, 924
3. Antonios, S. N. et al. (1989). Experimental trichinosis in alloxan induced diabetes in mice. J. Egypt. Soc. Parasitol., **19**, 149
4. Brown, P. J. and Bruce, R. G. (1989). Kinetics of IgA plasma cells in the intestine of NIH mice infected with Trichinella spiralis. Res. Vet. Sci., **46**, 187
5. Jasmer, D. P. (1991). Trichinella spp.: differential expression of acid phosphatase and myofibrillar proteins in infected muscle cells. Exp. Parasitol., **72**, 321
6. Kumar, V. et al. (1990). Characterization of a Trichinella isolate from polar bear. Ann. Soc. Belg. Med. Trop., **70**, 131

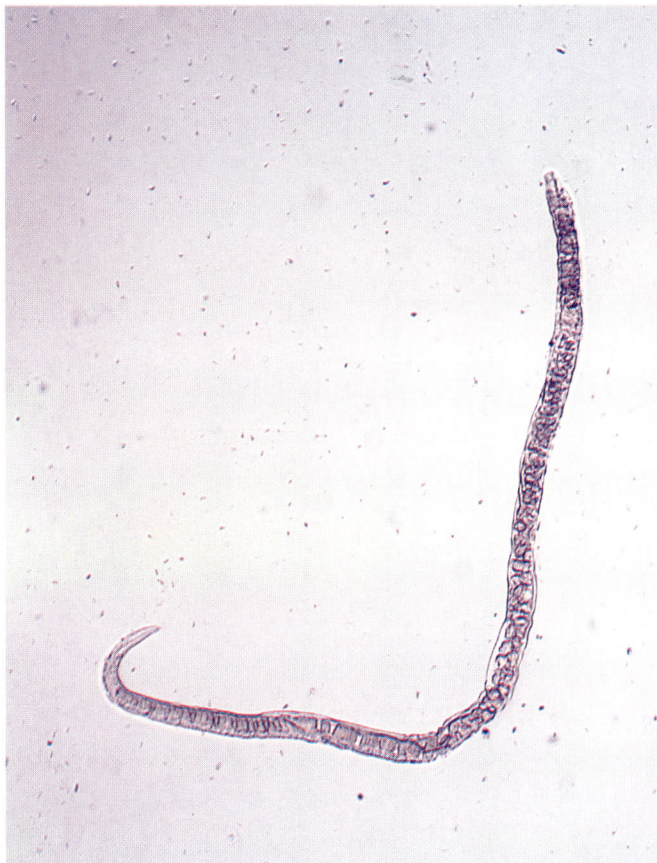

Fig. 25.1 Mature female worm of *Trichinella spiralis*

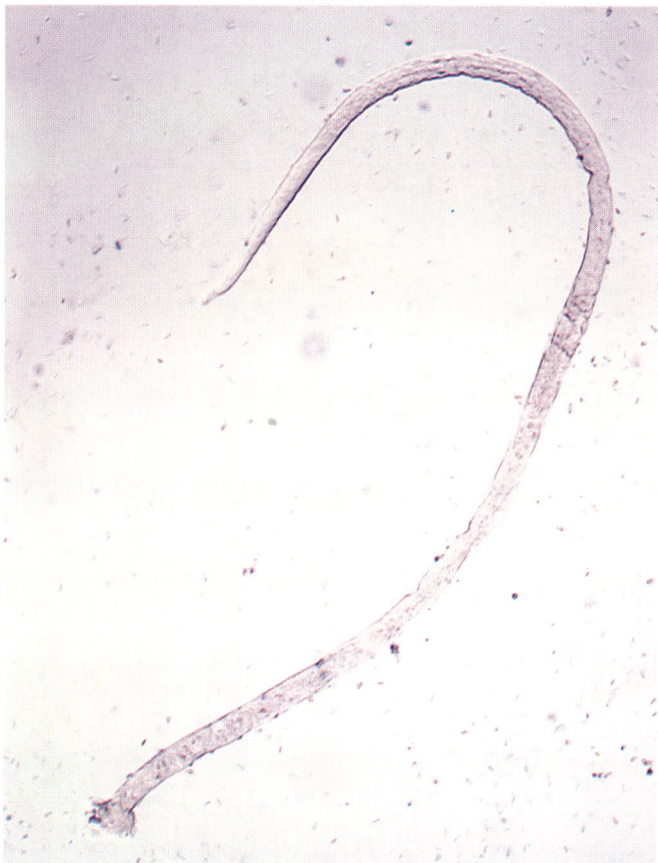

Fig. 25.2 Mature male worm of *Trichinella spiralis*

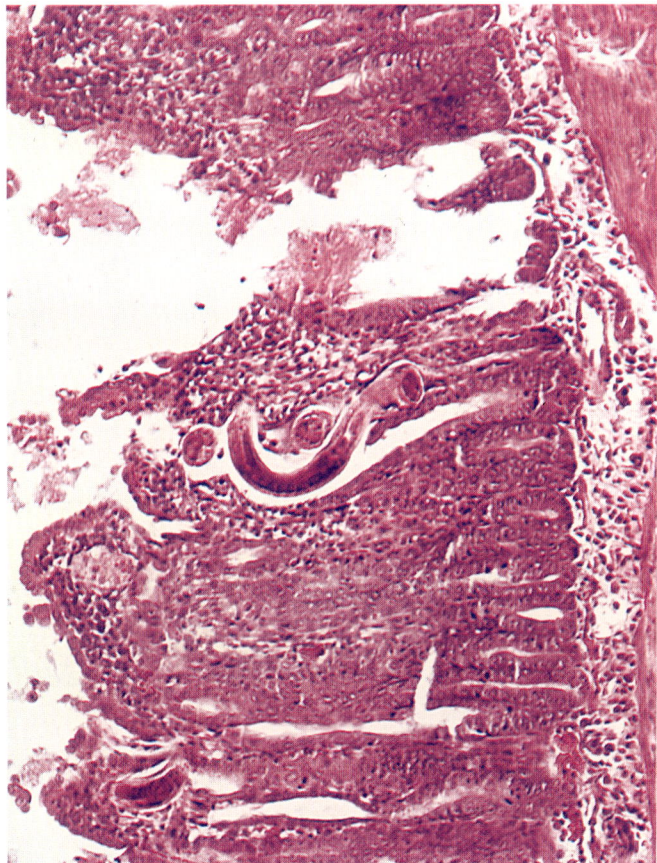

Fig. 25.3 *Trichinella spiralis* in the intestinal mucosa of a rat. H&E

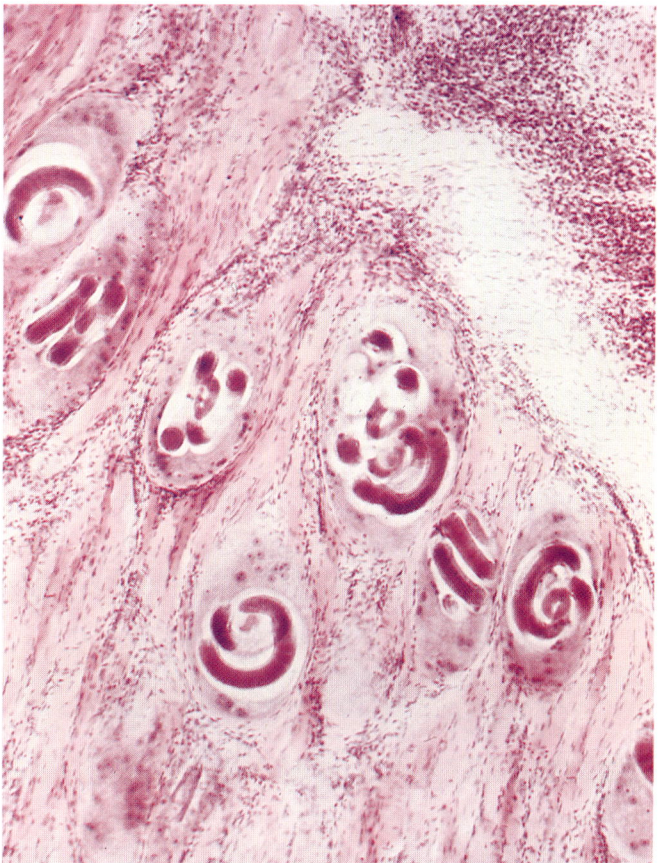

Fig. 25.4 *Trichinella spiralis* in the musculature of a rat. H&E

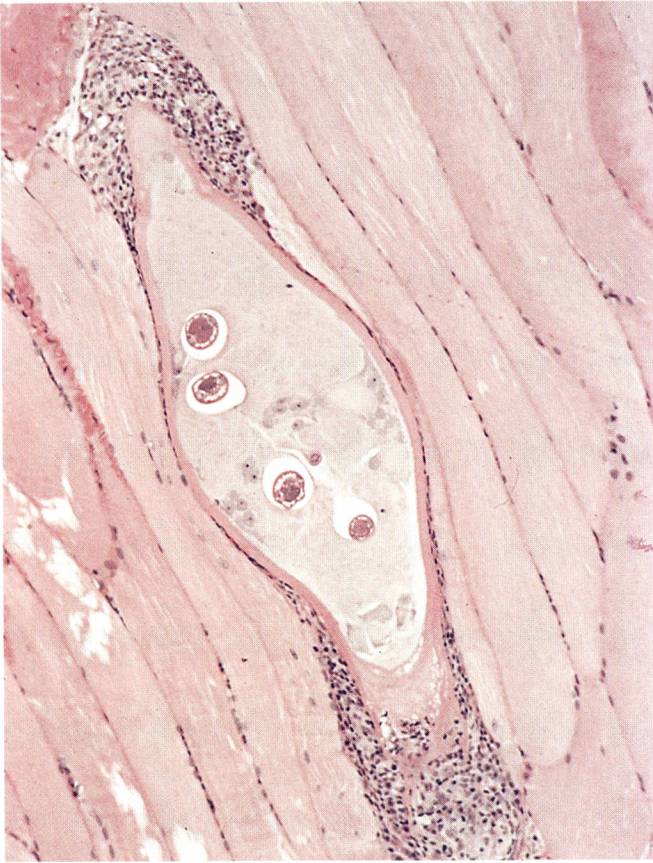

Fig. 25.5 Larvae of *Trichinella spiralis* in human musculature, 10 days after infection. A case from the 1982 epidemic in Germany. H&E

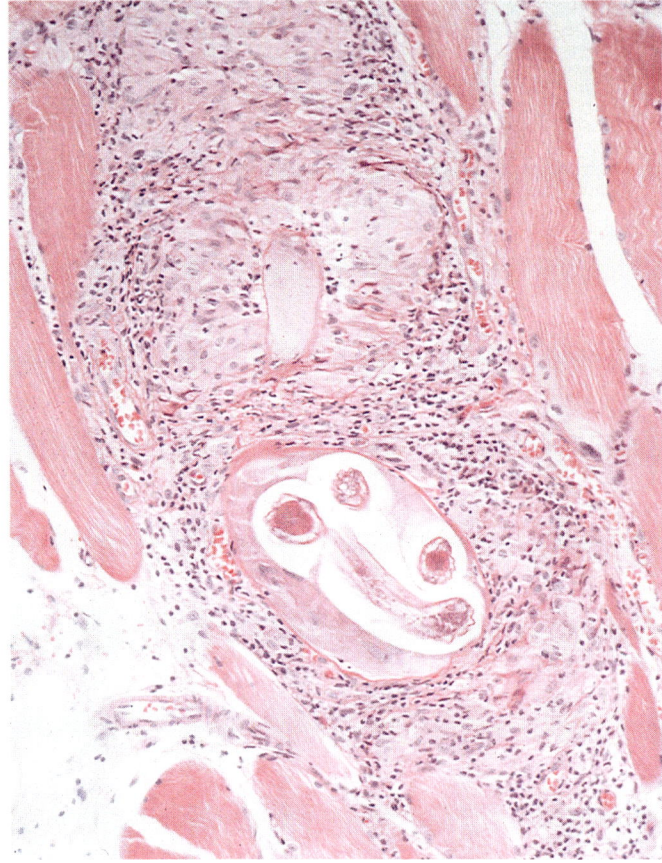

Fig. 25.6 Larvae of *Trichinella spiralis* in human musculature with marked inflammatory reaction, 4 weeks after infection. A case from the 1982 epidemic in Germany. H&E

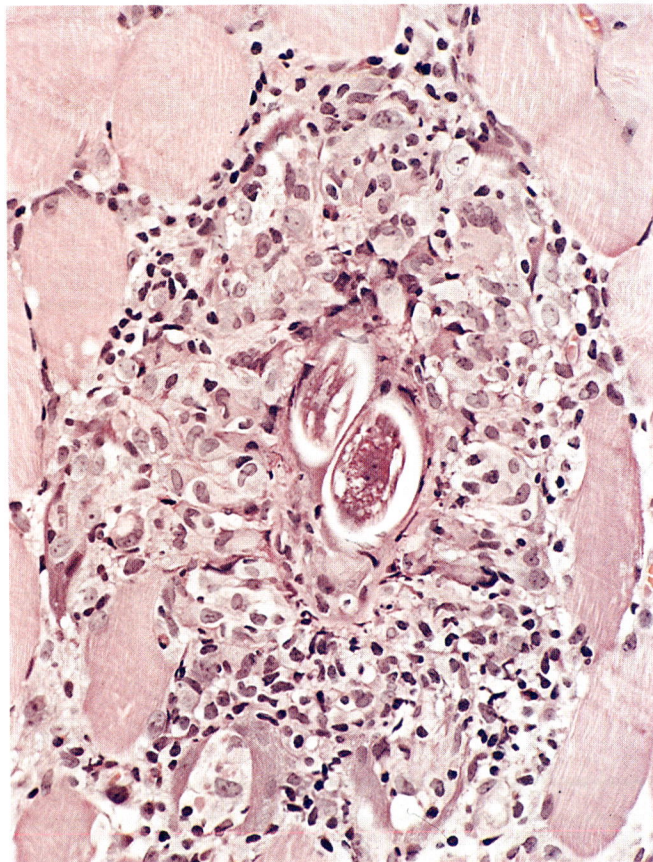

Fig. 25.7 Larvae of *Trichinella spiralis* in human musculature with marked inflammation, 3 months after infection. Same 1982 epidemic as cases in Figs. 25.5 and 25.6. H&E

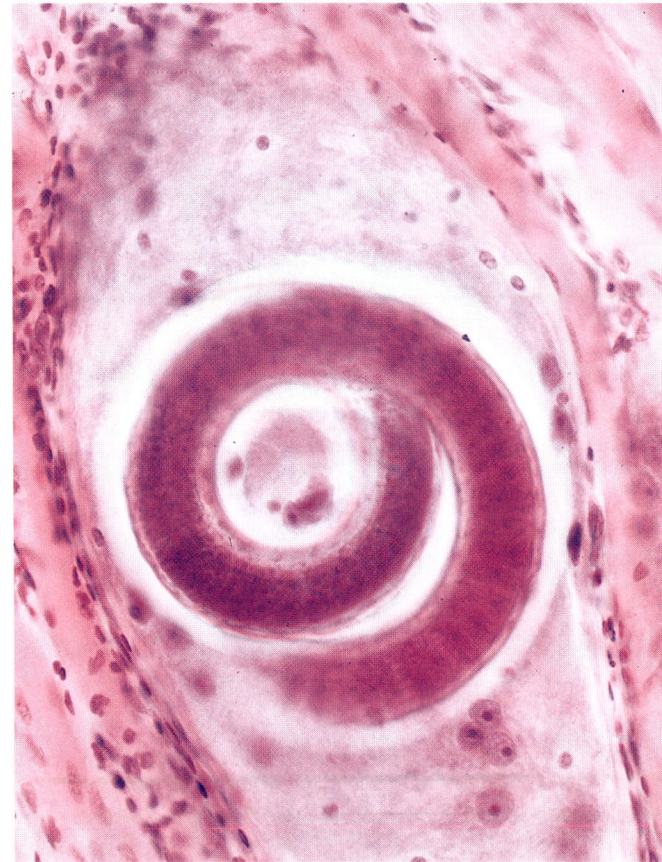

Fig. 25.8 Well developed larva of *Trichinella spiralis* in human tissue. H&E

7. Ancelle, T. *et al.* (1986). The 1985 trichinosis outbreaks due to horse meat in France. *IX. Int. Congr. Infect. Parasit. Dis. Muenchen.* Abstr. 757
8. Wright, K. A. (1979). Trichinella spiralis: An intracellular parasite in the intestinal phase. *J. Parasitol.,* **65**, 441
9. Campbell, W. C. (1988). Trichinosis revisited – another look at modes of transmission. *Parasitol. Today,* **4**, 83

26. TOXOCARIASIS

Introduction

This worm infection is also called visceral larva migrans[1]. But, since this entity also may be considered under other headings and another definition, it will be treated separately in Section 37.

Toxocariosis is becoming increasingly important. The number of pets in industrialized countries is increasing, and 20% of all dogs, especially pups, are said to be infected with *Toxocara canis*. The infection seems to occur worldwide[2,3]; children are most often affected, frequently by playing in sand boxes or play grounds[4]. In Venezuela, apparently, the consequences of this worm infection are found frequently.

Dogs and cats are carriers of this nematode worm (Fig. 26.1)[5,6], more often young animals than older ones. Man is a 'false' host. Pigs and mice may be used for experimental purposes[7-9].

Clinically, in man, the lungs, eyes[10] and central nervous system are the main organs to be involved and show clinical symptomatology[11]. Asthma, retinal detachment, blindness and epilepsy are the main manifestations of this worm infection.

For clinical diagnosis, persistent blood eosinophilia is a key sign. Antibodies may be demonstrated by a series of serological tests.

The parasites

Larvae of the nematode genus *Toxocara* (*T. canis, T. cati*) are the causal agents. Their characteristics in tissues will be discussed later. See above, under *Introduction*.

Pathogenesis

Eggs are ingested. Their larvae become liberated within the human gastrointestinal tract. They penetrate the intestinal wall and move randomly in the foreign host. However, their migration is blocked at some stage by inflammation and granuloma formation. Maturation will not be completed; the larvae die. Man, therefore, is a 'false' host. During migration, larvae may carry other micro-organisms to various sites[12].

Pathology

See Section 37.

References

1. Reotutar, R. (1990). Taking a close look at toxocariasis (news). *J. Am. Vet. Med. Assoc.,* **196**, 1009
2. Lamina, J. (1980). Larva-migrans-visceralis-Infektionen durch Toxocara-Arten. *Dtsch. Med. Wschr.,* **105**, 796
3. Gillespie, S. H. (1988). The epidemiology of Toxocara canis. *Parasitol. Today,* **4**, 180
4. Dubin, S. *et al.* (1975). Contamination of soil in two city parks with equine nematode ova including Toxocara canis: A preliminary study. *Am. J. Publ. Health,* **65**, 1242
5. Barron, C. N. and Saunders, L. Z. (1966). Visceral larva migrans in the dog. *Pathol. Vet (Basel),* **3**, 315
6. Parsons, J. C. *et al.* (1988). Disseminated granulomatous disease in a cat caused by larvae of Toxocara canis. *J. Comp. Pathol.,* **99**, 343
7. Done, J. T. *et al.* (1960). Experimental visceral larva migrans in the pig. *Res. Vet. Sci.,* **1**, 133
8. Parsons, J. C. and Grieve, R. B. (1990). Kinetics of liver trapping of infective larvae in murine toxocariasis. *J. Parasitol.,* **76**, 529
9. Higa, A. *et al.* (1990). Effects of Toxocara canis infection on haemopoietic stem cells and haemopoietic factors in mice. *Int. Arch. Allergy Appl. Immunol.,* **91**, 239
10. Maguire, A. M. (1990). Recovery of intraocular Toxocara canis by pars plana vitrectomy. *Ophthalmology,* **97**, 675
11. Glickman, L. T. *et al.* (1979). Epidemiological characteristics and clinical findings in patients with serologically proven toxocariasis. *Trans. R. Soc. Trop. Med. Hyg.,* **73**, 254
12. Frenkel, J. K., Dubey, J. P. and Miller, N. L. (1969). Toxoplasma gondii: fecal forms separated from eggs of the nematode Toxocara cati. *Science,* **164**, 432

27. ANISAKIASIS

Introduction

This infection, caused by larvae of the genus *Anisakis*, is also called herring worm disease. Its prevalence is increasing; up to 1983, more than 1000 cases had been reported from Japan. Anisakiasis is found in countries surrounding the North Sea and the Pacific Ocean. Most cases have been reported from Japan[1,2], the Netherlands and England, and infection also occurs in tourists to these places. Larvae of the herring worm, found in fish, caused a lot of hysterical publicity in Germany a few years ago. In Venezuela, no cases of this sort have been reported.

Natural definitive hosts are mammals from the sea, such as dolphins, whales, seals[3] etc. Man is a 'false' host. Laboratory animals may be used for experimental studies[4,5].

Clinically, symptoms from the gastrointestinal tract may be present. Obstruction of the small bowel may occur due to stenosis and require surgery.

Clinical diagnosis: the complement fixation test and skin test do not seem to be reliable tools. Duodenal endoscopy may be useful in cases of gastric involvement.

The parasite

Anisakis marina (Fig. 27.1), *A. simplex* and probably other *Anisakis* species, may be causal agents. Recently, *Pseudoterranova decipiens*, causing codworm anisakiasis, has also been described in Japan and USA.

In herring and mackerel, the third stage larva is said to reach 3 cm in length. For larvae in human tissues, see *Pathogenesis*.

Pathogenesis

The ingestion of raw fish, above all herring, causes lesions in the wall of the stomach and small bowel due to larvae of the genus *Anisakis*. An allergic reaction is thought to be responsible for these lesions.

The life cycle of these worms is not known completely. It is thought that larvae of this kind must live in sea water. The larvae, apparently, pass through several intermediate animal hosts living in the sea. Definitive hosts seem to be mammals which live in salt water. In man, as a 'false'

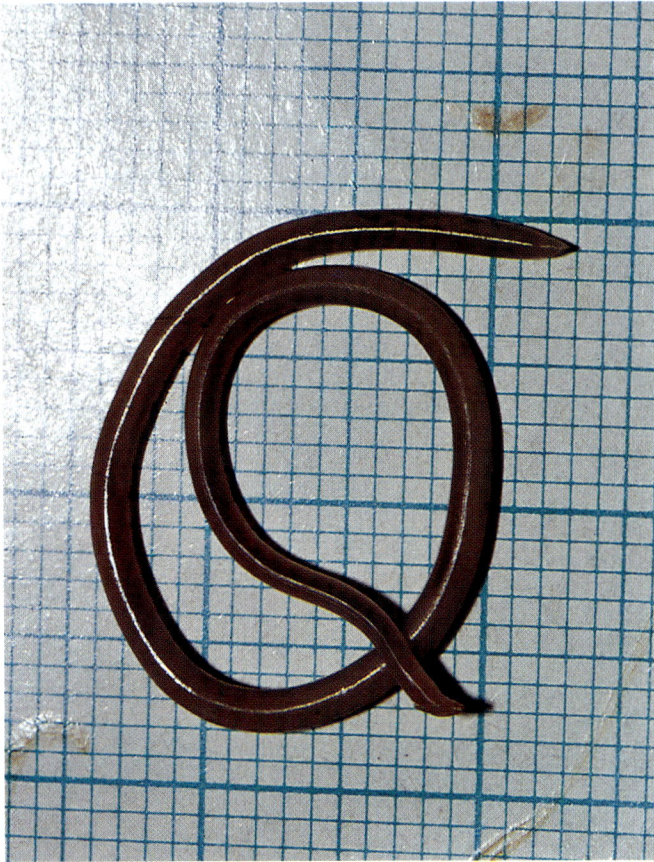

Fig. 26.1 Mature adult worm of *Toxocara* sp.

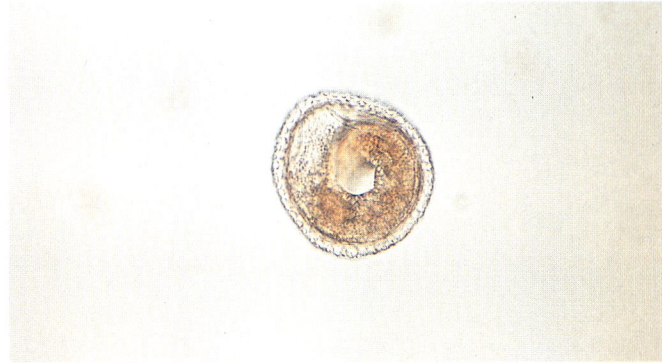

Fig. 26.2 Embryonated egg of *Toxocara* sp.

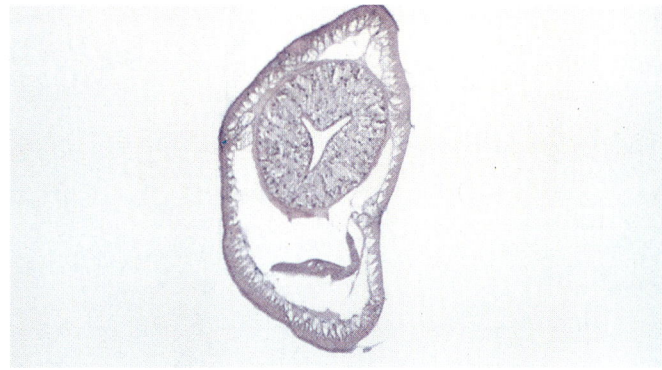

Fig. 27.1 Horizontal cut of an *Anisakis marina* worm. H&E

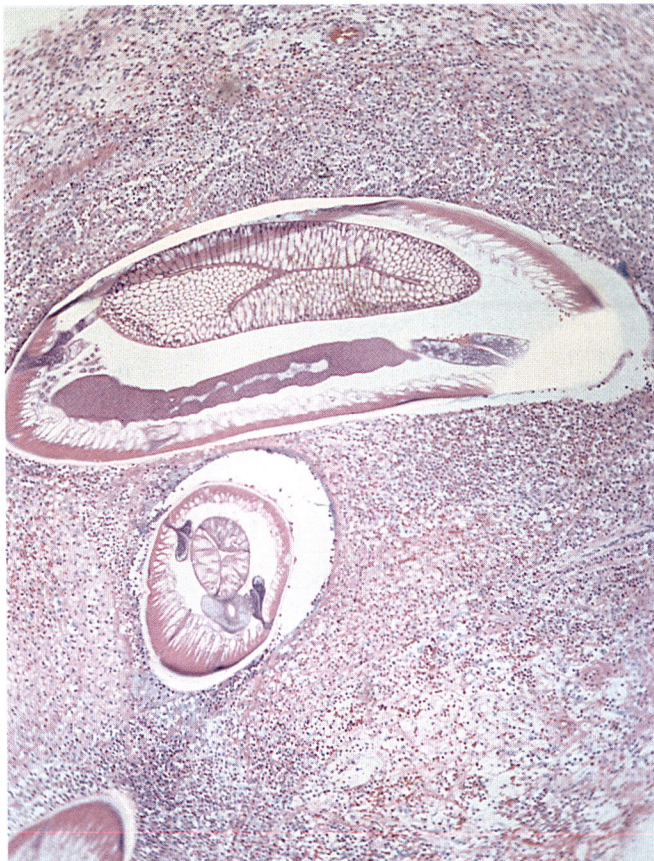

Fig. 27.2 *Anisakis marina* worms in human tissue with marked inflammatory reaction. H&E

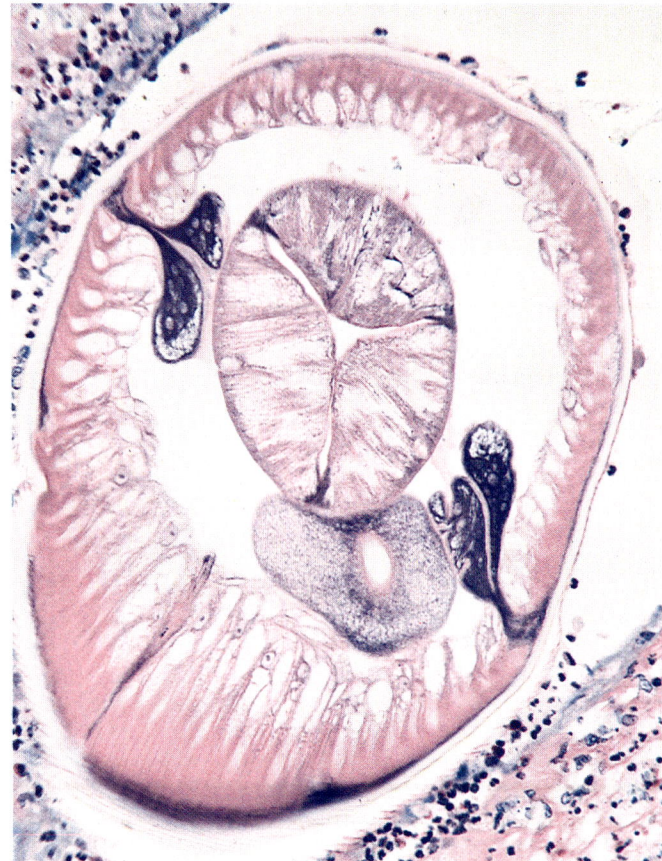

Fig. 27.3 Higher power of a transversally cut *Anisakis marina* worm in human tissue. The oesophagus with a triangular lumen is clearly seen, the same as the two typical fungus-like lateral cords. Beneath the oesophagus the excretory organ is visible. H&E

host, the larvae of these worms do not become sexually mature and do not complete migration and maturation. They may be found beyond the gastrointestinal tract[6,7].

Pathology

The lesions in the antral region of the stomach wall and/or in the small bowel wall consist of localized infiltrates (Figs. 27.2 and 27.3) of eosinophilic leukocytes and formation of eosinophilic granulomata. The localization in the small intestine may lead to obstruction and stenosis[8]. When larvae are not found in tissues, the lesions are believed to be due to an allergy. In the cases reported from Japan, localization of lesions in the stomach prevails, while, in cases from the Netherlands, the lesions are found predominantly in the small bowel.

References

1. Asami, K. *et al.* (1965). Two cases of stomach granulomas caused by Anisakis-like larvae nematodes in Japan. *Am. J. Trop. Med. Hyg.,* **14**, 119
2. Yokogawa, M. and Yoshimura, H. (1967). Clinico-pathologic studies on larval anisakiasis in Japan. *Am. J. Trop. Med. Hyg.,* **16**, 723
3. Popov, V. N. *et al.* (1989). Anisakiasis in the Caspian seal. *Parazitologiia,* **23**, 178
4. Jones, R. E. (1990). Anisakis simplex: histopathological changes in experimentally infected CBA/J mice. *Exp. Parasitol.,* **70**, 305
5. Sakanari, J. A. and McKerrow, J. H. (1990). Identification of the secreted neutral proteases from Anisakis simplex. *J. Parasitol.,* **76**, 625
6. Sakanari, J. A. and McKerrow, J. H. (1989). Anisakiasis. *Clin. Microbiol. Rev.,* **2**, 278
7. van Thiel, P. H. and van Houten, H. (1967). The localization of the herringworm Anisakis marina in and outside the human gastrointestinal tract. *Trop. Geogr. Med.,* **19**, 56
8. Morlier, D. *et al.* (1989). A rare etiology of acute occlusion of the small intestine: anisakiasis. Review of the literature apropos of a case. *Ann. Gastroenterol. Hepatol. Paris,* **25**, 99

28. GNATHOSTOMIASIS

Introduction

This parasitosis is less important since it is geographically limited, its prevalence is low and severe disease is not common. The infection occurs practically only in Eastern[1] and South-East Asia[2] and in Oceania. Major endemic foci have been reported from Thailand and Japan. The disease is not known in Venezuela.

Normally, dogs, cats, wild felines and numerous other lower animal species are infected and represent the normal definitive hosts. Experimentally, rats, mice and monkeys may be infected by giving them larvae orally[3].

Clinically, a wide variety of symptoms may be present since migration to any part of the body can take place[4,5]. The pattern observed is usually that of cutaneous or visceral larva migrans (Section 37), but aetiological diagnosis of gnathostomiasis is difficult. The mortality rate is high for gnathostoma encephalitis.

Clinical diagnosis is made by biopsy or when the worm is surgically recovered or erupts to the surface of skin. Eosinophilia is variable but generally not pronounced.

The parasite

Gnathostoma spinigerum is the most important of eight species of this genus belonging to the group Spirurids. Other members of this group include the nematodes, *Thelazia callipaeda, Gongylonema pulchrum, Physaloptera caucasica* and *Cheilospirura* sp. (but only single human cases of infection with the latter have been reported).

Adult worms occur in man rarely; when they do, they are sexually immature and ≤ 1 cm long. The head bulb is retractable and has rows of cuticular spines; the body is covered in spines. The larvae of *Gnathostoma spinigerum* in human tissues closely resemble the adult worms. The entire body surface is covered by minute cuticular spines (Fig. 28.1).

Pathogenesis

The ova of *Gnathostoma spinigerum* (Fig. 28.2) reach the water in the excrement of meat-consuming hosts. Larvae hatch from the eggs and reach, through two intermediate hosts (crustaceans and fish, frogs or snakes), other meat consumers, including man. Infection in man is accidental; this parasite does not mature in man.

Infection is acquired by eating parasitized raw[6], fermented or marinated fresh water fish or poorly cooked meat, especially chicken and duck. The larvae penetrate the wall of the digestive tract and move randomly into tissues of internal organs and subcutis. They cause damage by mechanical injury and toxic substances.

Pathology

Adult worms are found in nodules of the gastric wall in meat consumers, including exceptionally man. The larvae may reach practically all organs, and frequently the subcutis. The organs preferentially involved are liver, lungs, eyes, central nervous system, subcutis[7], and, exceptionally, the breast[8].

The tissue reaction in thoracic and abdominal organs has been studied mainly in experimentally infected animals. In the lungs, pneumothorax has been observed due to this worm infection; in abdominal organs, a tumour-like swelling may result. Histologically, necrosis, haemorrhages and acute, non-specific inflammation with few eosinophils have been described (Figs. 28.3 and 28.4). In skin biopsies, a minor tissue reaction is common. When the larvae become stationary, fibrosis and giant cells may be observed.

References

1. Miyazaki, I. (1960). On the genus Gnathostoma and human gnathostomiasis with special reference to Japan. *Exp. Parasitol.,* **9**, 338
2. Daengsvang, S. *et al.* (1964). Epidemiological observations on Gnathostoma spinigerum in Thailand. *J. Trop. Med. Hyg.,* **67**, 144
3. Koga, M. and Ishibashi, J. (1988). Experimental infection in a monkey with Gnathostoma hispidum larvae obtained from loaches. *Ann. Trop. Med. Parasitol.,* **82**, 383
4. Prijyanonda, K. B. *et al.* (1955). Pulmonary gnathostomiasis, a case report. *Ann. Trop. Med. Parasitol.,* **49**, 121
5. Bovornkitti, S. and Tandhanand, S. (1959). A case of spontaneous pneumothorax complicating gnathostomiasis. *Dis. Chest.,* **35**, 1
6. Taniguchi, Y. *et al.* (1991). Comment in: J. Cutan. Pathol. 1991 Apr.: 18 (2): 65–6. *J. Cutan. Pathol.,* **18**, 112
7. Nagao, M. (1955). A case of creeping disease caused in man by a larval Gnathostoma spinigerum. (Jap. text with Engl. abstract) *Fukuoka Acta Med.,* **46**, 207
8. Tesjaroen, S. *et al.* (1990). A breast mass caused by gnathostomiasis: brief report of a case. *S.E. Asian J. Trop. Med. Publ. Health,* **21**, 151

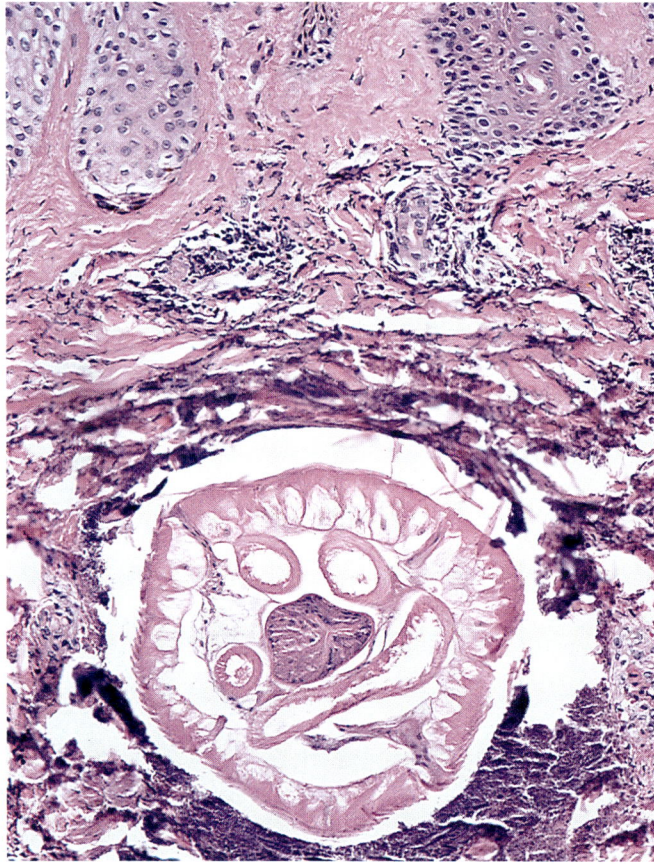

Fig. 28.1 Adult of *Gnathostoma spinigerum* in the human dermis causing 'creeping eruption' similar to cutaneous larva migrans. H&E

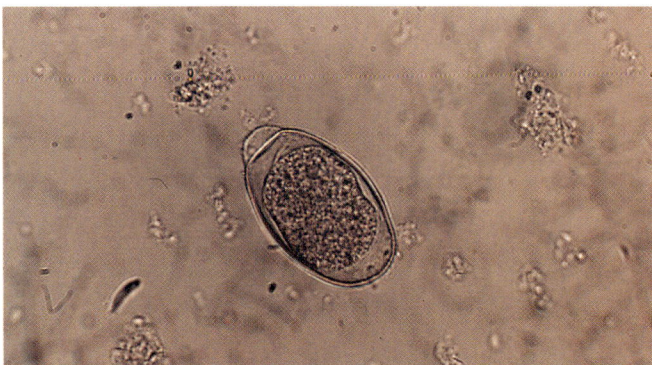

Fig. 28.2 Typical ovum of *Gnathostoma* sp.

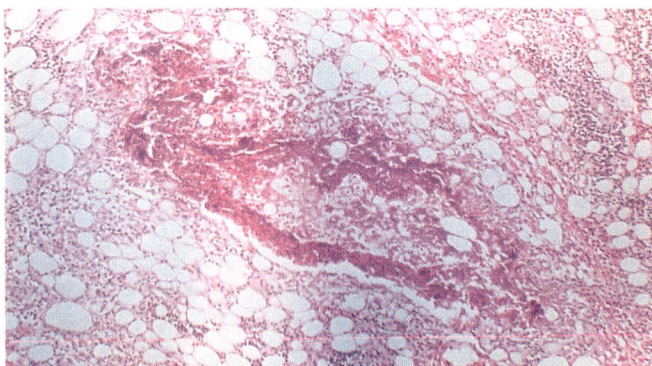

Fig. 28.3 This structure in the subcutis near the larva of *Gnathostoma spinigerum* in Fig. 28.1 may represent a dead parasite. H&E

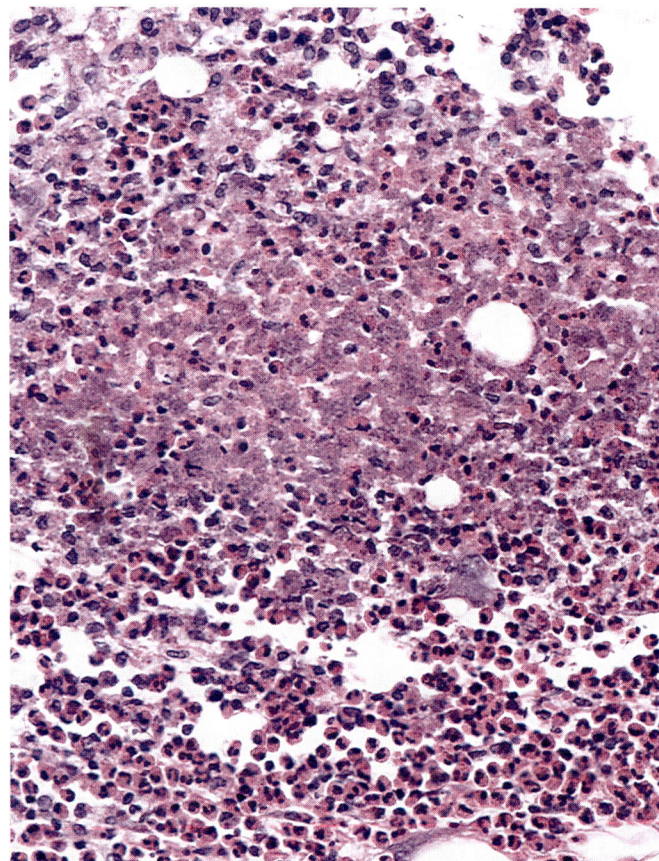

Fig. 28.4 Marked leukocytic reaction around the *Gnathostoma* larva of Fig. 28.1

29. ANGIOSTRONGYLOSIS

Introduction

Under this heading, two completely different parasitic diseases are considered (**A** and **B**). Both are caused by the same nematode genus, *Angiostrongylus*, and may result in a fatal outcome. Two different species are the causal agents, diverse organs are involved and the infections occur in distinct geographical areas.

A is the Asiatic type of angiostrongylosis, found in the region of the Pacific Ocean – India, China, South East Asia and Australia[1-6].

B is the American type, occurring in Central America, the South of North America, Colombia, Brazil and also in Venezuela[7-13]. Six cases have been found in Mérida and could be examined histologically. The disease is observed mainly in children.

In both **A** and **B**, the specific and definitive host is the rat. In **A**, cows, pigs, snails, crayfish, shrimp and captive non-human primates[6] are also infected; in **B**, snails and foals[14]. Experimentally, **A** may be produced by infecting monkeys; **B** by infecting rats.

Clinically, in **A**, there is a tropism for the parasites. They are disseminated haematogenously and cause lesions in the brain and meninges. In **B**, the ileocaecal region is affected with tumour-like lesions which often require surgery.

Clinical diagnosis is difficult in both types. In **A**, a skin test is available for man; occasionally, parasites are found in spinal fluid. Eosinophilia may be present in liquids and in tissues. In **B**, intestinal biopsy is recommended for clinical diagnosis[15].

The parasite

Two of the sixteen species of *Angiostrongylus* are pathogenic for man:

Causing **A**, *Angiostrongylus cantonensis* or *Parastrongylus cantonensis*, also called rat lung worm.
Causing **B**, *Angiostrongylus costaricensis* or *Morerastrongylus costaricensis*.

In **A**, the rat is the specific host with 20–25 mm-long adult worms in the pulmonary arteries. Snails are intermediate hosts. Cow, pig, crab, crayfish, and shrimp are nonspecific hosts; man is an accidental host. In **B**, the rat is the definitive host with parasites in the mesenteric arteries. The rat is infected by snails. Also man is a definitive host.

Pathogenesis

In **A**, human infection takes place by consumption of infected intermediate hosts (shrimps and crustaceans). The larvae penetrate the wall of the digestive tract and reach, by haematogenous dissemination, the central nervous system. Man is a false dead-end host.

In **B**, infection occurs by digestion of snails (intermediate hosts). The ova reach the ileocaecal region. Rat and man are dead-end hosts.

Pathology

In **A**, larvae of *A. cantonensis* may be found at any site but mainly in the central nervous system. Histologically, proven cases are rare. The findings in experimentally infected monkeys seem to be similar to those in man. Grossly, abnormalities may be lacking. Microscopically,

a diffuse meningoencephalitis with dense infiltrates of numerous eosinophils is found. Fragments of dead parasites may be surrounded by giant cells.

In human **B** infections, with *Morerastrongylus costaricensis*, the terminal ileum, caecum, ascending colon and appendix may be involved.

Grossly, inflammatory lesions with tumour-like enlargement and thickening of the wall of the intestine may be seen, as well as obstruction with mechanical ileus. Ulceration of the mucosa is common.

Histologically, ova, larvae and mature worms (they do become sexually mature in man) may be encountered, accompanied by diffuse infiltrates of eosinophils, lymphocytes, plasma cells and neutrophils. Additionally, a granulomatous reaction, eosinophilic granuloma, vasculitis and thrombosis may be observed.

Figures 29.1–29.6 illustrate *Angiostrongylus cantonensis* (**A**) in man; Figures 29.7–29.10 *Angiostrongylus costaricensis* (**B**) in the rat and Figures 29.11–29.19 *Angiostrongylus costaricensis* (**B**) in man.

References

1. Alicata, J. E. (1965). Biology and distribution of the rat lungworm, Angiostrongylus cantonensis and its relationship to eosinophilic meningoencephalitis and other neurological disorders of man and animals. *Adv. Parasit.*, **3**, 223

2. Alicata, J. E. and Jindrak, K. (1970). *Angiostrongylosis in the Pacific and Southeast Asia*. Thomas C C, Springfield

3. Beaver, P. C. and Rosen, L. (1964). Memorandum on the first report of Angiostrongylus in man by Nomura and Lin, 1945. *Am. J. Trop. Med. Hyg.*, **13**, 589

4. Rosen, L. *et al.* (1967). Studies on eosinophilic meningitis. III. Epidemiologic and clinical observations on Pacific Islands and the possible etiologic role of Angiostrongylus cantonensis. *Am. J. Epidemiol.*, **85**, 17

5. Punyagupta, S. (1965). Eosinophilic meningoencephalitis in Thailand: Summary of nine cases and observations on Angiostrongylus cantonensis as a causative agent and Pila ampullacea as a new intermediate host. *Am. J. Trop. Med. Hyg.*, **14**, 370

6. Gardiner, D. H. *et al.* (1990). Eosinophilic meningoencephalitis due to Angiostrongylus cantonensis as the cause of death in captive non-human primates. *Am. J. Trop. Med. Hyg.*, **42**, 70

7. Morera, P. (1970). Investigación del huésped definitivo de Angiostrongylus costaricensis. *Bol. Chil. Parasit.*, **25**, 133

8. Morera, P. and Ash, L. R. (1970). Investigación del huésped intermediario de Angiostrongylus costaricencis. *Bol. Chil. Parasit.*, **25**, 135

9. Morera, P. and Céspedes, R. (1971). Angiostrongylus costaricensis n. sp. (Nematoda: Metastrongyloidea), a new lungworm occurring in man in Costa Rica. *Rev. Biol. Trop.*, **18**, 173

10. Zambrano, P. Z., Diaz, P. I. and Salfelder, K. (1975). Ileocolitis seudotumoral eosinofílica de origen parasitario. *GEN (Caracas)*, **29**, 87

11. Loria-Cortés, R. and Lobo-Sanahuja, J. F. (1980). Clinical abdominal angiostrongylosis. A study of 116 children with intestinal eosinophilic granuloma caused by Angiostrongylus costaricensis. *Am. J. Trop. Med. Hyg.*, **29**, 538

12. Malek, E. A. (1981). Presence of Angiostrongylus costaricensis Morera and Cespedes 1971 in Colombia. *Am. J. Trop. Med. Hyg.*, **30**, 81

13. Salfelder, K. *et al.* (1970). Ileitis regional eosinofílica de origen parasitario. *GEN (Caracas)*, **25**, 132

14. Wright, J. D. *et al.* (1991). Equine neural angiostrongylosis. *Aust. Vet. J.*, **68**, 58

15. Fauza, D. de O. *et al.* (1990). Abdome agudo na infancia por angiostrongiliase intestinal: relato de um caso. *AMB Rev. Assoc. Med. Bras.*, **36**, 150

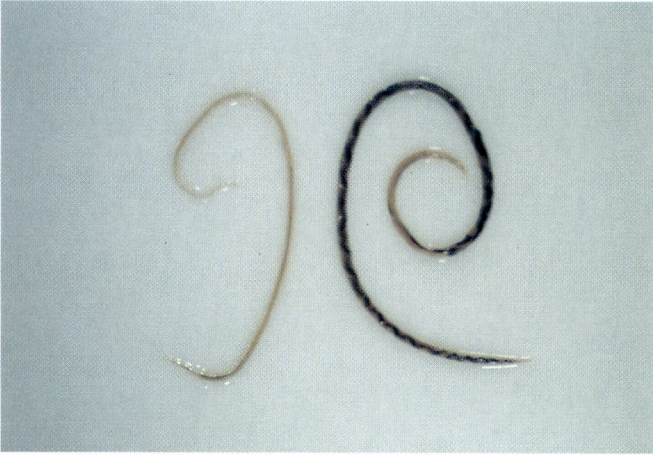

Fig. 29.1   Two adult worms of *Angiostrongylus cantonensis*

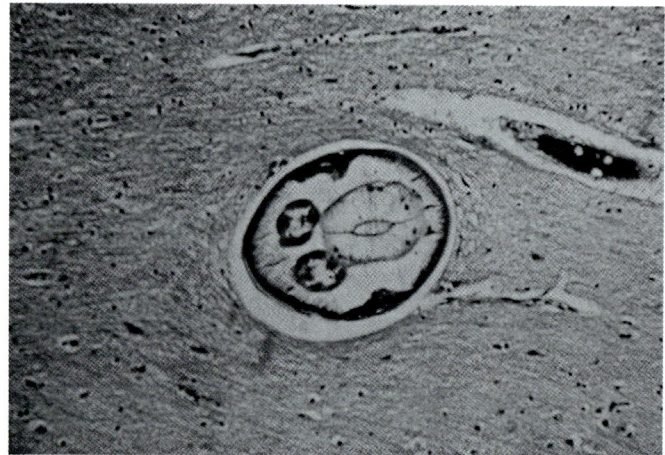

Fig. 29.2   Young adult roundworm of *Angiostrongylus cantonensis* in human brain tissue. H&E

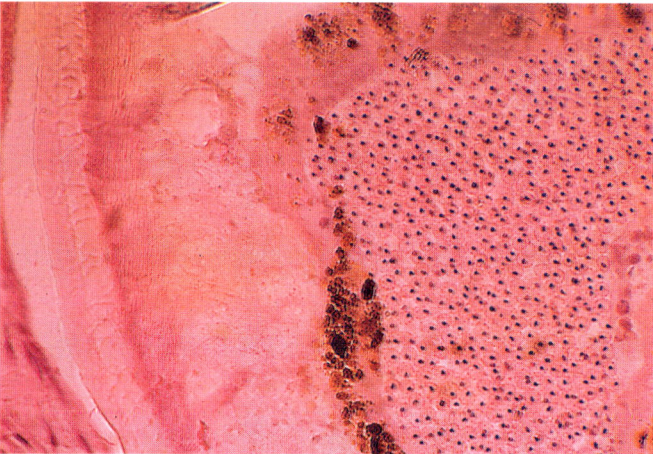

Fig. 29.3   Adult *Angiostrongylus cantonensis* roundworm in human lung tissue. Testicle with spermatozoa is seen. H&E

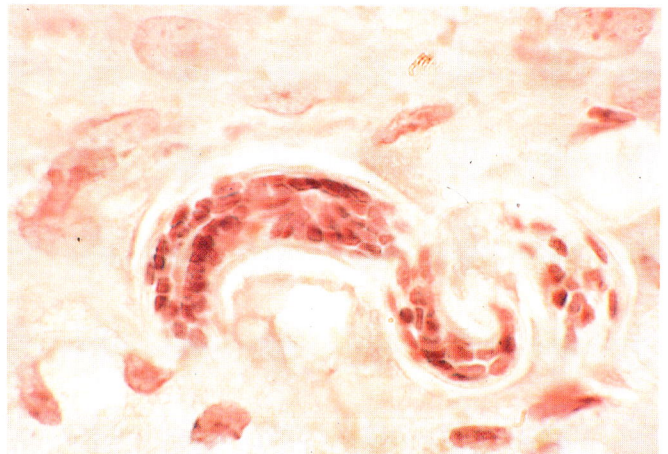

Fig. 29.4   Larva of *Angiostrongylus cantonensis* in human lung tissue. H&E

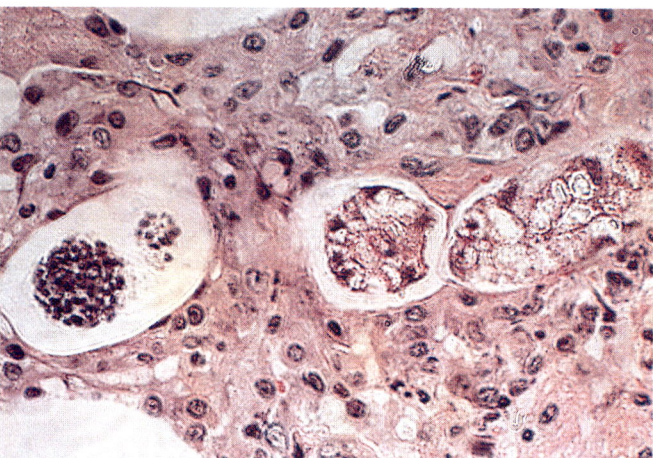

Fig. 29.5   Two types of eggs of *Angiostrongylus cantonensis* in human lung tissue. H&E

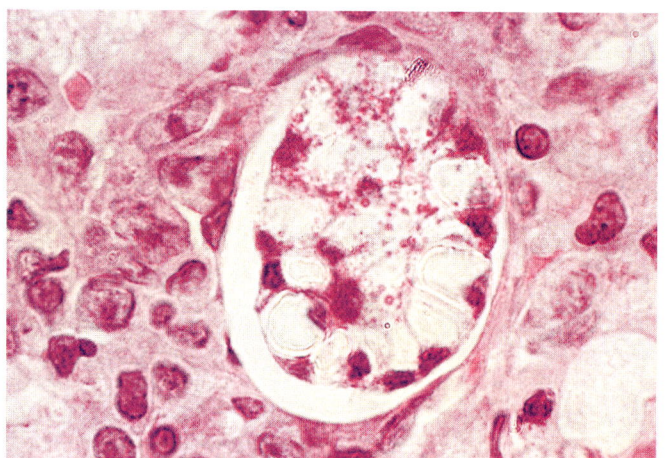

Fig. 29.6   Egg of *Angiostrongylus cantonensis* in human lung tissue at high power. H&E

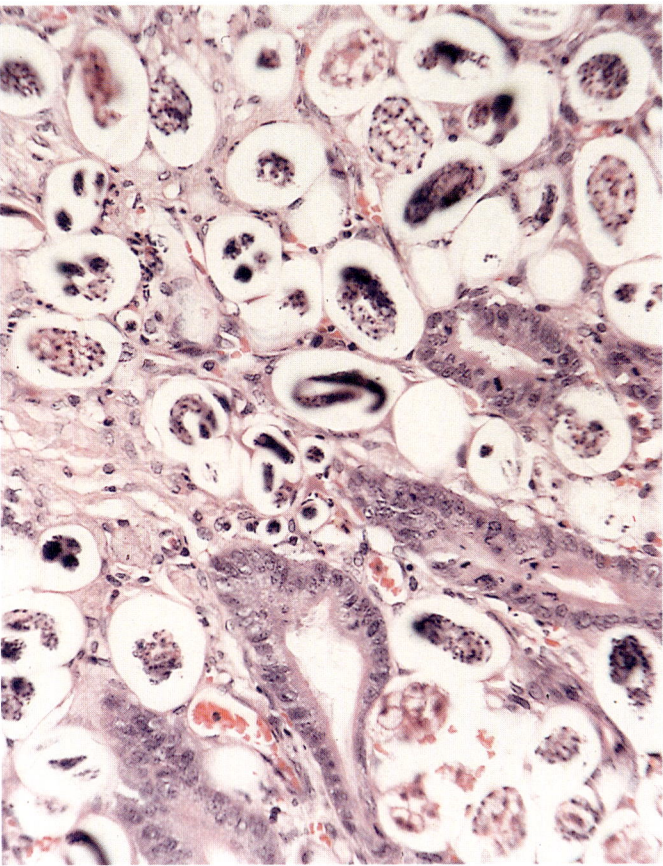

Fig. 29.7 Numerous larvae and eggs of *Angiostrongylus costaricensis* in the intestinal mucosa of a rat. Experimental inoculation. H&E

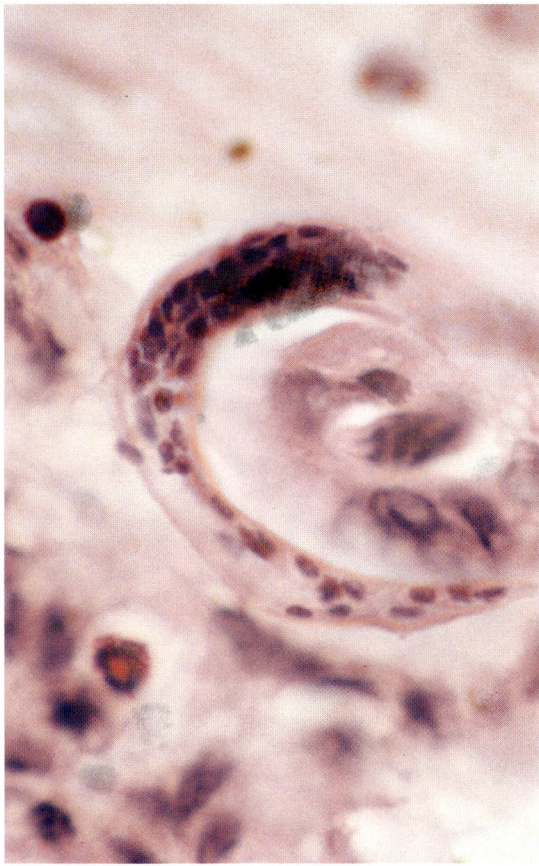

Fig. 29.8 Larva of *Angiostrongylus costaricensis* in tissues of a rat. Experimental inoculation. H&E

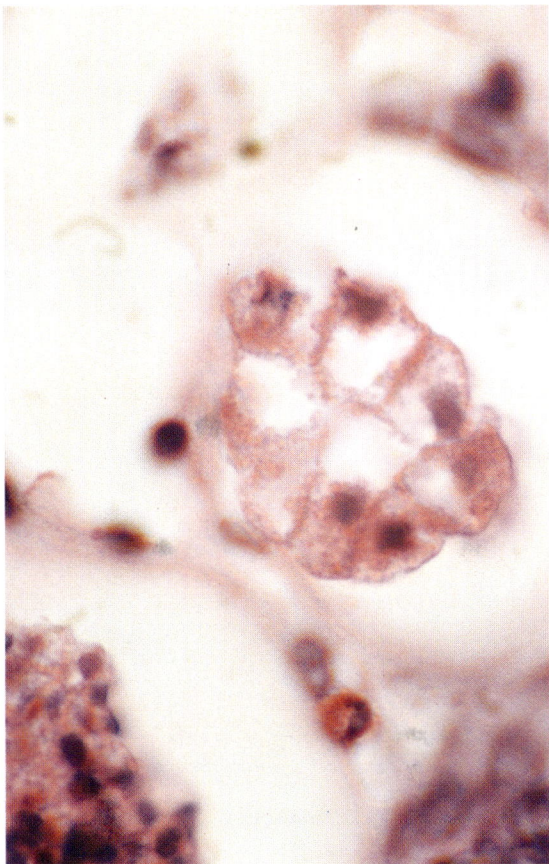

Fig. 29.9 Ovum of *Angiostrongylus costaricensis* in tissue of a rat in later stage of evolution. Experimental inoculation. H&E

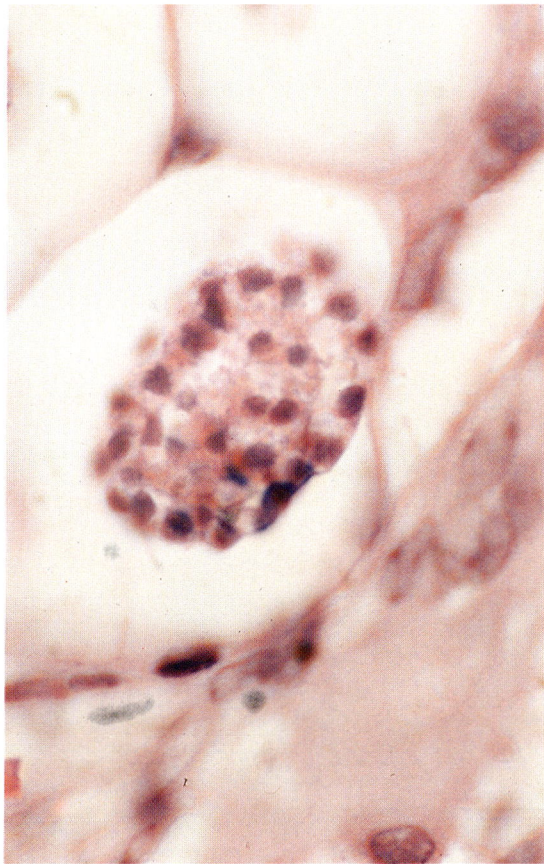

Fig. 29.10 Ovum of *Angiostrongylus costaricensis* of a rat in still later stage of evolution. Experimental inoculation. H&E

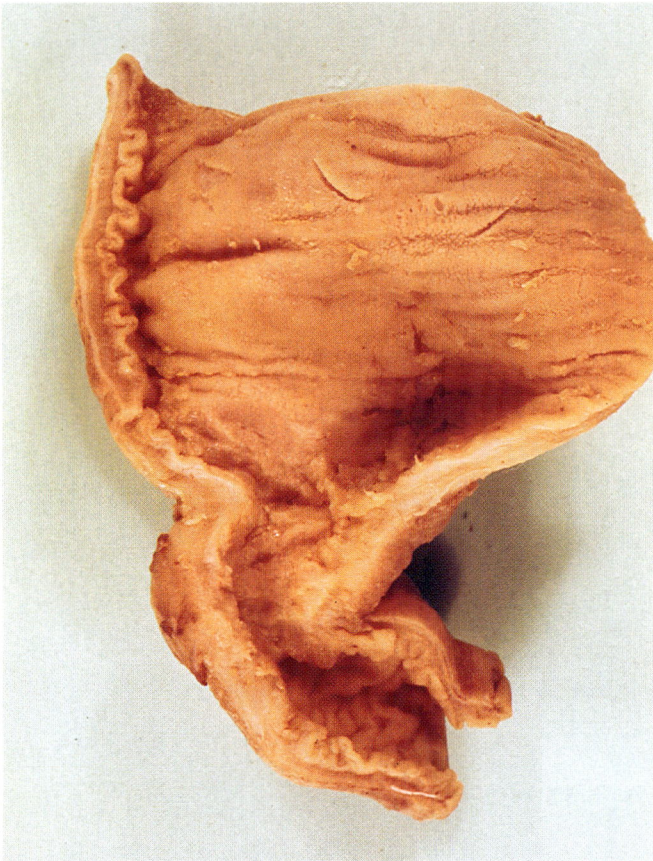

Fig. 29.11 Ileocaecal involvement of human *Angiostrongylus costaricensis* infection with marked thickening of the intestinal wall. A case from Mérida, Venezuela

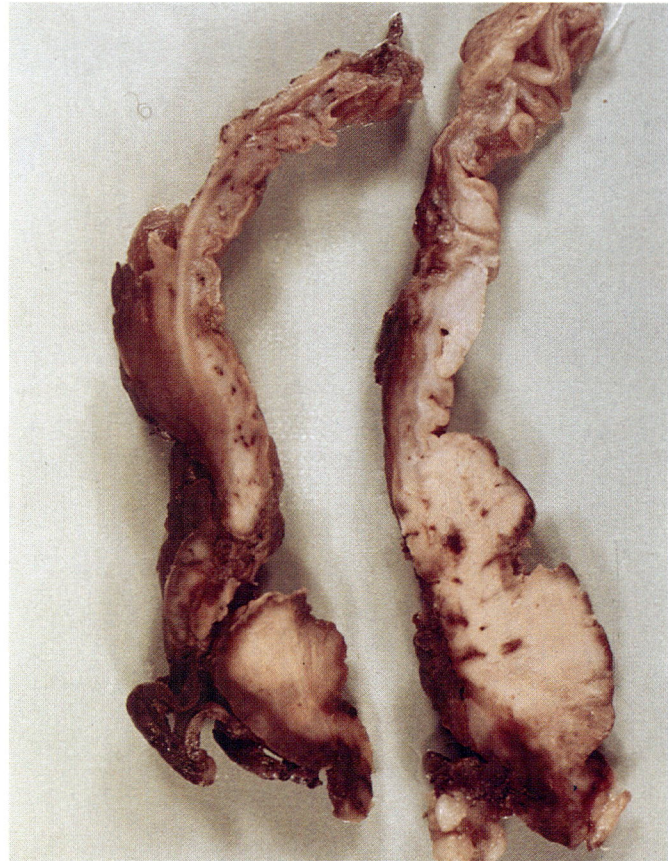

Fig. 29.12 Another case of human *Angiostrongylus costaricensis* infection from Mérida, showing marked thickening of the intestinal wall. Surgical specimen; resection because an intestinal cancer was suspected

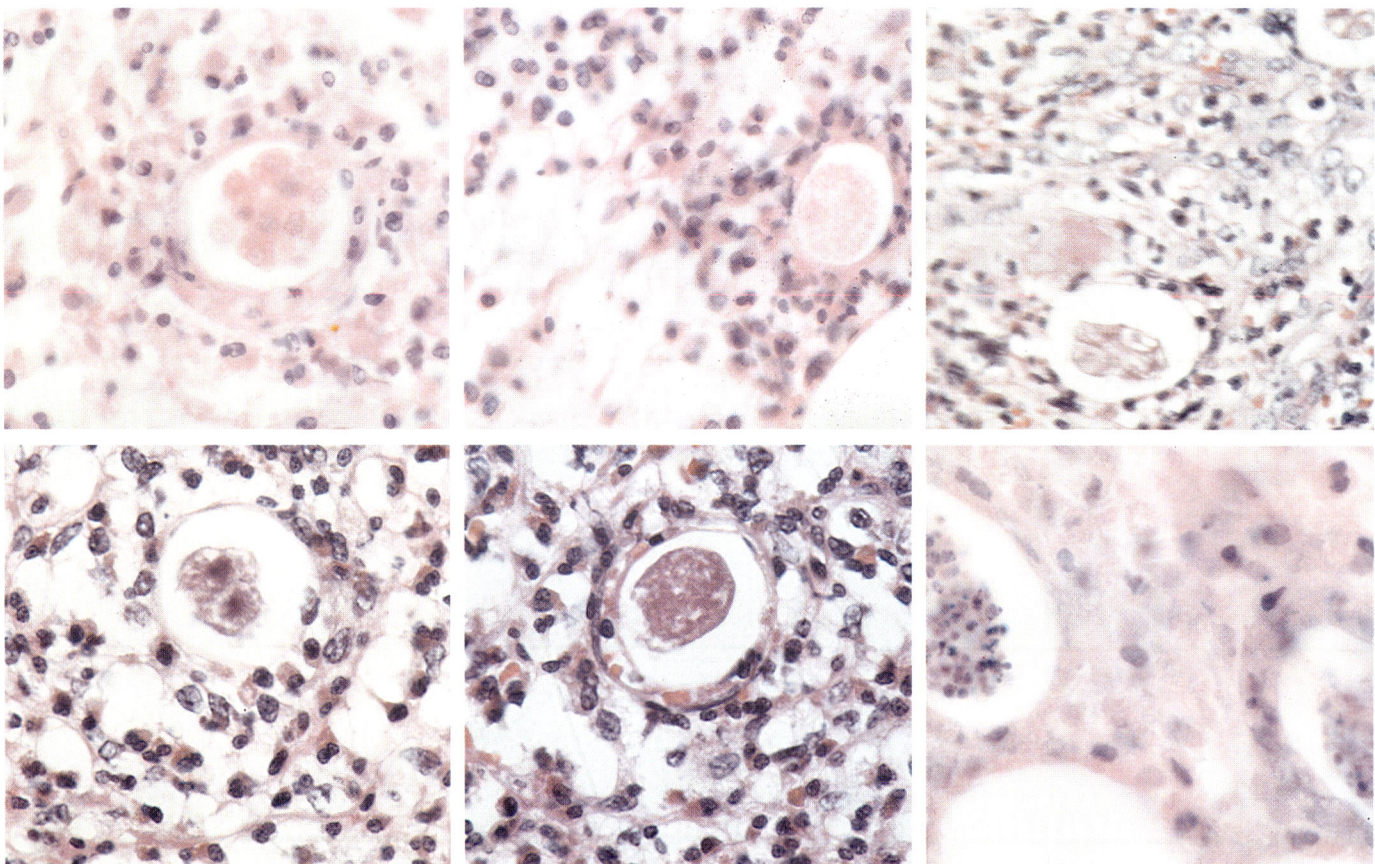

Fig. 29.13 Several ova of *Angiostrongylus costaricensis* in tissues of the human cases of Figs. 29.11 and 29.12. H&E

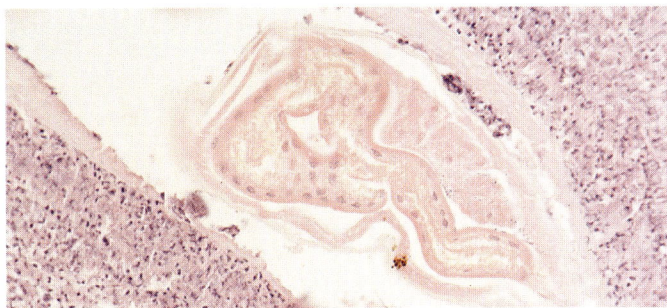

Fig. 29.14 Adult worm of *Angiostrongylus costaricensis* in tissues of the human cases in Mérida, low power. H&E

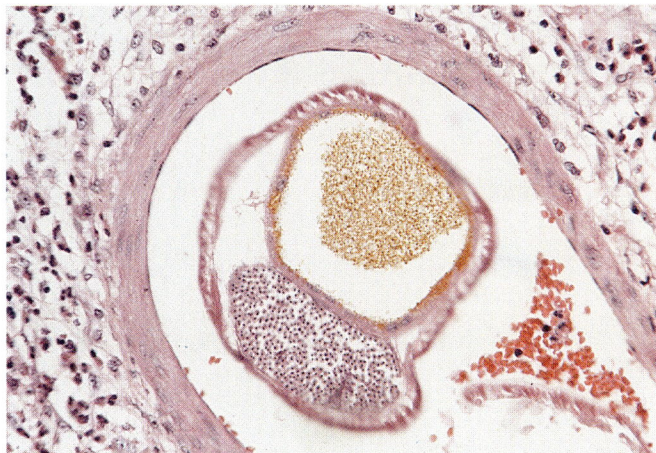

Fig. 29.15 Male *Angiostrongylus costaricensis* worm in human tissues, high power. Testicle with spermatozoa is clearly visible. H&E

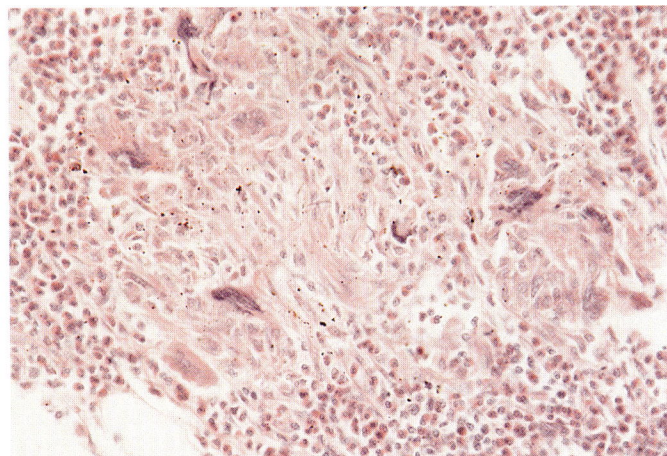

Fig. 29.16 *Angiostrongylus costaricensis* with eosinophilic and granulomatous tissue reaction. H&E

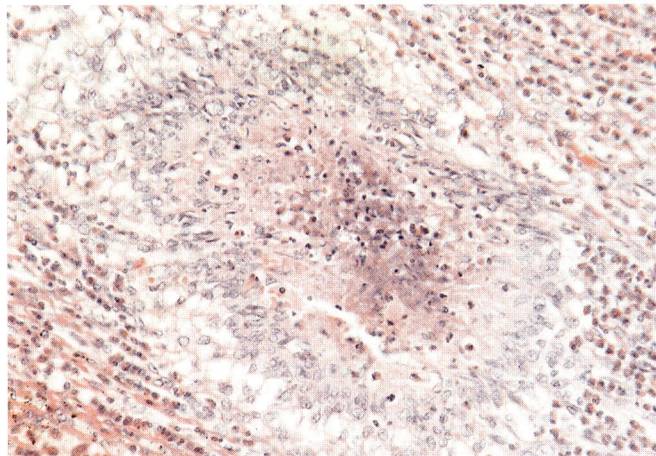

Fig. 29.17 *Angiostrongylus costaricensis* with eosinophilic tissue reaction and granuloma formation. H&E

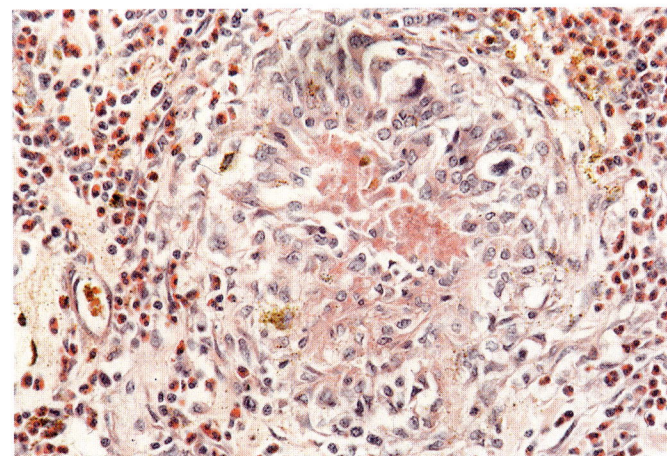

Fig. 29.18 *Angiostrongylus costaricensis*. Eosinophilic and granulomatous reaction at high power. H&E

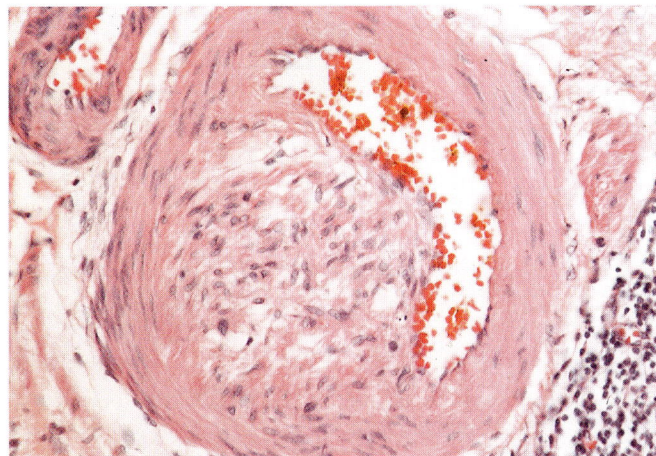

Fig. 29.19 *Angiostrongylus costaricensis*. Intestinal lesions with vasculitis. H&E

30. CAPILLARIASIS

Introduction

Again, a nematodiasis of minor importance is produced by two different species of a sole genus (**A**, *Capillaria hepatica* and **B**, *Capillaria philippensis*). The species occur in different geographical areas.

A has a large geographical distribution in the USA, the region of the Pacific Ocean, South Africa and South America, but not in Europe[1-5], while **B** has been found only in the Philippines[6-9]. Worm infections of this sort have not been reported in Venezuela.

A is observed in numerous lower animal species (rodents, mostly rats, and domestic animals)[10]. **B** is seen in fish and domestic animals.

Clinically, only a few fatal cases have been reported in **A**, while, in **B**, epidemics with a high mortality rate have been noted, accompanied by severe diarrhoea. Cardiac failure and secondary infections were the causes of death.

Clinical diagnosis can be made only by biopsy of the liver or small intestine.

The parasite

Structurally, this parasite is similar to the genus *Trichinella*, at least regarding morphology of the oesophagus.

In **A**, adult worms of *Capillaria hepatica* or *Hepaticola hepatica* reach 2 cm in length and are very thin. The typical ova, in the liver of the host, reach the soil when the host dies, via the decaying carcass. They then become infective in the soil.

In **B**, the adult *C. philippensis* reaches only 5 mm in length. The development cycle, through one or more intermediate hosts, is unknown. The ova show characteristic structures.

Pathogenesis

In **A**, infection takes place by ingesting ova from uncooked livers of rodents or contaminated food and water. The larvae hatch from the ova in the caecum and reach the liver via the portal vein.

In **B**, people become infected by eating raw fish or meat. The parasites penetrate into the mucosa of the small bowel, causing inflammation[11].

Pathology

In **A**, nodules up to 2–3 cm in diameter may be found in the enlarged liver. Histologically, preserved or disintegrated parasites and ova are present in large numbers. Abscess-like foci, eosinophilic infiltrates and a marked granulomatous reaction with numerous giant cells, are observed.

In **B**, only the mucosa of the small intestine is invaded by the small nematodes; they do not penetrate into deeper layers. The tissue reaction consists of a non-specific inflammation with occasional eosinophils (Figs. 30.1–30.3).

References

1. Ward, R. L. and Dent, J. H. (1959). Capillaria hepatica infection in a child. *Bull. Tulane Med. Fac.*, **19**, 27
2. Calle, S. (1961). Parasitism by Capillaria hepatica. *Pediatrics*, **27**, 648
3. García, F. R. *et al.* (1962). Eosinofilia elevada con manifestaciones viscerales. Primer caso de infección por Capillaria hepática en Mexico. *Bol. Med. Hosp. Inf. (Mex.)*, **19**, 179
4. Piazza, R., Correa, M. A. and Fleury, R. V. (1963). Sobre um caso de infestacao humana por Capillaria hepatica. *Rev. Inst. Med. Trop. S. Paulo*, **5**, 37
5. Kokai, G. K. *et al.* (1990). Capillaria hepatica infestation in a 2-year-old girl. *Histopathology*, **17**, 275
6. Chitwood, M. B. *et al.* (1968). Capillaria philippensis sp. n. (Nematoda: Trichinellida) from the intestine of man in the Philippines. *J. Parasitol.*, **54**, 368
7. Cabrera, B. D. *et al.* (1968). Human intestinal capillariasis. III. Parasitological features and management. *Acta Med. Philippina*, **4**, 92
8. Detels, R. *et al.* (1969). An epidemic of intestinal capillariasis in man. A study in a barrio in Northern Luzon. *Am. J. Trop. Med. Hyg.*, **18**, 676
9. Whalen, G. E. *et al.* (1969). Intestinal capillariasis. A new disease in man. *Lancet*, **1**, 13
10. Brander, P. *et al.* (1990). Capillaria hepatica bei einem Hund und einem Igel. *Schweiz. Arch. Tierheilkd.*, **132**, 365
11. Diaz, U. *et al.* (1967). Human intestinal capillariasis. I. Clinical features. *Acta Med. Philippina*, **4**, 72

31. DRACUNCULOSIS

Introduction

This threadworm infection, also called dracunculiasis or dracontiasis, is widespread in endemic areas of Africa, the Near East and Asia[1,2]. Millions of people were said to be infected but the prevalence has reduced during recent years. In Venezuela, autochthonous infections of this sort are unknown.

Dogs, wolves and cats may be infected and serve as reservoir hosts.

Clinically, during migration of the larvae in man (prepatent period 10–14 months), symptoms may be lacking or be of a non-specific or allergic type. One to four worms may be present per patient.

Clinical diagnosis during migration may be made by an indirect fluorescence method or skin test. Commonly, eosinophilia is present. When the mature female long worm appears on a ruptured skin blister, diagnosis is easily made.

The parasite

Dracunculus medinensis, Medina, Guinea or Dragon worm, is the longest threadworm in man. Mature male worms reach 3–4 cm and females are up to 1 m long. Males and females have different tail ends. The larvae of *D. medinensis* (Fig. 31.1) are 0.5–1 cm long with a digestive tract. They reach drinking water and are eaten by small crustacean species of the genus *Cyclops*, which act as intermediate hosts. Two moults take place in these copepods. Man or animals ingesting the small crustaceans are the definitive hosts.

Pathogenesis

The minute *Cyclops* species (containing infective larvae of *D. medinensis*) are ingested with the drinking water. The larvae are liberated, penetrate the mucosa of the duodenum and reach the bloodstream. During haema-

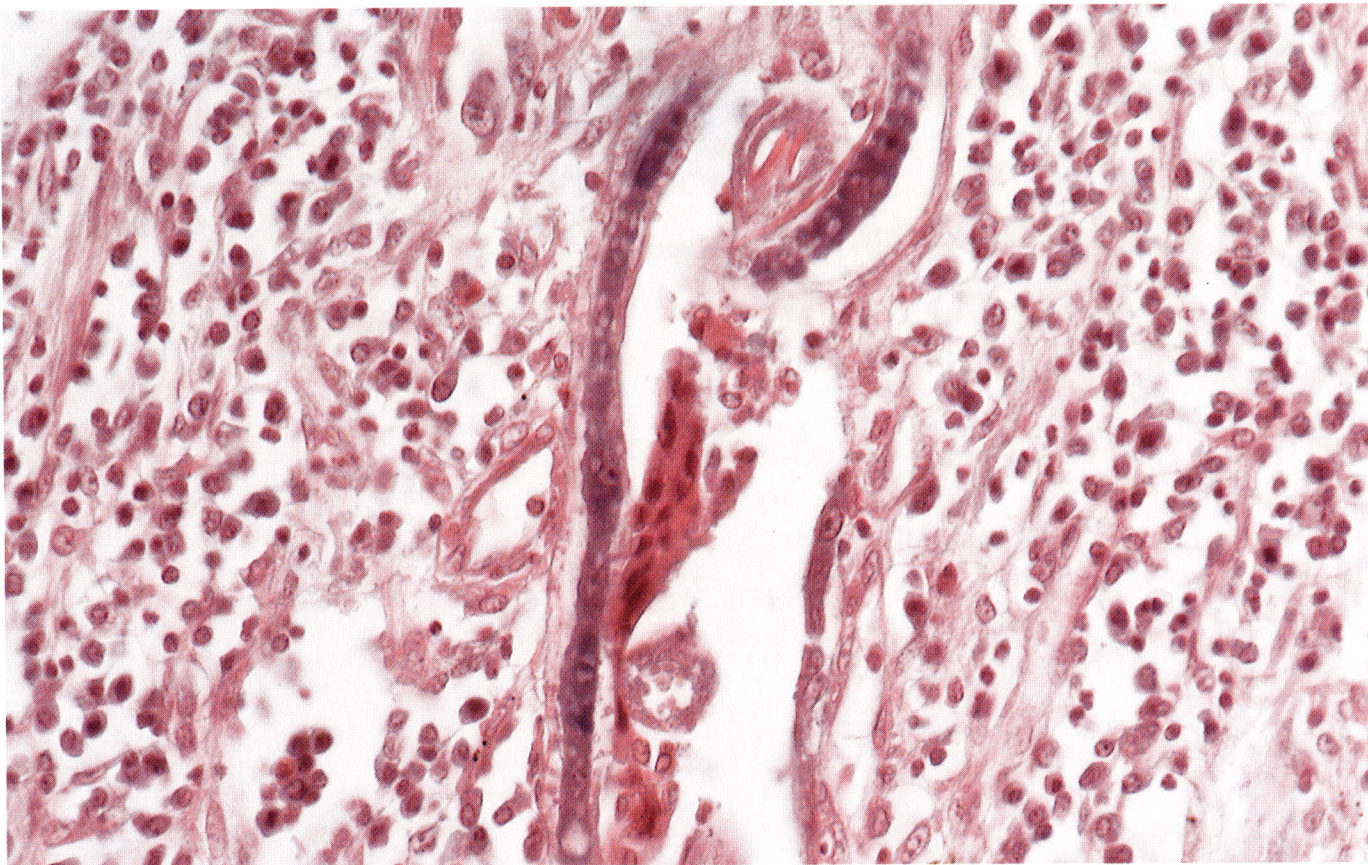

Fig. 30.1 *Capillaria philippensis* worms in the mucosa of the small intestine with marked non-specific inflammation. H&E

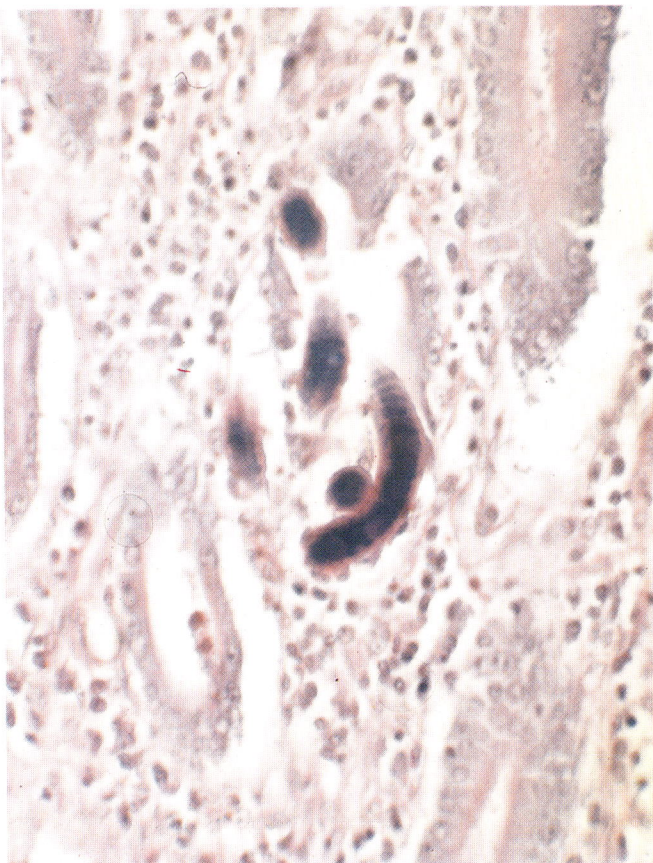

Fig. 30.2 Fragments of *Capillaria philippensis* worms in human tissue. H&E

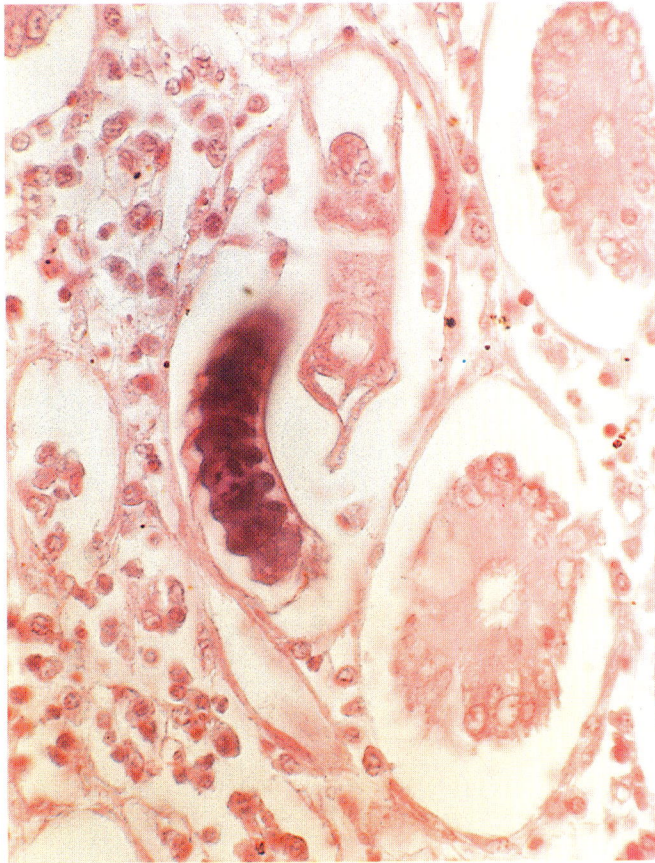

Fig. 30.3 *Capillaria philippensis* worm in the mucosa of small intestine at high power. H&E

togenous dissemination, maturation of the larvae takes place. It is completed in the tissues of the subcutis where copulation occurs with formation of new larvae.

Haematogenous migration until formation of mature adult worms, and reproduction with formation of larvae in the subcutis, takes about one year. The long female worm may penetrate the skin and remain just under the surface forming a blister after one month. When the blister ruptures, the worm appears outside the body. The larvae are liberated into the content of the blister, and, from there, to a watery environment in order to be ingested by the *Cyclops* species once more.

Pathology

During migration and before coming to the subcutis, the larvae may cause encephalitis, pericarditis, lymphadenitis, myositis, and may involve urogenital organs and other sites[3-7], causing abscesses which heal, leaving calcified foci.

Skin lesions are found in legs and feet preferentially, but also at other sites of the body. They may consist of:

palpable moving worms; cutaneous allergic reactions; or a blister of 3–5 cm long which, after rupture, reveals a long female worm (Fig. 31.2).

References

1. Ansari, A. R. and Nasir, A. S. (1963). A survey of guinea worm disease in the Sind desert (Tharpaikar District) of West Pakistan. *Pakistan J. Health*, **13**, 156
2. Elgart, M. L. (1989). Onchocerciasis and dracunculosis. *Dermatol. Clin.*, **7**, 323
3. Kinare, S. G. *et al.* (1962). Constrictive pericarditis resulting from dracunculosis. *Br. Med. J.*, **1**, 845
4. Lacombe, M. and Gentilini, M. (1963). A propos des localizations intra-scrotales du verm de Guineé (Filaire de Medine). *Presse Med.*, **71**, 1862
5. Reddy, C. R. R. M. and Valli, V. V. (1967). Extradural Guinea worm abscess. *Am. J. Trop. Med. Hyg.*, **16**, 23
6. Smith, D. J. and Sindique, F. H. (1965). Calcified Guinea-worm in the broad ligament of a pregnant mother. *J. Obstetr. Gynaec. Br. Comm.*, **72**, 808
7. Verma, A. K. (1966). Ocular dracunculosis. *J. Ind. Med. Assoc.*, **47**, 188

FILARIA INFECTIONS (Sections 32–35)

There are ten important worm species in the group of Filaria: *Wuchereria bancrofti, Brugia malayi, Brugia timori, Loa loa, Onchocerca volvulus, Dirofilaria immitis, Dipetalonema perstans, Dipetalonema streptocerca, Mansonella ozzardi* and *Microfilaria bolivariensis*. Six of these filarial worms produce more or less significant diseases, while four are practically non-pathogenic for man. The diseases are: **filariasis** caused by *W. bancrofti, B. malayi* and *B. timori*; **loiasis** by *L. loa*; **onchocerciasis** by *O. volvulus*; and **dirofilariasis** by *D. immitis*.

D. perstans, D. streptocerca, M. ozzardi and *M. bolivariensis* are widely distributed in Africa and South America (*M. bolivariensis* in Venezuela). They are transmitted by insects of the genus *Culicoides* (small midges) but do not lead to any serious disease. The microfilariae are unsheathed.

Filarial worms are very thin; the mature forms (adults or macrofilariae) may be more than 10 cm long. The larvae of the filariae are called also microfilariae, reach 150–350 μm long and often cause more damage than the mature worms. They may be found in lymphatic or blood vessels, in the subcutis and, occasionally, in other organs and tissues (larva migrans).

Infection occurs through the bite of a blood-sucking insect in which the microfilariae have reached maturation. They go through 4 moults. Man is the final host. Adults measure from 1 cm (*Loa loa*) to 50–100 cm (*D. volvulus*). In almost all cases of filarial infections, blood eosinophilia is present. Many infections remain asymptomatic. Ocular lesions are found in loiasis and onchocerciasis, and may lead to blindness.

For diagnosis of microfilariae, see Tables 15 and 16.

Table 15 Diagnosis of microfilariae

Schema of a microfilaria (shortened)

Head Nerve ring Tail

Sheath

Microfilariae **with** sheaths (in blood)

Wuchereria bancrofti	240–300 μm	
Brugia malayi	180–230 μm	
Loa loa	250–300 μm	

Microfilariae **without** sheaths (in blood)

Dipetalonema perstans	< 200 μm	
Mansonella ozzardi	170–240 μm	
Onchocerca volvulus	250–330 μm	
Dipetalonema streptocerca	180–240 μm	

Important: H&E stain is recommended for microfilariae. Giemsa stain and other techniques do not always stain the sheaths, especially in *Loa loa*. Microfilariae, when drying, lose their sheaths, either partially or totally.

32. FILARIASIS

Introduction

This infection by three filarial species is called also lymphatic filariasis or tropical elephantiasis. It is an important disease, because many millions of people are parasitized. Infection by *Wuchereria bancrofti* is most frequent and occurs in tropical regions of Africa[1], America[2,3], Asia[4,5], Australia and the Mediterranean countries. They have been observed also in Venezuela.

Brugia malayi is limited to Southeast Asia and *B. timori* to a small focus in Indonesia.

Dogs, cats and other animal species[6] have been found to be infected with these species of filarial worms. Ferrets are used for experimental purposes[7].

Clinically, microfilariae of these species may remain for years in the blood of practically symptomless human carriers. Mature worms may cause allergic reactions,

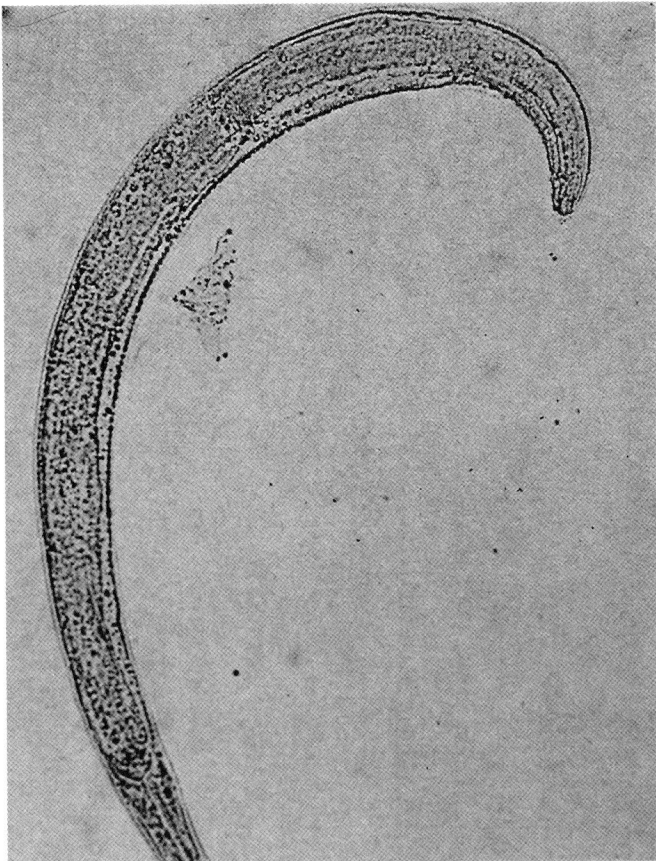

Fig. 31.1   First stage larva of *Dracunculus medinensis*

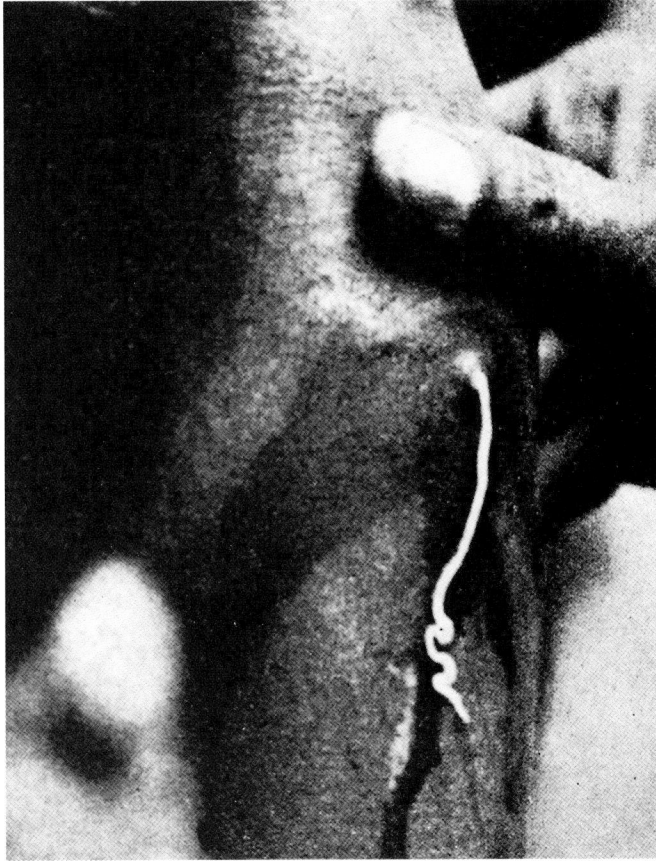

Fig. 31.2   Adult female worm of *Dracunculus medinensis* perforating the skin and appearing outside the human body

Table 16 *Wuchereria bancrofti* microfilaria from a thick blood smear, stained with haematoxylin (Delafield).

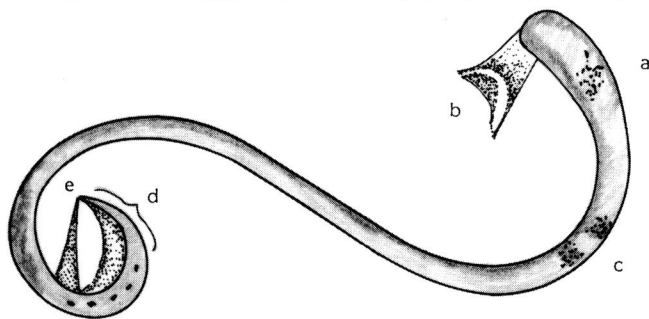

a. head, **b**. multifolded 'sheath', **c**. space within the succession of nuclei = nerve ring, **d**. area free of nuclei, **e**. tail

lymphangitis and lymphadenitis with hydrocele, elephantiasis and chyluria.

For a clinical diagnosis, mobile microfilariae may be seen in fresh blood samples taken at night and in fine needle aspirates[8]. For serological diagnostic methods[9], see also Section 33.

The parasite

Adult worms of these three species have a nocturnal periodicity. *Wuchereria bancrofti* reaches 10 cm long; the other species are somewhat shorter.

Female filarial worms are ovoviviparous. The larvae are coiled up in the ova situated in the uterus. When they are released from the female, the larvae are liberated from the eggs as microfilariae.

Microfilariae may be found in lungs and lymph nodes of man. They are sheathed and measure 220–320 μm long on average. They may be differentiated by the nuclei at the end of the tail; see Tables 15 and 16 as well as Figs. 32.1–32.3.

Microfilariae are taken up in blood meals by mosquitos of the genera *Culex, Aedes, Mansonia* and *Anopheles*. In the insect, there are two moults before infective microfilariae reach the labium of the mosquito.

Pathogenesis

When the mosquitos bite, the infective microfilariae burst out of the labium and enter the human skin. The incubation period is 8–16 months. The prepatent period, i.e. the development from the embryonic stage (microfilariae) to sexually mature worms, is different for each species. The filarial worms of these species have a tendency to situate themselves inside lymph vessels.

Congenital transmission is also known to occur.

Pathology

Grossly, splenomegaly and enlargement of lymph nodes may be noted. The filarial worms are located in the connective tissue, lymph vessels and lymph nodes (Figs. 32.4 and 32.5), and produce, due to obstruction of the lymphatic vessels, chronic oedema and fibrosis leading to elephantiasis of certain regions or organs. The latter is often complicated by bacterial super-infection. Obviously, in the tissues of long-standing elephantiasis, the parasites are no longer found.

In lungs and lymph nodes, eosinophilic granulomas caused by microfilariae may be observed. This feature is also called tropical eosinophilic syndrome and belongs to the larva migrans syndrome (Section 37).

References

1. Jordon, P. (1960). Epidemiology of Wuchereria bancrofti in Africa. *Indian J. Malariol.*, **14**, 353
2. Markell, E. K. (1964). Filarial infections in a Californian clinic. *Ann. Int. Med.*, **61**, 1065
3. Baird, J. K. and Neafie, R. C. (1988). South American brugian filariasis: report of a human infection acquired in Peru. *Am. J. Trop. Med. Hyg.*, **39**, 185
4. Liekian, J. *et al.* (1960). Wuchereria bancrofti infection in Djakarta, Indonesia. A study of some factors influencing its transmission. *Indian J. Malariol.*, **14**, 339
5. Trent, S. (1963). Reevaluation of World War II veterans with filariasis acquired in the South Pacific. *Am. J. Trop. Med. Hyg.*, **12**, 877
6. Hines, S. A. *et al.* (1989). Lymphatic filariasis. Brugia malayi infection in the ferret (Mustela putorius furo). *Am. J. Pathol.*, **134**, 1373
7. Crandall, R. B. *et al.* (1990). Injection of microfilariae induces resistance of Brugia malayi infection in ferrets and accelerates development of lymphostatic disease. *Parasite-Immunol.*, **12**, 229
8. Kapila, K. and Verma, K. (1989). Gravid adult female worms of Wuchereria bancrofti in fine needle aspirates of soft tissue swellings. Report of three cases. *Acta Cytol.*, **33**, 390
9. Carvalho, P. A. *et al.* (1990). Evaluation of in vitro released Wuchereria bancrofti third stage larval antigens for detection of bancroftian filariasis. *Trop. Med. Parasit.*, **41**, 71

33.　LOIASIS

Introduction

This infection with the filarial species (*Loa loa*) is limited to Western Central Africa from Sierra Leone to Angola, and occurs predominantly in the region of the great rivers. The number of carriers of *Loa loa* is estimated at 20–40 million. Obviously, there are no autochthonous infections of this kind in Venezuela.

Loiasis may occur in monkeys as reservoir hosts[1].

Clinically, usually a mild disease is present, but its manifestations may be severe[2]. An allergic swelling, which may recur and cause severe itching, may be present, and, in addition, marked pain in muscles and joints, as well as conjunctivitis and blindness may be observed.

When making a clinical diagnosis, there is a marked blood eosinophilia. In fresh blood drops, few microfilariae may be found in the peripheral blood during the day time, and 1–4 years after infection. This phenomenon of the day and night periodicity of the filarial species has not been elucidated satisfactorily.

Serological and skin tests are only group specific (i.e. for all species of filariae).

The parasite

Loa loa is also called migrating filaria, loa worm or eye worm. Mature female worms of *Loa loa* are up to 70 mm long and 0.5 mm wide; males are up to 35 mm long. Their life-span may be 15 or more years. Adult worms are thin, whitish, filamentous and cylindrical. The sheathed microfilariae measure 275 × 7 μm. The sheaths on the microfilariae are better seen with H&E than with Giemsa stain (Figs. 33.1 and 33.2). The larvae of *Loa loa* are located in peripheral blood vessels during the day. They are taken up by fly species of the genus *Chrysops* (mango fly) in a blood meal. The microfilariae reach the thoracic muscles of the fly and mature, passing finally into the head in the region of the mouth.

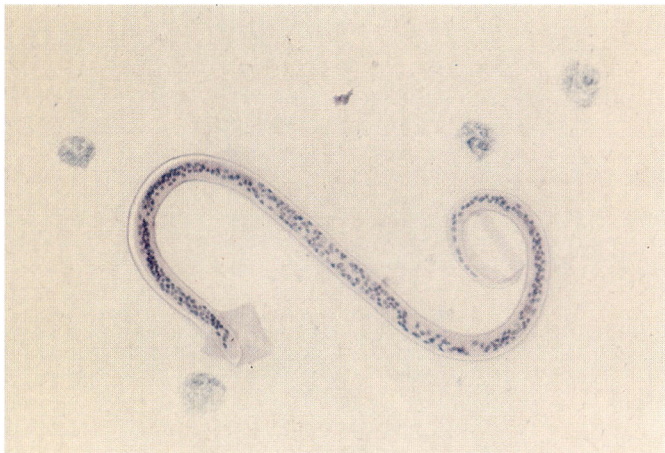

Fig. 32.1 Microfilaria of *Wuchereria bancrofti* in blood smear. Note tail without nuclei. Giemsa

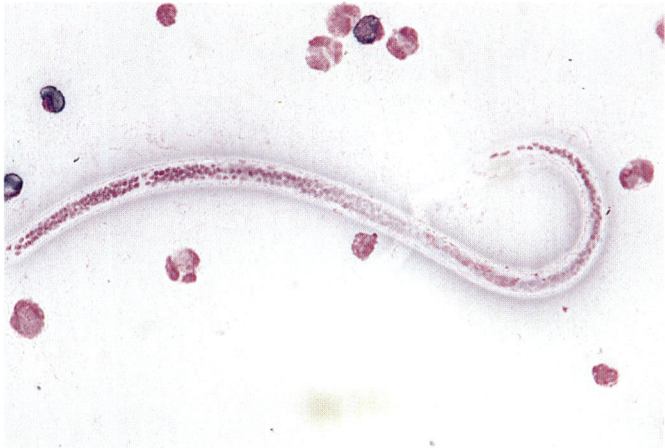

Fig. 32.2 Microfilaria of *Wuchereria bancrofti* in blood smear. The sheath is clearly visible. The dark dots are nuclei. H&E

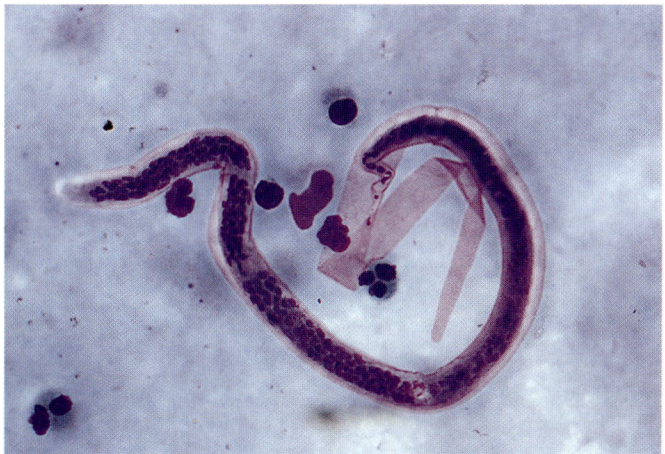

Fig. 32.3 Microfilaria of *Brugia malayi* in blood smear. The sheath is recognizable. H&E

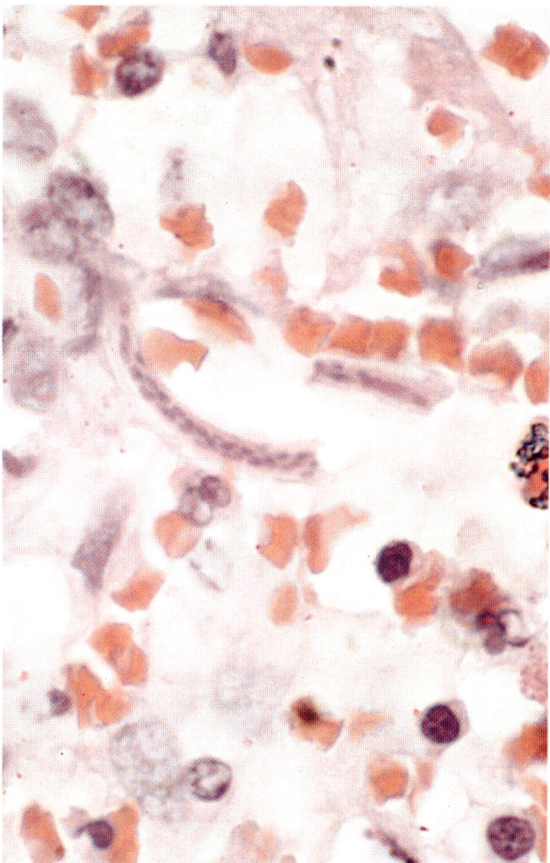

Fig. 32.4 Microfilariae of *Brugia malayi* in lymph node. The dark dots are nuclei. H&E

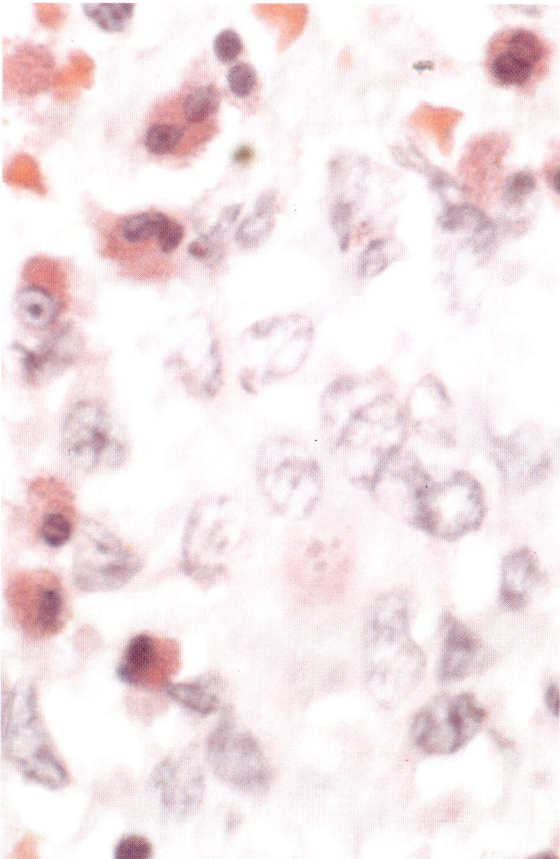

Fig. 32.5 Eosinophilic lymphadenitis. One microfilaria of *Brugia malayi*, transversally cut, surrounded by macrophages. H&E

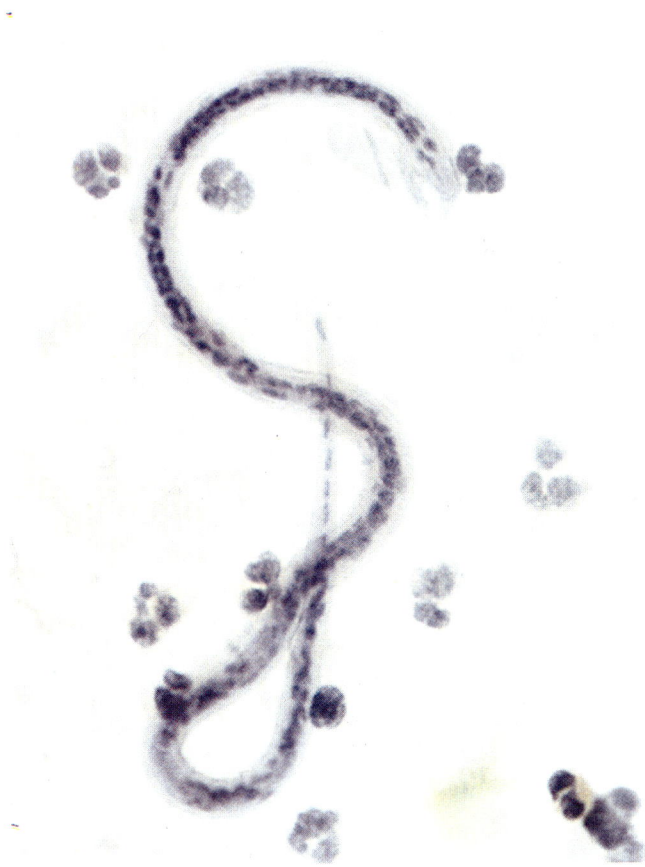

Fig. 33.1 Microfilaria of *Loa loa* in a thick blood smear. The sheath is clearly seen with this staining method. H&E

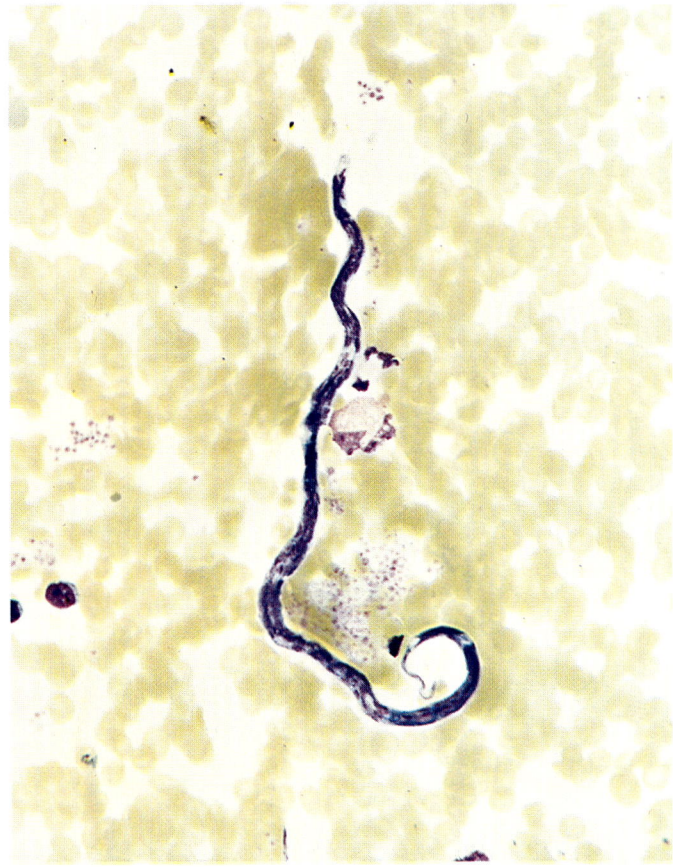

Fig. 33.2 Microfilaria of *Loa loa*; same case as Fig. 33.1 but with another staining method. Here, the sheath cannot be recognized. Giemsa

Pathogenesis

During the bite of the *Chrysops* fly, the microfilariae burst out of the insect and enter the human skin. The incubation period is usually several months. The development from the microfilariae to mature worms of *Loa loa* takes from 1–4 years (prepatent period).

Pathology

The sexually mature worms of *Loa loa* may be found in all parts of the subcutaneous connective tissue, but preferentially at uncovered sites of the body. Live moving worms may be seen beneath the skin or conjunctiva[3]. They may cause oedema and swelling. Histologically, the live worms cause non-specific inflammation with a few giant cells and a fibroplastic reaction. A marked tissue reaction usually is due to dead worms which also produce chronic abscesses.

Microfilariae may be found occasionally at numerous sites[4–6], such as central nervous system, spinal cord, choroid and retina, lungs, myocardium, spleen and kidneys. Usually, eosinophilic granulomas are seen, similar to those in visceral larva migrans (Section 37).

References

1. Duke, B. O. L. and Wijers, D. J. B. (1958). Studies on loiasis in monkeys. I. The relationship between human and simian Loa in the rain-forest zone of the British Cameroons. *Am. Trop. Med. Parasit.*, **52**, 158
2. Noireau, F. *et al.* (1990). Clinical manifestations of loiasis in an endemic area in the Congo. *Trop. Med. Parasit.*, **41**, 37
3. Pinder, M. *et al.* (1988). Identification of a surface antigen on Loa loa microfilariae the recognition of which correlates with the amicrofilaremic state in man. *J. Immunol.*, **141**, 1480
4. van Bogaert, L. *et al.* (1955). Encephalitis in Loa loa filariasis. *J. Neurol. Psychiatr.*, **18**, 10
5. Morel, L. *et al.* (1967). Infiltrats pulmonaires éosinophiliques au cours de filarioses de type Loa-loa. *Poumon Coeur*, **23**, 685
6. Toussaint, D. and Danis, P. (1965). Retinopathy in generalized Loa-loa filariasis. A clinico-pathological study. *Arch. Ophthal. (Chicago)*, **74**, 470

34. ONCHOCERCIASIS

Introduction

This filarial worm disease is also named river blindness. In endemic regions, it represents a significant social and economic problem. Onchocerciasis occurs in Central and West Africa[1–3], the Nile Valley and Yemen; also in the Caribbean region, Central America, Colombia and in the North East of Venezuela[4].

Some species of monkeys may be reservoir hosts. Another species, *Onchocerca armillata* is found in cattle[5].

Clinically, skin nodules are the typical manifestation of this nematodiasis, but they are normally harmless and may even be absent. Ocular lesions are a severe complication; the blindness rate in parasitic carriers is 10%.

For clinical diagnosis, microfilariae may be found in small skin 'snips' taken from the areas surrounding the skin nodules with bleeding[6]. Sometimes, microfilariae may be found in the urine. Eosinophilia is present, as in other worm infections.

The parasite

Onchocerca volvulus or *O. caecutiens*, a very thin filarial worm, is the causal agent. The females are up to 70 cm long and 0.4 mm wide but the males only up to 2–4 cm long. Their lifespan is usually less than 10 years. The microfilariae measure 250–330 μm in length and do not have a sheath[7].

The viviparous females may give birth to up to 1000 larvae or so-called microfilariae, daily (Fig. 34.1). Numerous species of *Simulium* flies (buffalo gnats or black flies) are blood sucking and take up microfilariae with a blood meal. If one fly takes up more than about 20 microfilariae, it will perish. Inside the fly, the microfilariae develop and migrate to the mouth region where infective microfilariae are found.

Pathogenesis

An infected gnat bites man and the microfilariae may penetrate the skin. Here, mature worms develop producing new microfilariae (larvae). Skin nodules may form 3–4 months after the bite. The prepatent period, from infection until formation of new microfilariae, is 12–15 months.

Male worms and microfilariae may wander in dermis and subcutis and do not always form nodules.

Adult worms are of less clinical significance than microfilariae. The latter may invade the cornea of the eyes, causing damage to all parts of the ocular bulb and thus lead to blindness[8].

Pathology

Cutaneous lesions. Typical lesions are palpable nodules in the skin, also called onchocercomas. They may be found on the trunk, head and shoulders or at other sites[9,10]. In each country or region, a different or specific localization of onchocercomas may prevail. Up to 50 nodules may be present in one patient. In each nodule, several mature worms may be present, and when the nodules perforate or break up, loops of thin worms may be seen. In addition to the typical nodular lesions in the skin, there may be eczema-like, sclerodermiform and hypo- or depigmented cutaneous lesions.

Histologically, in the nodules, three zones may be distinguished:

1. A fibrous capsule on the periphery with few cells and numerous collagen fibres.
2. A non-specific granulation tissue with infiltrates of neutrophils, eosinophils, lymphocytes, plasma cells and histiocytes in variable amounts.
3. A central region where adult worms are situated coiled up; thus, they will be cut in various directions. Also microfilariae are found in these regions. Histiocytes, epithelioid cells and multinucleated giant cells may be seen. Adult worms may be examined by special methods[11,12] (Figs. 34.2–34.8).

Older nodular lesions show more fibrous tissue. Cellular infiltrates and microfilariae may also be present, outside the onchocercomas. Active inflammation is found mostly after the microfilariae have died.

Summarizing, microfilariae are found in the uteri of the worms, free in the surrounding tissues and, occasionally, in the peripheral blood. There is no periodicity as in other filarial worm infections. Microfilariae may survive in the skin for 6–10 months.

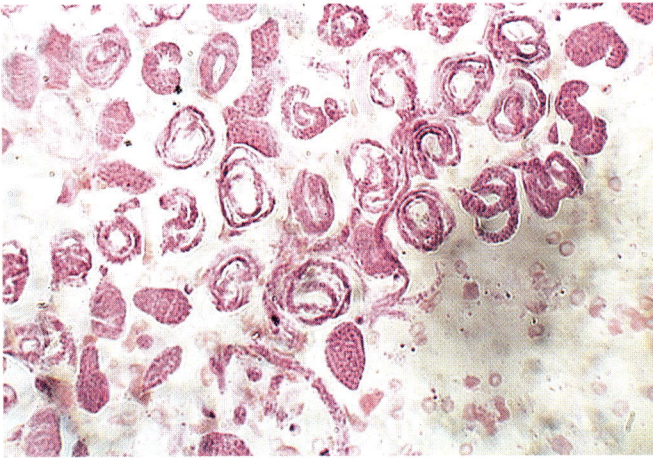

Fig. 34.1 Cluster of young larvae (microfilariae) of *Onchocerca volvulus* in smear of the cut surface of a fresh nodule in the skin. H&E

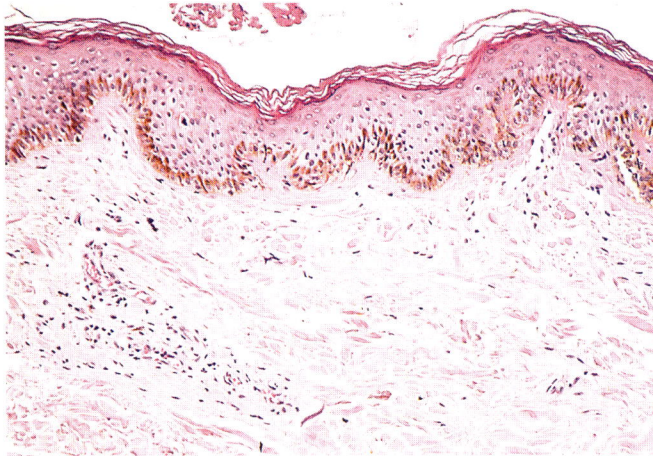

Fig. 34.2 Onchocerciasis. Microfilariae of *Onchocerca volvulus* are difficult to recognize in the dermis at this magnification. H&E

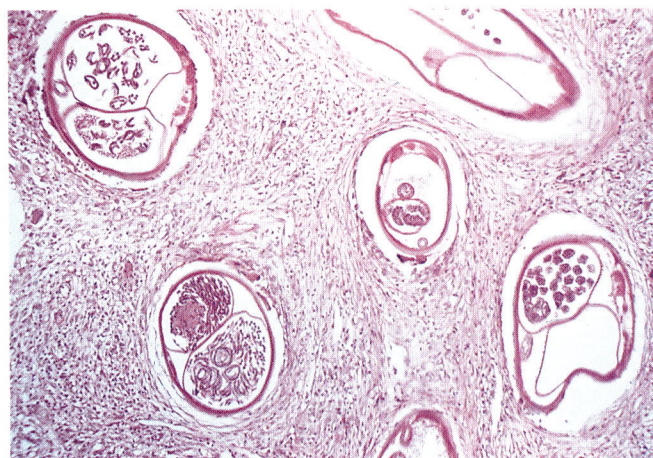

Fig. 34.3 *Onchocerca volvulus* worms in skin nodule containing microfilariae. Low power. H&E

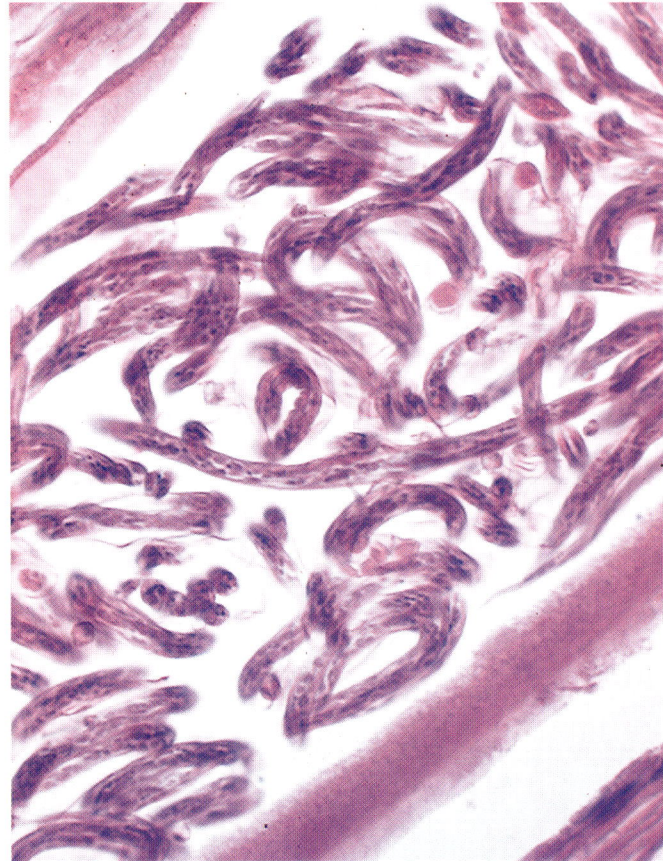

Fig. 34.4 Microfilariae of *Onchocerca volvulus* in an adult female worm. H&E

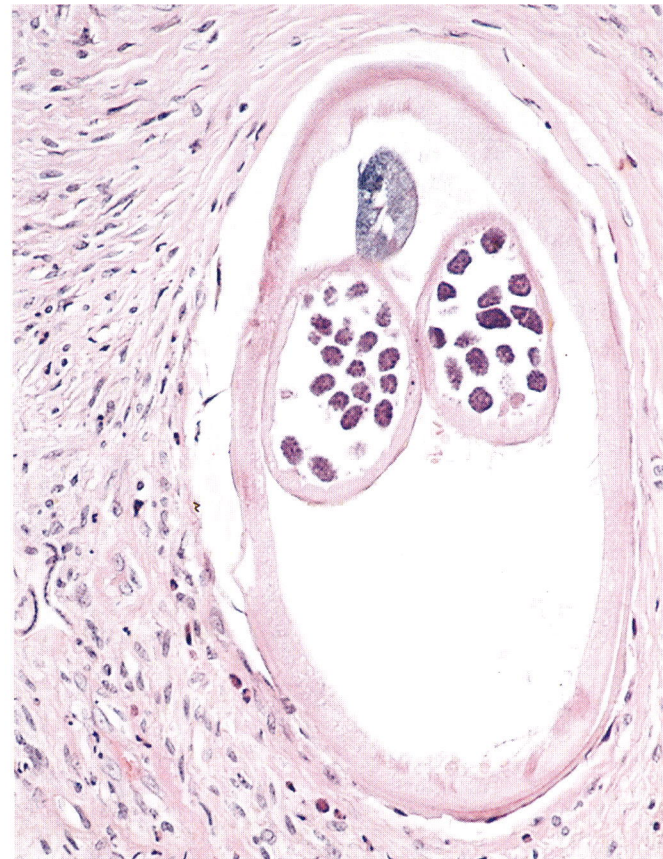

Fig. 34.5 Female *Onchocerca volvulus* worm in skin nodule showing eggs. H&E

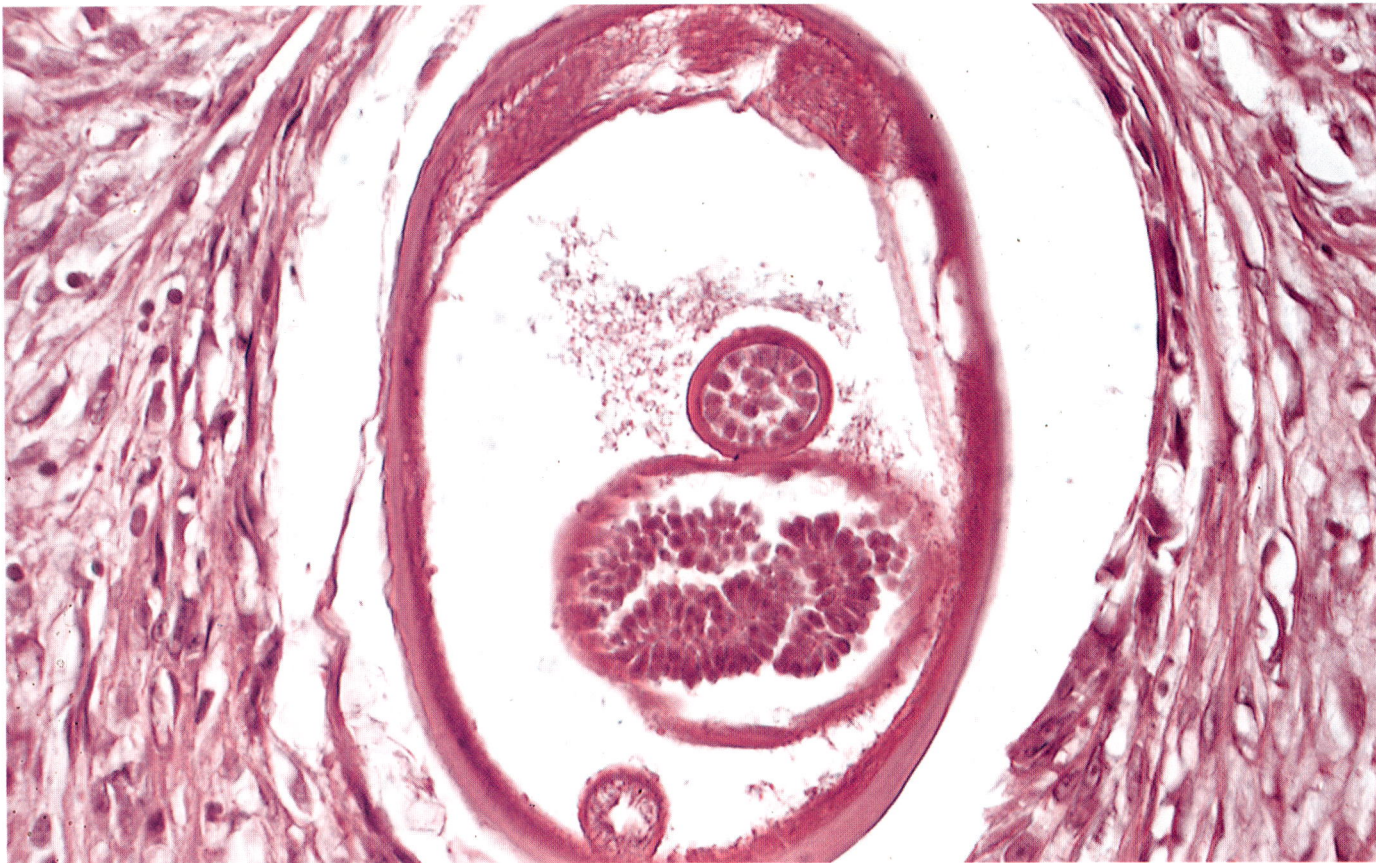

Fig. 34.6 Adult *Onchocerca voluvlus* filaria in skin lesion, cut in another direction. H&E

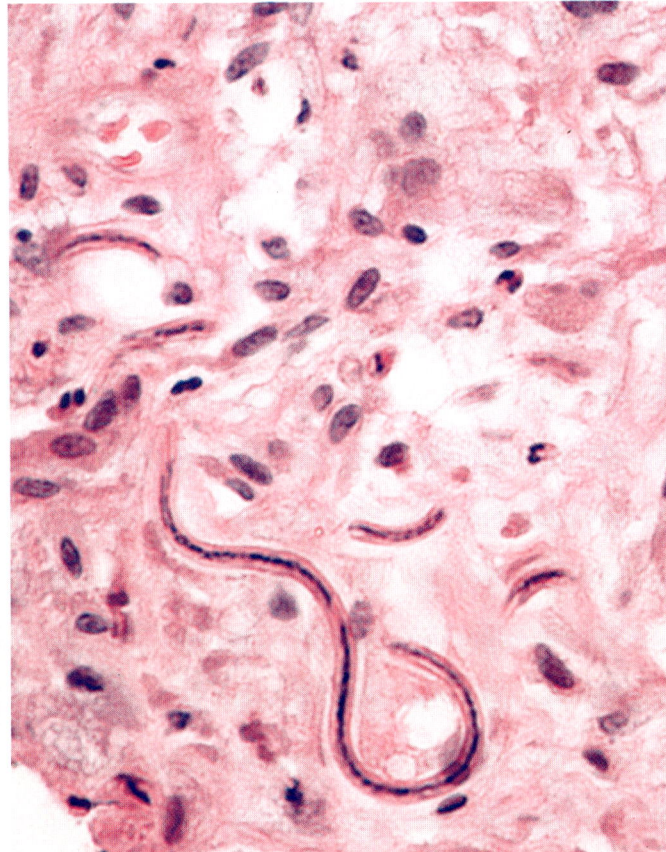

Fig. 34.7 Microfilariae of *Onchocerca volvulus* in skin lesion with scarce inflammatory reaction. H&E

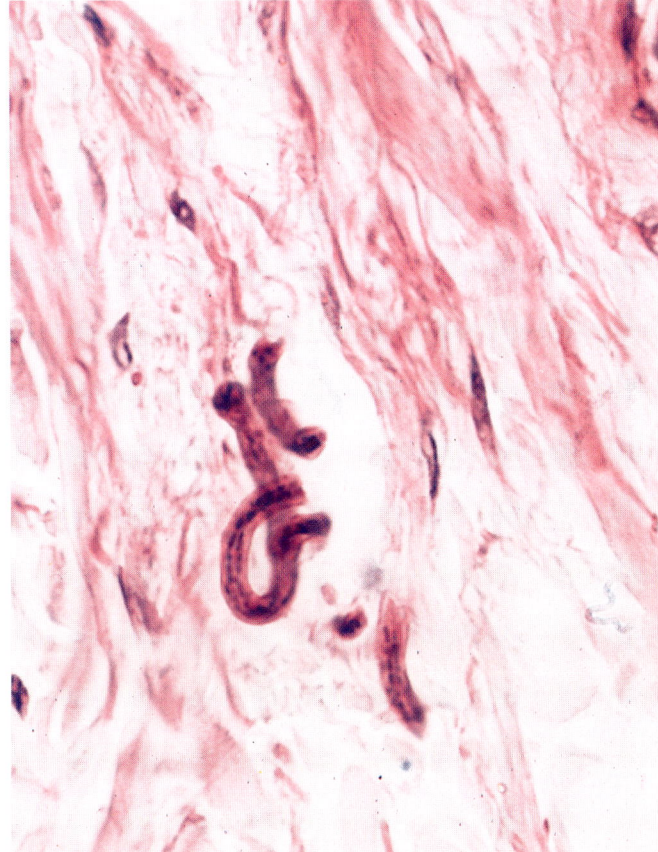

Fig. 34.8 Microfilariae of *Onchocerca volvulus* in skin lesion at high power. H&E

Ocular lesions. These are due to invasion of microfilariae. They may be found microscopically, as living micro-organisms, as dead ones or as fragments[13-15]. Features which may be present include oedema of the eyelids, conjunctivitis, keratitis and panophthalmitis in different stages of evolution. The inflammatory reaction will be more marked when the microfilariae are dead.

References

1. Albiez, E. J. et al. (1984). Studies on nodules and adult Onchocerca volvulus during a nodulectomy trial in hyperendemic villages in Liberia and Upper Volta. II. Comparison of the macrofilaria population in adult nodule carriers. Tropenmed. Parasit., **35**, 163
2. De Sole, G. (1990). Migration studies in the onchocerciasis controlled areas of West Africa. Trop. Med. Parasit., **41**, 33
3. Vuong, P. N. et al. (1988). Forest and savanna onchocerciasis: comparative morphometric histopathology of skin lesions. Trop. Med. Parasitol., **39**, 105
4. Botto, C., Arango, M. and Yarzabal, L. (1984). Onchocerciasis in Venezuela: prevalence of microfilaraemia in Amerindians and morphological characteristics of the microfilariae from the Upper Orinoco focus. Tropenmed. Parasit., **35**, 167
5. Mtei, B. J. and Sanga, H. J. (1990). Aortic oncocercosis and elaeophorosis in traditional TSZ-cattle in Tabora (Tanzania): prevalence and pathology. Vet. Parasitol., **36**, 165
6. Rivas Alcala, A. R. et al. (1990). Correlación entre oncocercomas y positividad para microfilarias en oncocercosis. Salud Pública Mex., **32**, 658
7. Eichner, M. and Renz, A. (1990). Differential length of Onchocerca volvulus infective larvae from the Cameroon rain forest and savanna. Trop. Med. Parasit., **41**, 29
8. Duke, B. O. (1990). Human onchocerciasis – an overview of the disease. Acta Leiden, **59**, 9
9. Guderian, R. H. and Kerrigan, K. R. (1990). Onchocerciasis and acquired groin hernias in Ecuador. Trop. Med. Parasit., **41**, 69
10. Albiez, E. J. and Buettner, D. W. (1984). Corium attached onchocercomata: clinical and histological findings. Zbl. Bakt. Hyg. A., **258**, 388
11. Duke, B. O. (1990). An improved method of examining adult Onchocerca volvulus worms. Trop. Med. Parasitol., **41**, 25
12. Duke, B. O. et al. (1990). On the reproductive activity of the female Onchocerca volvulus. Trop. Med. Parasitol., **41**, 387
13. Semba, R. D. et al. (1990). Longitudinal study of lesions of the posterior segment in onchocerciasis. Ophthalmology, **97**, 1334
14. Rothova, A. et al. (1990). Ocular involvement in patients with onchocerciasis after repeated treatment with ivermectin. Am. J. Ophthalmol., **15**, 110
15. Newland, H. S. et al. (1991). Ocular manifestations of onchocerciasis in a rain forest area of west Africa. Br. J. Ophthalmol., **75**, 163

35. DIROFILARIASIS

Introduction

Dirofilariasis, also called human zoonotic filariasis, is another filarial worm infection of minor importance; only sporadic reports of human dirofilariasis exist.

Worm infections of this sort have been found in Southern Europe, the Eastern Mediterranean countries and the USA, mainly in the southern regions[1]. Infection is also known in Venezuela. One human case has been reported from Mérida[2]; this was a fortuitous finding at autopsy.

In numerous cases of human dirofilariasis, diagnosis is not confirmed; other filarial worms are discussed as possible causative agents.

There is a large animal reservoir of hosts, mostly domestic animals, such as dogs[3] and cats, but also wild carnivores from all over the world. Dogs and cats may be used for experimental work[4-8]. Aedes aegypti has been found to transmit microfilariae to dogs[9].

Few human cases are known. They show subcutaneous or conjunctival nodular lesions, or pulmonary and cardiovascular involvement, with variable and non-specific symptoms. In some cases, 'coin lesions' have been found in the lungs with X-ray.

Clinical diagnosis has been made mostly by examination of surgical specimens. ELISA has been found lately to be useful for diagnosis[10].

The parasite

Dirofilaria immitis is also called dog heartworm. This species is found mainly in cases with involvement of viscera, while, in cases of cutaneous lesions, other species of the genus *Dirofilaria* are observed (*D. tenuis, D. repens, D. conjunctivae*).

The morphology of adult worms has not been studied completely because only dead worms, fragments of them or immature parasites have been examined in tissues. Female worms have been found to reach 10 cm in length, contain unfertilized ova, and also microfilariae in the uterus. A characteristic feature seems to be the thick laminated cuticle of the adult worms with spines.

The cycle of development of these filarial species is unknown. Man seems to be a false unsuitable dead-end host. Mosquitos (*Aedes, Anopheles, Culex*) and fleas are carriers, vectors or intermediate hosts.

Pathogenesis

Details of transmission and infection are not available. When isolated parasites have been found, they have been young. Free microfilariae have not been found in tissues of man, only in blood (Fig. 35.1).

Pathology

Cutaneous lesions. Nodular subcutaneous lesions are present at various sites and also in the conjunctiva. Subjacent musculature and bones are not usually involved. The nodules reach 1–6 cm in diameter. Only once, has more than one parasite been found in a nodule. Nodular lesions have also been reported in lymph nodes.

Pulmonary and cardiovascular lesions. Grossly, infarct-like foci have been noted in the lungs. Female worms are usually noted in pulmonary arteries, the inferior vena cava, cardiac cavities and peripheral arteries. Immature and dead worms, larger than microfilariae, are situated coiled up in thrombotic masses; they are seen cut in various directions. At these sites, parasites are found rarely and usually fortuitously in surgical or autopsy specimens (Figs. 35.2–35.7). The structural details of the worm's cuticle leads to diagnosis. An eosinophilic pneumonia is noted surrounding the intra-arterial parasites and sometimes a foreign body reaction is seen (Fig. 35.8).

References

1. Risher, W. H. et al. (1989). Pulmonary dirofilariasis. The largest single-institution experience. J. Thorac. Cardiovasc. Surg., **97**, 303
2. Salfelder, K., de Arriaga, A. D. and Rujano, J. J. (1976). Caso humano de dirofilariasis pulmonar. Acta Med. Venezol., **23**, 87
3. Ward, J. W. (1965). Prevalence of Dirofilaria immitis in the heart of

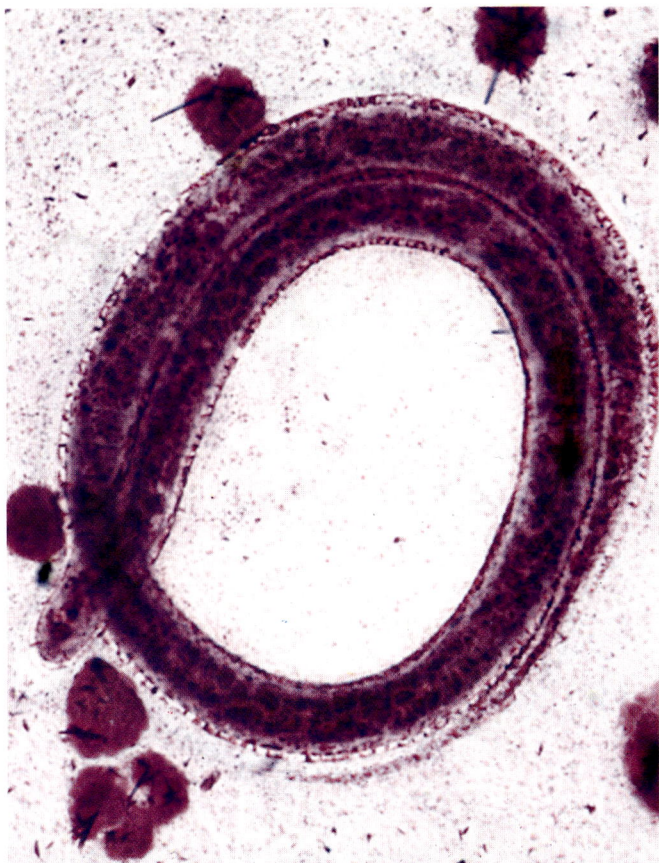

Fig. 35.1 Microfilaria of *Dirofilaria immitis* in blood smear. H&E

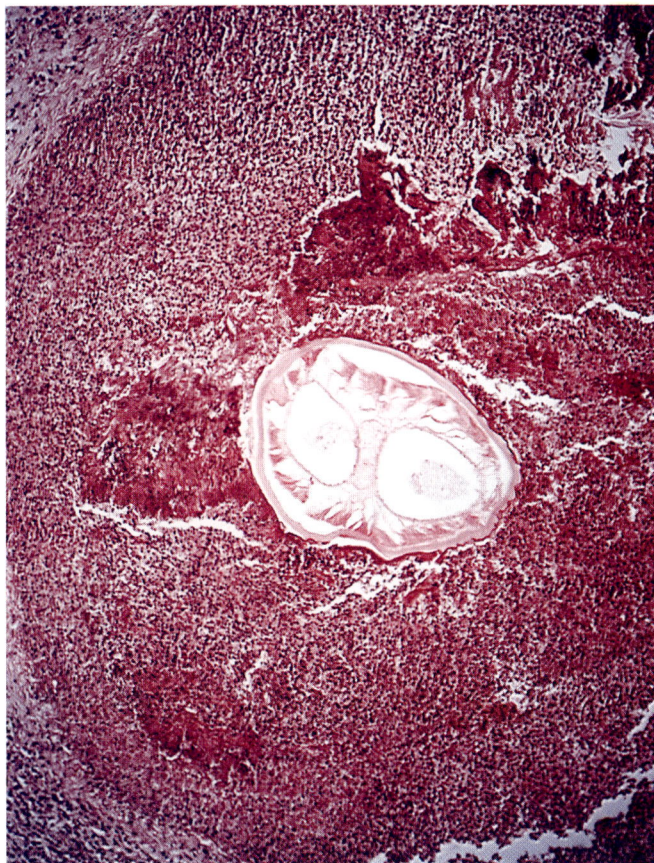

Fig. 35.2 Adult *Dirofilaria immitis* filaria in a lung focus surrounded by numerous leukocytes. Human case. H&E

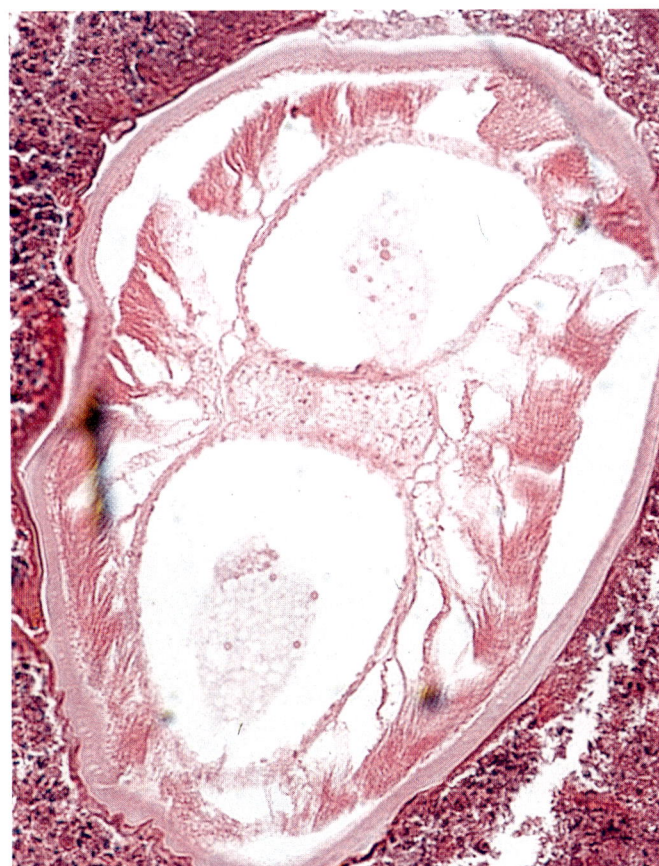

Fig. 35.3 High power of Fig. 35.2. H&E

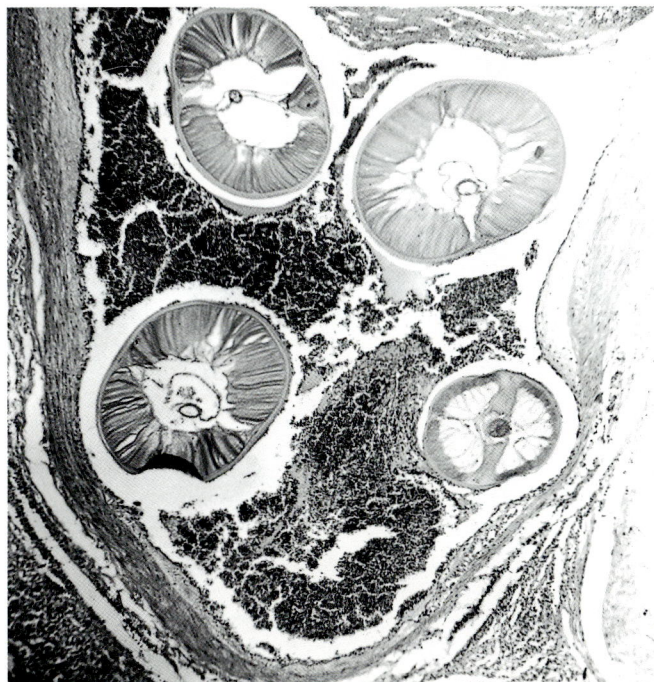

Fig. 35.4 Four filariae of *Dirofilaria immitis* in a pulmonary artery. Human case. H&E

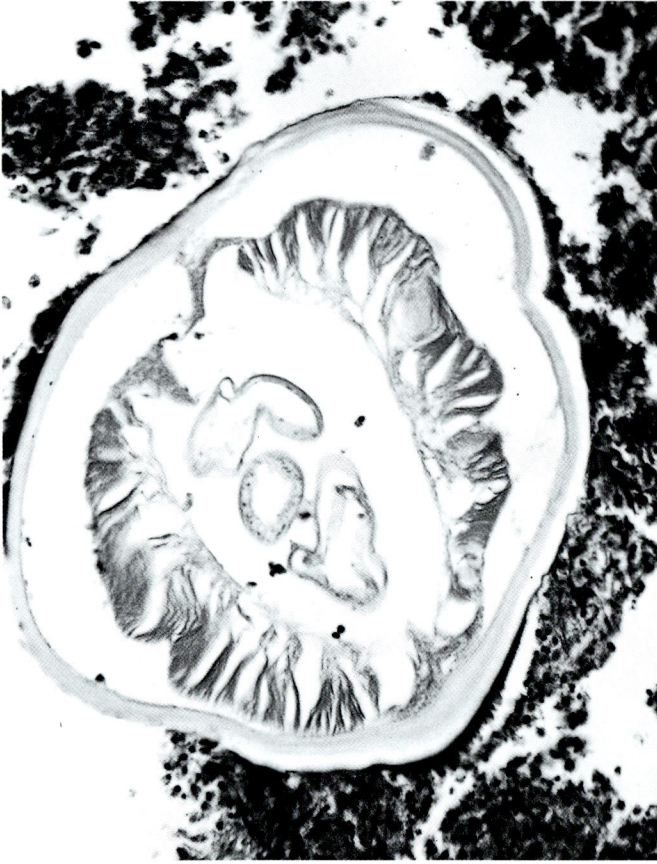

Fig. 35.5 Adult filaria of *Dirofilaria immitis* in a human lung at high power. H&E

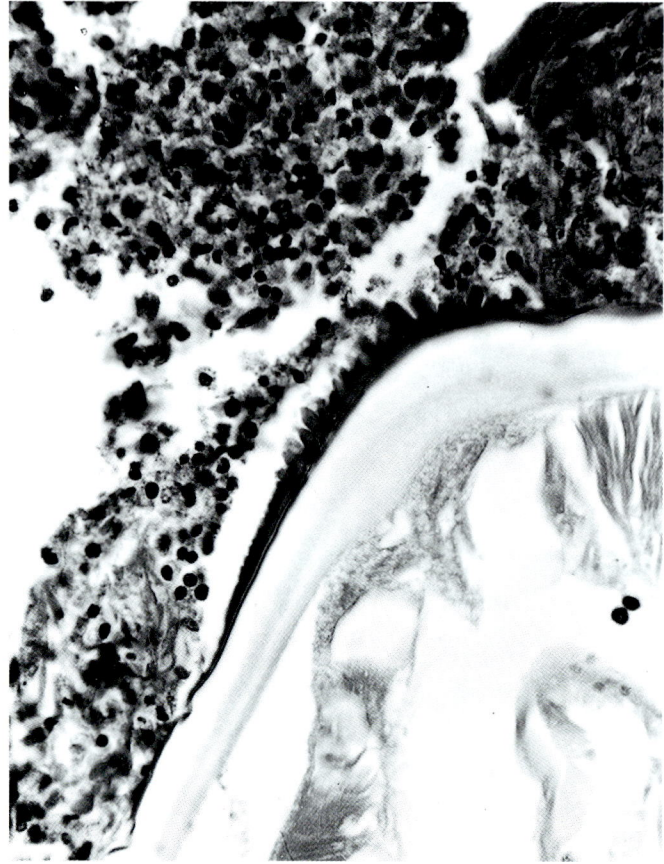

Fig. 35.6 Transversally cut *Dirofilaria immitis* filaria in human pulmonary artery with Hoeppli–Splendore phenomenon. H&E

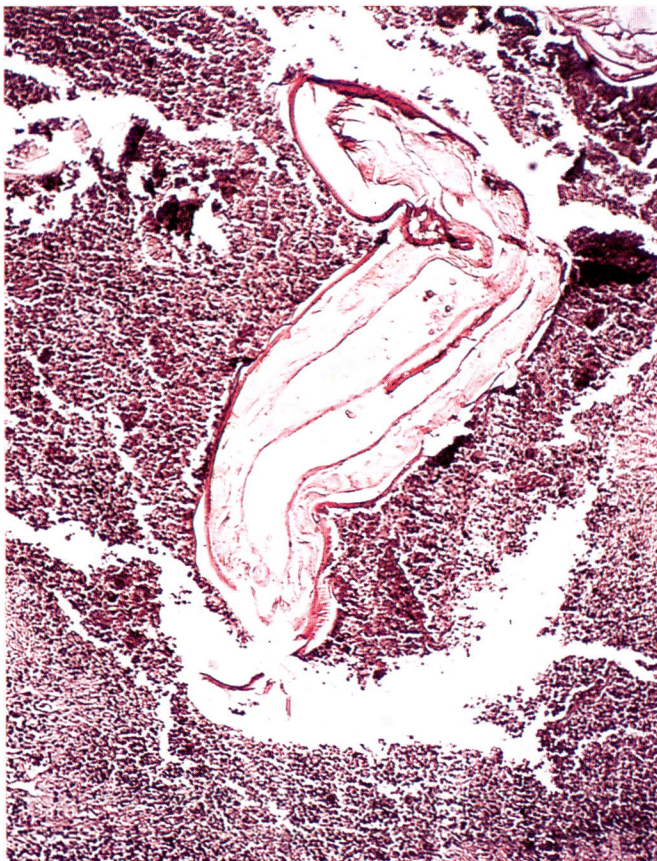

Fig. 35.7 Deformed filaria of *Dirofilaria immitis*, longitudinally cut, in a lung focus. H&E

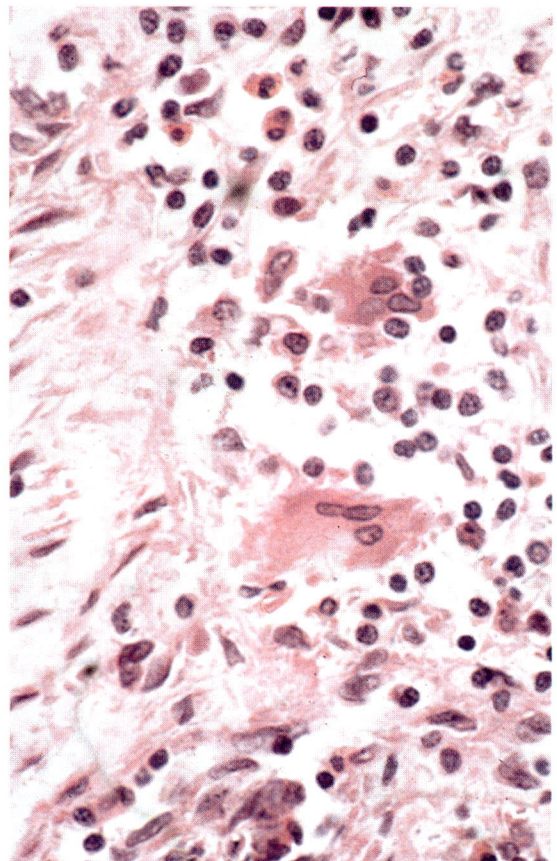

Fig. 35.8 Foreign body reaction near filaria of *Dirofilaria immitis* in a human lung. H&E

dogs examined in Mississippi. *J. Parasit.*, **51**, 404
4. Eaton, K. A. and Rosol, T. J. (1989). Caval syndrome in a Dirofilaria immitis-infected dog treated with dichlorvos. *J. Am. Vet. Med. Assoc.*, **195**, 223
5. Ludders, J. W. *et al.* (1988). Renal microcirculatory and correlated histologic changes associated with dirofilariasis in dogs. *Am. J. Vet. Res.*, **49**, 826
6. Grauer, G. F. *et al.* (1989). Experimental Dirofilaria immitis-associated glomerulonephritis induced in part by in situ formation of immune complexes in the glomerular capillary wall. *J. Parasitol.*, **75**, 585

7. Sasaki, Y. *et al.* (1990). Improvement in pulmonary arterial lesions after heartworm removal using flexible allegator forceps. *Nippon Juigaku Zasshi*, **52**, 743
8. Rawlings, C. A. *et al.* (1990). Morphologic changes in the lungs of cats experimentally infected with Dirofilaria immitis. Response to aspirin. *J. Vet. Intern. Med.*, **4**, 292
9. Hendrix, C. M. *et al.* (1986). Natural transmission of Dirofilaria immitis by Aedes aegypti. *J. Am. Mosq. Control Assoc.*, **2**, 48
10. Sato, M. *et al.* (1985). Human pulmonary dirofilariasis with special reference to the ELISA for the diagnosis and follow-up study. *Z. Parasitenkd.*, **71**, 561

36. RARE AND UNCOMMON NEMATODIASES

Six roundworm infections have been reported in man rarely and/or in limited geographical areas.

Acanthocephaliasis

Moniliformis moniliformis and *Macracanthorhynchus hirudinaceus* belong to the class Acanthocephala or thorn-head worms of nematodes. They have a retractable head with thorn-like recurved spines and attack the digestive tract. They are found only occasionally in man in the Far East and South East Asia[1]. There were only nine recorded human infections with *M. hirudinaceus* in Thailand up to 1989[2].

Dioctophymatosis

Dioctophyma renale, the giant renal worm, is a roundworm, the female being up to 1 m long. This infection has been reported in Europe, Asia and the Americas. The renal pelvis and the abdominal cavity may be invaded by the adult worm. Carnivorous animals may be infected.

Lagochilascariasis

Lagochilascaris minor is a roundworm species in which the females measure up to 1.5 cm in length. Human infection is limited to the Caribbean region. Draining subcutaneous abscesses are formed. It is possible that the reservoir hosts are wild animals with intestinal infections[3–5].

Micronemiasis

Micronema deletrix is a free-living saprophagous roundworm. The adult worms have the dimensions of a microfilaria. One human case with meningo-encephalomyelitis has been reported and infection is known in horses[6–8].

Oesophagostomiasis

Several species of the genus *Oesophagostomum* may infect man. Female worms are up to 22 mm long. Human cases have been found in Brazil, Indonesia and tropical Africa. The caecum and large intestine are involved. Infection occurs through contaminated food and water. Domestic animals and simians may also be infected[9–11].

Trichostrongyliasis

Eight species of the genus *Trichostrongylus* are pathogenic for man. Infections are generally encountered in the warm countries of the Near East, Africa and Asia; the prevalence of human infection varies considerably but millions of cases are estimated worldwide. Infection takes place orally via contaminated food and water or migration like the hookworms and the adult worms measure up to 9 mm. Domestic animals, especially ruminants, may be infected. The digestive tract is affected, but with relatively little clinical significance. Poisoning of the host by metabolic products of the parasite may occur in severe infections[12–16].

References

1. Zhao, B. *et al.* (1990). Licht-und elektronenmikroskopische Untersuchungen zur Histopathogenität von Macracanthorhynchus hirudinaceus in experimentell infizierten Hausschweinen. *Parasitol. Res.*, **76**, 355
2. Radomyos, P. *et al.* (1989). Intestinal perforation due to Macracanthorhynchus hirudenaceus infection in Thailand. *Trop. Med. Parasit.*, **40**, 476
3. Draper, J. W. (1963). Infection with Lagochilascaris minor. *Br. Med. J.*, **1**, 931
4. Little, M. D. (1964). Life cycle of Lagochilascaris minor. *J. Parasit.*, **50**, 34
5. Oostburg, B. F. J. and Varma, A. A. O. (1968). Lagochilascaris minor infection in Surinam. *Am. J. Trop. Med. Hyg.*, **17**, 548
6. Ferris, D. H. *et al.* (1972). Micronema deletrix in equine brain. *Am. J. Vet. Res.*, **33**, 33
7. Hoogstraten, J. and Young, W. G. (1973). Meningo-encephalitis due to the saprophagous nematode Micronema deletrix. *Can. J. Neurol. Sci.*, **2**, 121
8. Rubin, H. L. and Woodward, J. C. (1974). Equine infection with Micronema deletrix. *J. Am. Vet. Med. Assoc.*, **165**, 256
9. Haaf, E. and van Soest, A. H. (1964). Oesophagostomiasis in man in North Ghana. *Trop. Geogr. Med.*, **16**, 49
10. Anthony, P. P. and McAdam, I. W. (1972). Helminthic pseudotumours of the bowel: thirty four cases of helminthoma. *Gut*, **13**, 8
11. Chang, J. and McClure, H. M. (1975). Disseminated oesophagostomiasis in the rhesus monkey. *J. Am. Vet. Med. Assoc.*, **167**, 628
12. Biocca, E. *et al.* (1960). Further studies on Trichostrongyliasis in Jewish communities in Iran. *Parasitology*, **2**, 345
13. Tejada, A. and Burstein, Z. (1964). Primer caso autóctono de trichostrongylosis en Perú. *Bol. Chil. Parasitol.*, **19**, 125
14. Markell, E. K. (1968). Pseudohookworm infection – Trichostrongyliasis. *N. Engl. J. Med.*, **278**, 831
15. Sabka *et al.* (1967). Intestinal helminthiasis in the rural area of Khuzestan, South West Iran. *Am. Trop. Med. Parasitol.*, **61**, 352
16. Lawless, D. K. *et al.* (1956). Intestine parasites in an Egyptian village of the Nile Valley with emphasis on the Protozoa. *Am. J. Trop. Med. Hyg.*, **5**, 1010

37. LARVA MIGRANS

Two definitions have been proposed for this clinical entity:

1. The presence of larvae in tissues of a 'false' host, or infection due to larvae which do not mature in man.

   Aberrant nematode larvae may move aimlessly for a prolonged time; are not able to reach sexual maturity in man and are not transmitted further. Man is infected fortuitously, being a 'false' dead-end host. This group also includes worms which become mature, but the eggs or larvae remain in the tissues or the intestine and are not excreted. Apart from the skin, the liver, lungs, central nervous system and eyes are the main organs to be involved, but other organs and tissues may be affected. Larvae of the species of the genera *Toxocara*, *Anisakis* and *Angiostrongylus* may behave in this way. It is admitted that larvae of the nematode genera, *Strongyloides*, *Dirofilaria* and *Gnathostoma*, cause a similar clinical picture.

2. The often fortuitous finding in tissues of larvae whose species cannot be determined on morphological grounds.

   By this definition, larva migrans includes all cases of larvae, microfilariae, or fragments of them, in human tissue, in which histological diagnosis of the worm species is impossible to make. In a case of microfilariae of filarial worms in tissues, for instance, it cannot often be determined whether or not they possess sheaths, a feature which allows classification. Thus, this definition is of practical significance for pathologists.

Two clinical entities are considered: **cutaneous LM** and **visceral LM**.

Cutaneous larva migrans (creeping eruption)

This localization of migrating larvae or microfilariae is found mainly in the tropics or subtropics[1]. The wandering larvae in the superficial layers of the skin do not commonly get into the circulation nor do they invade viscera.

The best known agents of creeping eruption are the canine hookworms, *Ancylostoma braziliense* and *A. caninum*. On the feet, hands or any other part of the body, a slight irritation results with papules and linear skin lesions (Fig. 37.1). These mark the route of the larvae and may be infected secondarily. They are active for up to a few weeks only advancing 3–5 cm per day, and then they die.

The larvae of human hookworms, *Strongyloides*, *Gnathostoma* and the microfilariae of filarial worms, also may cause creeping eruption[2-4].

A picture similar to cutaneous larva migrans is called 'swimmer's itch', but, in this infection, there is no migration. Cercariae of trematode species produce the cercarial dermatitis, and sparganum stages of fish tapeworm species cause sparganosis. Fly larvae may provoke cutaneous myiasis.

Visceral larva migrans

Introduction

When infection with larvae of the genera, *Toxocara*, *Anisakis*, *Angiostrongylus* or others, can be demonstrated, the disease should be named toxocariasis or after the name of the causal nematode. The denomination visceral larva migrans is better reserved for cases without an exact diagnosis of the species of worm.

Visceral larva migrans occurs worldwide, but preferentially in tropical countries. In Europe and North America, an increasing number of pets (dogs and cats) is maintained in urban centres and this, possibly, is the reason why an increasing number of cases of visceral larva migrans is reported in these parts. Mostly infants are affected.

Clinically, hepatomegaly, pulmonary disorders and symptoms like asthma, pyrexia, granulomatous ophthalmitis[5], retinal detachment and blindness, and epilepsy, may be due to visceral larva migrans.

Clinical diagnosis: almost always a high blood eosinophilia is present. Serological tests may be useful.

The parasite

In addition to larvae of the above-mentioned genera, those of *Ascaris lumbricoides*, *Strongyloides*, *Capillaria hepatica*, *Trichostrongylus* spp. filarial worms and species of *Pentastomida* and *Spirometra*, belong to this group, since, when found in tissues, species diagnosis cannot be made on structural grounds. Exceptionally, *Trichuris vulpis* may cause visceral larva migrans[6].

Pathogenesis

Visceral LM occurs when the larvae or microfilariae of filarial worms do not follow their normal cycle of development but wander around and come to organs and sites out of their usual way. There, they may be blocked by an inflammatory reaction with granuloma formation. The larvae may still be visible in these lesions, they may have disappeared, following their migratory route, or they may have disintegrated after producing the inflammation. Migrating nematode larvae may spread micro-organisms.

Pathology

The damage caused by visceral larva migrans is more pronounced than that resulting from the creeping eruption. Grossly, miliary granulomas may be seen in the viscera. The localization of tissue lesions is fortuitous, and they may be found in several organs of a single person (Figs. 37.2–37.6).

The following entities belong more or less to the disease under discussion.

1. **Allergic granulomas** with manifestations in several organs[7-11].

2. **Loeffler syndrome** is due to larvae of *Ascaris lumbricoides* in the lungs which cause fast-vanishing infiltrates of eosinophilic leukocytes. After a few days, these are invisible to X-ray and are found only fortuitously at autopsy.

3. **Tropical pulmonary eosinophilia (TPE)** and the **syndrome of Meyers–Koumenaar** may be due to filariasis with granulomas in liver, spleen and lymph nodes.

4. **Visceral eosinophilic granulomas**, in various organs, also possibly belong to this group of lesions[12,13]. Larvae or microfilariae are usually no longer seen in these granulomas (see *Pathogenesis*) (Figs. 37.7–37.9). The latter, however, for instance in the liver, may also be produced by ova of *Schistosoma* or by other parasites.

References

1. Scheiner, R. B. *et al.* (1990). Lesions on the feet of a scuba diver. Cutaneous larva migrans. *Arch. Dermatol.*, **126**, 1092
2. Caplan, J. P. (1949). Creeping eruption and intestinal strongyloidiasis. *Br. Med. J.*, **1**, 396
3. Nagao, M. (1955). A case of creeping disease caused in man by a larval Gnathostoma spinigerum. *Fukuoka Acta Med.*, **46**, 2013

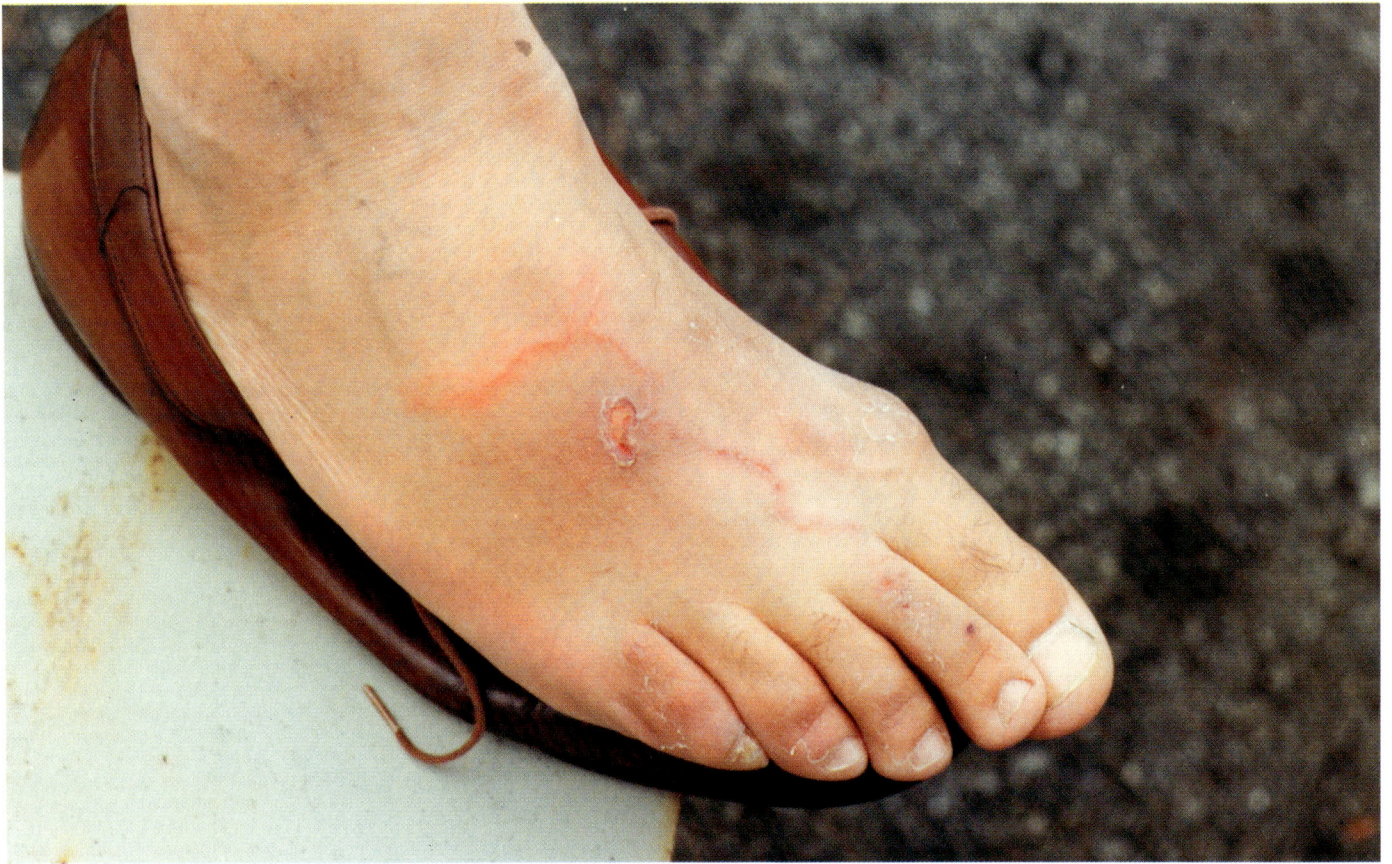

Fig. 37.1 Cutaneous larva migrans ('creeping eruption').

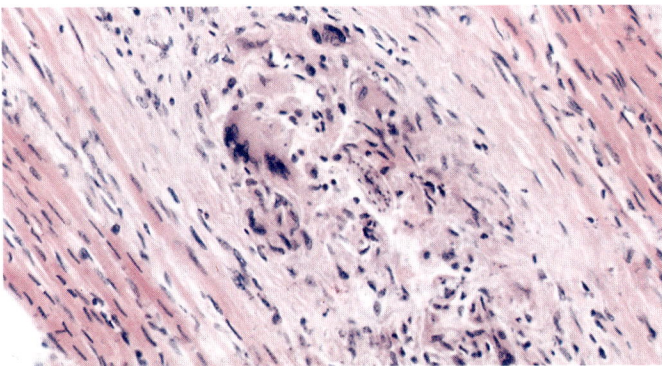

Fig. 37.2 Visceral larva migrans in the myocardium with foreign body giant cell and focal inflammation. H&E

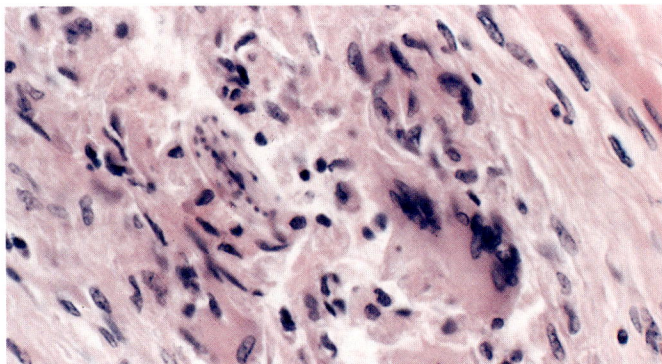

Fig. 37.3 The same case as Fig. 37.2 at medium power. H&E

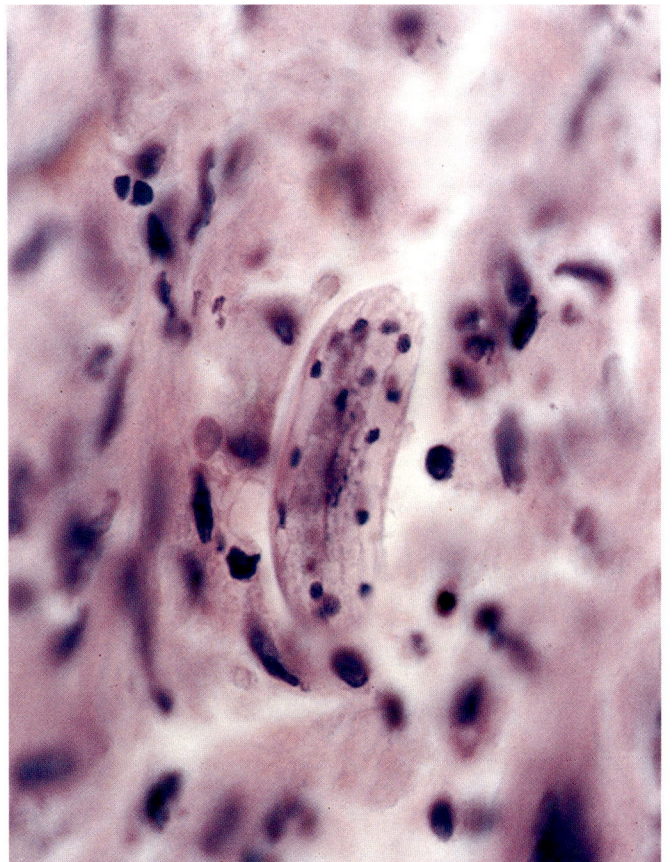

Fig. 37.4 The same case as Figs. 37.2 and 37.3. The microfilaria-like larva is clearly visible at high power. H&E

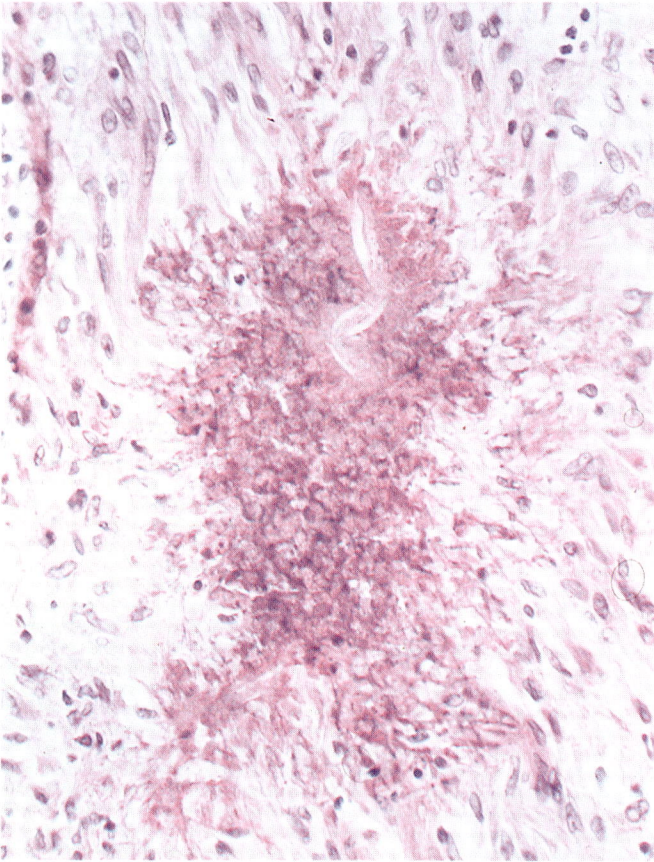

Fig. 37.5 Granuloma due to larva migrans in the mesocolon. The larva is not seen at this magnification. H&E

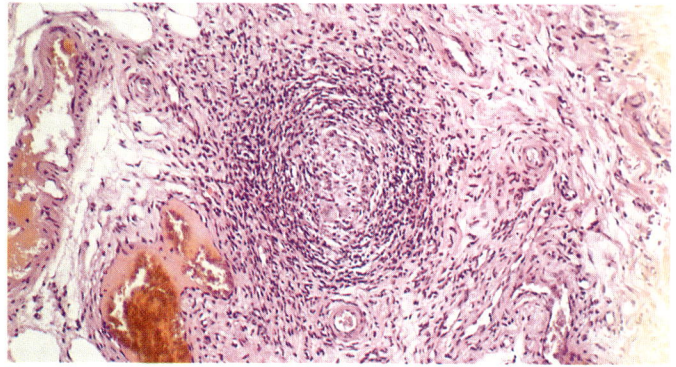

Fig. 37.6 Larva migrans with focal inflammation in the wall of the duodenum. The necrobiotic larva is faintly seen in the upper part. H&E

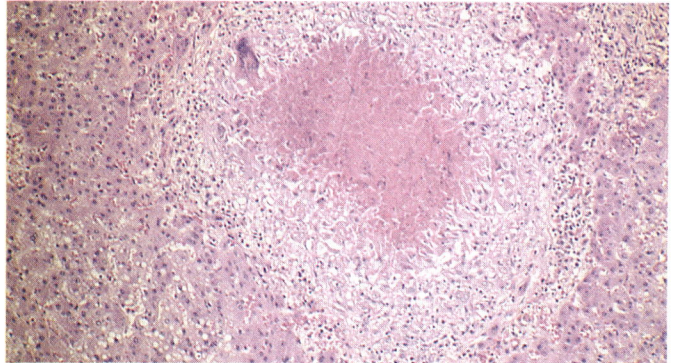

Fig. 37.7 Visceral eosinophilic granuloma with central necrosis in the liver, probably due to visceral larva migrans. H&E

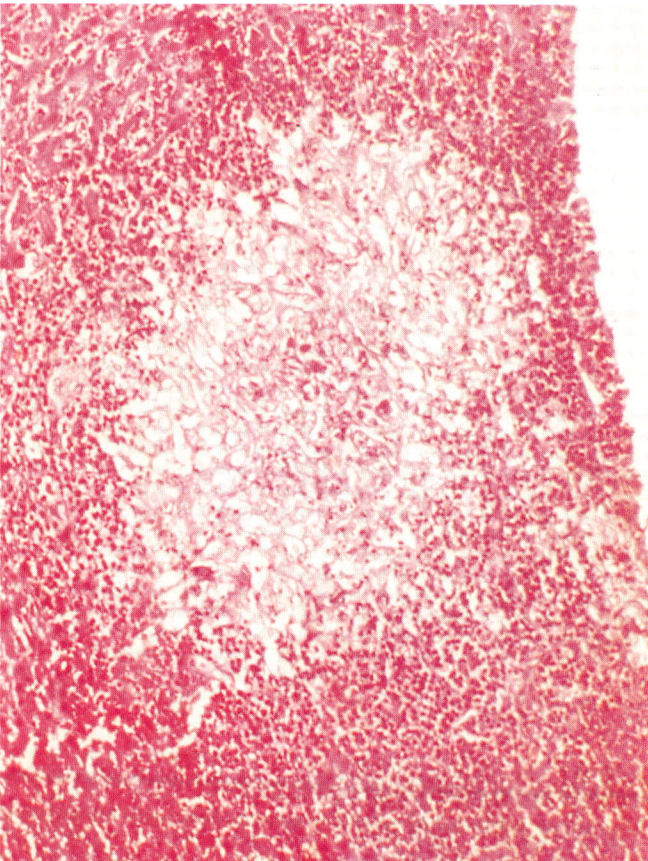

Fig. 37.8 Visceral eosinophilic granuloma in the liver. A larva is not seen (anymore?). H&E

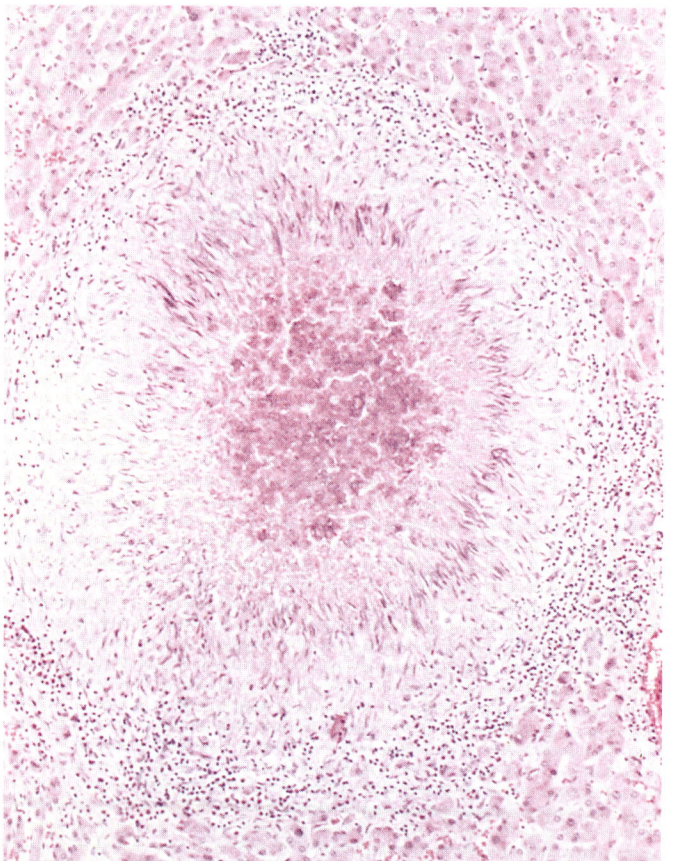

Fig. 37.9 Visceral eosinophilic granuloma in the liver with palisading epithelioid cells. A larva is not seen, the same as in Figs. 35.7 and 35.8. H&E

4. Kaminsky, C. A. *et al.* (1989). Eosinophilic migratory nodular panniculitis (human ganthostomiasis). *Med. Cutan. Ibero. Lat. Am.*, **17**, 158
5. Wilder, H. B. (1950). Nematode endophthalmitis. *Trans. Am. Acad. Ophthalmol. Otolaryng.*, **55**, 99
6. Sakano, T. *et al.* (1980). Visceral larva migrans caused by Trichuris vulvis. *Arch. Dis. Child.*, **55**, 63
7. Brill, R. *et al.* (1953). Allergic granulomatosis associated with visceral larva migrans. *Am. J. Clin. Path.*, **23**, 1208
8. Stout, C. (1970). Allergic granulomas of gut (to the editor). *N. Engl. J. Med.*, **282**, 1324

9. Churg, J. and Strauss, L. (1951). Allergic granulomatosis, allergic angiitis and periarteritis nodosa. *Am. J. Path.*, **27**, 277
10. Vanek, J. (1964). Granulomata of the liver, probably of allergic origin. *Acta Morph.*, **XIII**, 411
11. Abell, M. *et al.* (1970). Allergic granulomatosis with massive gastric involvement. *N. Engl. J. Med.*, **282**, 665
12. Liscano, T. R. de (1972). Granulomas hepáticos en autopsias con especial referencia a los granulomas 'eosinofílicos'. *Tesis doctoral.* ULA (Mérida, Venezuela)
13. Salfelder, K., Liscano, T. R. de and Mendelovici, M. de (1973). Visceral eosinophilic granulomas. *Beitr. Path.*, **149**, 420

B. CESTODIASIS

Cestodes or tapeworms have a small head (scolex with suckers and hooks), a short neck (proliferation zone) and the main body has a chain of flat bands (proglottids) (Table 17). Tapeworms measure from a few cm up to 20 m long.

Nutrition takes place by percutaneous absorption; there is no digestive tract. Since tapeworms are hermaphroditic, male and female genital organs are found together in the posterior proglottids of mature worms. Scolex and form of uteri allow differentiation of species.

Man is the definitive host for **mature tapeworms** (in the digestive tract) of the genera *Taenia, Diphyllobothrium, Dipylidium* and *Hymenolepis*. Man may also be the intermediate host for *Taenia solium*. Transmission occurs by consumption of meat (*Taenia*), fish (*Diphyllobothrium*), swallowed insects (*Dipylidium*) and, directly, via eggs from man to man (*Hymenolepis*).

Cysticercosis and echinococcosis are diseases caused by the **larvae** of tapeworms. In these cases, transmission occurs by ingestion of eggs.

Damage to man by mature tapeworms is minimal, and never directly fatal. The possible toxicity of these worms is difficult to ascertain. In contrast, the larvae of tapeworms may lead to serious disease and cause death.

Certain infections will **not** be discussed in this atlas. These are:

1. Rare infections in man by the Cestodes larvae of:
   Taenia multiceps (coenurosis) which affect CNS, subcutis and eyes,
   Mesocestoides spp. with lesions in subcutis and musculature,
   Spirometra spp. (sparganosis) in subcutis, and
   Sparganum proliferum with lesions of numerous larvae in subcutis and viscera.

2. The rare infections reported only in certain countries in South America by:
   Echinococcus oligarthus,
   Echinococcus vogeli and
   Echinococcus patagonicus.

Table 17 Cestodes. Head and proglottids of: **1** Taenia saginata; **2** Taenia solium; **3** Diphyllobothrium latum

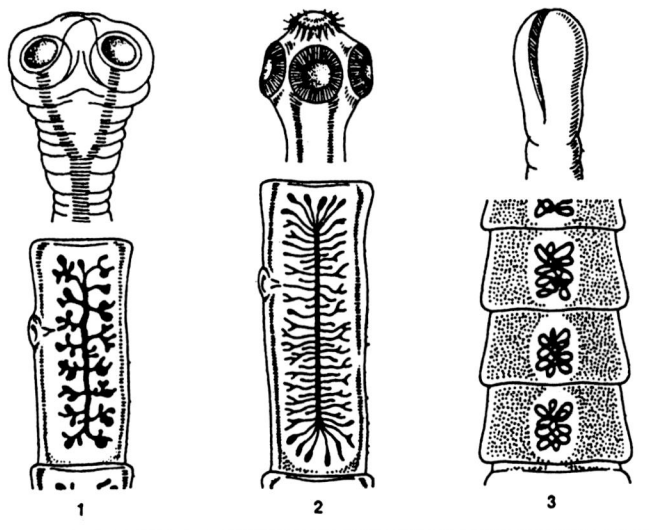

38. TAENIASIS

Introduction

This infection with adult worms may be caused by the beef or pork tapeworms (*Taenia saginata* or *Taenia solium* respectively), which are the best known worm species of this sort in man. Carriers of these two worm species in the digestive tract are found worldwide. Millions of people, mostly children[1,2], are carriers. Now, infection with *Taenia solium* in many countries has become rare because of systematic meat inspection.

Taeniasis is well known in Venezuela and cysticercosis has been found frequently in autopsy material in Mérida.

It must be emphasized here that infection with eggs of *Taenia solium* leads to the formation of larvae (cysticerci) in tissues. This disease, called cysticercosis (see Section 42), is much more dangerous than the presence of pork tapeworms in the gut (taeniasis). The latter is due to consumption of infected raw meat. *Taenia saginata* does not produce cysticercosis[3-5].

The intermediate hosts for *Taenia saginata* are cattle and, less frequently, zebra, buffalo, reindeer and antelopes. *Taenia solium* is found in pigs; *Taenia teniforme* occurs only in rats (Fig. 38.1).

Clinically, people in contact with raw meat are liable to get tapeworm infection. These worms seldom produce serious clinical symptoms in man, mostly general symptoms of the digestive tract and loss of appetite or weight[6,7].

Clinical diagnosis: there may be a slight blood eosinophilia. Eggs of *Taenia* are found only occasionally in stools. For diagnosis, yellow-white tapeworm segments or proglottids must be looked for in stools. They may also occur spontaneously in the anal region.

The parasite

The best known tapeworms in man are *Taenia saginata*, or beef, and *Taenia solium*, or pork tapeworm. They are flat, segmented worms which reach, in case of *T. saginata*, 6–10 m and, in case of *T. solium*, 3–4 m in length.

The head (scolex) is small, measuring only 1–2 mm with 4 suckers and, in the pork tapeworm, two circles of hooks. The segments or proglottids measure up to 20 mm and are larger in the beef tapeworm. In the gravid

Fig. 38.1 Head of *Taenia teniforme*,
tapeworm of the rat. H&E

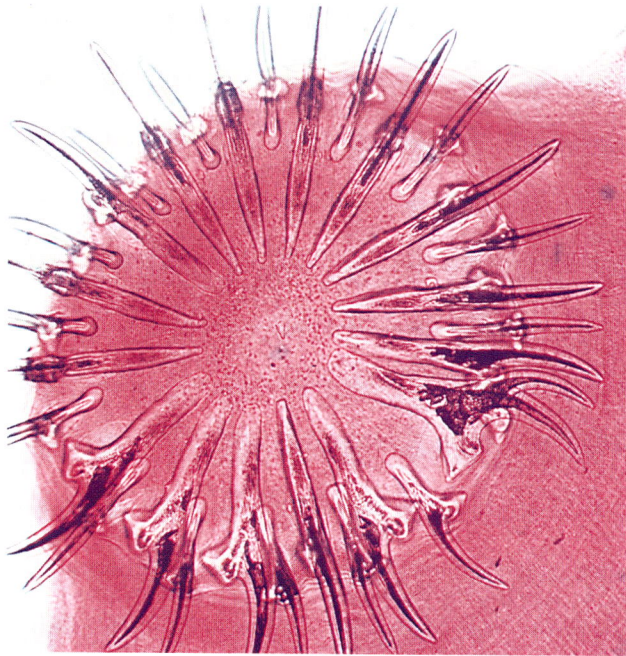

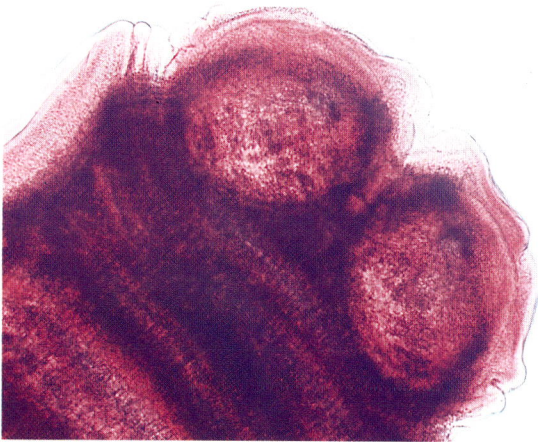

Fig. 38.2 Head of *Taenia saginata*. H&E

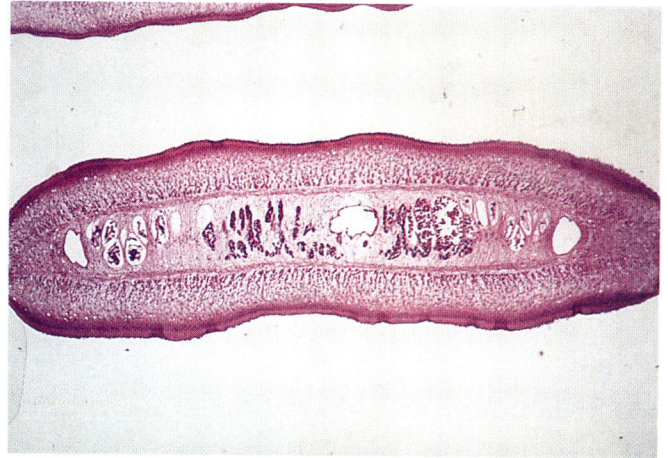

Fig. 38.3 Proglottid of *Taenia saginata*. H&E

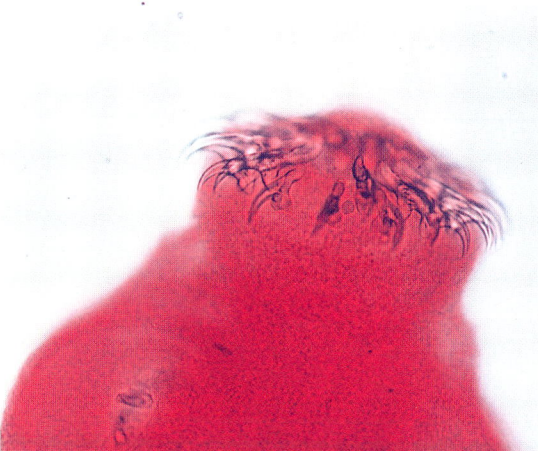

Fig. 38.4 Head of *Taenia solium*. H&E

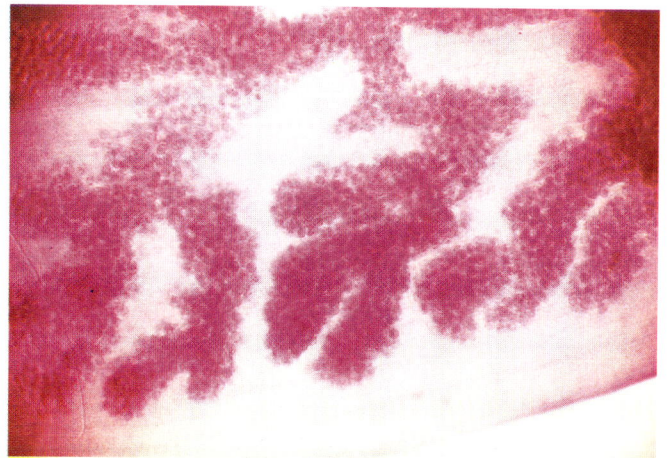

Fig. 38.5 Proglottid of *Taenia solium* at high power. H&E

proglottids, the number of uterine branches is higher in *T. saginata* than in *T. solium*[8] (Figs. 38.2–38.5).

In the intermediate host – and this may happen in man too (see *Cysticercosis*, Section 42) – eggs containing larvae (38 × 32 μm) are ingested[9]. They are released into the gastrointestinal tract, penetrate the wall of the small intestine, reach the main circulation via venous bloodstream, liver, heart and lung and are carried into almost all organs, but mainly into the skeletal musculature. In the tissues, the cysticercus stage of the larvae (sexless juvenile form) develops after 2–4 months and reaches a size of up to 10 mm in diameter. The cysticerci in tissues of the intermediate host show as white nodules and the meat appears measled. Under the microscope, a connective tissue capsule surrounds the cysticercus vesicle with liquid which contains the inverted scolex.

The larval stage of *Taenia saginata* (cysticercus bovis) develops very rarely in the intermediate host while the cysticercus cellulosae of *Taenia solium* is a common finding.

Pathogenesis

If raw infected meat, containing cysticerci, is ingested, the gastric juice dissolves the capsule and the scolex is everted into the lumen of the small intestine. Here, the parasite anchors itself in the superior part of the small bowel with the help of its suckers and/or hooks. Directly behind the scolex, the development of a chain of proglottids begins, reaching, within 3–4 months, the full length of the mature worms (6–10 m in *Taenia saginata* and 3–4 m in *Taenia solium*). The mature tapeworms may remain live in the human gut for many years.

Pathology

Both species of *Taenia* are found in the small intestine of man. They do not invade tissues and the intestinal mucosa remains intact, although it is sometimes said to show slight inflammation.

Quite a few cases of intestinal obstruction, perforation or appendicitis have been reported[6]. Since hundreds of thousands of eggs may be produced and shed, infection from man to man may lead to cysticercosis.

References

1. Hornbostel, H. (1959). *Bandwurmprobleme in Neuer Sicht*. Ferdinand Enke, Stuttgart
2. Beier, A. (1983). Sozialmedizinische Aspekte der Bandwurmbefalls (Taenia saginata) bei türkischen Mitbürgern in Berlin (West). *Bundesgesundheitsblatt*, **26**, 168
3. Rees, G. (1967). Pathogenesis of adult cestodes. *Helminthology Abstr.*, **36**, 1
4. Abudladze, K. E. (1970). *Taeniata of Animals and Man and Diseases Caused by Them*. Israel program for scientific translations: Jerusalem
5. Pawlowski, Z. and Schultz, M. G. (1972). Taeniasis and cysticercosis (Taenia saginata). *Adv. Parasitol.*, **10**, 269
6. Upton, A. C. (1950). Taenial proglottids in the appendix: Possible association with appendicitis. *Am. J. Clin. Path.*, **20**, 1117
7. Hurst, D. M. and Robb-Smith, A. H. J. (1942). Fatal tapeworm enteritis. *Guys Hosp. Rep.*, **91**, 58
8. Mehlhorn, H. *et al.* (1981). On the nature of proglottids in cestodes. *Z. Parasitenkd.*, **65**, 343
9. Slais, J. (1973). Functional morphology of cestodes larvae. *Adv. Parasit.*, **11**, 395

39. DIPHYLLOBOTHRIASIS

Introduction

This worm disease, also called fish tapeworm infection, is of relatively minor importance since it may be avoided by changing eating habits. Infections of the fresh water tapeworm (*D. latum*) are found in certain regions of river systems and lakes in Europe, the Near and Far East and in North America. The salt water tapeworm (*D. pacificum*) occurs on the coasts of South America, above all in the north of Peru. Fishermen and people eating uncooked fish, like eskimos, are carriers of mature fish tapeworms[1]. Infections of this kind are not known in Venezuela.

Man is the definitive and principal host, but others include dogs, cats, foxes and other fish-eating domestic and wild animals as well as seals. The first intermediate hosts are crustaceans; the second intermediate hosts are carp and carnivorous fish.

Carriers of fish tapeworms may have slight disorders of the gastrointestinal tract, as in taeniasis. Since fish tapeworms take up vitamin B_{12}, an anaemia of the pernicious type may be observed, especially in eskimos. A microcytic hypochromic anaemia has also been noted[2,3].

Clinical diagnosis is made by detecting characteristic eggs in the stools.

The parasite

The broad or fish tapeworm *Diphyllobothrium latum*, found in fresh water, and *Diphyllobothrium pacificum*[4] in salt water are the principal worms of this sort in man. They may become 20 m long and are the largest tapeworms (Fig. 39.1). The small scolex measures 2–3 mm across and is spatula-shaped with two sucker-like structures (Fig. 39.2). The mature segments (proglottids) are 10–15 mm broad and 3–5 mm long. In mature proglottids, a small rosette-shaped uterus is found. Eggs reach 70 × 50 μm in diameter, have a smooth surface and have at one end, an operculum and, at the other, a small knob (Fig. 39.3). Those of *Diphyllobothrium pacificum* are somewhat smaller.

The first intermediate hosts are small crustaceans, e.g. the genus *Cyclops*, which eat the eggs and produce ciliate larvae with hooks inside of them. The crustaceans are eaten by the second intermediate host (carp species or carnivorous fishes) and the larvae of the tapeworms reach the muscles of these fishes.

Pathogenesis

Man and other definitive hosts (for instance dogs, cats, foxes and other fish-eating animals) become infected by consuming uncooked fish which may contain numerous larvae.

Pathology

Fish or broad tapeworms inhabit the small intestine. They do not invade tissues.

Rarely, related species of tapeworms fail to become sexually mature in man (plerocercoids or spargana) and migrate, as in the second intermediate host, into the abdominal cavity and musculature where they may produce sparganosis (Figs. 39.4 and 39.5). Lesions of this kind consist of clusters of parasites surrounded by granu-

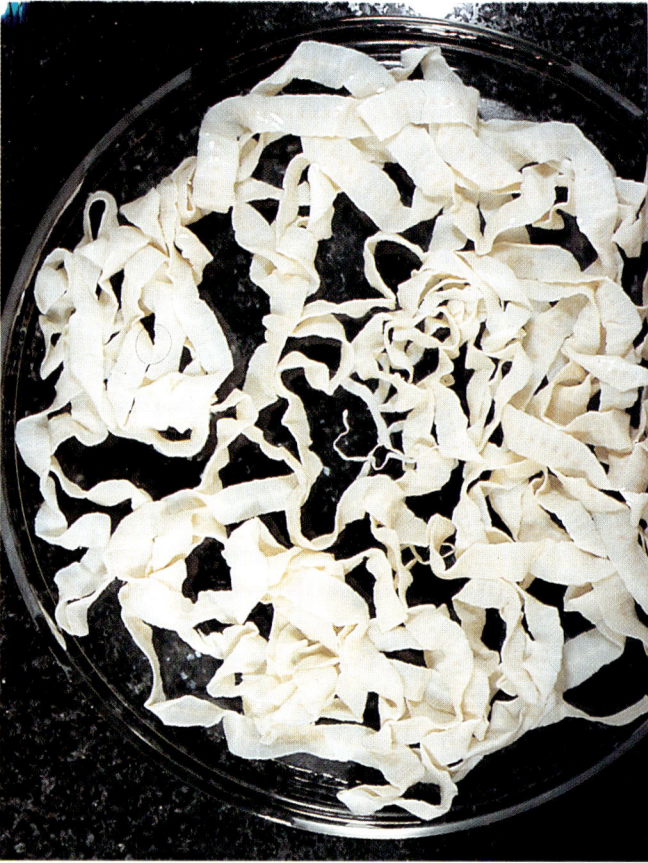

Fig. 39.1 *Diphyllobothrium latum* or fish tapeworm, entire adult worm, expelled after treatment

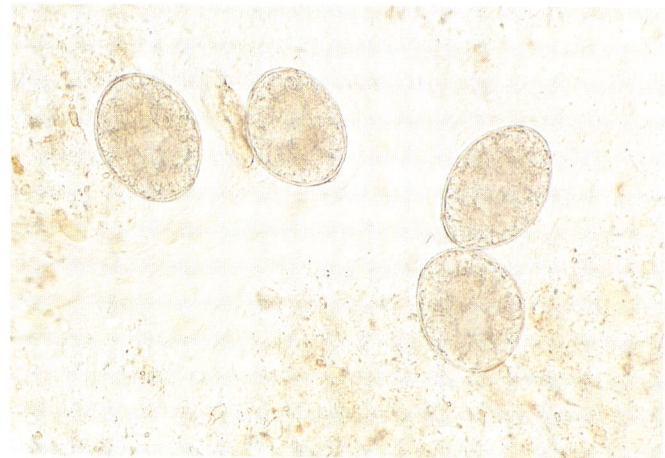

Fig. 39.3 Eggs of the fish tapeworm

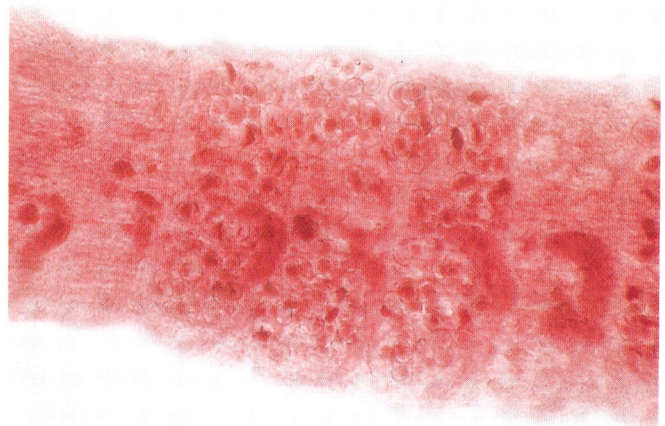

Fig. 39.4 Proglottids of *Spirometra* sp.

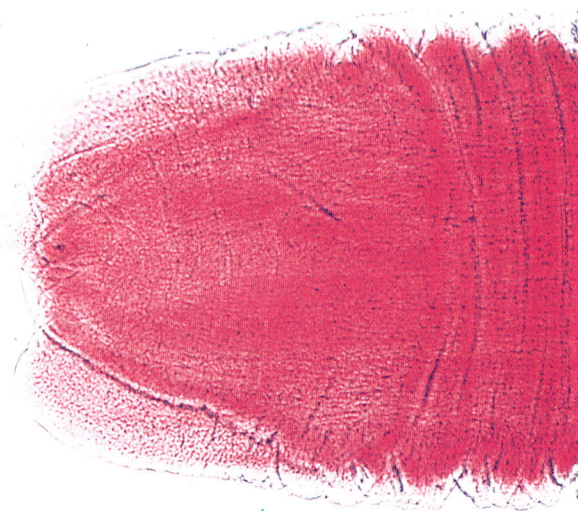

Fig. 39.2 Head of *Diphyllobothrium latum* with two sucker-like structures (sucking grooves or bothria)

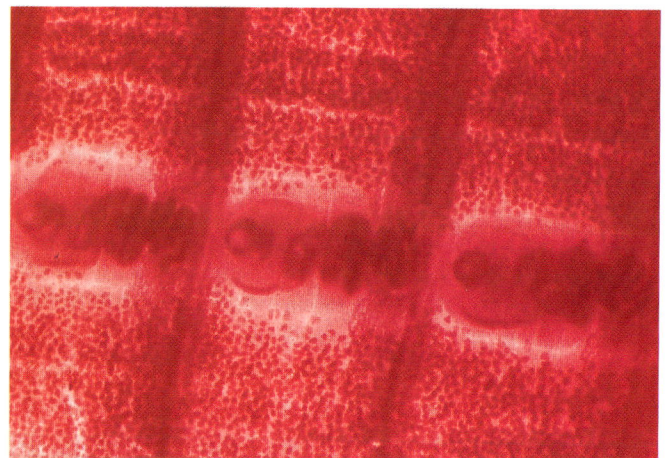

Fig. 39.5 Proglottids of *Spirometra* sp.

lation tissue rich in eosinophils. Sparganosis is observed in the USA[5], the former USSR, the Far East and South East Asia.

References

1. Rausch, R. L. *et al.* (1967). Helminths in Eskimos in Western Alaska, with particular reference to Diphyllobothrium infection and anaemia. *Trans. R. Soc. Trop. Med. Hyg.*, **61**, 351

2. Saarni, N. (1963). Symptoms of carriers of Diphyllobothrium latum and in non-infected controls. *Acta Med Scand.*, **173**, 147
3. Bonsdorff, B. (1977). *Diphyllobothriasis in Man*. Academic Press, London
4. Lumbreras, H. *et al.* (1982). Single dose treatment with Praziquantel of human cestodiasis caused by Diphyllobothrium pacificum. *Tropenmed. Parasit.*, **33**, 5
5. Swartswelder, J. C. *et al.* (1964). Sparganosis in Southern United States. *Am. J. Trop. Med. Hyg.*, **13**, 43

40. DIPYLIDIASIS

Introduction

This dog tapeworm infection is relatively rare in man and occurs worldwide, mostly in children[1]. The mode of transmission of these worms is of particular interest. Tapeworms of the genus *Echinococcus* occur also in dogs as definitive hosts, but, in man, only the larvae cause disease (echinococcosis).

Dipylidiasis is noted, also, in canine and feline species. Fleas and dog hair lice are the intermediate hosts, in which the dog tapeworm is observed in its cysticercoid stage.

Clinically, symptoms, when present, are general and observed only in massive infections or in especially sensitive individuals.

Clinical diagnosis is made looking for proglottids and eggs in the stools. The worm segments appear as structures similar to rice grains; they swell in water and then show the form of proglottids. Eggs are arranged in packets.

The parasite

Dipylidium caninum or the dog tapeworm is also called the cucumber tapeworm due to the shape of proglottids found in faeces.

Adult worms are 15–50 cm long and 2–4 mm wide. The scolex is 0.5 mm broad with 4 suckers and 3–7 small rows of hooks on a retractable rostellum. The elongated segments measure about 20 mm, are yellowish-reddish in colour and are similar to cucumber seeds.

Individual eggs measure 25–30 μm in diameter and contain larvae with six hooks. They are excreted with faeces in packets of 30–40 in number and are eaten by flea larvae or dog lice (Fig. 40.1). Here the larvae hatch out of the eggs, enter the gut of the insect, penetrate the gut wall and reach the fat tissue. During migration in the insect, the larva develops into a cysticercoid.

Pathogenesis

The infected fleas or lice may be ingested by the definitive host. The scolex evaginates from the cysticercoid in the gut and attaches itself to the gut wall where it develops within 15–20 days into an adult worm.

Pathology

As in other cases of tapeworm infection, the worms remain in the lumen of the digestive tract and do not invade tissues.

References

1. Schmidt, G. D. and Roberts, L. S. (1977). *Foundations of Parasitology*. The C. B. Mosby Company, Saint Louis

41. HYMENOLEPIASIS

Introduction

Worm infection by two species of the genus *Hymenolepis* may be found in man. The infection produced by *Hymenolepis nana* is the most important one and will be discussed in the following, while infection with *Hymenolepis diminuta* will be described summarily at the end of this Section.

The *Hymenolepis nana*, or dwarf tapeworm infection, more often affects children than adults. Although this worm disease occurs worldwide, it is more frequent in hot countries. It is said to be found in South America too. Rates of infection run from 1% in the Southern United States to 9% in Argentina. Cases have been described in Venezuela[1].

In addition to man, dogs and rodents may be definitive hosts[2]. Fleas and beetles may be intermediate hosts. Mice are used for experimental purposes[3–6].

Carriers of dwarf tapeworms commonly show minimal symptoms, as with other tapeworm infections. Only in heavy infections do abdominal pain and other non-specific symptoms occur. Immunosuppression favours the development in man of this worm disease, as with

Strongyloides infection.

Clinical diagnosis is made quite easily by confirming the presence of the characteristic eggs in the stools.

The parasite

Hymenolepis nana or dwarf tapeworm is the smallest tapeworm living in the digestive tract of man. Commonly, it reaches only 10–45 mm in length and 0.5–1 mm in width. Isolated tapeworms of this sort, however, can become quite long, although, in the presence of numerous tapeworms, the size of each individual is small.

The scolex, measuring about 0.15–0.5 mm, has a small rostellum with a single row of 20–30 hooklets and four suckers. The proglottids are wider than they are long[7,8] (Fig. 41.1).

The eggs measure 30–50 μm, are oval or spherical and almost colourless. They occur individually in the faeces and contain a larva with six hooks. These eggs may be eaten by insects as intermediate hosts. When the insects are swallowed, cysticercoids of *Hymenolepis nana* reach the duodenum.

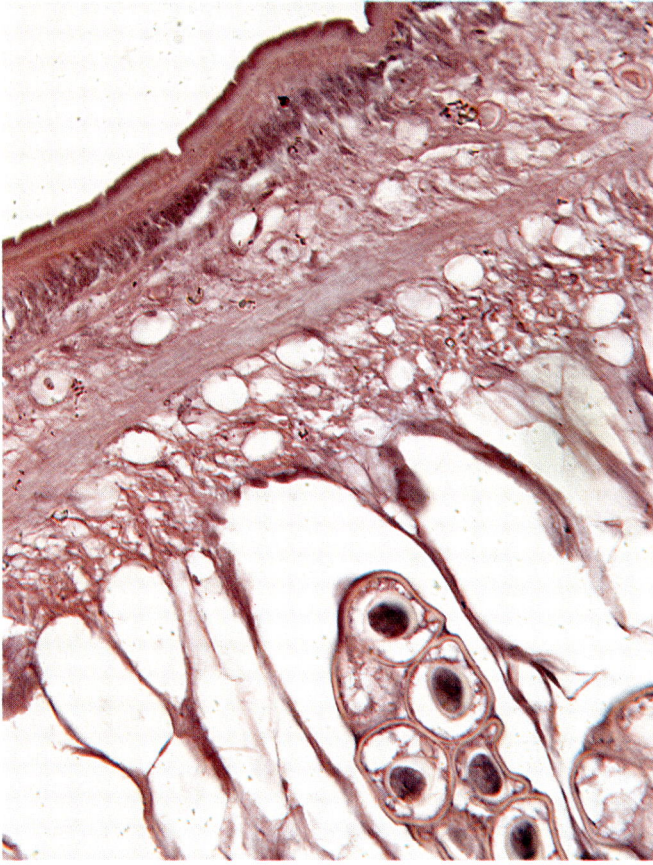

Fig. 40.1 Small packet of eggs in the uterus of *Dipylidium caninum*. H&E

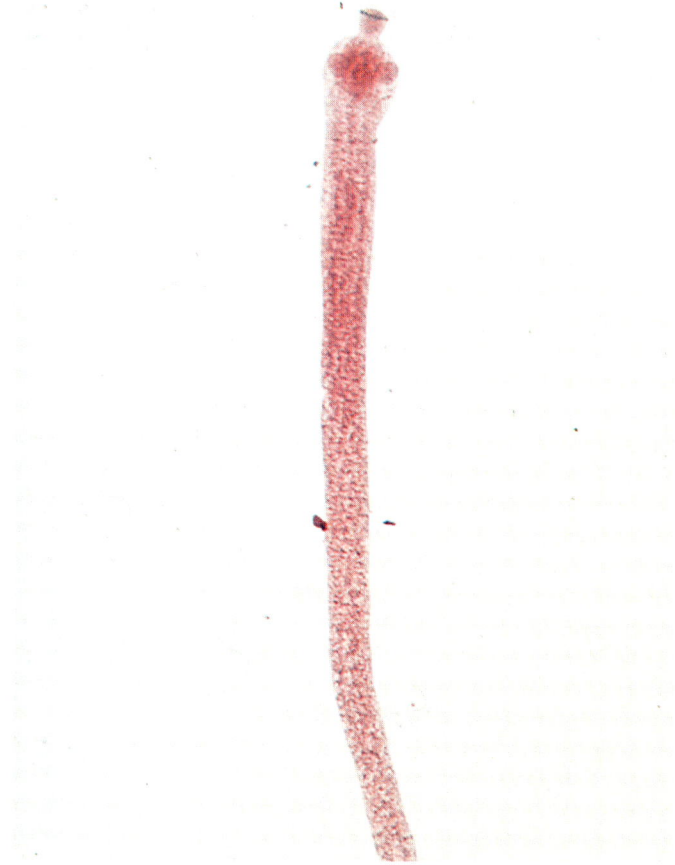

Fig. 41.1 *Hymenolepis nana* or dwarf tapeworm. H&E

Pathogenesis

There are two principal means of transmission of *Hymenolepis nana*: that mentioned above, via intermediate hosts; and direct infection, by ingestion of contaminated food or by autoinfection. Here, the larval stage (cysticercoids) may develop from the eggs in the small intestine of the definitive host. After 2–4 weeks, tapeworms may develop from the cysticercoids.

Pathology

Dwarf tapeworms inhabit the human small intestine. Occasionally, cysticercoids may be found inside villi of the mucosa.

Hymenolepis diminuta, or rat tapeworm, is a cosmopolitan parasite. Numerous cases of human infections are observed, preferentially in children. The scolex does not have hooklets. The eggs measure 65–75 μm in diameter. Sexually mature rat tapeworms reach up to 90 cm in length. Transmission occurs always and exclusively through intermediate hosts (insects) which are swallowed.

References

1. Soto Urribarri, R. and Torazon, S. S. de (1988). Efecto terapéutico de Praziquantel sobre Hymenolepis nana. *Kasmera*, **16**, 51
2. Hauff, P. and Arnold, W. (1990). Spontaneous Hymenolepis nana infection in a breeding colony of nude mice. *Z. Versuchtstierkd.*, **33**, 133
3. Kilkinov, G. T. (1967). Unusual cases of Hymenolepis nana localization in experimental Hymenolepsis infection. *Trop. Dis. Bull.*, **64**, 994
4. Novak, M. and Nombrado, S. (1988). Mast cell responses to Hymenolepis microstoma infection in mice. *J. Parasitol.*, **74**, 81
5. Novak, M. *et al.* (1990). Effects of cyclophosphamide and dexamethasone on mast cell population in Hymenolepis microstoma-infected mice. *Parasitology*, **100**, 337
6. Van der Vorst, E. *et al.* (1990). Hymenolepis diminuta: intestinal mast cells and eosinophil response of the mouse to infection. *Ann. Soc. Belg. Med. Trop.*, **70**, 113
7. Becker, B. *et al.* (1980). Scanning and transmission electron microscope studies on the efficacy of praziquantel on Hymenolepis nana (Cestoda) in vitro. *Z. Parsitenkd.*, **61**, 121
8. Becker, B. *et al.* (1980). Ultrastructural investigations on the effect of praziquantel on the tegument of five species of Cestodes. *Z. Parasitenkd.*, **64**, 257

42. CYSTICERCOSIS

Introduction

This disease, due to larvae (cysticerci) of *Taenia solium* or the pork tapeworm, is very important, while cysticerci bovis, due to larvae of *Taenia saginata* or the beef tapeworm, occur very rarely in man[1]. In cysticercosis, man is the accidental intermediate host after consumption of the tapeworm eggs. The cysticerci are located in internal organs, causing serious and dangerous disease; 50 000 deaths are said to occur each year due to cysticercosis. Only in a small percentage of cases are adult pork tapeworms observed in the digestive tract of man (taeniasis solium, see Section 38) simultaneously with cysticercosis.

Cysticercosis occurs mainly in Central and South America, Africa, India[2] and the former USSR. It is well known in Venezuela. In Mérida, numerous cases have been observed in biopsy and autopsy material[3].

Pigs are also intermediate hosts. In these animals, cysticerci are found preferentially in the tongue, larynx, diaphragm, and muscles of the back and thigh, as well as in the heart and peritoneum. The parasite is said to occur in the liver, lungs and brain. Experimentally, cysticercosis may be induced in rhesus monkeys[4].

Clinically, CNS symptoms are the most frequent and important in man. Often, epileptiform convulsions occur, or disorders, apparently due to tumour-like lesions, prevail. Neurological and mental symptoms depend on the location of the brain lesions. The direct cause of death is usually internal hydrocephalus. Involvement of the musculature is often symptomless, but rheumatic pain may occur. Ocular cysticercosis may lead to blindness.

Clinical diagnosis is possible by confirming the presence of calcified cysticerci with X-ray. Immunological methods and computed tomography are useful[5–8], but there are only group-specific antigens available. Lately, MR (magnetic resonance) has been applied successfully in neurocysticercosis[9–11].

The parasite

Larvae of the pork tapeworm (*Taenia solium*) represent the sexless juvenile forms and are called cysticerci, *Cysticercus cellulosae* or *Taenia solium* cysticercus. Their structure is the same in tissues of man and pig.

On average, they measure 1 cm in diameter and consist of a vesicle, which contains liquid, and a connective tissue capsule surrounding the vesicle. The larva swims in the liquid and presents an inverted scolex with hooks. *Cysticercus bovis* does not have hooks (Fig. 42.1).

Pathogenesis

Eggs of *Taenia solium* are ingested by man with contaminated food, often salad vegetables. They transform in the lumen of the digestive tract into larvae, penetrate the intestinal wall and reach the internal organs via the bloodstream. They remain in the tissues and grow up to a certain size for 2–4 months. They then remain infectious in the tissues for 1–2 years. Theoretically, when antiperistalsis occurs in carriers of *Taenia solium*, so-called retroinfection may take place and the proglottids will shed eggs into the stomach making development of cysticercosis possible. Intrauterine infection of a fetus may occur from the third month of pregnancy onwards.

In the other intermediate host, the pig, pathogenesis is the same when eggs of *Taenia solium* are ingested. The pork meat then appears measly with white nodules. When this meat is eaten raw, adult tapeworms will develop in the human gut (taeniasis solium, Section 38).

Pathology

In man, there is a kind of tropism regarding involvement of organs. Cysticerci are located mainly in the central nervous system[12–14] (Figs. 42.2–42.5), the skeletal musculature (Fig. 42.6) and subcutis, in descending order of frequency.

Occasionally, the eyes may be involved, and, rarely, cysticerci may be found in other organs, such as the heart (Fig. 42.7), peritoneum, tongue[15], lips[16] and orbital muscles[17].

In the brain, exceptionally, cysticercus racemosus may be observed; this has the appearance of large thin-walled cysticercus cysts, up to 10 cm in diameter, arranged in clusters, like bunches of grapes.

Histologically, when the inverted scolex is cut appropriately, hooks may be seen clearly in the sections (Figs. 42.8–42.10). After the death of the larva, a slight nonspecific inflammatory reaction appears and, later, calcification takes place. Sometimes, calcified deposits which mimic spherical structures, i.e. eggs, are observed. However, eggs are not formed by larvae. Concomitant infections of cysticerci are rare[18]. Occasionally, a foreign body reaction may be observed (Fig. 42.11).

References

1. Froyd, G. (1965). The incidence of Cysticercus bovis. *Bull. Off. Int. Epiz.*, **63**, 311
2. Venkataraman, S. *et al.* (1990). Cysticercal meningoencephalitis. Clinical presentation and autopsy findings. *J. Assoc. Physicians India*, **38**, 763
3. Rada Fangher, R. G. (1964). *Neurocysticercosis*. Universidad de Los Andes, Facultad de Medicina, Centro Neurológico, Mérida/Venezuela
4. Saleque, A. *et al.* (1988). Induced Taenia solium cysticercosis in rhesus monkeys (Macaca mulatta): a clinico-pathological study. *Ann. Trop. Med. Parasitol.*, **82**, 103
5. Proctor, E. M. (1966). The serological diagnosis of cysticercosis. *Ann. Trop. Med. Parasitol.*, **60**, 146
6. Gottstein, B. *et al.* (1986). Antigenanalyse von Taenia solium und spezifische Immundiagnose der Zystizerkose beim Menschen. 12. *Tg. Dtsch. Ges. Parasit: Referat Nr.*, **32**, Wien
7. Hoffman, P. *et al.* (1990). Atteinte isolée du système nerveux central au cours d'une cysticercose. Etude anatomo-clinique d'une observation. *Ann. Pathol.*, **10**, 122
8. Dhamija, R. M. *et al.* (1990). Computed tomographic spectrum of neurocysticercosis. *J. Assoc. Physicians India*, **38**, 566
9. Jena, A. *et al.* (1988). Cysticercosis of the brain shown by magnetic resonance imaging. *Clin. Radiol.*, **39**, 542
10. Zee, C. S. *et al.* (1988). MR imaging of neurocysticercosis. *J. Comput. Assist. Tomogr.*, **12**, 927
11. Lotz, J. *et al.* (1988). Neurocysticercosis: correlative pathomorphology and MR imaging. *Neuroradiology*, **30**, 35
12. Alarcon Egas, F. *et al.* (1988). Neurocisticercosis: a review of 65 patients. *Arch. Neurobiol. Madr.*, **51**, 252
13. Esberg, G. and Reske-Nieksen, E. (1988). Sudden death from cerebral cysticercosis. *Scand. J. Infect. Dis.*, **20**, 679
14. McKelvie, P. A. and Goldsmid, J. M. (1988). Childhood central nervous system cysticercosis in Australia. *Med. J. Aust.*, **149**, 42
15. Rao, P. L. *et al.* (1990). Cysticercosis of the tongue. *Int. J. Pediatr. Otorhinolaryngol.*, **20**, 159
16. Fazakerley, M. W. and Woolgar, J. A. (1991). Cysticercosis cellulosae. An unusual cause of a labial swelling. *Br. Dent. J.*, **170**, 105
17. DiLoreto, D. A. *et al.* (1990). Infestation of extraocular muscle by Cysticercus cellulosae. *Br. J. Ophthalmol.*, **74**, 751
18. Walus, M. A. and Young, E. J. (1990). Concomitant neurocysticercosis and brucellosis. *Am. J. Clin. Pathol.*, **94**, 790

43.   ECHINOCOCCOSIS

Introduction

This disease is produced by two main tapeworm species and may be called echinococcosis, hydatidosis, hydatid worm infection or alveolar echinococcosis[1]. Man may become infected as an intermediate host. The tapeworm species are **A** *Echinococcus granulosus* and **B** *Echinococcus multilocularis*; each produces a disease, with different features, by ingestion of worm eggs. Adult tapeworms of the genus *Echinococcus*, however, occur only in animals, mainly dogs and foxes, as definitive hosts. Echinococcosis is the most dangerous tapeworm infection in man. It is caused by the larvae of these worms producing cyst-like or tumour-like lesions.

A is more frequent than **B**. It occurs in parts of Europe, South America, mostly the south, Africa and South Australia. Single autochthonous infections have also been noted in Venezuela[2,3]. **B** is endemic in parts of the northern hemisphere, Europe, the former USSR, USA and Canada[4–9].

In **A** the definitive hosts, with adult worms, are dogs, cats and canine species. **B** occurs only in wild animals. The intermediate hosts, with lesions due to larvae, are, in addition to man, sheep, camels, domestic animals and small rodents[10]. Experimentally mice may be used[11,12].

Clinically, symptoms develop according to the location of lesions. In liver and lungs, the most affected organs, lesions may remain asymptomatic for a long time. They grow and increase in size slowly. As they enlarge, they cause atrophy of the surrounding tissues by compression and may be painful. Care must be taken when removing lesions surgically because the parasitic elements within the cyst content may be disseminated after the rupture of the cystic wall, producing local or disseminated metastases by lymphogenous or haematogenous spread. Consequently, new hydatid cysts (secondary hydatidosis)[13] or tumour-like lesions may be formed. Furthermore, fatal anaphylactic shock may occur as a result of the proteinogenous liquid spilled into the body cavity during surgical removal of the cyst.

Clinical diagnosis: cavitary lesions may be seen by tomography and sonography, and calcified cysts by X-ray. Scolices and isolated hooks may be confirmed by cytology and histology for instance in sputum after rupture of cysts into the airways. In lesions with multiple cysts in **B**, caused by *E. multilocularis*, scolices are mostly absent. With immunological methods, cross reaction with *Taenia cysticercus* must be taken into consideration. Frequently, the most difficult differential diagnosis to make is with malignant tumour.

The parasite

This disease is caused by larvae of the two main *Echinococcus* species found in man (see Pathology below);

> **A** *Echinococcus granulosus, Echinococcus cysticus* or *Echinococcus hydatidicus* is also called hydatid worm or dog tapeworm (Figs. 43.1 and 43.2).
> **B** *Echinococcus (Alveococcus) multilocularis* or *Echinococcus alveolaris* is also called fox tapeworm.

The mature worms are never seen in man. They reach < 1 cm long in the small intestine of the definitive hosts (**A** is a little longer than **B**). There are only 3–4 proglottids. Occasionally, single proglottids are shed, containing numerous eggs; the segments are then replaced.

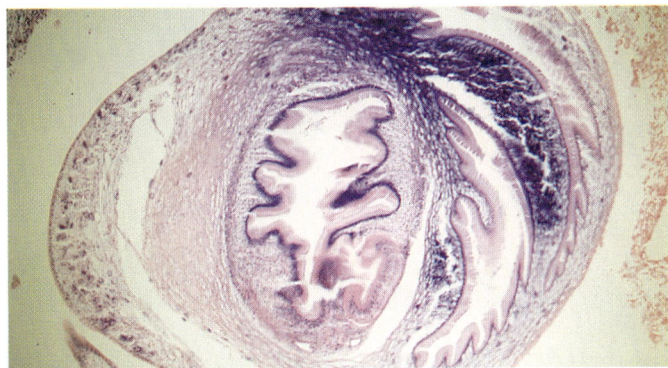

Fig. 42.1 *Cysticercus bovis.* H&E

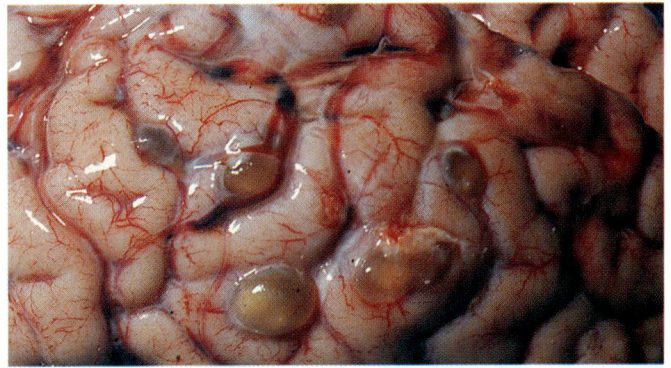

Fig. 42.2 *Cysticercus cellulosae* visible in the surface of the human brain

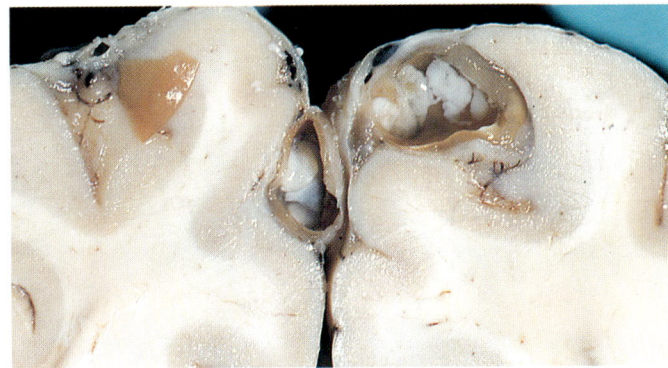

Fig. 42.3 *Cysticercus cellulosae* at the cut surface of the human brain

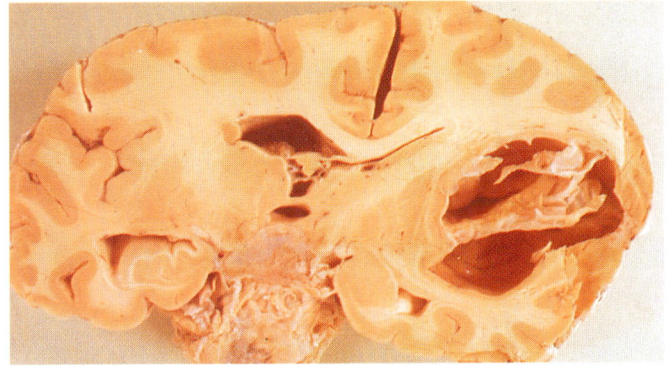

Fig. 42.4 Cysticercosis with marked deformation at the cut surface of the human brain

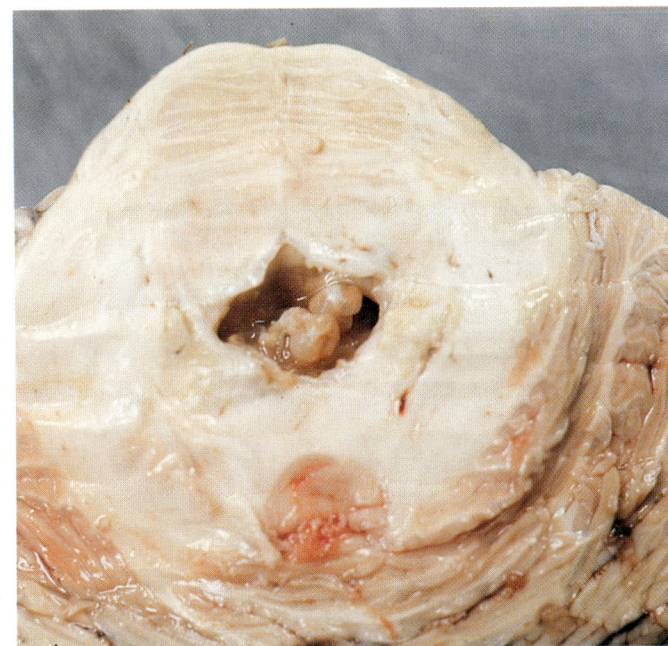

Fig. 42.5 *Cysticercus cellulosae* obstructing the Aquaeductus Sylvii

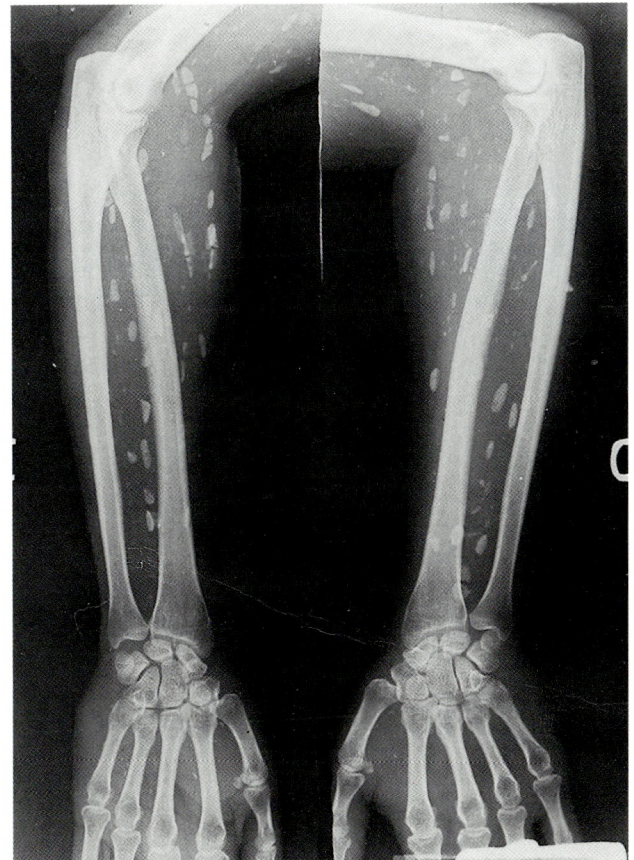

Fig. 42.6 Numerous *Cysticercus cellulosae* in the skeletal musculature of both forearms

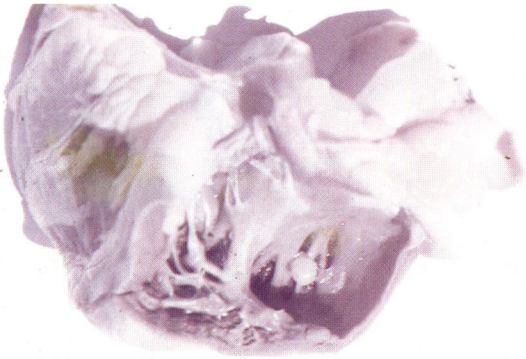

Fig. 42.7 Small subendocardial *Cysticercus cellulosae* in the left ventricle

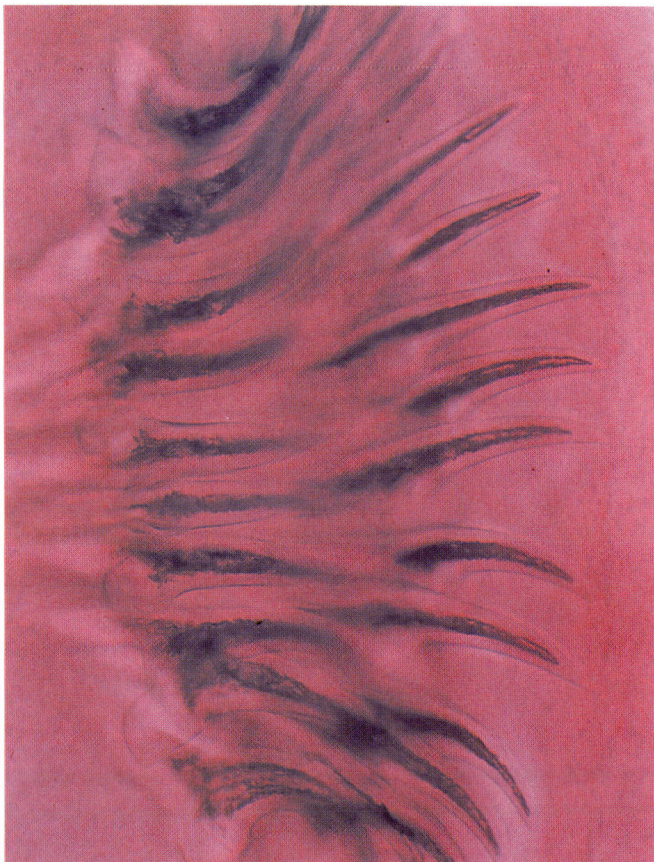

Fig. 42.8 Inverted scolex of *Cysticercus cellulosae* with hooks in the centre. H&E

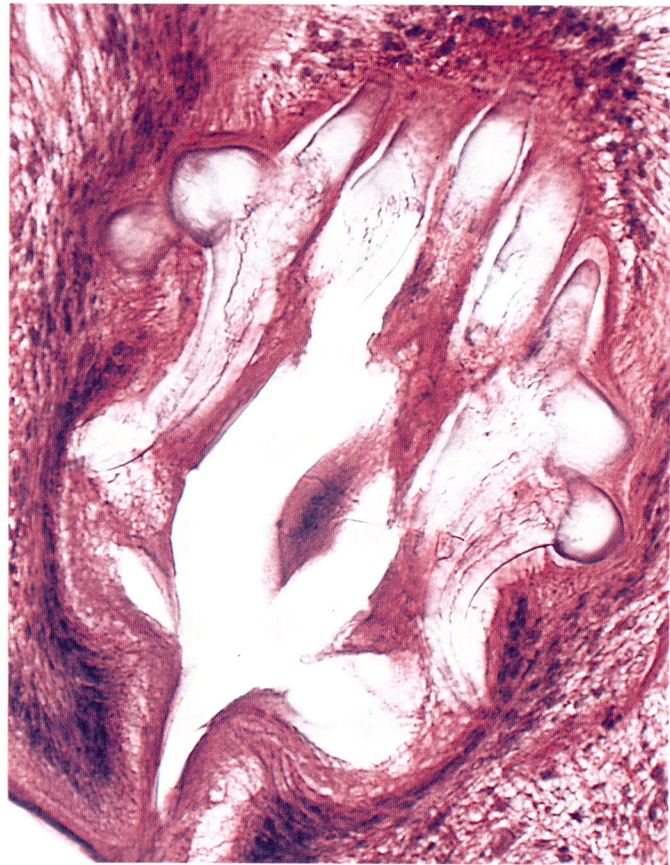

Fig. 42.9 High magnification of Fig. 42.8 with the hooks clearly visible. H&E

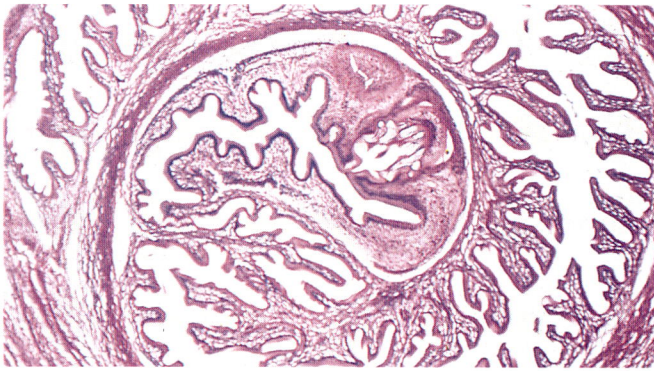

Fig. 4.10 The hooks of scolex of *Cysticercus cellulosae* in another projection

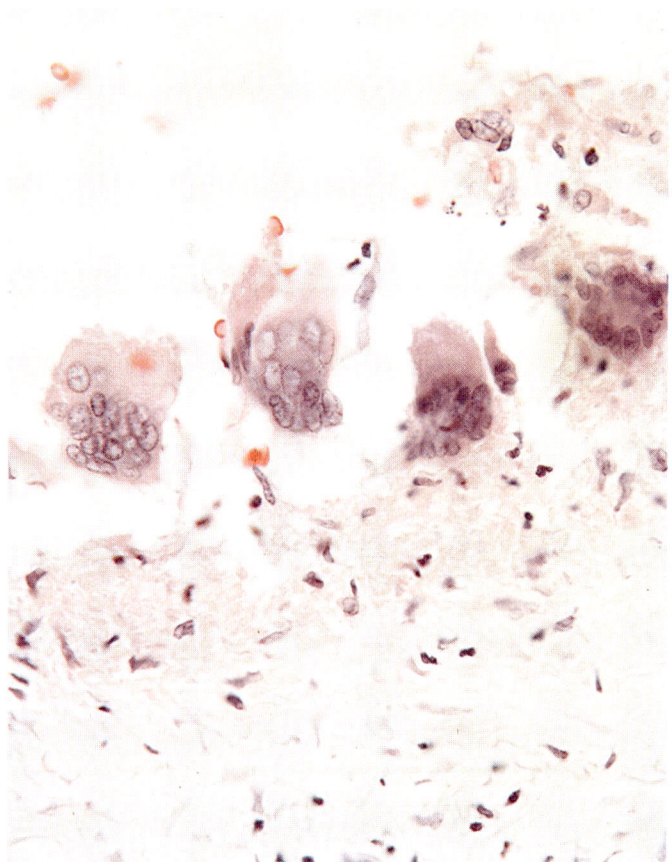

Fig. 42.11 Foreign body reaction around a cysticercus in the meninges. H&E

Pathogenesis

This is similar in **A** and **B**. The eggs of *Echinococcus* worms are ingested by man and reach the liver, lungs and other organs after penetrating the wall of the small intestine. Here, they grow, in a kind of larval stage, very slowly over the course of years never reaching maturity, i.e. formation of adult worms. Instead, they form solitary cystic lesions in **A** and tumour-like lesions in **B**. In the latter, they remain a long time in the liver and eventually disseminate from this organ to others in a tumour-like manner.

Pathology

During infection with **A**, solitary unilocular hydatid cysts may be found in liver (Figs. 43.3–43.8), spleen, lungs, CNS[14–16], bones[17,18] (Figs. 43.9–43.11) and other organs[19] (Figs. 43.12 and 43.13). From the liver, there may be extension to thoracic organs[20]. On average they measure 5 cm in diameter and are filled with fluid. Frequently, in the liver they reach larger dimensions up to more than 20 cm. The cyst is surrounded by a connective tissue capsule formed by the host. The internal surface is lined by a germinal layer with daughter cysts or brood capsules showing scolices. In the fluid of the cysts, entire scolices may be found (Fig. 43.14).

Lesions due to infection with *Echinococcus multilocularis* (**B**) are quite different from those due to *Echinococcus granulosus* (**A**). They are found mainly in the liver and consist of a focal tumorous lesion with numerous small vesicles filled with a gelatinous substance. Scolices are not always present since lesions may be sterile. Often, cystic cavities can no longer be recognized, but a fibrous network prevails with partly tubular or rope-like structure. Further, areas with marked necrosis, forming cavities, calcifications and haemorrhages, may be observed. Grossly, these lesions very much resemble malignant tumours. Secondary metastatic lesions may be found in lymph nodes, lungs and other organs. In laboratory animals, metastases have been observed, apparently due to detached cells which have been disseminated by lymphogenous or haematogenous spread.

References

1. Miguet, J. P. and Bresson-Hadni, S. (1989). Alveolar echinococcosis of the liver. *J. Hepatol., **8**,* 373

2. Salfelder, K. *et al.* (1967). Caso de equinococcosis autóctona en Venezuela. *Tribuna Med. Venezuela, **204**,* 1

3. Bont de, F. P. and Sauerteig, E. (1970). A propósito de un caso de equinococcosis autóctona del Estado Barinas/Venezuela. *Rev. Col. Med. Edo. Mérida, **XI**,* 75

4. Blood, B. D. and Leilijveld, J. L. (1969). Studies on sylvatic echinococcosis in Southern South America. *Z. Tropenmed. Parasit., **20**,* 475

5. Lukashenko, N. P. (1971). Problems of epidemiology and prophylaxis of alveococcosis (Multilocular echinococcosis): a general review – with particular reference to the USSR. *Int. J. Parasit., **1**,* 125

6. Williams, J. F. *et al.* (1971). Current prevalence and distribution of hydatidosis with special reference to the Americas. *Am. J. Trop. Med. Hyg., **20**,* 224

7. Hagedorn, H. J. (1982). Zystische Echinococcose. *Dtsch. Ärzteblatt, **44**,* 34

8. Chi, P. *et al.* (1990). Cystic echinococcosis in the Xinjiang/Uygur Autonomous Region, People's Republic of China. I. Demographic and epidemiologic data. *Trop. Med. Parasit., **41**,* 157

9. Auer, H. *et al.* (1990). First report on the occurrence of human cases of alveolar echinococcosis in the Northeast of Austria. *Trop. Med. Parasit., **41**,* 149

10. Gusbi, A. M. *et al.* (1990). Echinococcosis in Libya. IV. Prevalence of hydatidosis (Echinococcous granulosus) in goats, cattle and camels. *Ann. Trop. Med. Parasitol., **84**,* 477

11. Eckert, J. *et al.* (1983). Proliferation and metastases formation of larval Echinococcus multilocularis. I. Animal model, macroscopical and microscopical findings. *Z. Parasitenkd., **69**,* 737

12. Richards, K. S. *et al.* (1988). Echinococcus granulosus: the effects of praziquantel, in vivo and in vitro, on the ultrastructure of equine strain murine cysts. *Parasitology, **96**,* 323

13. Felice, C. *et al.* (1990). A new therapeutic approach for hydatid liver cysts. Aspiration and alcohol injection under sonographic guidance. *Gastroenterology, **98**,* 1366

14. Richards, K. S. and Morris, D. L. (1990). Effect of albendazole on human hydatid cysts: an ultrastructural study. *HPB Surg., **2**,* 105

15. Jena, A. *et al.* (1991). Primary spinal echinococcosis causing paraplegia: case report with MR and pathologic correlation. *AJNR Am. J. Neuroradiol., **12**,* 560

16. Altinors, N. *et al.* (1991). CT findings and surgical treatment of double intracranial echinococcal cysts. *Infection, **19**,* 110

17. Akyildiz, A. N. *et al.* (1991). Hydatid cyst of the pterygopalatine fossa. *J. Oral Maxillofac. Surg., **49**,* 87

18. Fyfe, B. *et al.* (1990). Intraosseous echinococcosis: a rare manifestation of echinococcal disease. *South Med. J., **83**,* 66

19. Gilevich, Miu *et al.* (1990). Clinico-morphological bases of selection of the methods of treatment of echinococcosis of the abdominal organs and retroperitoneal space. *Khirurgiia Mosk., **11**,* 116

20. Pinna, A. D. *et al.* (1990). Thoracic extension of hydatid cysts of the liver. *Surg. Gynecol. Obstet., **170**,* 233

C. TREMATODIASIS

Trematodes or flukes are flat or tongue-shaped worms with an oral orifice and digestive tract, and without segmentation. Many species possess suckers. All are hermaphrodites, with the exception of the schistosomes. In the definitive hosts, they occur as mature worms; larval development occurs in one or two intermediate hosts, mainly snails or aquatic animals.

Adult trematode worms in man, as the definitive host, are found in blood, lungs, liver and intestine. Only schistosomes cause damage in man by their eggs. The medicinal blood fluke, *Hirudo medicinalis*, used for bleeding, is segmented and is not a pathogen.

Only three of the fifteen medically important trematode species occur in countries of the New World, mostly in South America.

44. BLOOD FLUKE INFECTION

Introduction

Infection by blood trematodes or blood flukes is also called schistosomiasis, bilharziasis or 'water snail fever' It is an important disease because 200–300 million people in warm countries, mostly children and young people, are infected; also, in non-tropical regions, an increasing

number of 'imported' cases is found.

From the five different species of the genus *Schistosoma*, only three are medically important, namely *S. haematobium*, *S. mansoni* and *S. japonicum*. They occur in Africa and the Near and Middle East (*S. haematobium*), in central Africa (*S. intercalatum*), in the Far East and

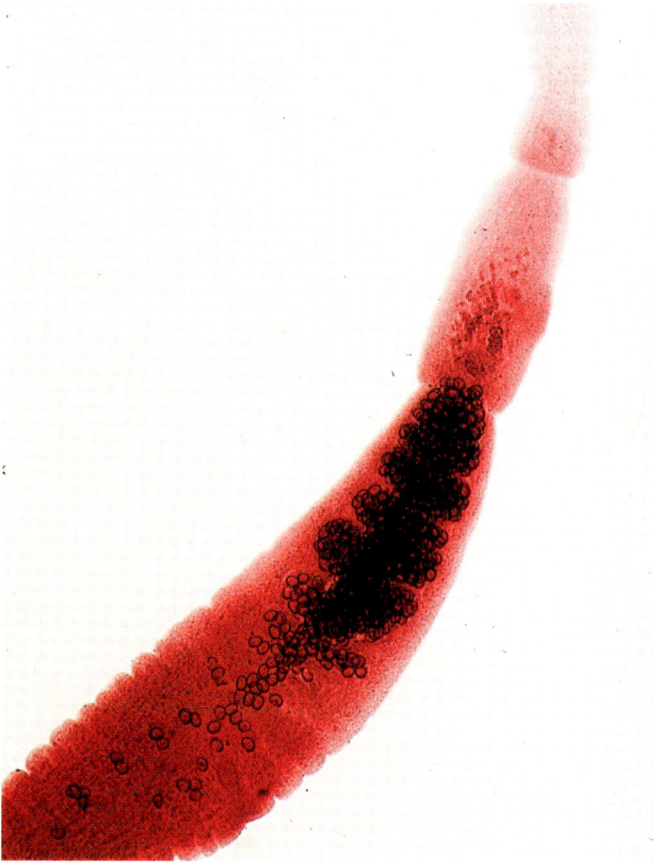

Fig. 43.1 *Echinococcus granulosus.* Carmine

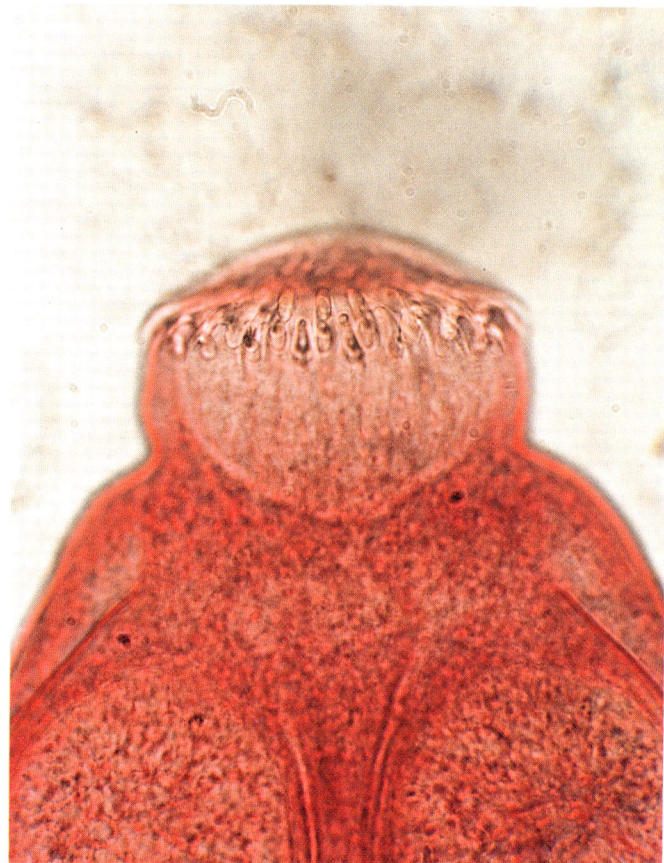

Fig. 43.2 Hooks on the scolex of *Echinococcus granulosus.* Carmine

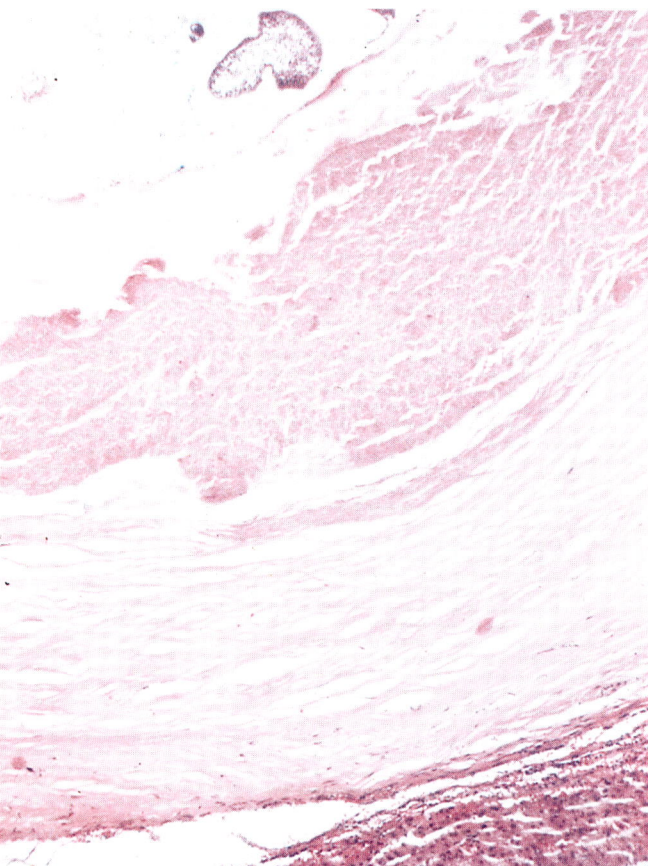

Fig. 43.3 Wall of a hydatid cyst in the liver. H&E

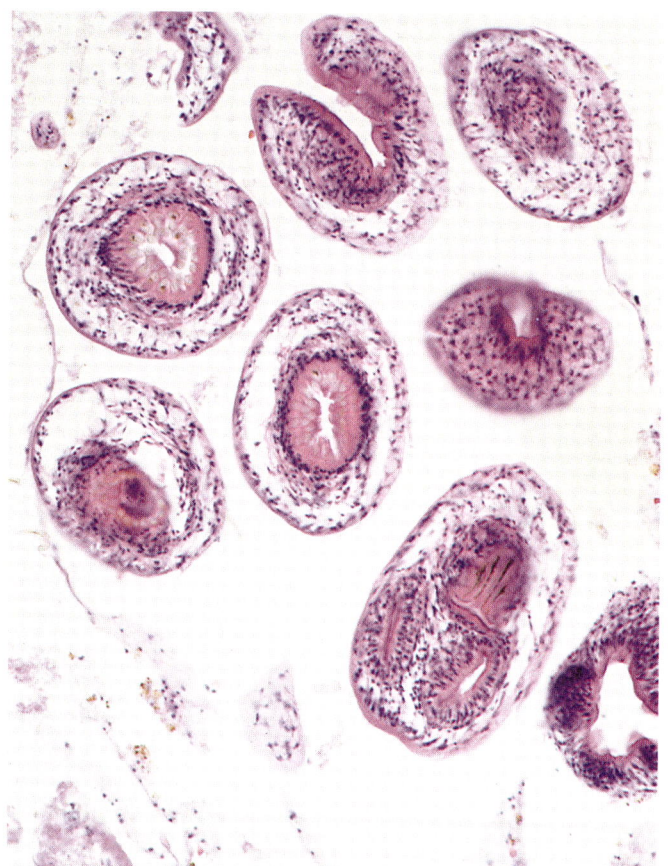

Fig. 43.4 Brood capsule containing several scolices of *Echinococcus granulosus* in a hydatid cyst of the liver. The thin capsule of the brood capsule is faintly visible. H&E

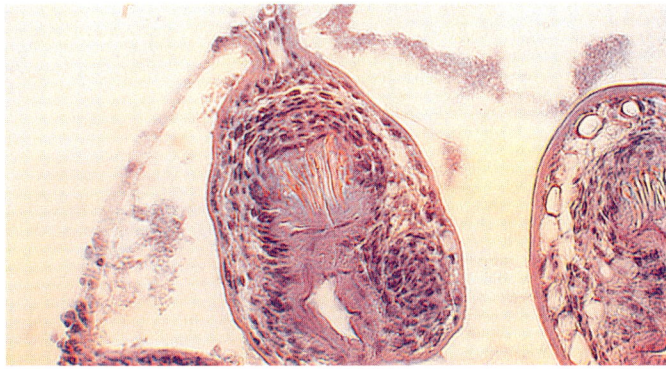

Fig. 43.5 Scolex of *Echinococcus granulosus* attached to the membrane of the brood capsule. H&E

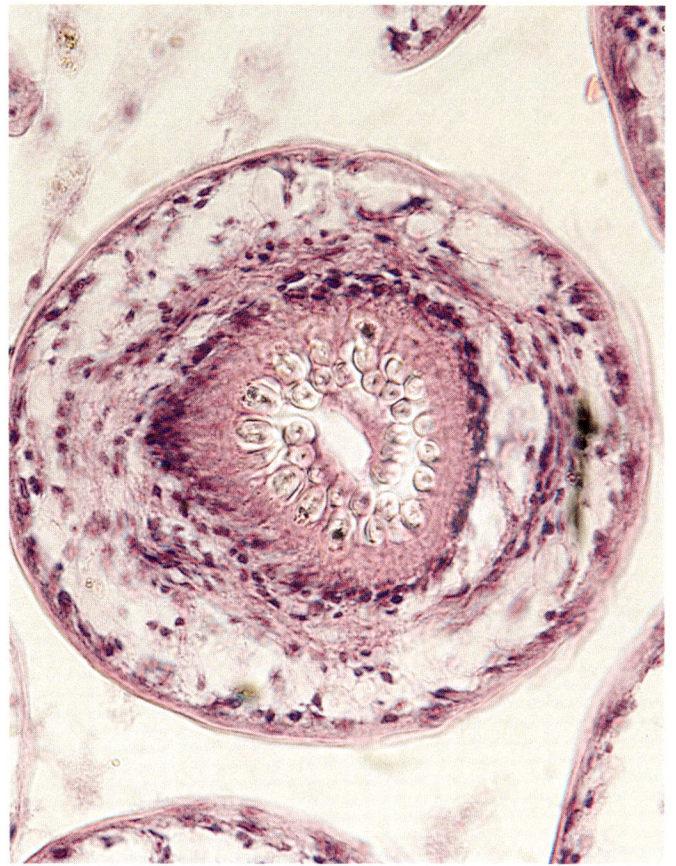

Fig. 43.6 Scolex of *Echinococcus granulosus* in hydatid cyst of the liver. Note the hooks. H&E

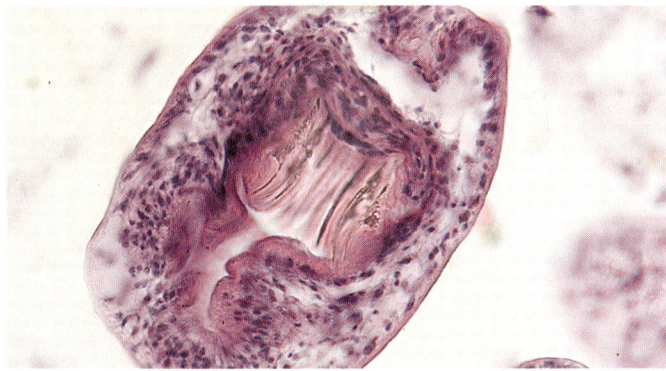

Fig. 43.7 Scolex of *Echinococcus granulosus* in hydatid cyst of the liver. Note the hooks cut horizontally. Compare with Fig. 43.5. H&E

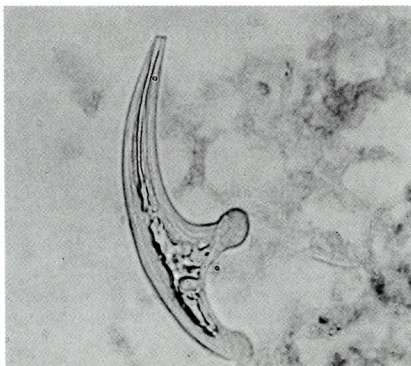

Fig. 43.8 Single hook of scolex of *Echinococcus granulosus* from the contents of hydatid cyst of the liver. H&E

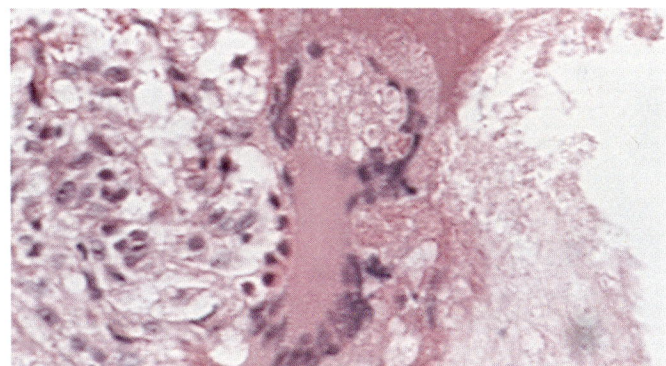

Fig. 43.9 Foreign body reaction with hooks of *Echinococcus granulosus* in a giant cell from a lesion in the ribs. H&E

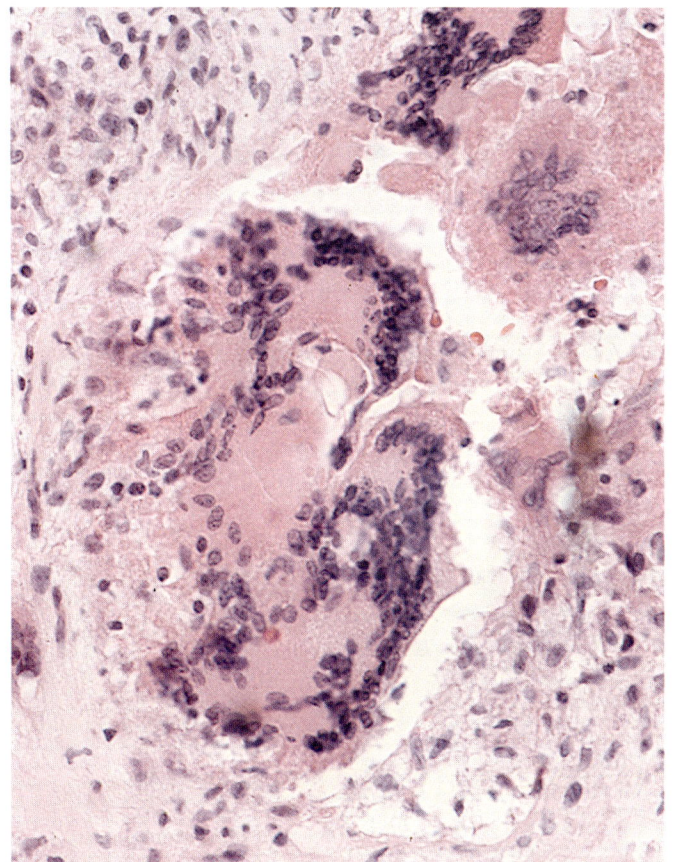

Fig. 43.10 Same case as Fig. 43.9. Fragments of hooks in giant cells. H&E

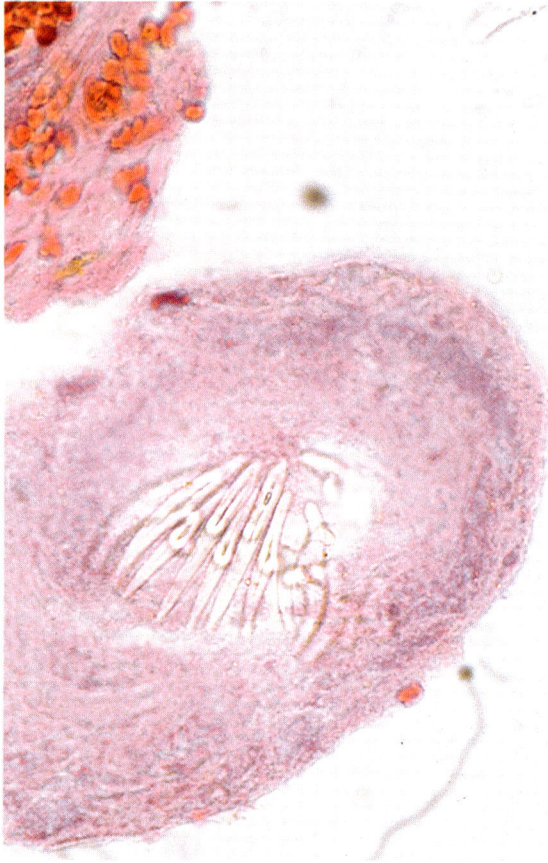

Fig. 43.11 Same case as Fig. 43.8. Crown of hooks in the contents of a cyst. H&E

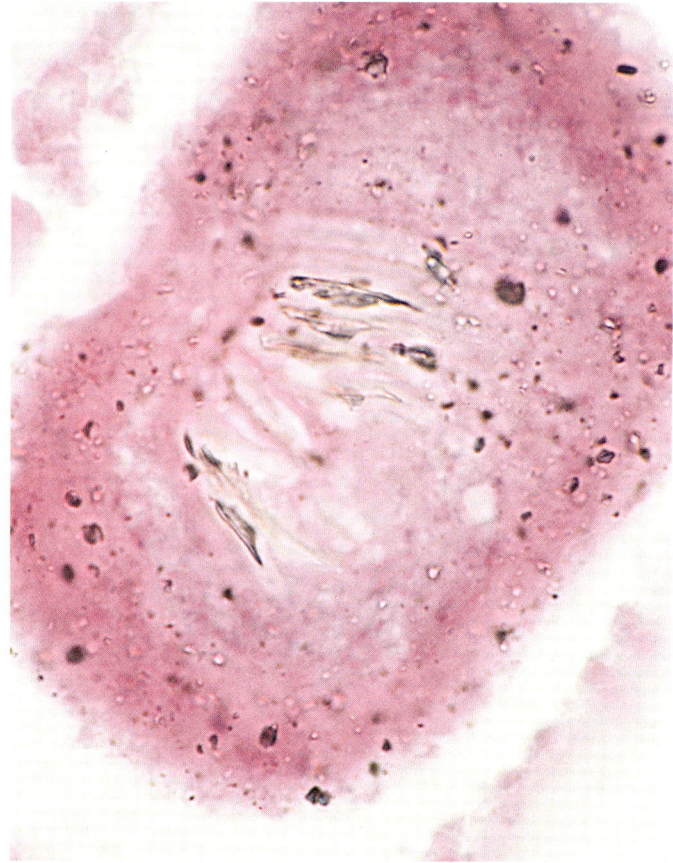

Fig. 43.12 Deformed scolex of *Echinococcus granulosus* with faintly visible hooks in the peritoneal exudate. A case with involvement of peritoneum. H&E

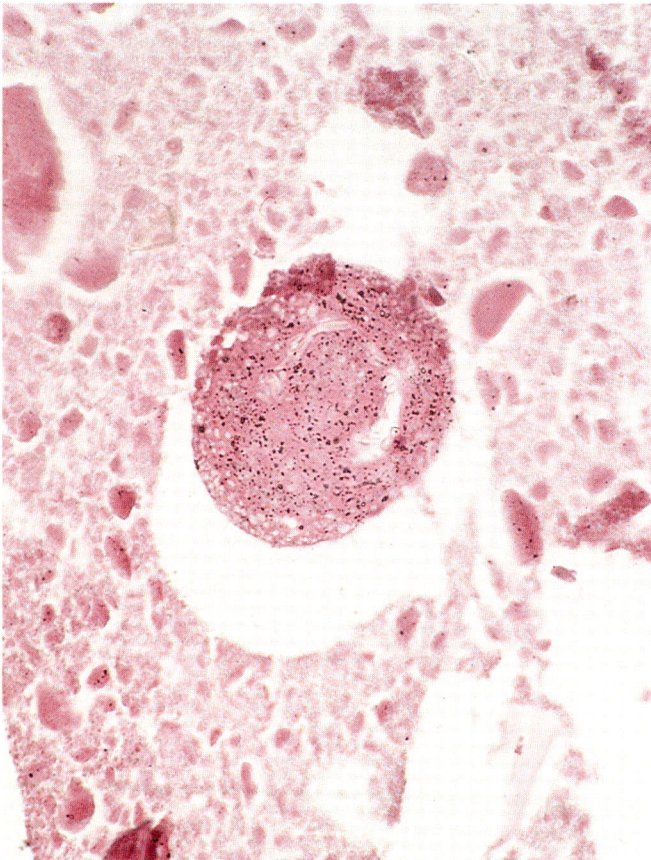

Fig. 43.13 Necrobiotic scolex of *Echinococcus granulosus* with faintly visible hook. Same case as Fig. 43.12. H&E

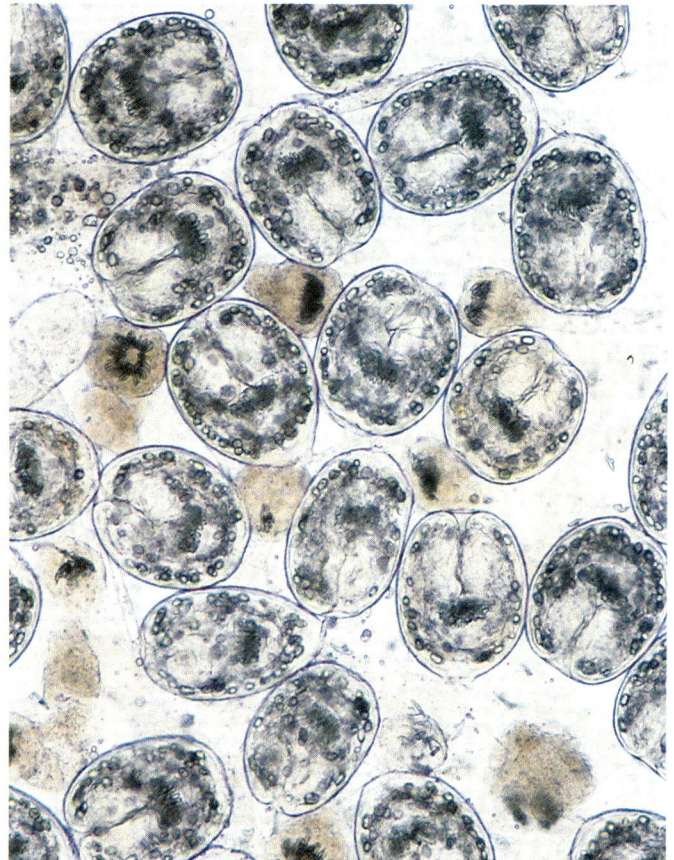

Fig. 43.14 Numerous scolices of *Echinococcus granulosus* in unstained smear of the fluid in a cyst. They appear bluish because photography was done with a filter

South East Asia (*S. japonicum*), in Laos and Cambodia (*S. mekongi*) and in Africa and South America (*S. mansoni*)[1-4]. Areas endemic for schistosomiasis are known in the central regions of Venezuela.

Definitive hosts, in addition to man, and reservoir hosts are, depending on parasite species, monkeys, rodents and several species of domestic animals[5]. Intermediate hosts are water snails. For experimental studies, mice, hamsters and rats may be used[6-11].

Clinically, an allergic dermatitis may be observed (cercarial dermatitis). Four to seven weeks after infection, clinical manifestations caused by worms and worm eggs may be noted. Many cases, however, remain asymptomatic for a long time. Symptoms appear according to the location of the lesions: in the digestive tract (sometimes with dysenteric-like bloody diarrhoea), in the liver, or in the urogenital region. Exceptionally, other organs may be involved. In chronic infections, carcinoma of the bladder may be observed.

Clinical diagnosis is made by confirmation of the characteristic worm eggs in stools or urine. Biopsy of the rectal mucosa may be helpful[12,13], and, serologically, different antigens exist for diagnosis of acute and chronic infections[14].

The parasite

The five species, *Schistosoma haematobium, S. intercalatum, S. japonicum, S. mansoni* and *S. mekongi*, occur in different geographical areas (see above). *S. mekongi* is very similar to *S. japonicum*. Recently, *Schistosoma curassoni* has been found to be an important species in Senegal[15].

Adult male and female worms of the genus *Schistosoma* measure from 6–24 mm in length with slight variations according to the species. Females are somewhat longer and thinner. In the blood vessels of the definitive host, female worms are found within a longitudinal (gynaecophoric) canal of the male worm. The latter has a similar appearance to a rowing boat. Therefore they are also named 'paired flukes' (Fig. 44.1).

The worm eggs have particular characteristic features and sizes which allow differentiation of the five species (Fig. 44.2).

S. haematobium – elliptical, terminal spine, 150 × 55 μm
S. intercalatum – elliptical, slimmer than *S. haematobium*, terminal spine, 140 × 150 μm
S. japonicum – oval, small lateral kob, 90 × 55 μm
S. mansoni – elliptical, lateral spine, 150 × 60 μm
S. mekongi – spherical, lateral knob, 40 × 45 μm

Development of the different *Schistosoma* species is similar. Eggs are excreted in stools or urine and reach the water. There, a larva with cilia, called a miracidium, hatches out from the egg and penetrates into a snail. Here, the larvae become infectious, transform into fork-tailed cercaria (Fig. 44.3) and reproduce copiously. After being released into water again, they can infect a definitive host.

Pathogenesis

There is no transmission from man to man or animal or man. Infection takes place only in water.

The fork-tailed cercaria penetrates through the intact skin of the definitive host, quickly loosing its tail. Through lymph and bloodstream, it reaches the mesenteric, liver and bladder veins (only *S. haematobium*) where the flukes become mature. Here, copulation of male and female worms takes place and production of eggs begins. The eggs pass through the intestinal and bladder walls

into the lumina of these organs and the developmental cycle begins again outside of the human body.

The eggs produce tissue lesions in the intestinal and bladder wall, and they may be disseminated, haematogenously, to almost all organs, causing further tissue alterations. Damage to human tissue caused by adult *Schistosoma* worms is of minor importance.

Pathology

Skin, intestine, liver, spleen, the urogenital tract, lungs, CNS and other organs (exceptionally) may be involved.

Grossly, cercarial dermatitis (Fig. 44.4) may manifest itself with red areas and transient papulomatous skin lesions.

Intestinal schistosomiasis, caused by *S. mansoni, S. japonicum, S. mekongi* and *S. intercalatum*, shows manifestations in the ileocaecal region and the large bowel. In the intestinal mucosa and peritoneum, nodular tubercle-like lesions may be present (Fig. 44.5). A marked acute or chronic colitis, with haemorrhages, ulceration and polypoid lesions, may be observed, as well as appendicitis[16].

Hepato- and splenomegaly, as well as hepatitis, pipe stem fibrosis of the liver and portal hypertension, due to portal vein obstruction may occur. These alterations may cause fatal oesophageal bleeding from varices produced by the *Schistosoma* species mentioned above, with the exception of *Schistosoma intercalatum*[17,18]. Fig. 44.6 shows liver granulomas due to *Schistosoma* infection.

Urogenital schistosomiasis, caused only by *S. haematobium*, may show acute and chronic cystitis, pyelonephritis, urolithiasis and hydronephrosis[19,20]. Furthermore, female (Fig. 44.7) and male genital organs[21] may be involved. In severe and chronic infections, cancer of the bladder may develop. Squamous cell carcinomas are more common than transitional carcinomas (Figs. 44.8 and 44.9).

In the lungs, obstructive arteritis may lead to cor pulmonale (Figs. 44.10 and 44.11).

In the central nervous system[22-24] and other organs, lesions caused by blood flukes are (Figs. 44.12–44.14) rare and not characteristic.

Histologically, *Schistosoma* eggs produce eosinophilic granulomas in the intestinal wall, liver, urogenital tract and elsewhere. These granulomas later undergo fibrosis. The eggs disintegrate and may be calcified. Granulomas of this type may be confused with those due to larva migrans, see Section 37. Surrounding the eggs, the Hoeppli–Splendore phenomenon may be observed[25].

Pipe stem fibrosis in the liver is rather typical and occurs without active schistosomiasis lesions.

When there is pulmonary involvement, the worm eggs produce granulomas situated in the vicinity and adventitia of pulmonary arteries which, consequently, lead to their obliteration, followed by pulmonary hypertension and hypertrophy of the right heart ventricle (cor pulmonale).

The glomerulonephritis found in patients with schistosomiasis is of an immunological type (without the presence of a causal agent)[26-28].

References

1. Doumenge, J. P. *et al.* (1987). *Atlas de la Repartition Mondiale des Schistosomiases.* CEGET-CNRS/OMS-WHO, Presses Universitaires de Bordeaux

2. Butterworth, A. E. *et al.* (1988). Longitudinal studies on human schistosomiasis. *Philos. Trans. R. Soc. Lond. Biol.*, **321**, 495

3. Vargas, M. *et al.* (1990). Schistosomiasis mansoni in the Dominican Republic; prevalence and intensity in various urban and rural communities, 1982–1987. *Trop. Med. Parasitol.*, **41**, 415

4. Hatz, C. *et al.* (1990). Ultrasound scanning for detecting morbidity

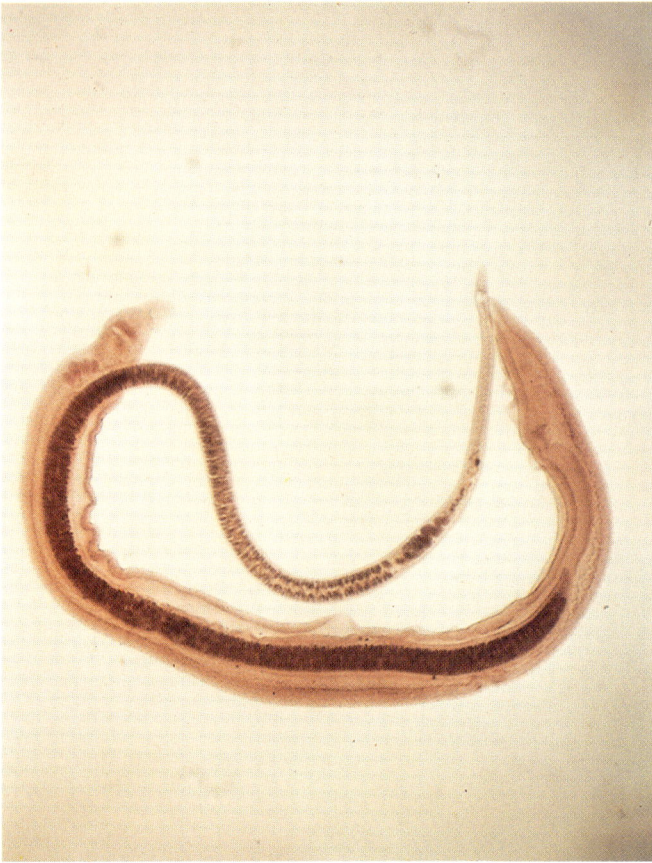

Fig. 44.1 Female worm of *Schistosoma mansoni* within a longitudinal (gynaecophoric) canal of the male. Carmine

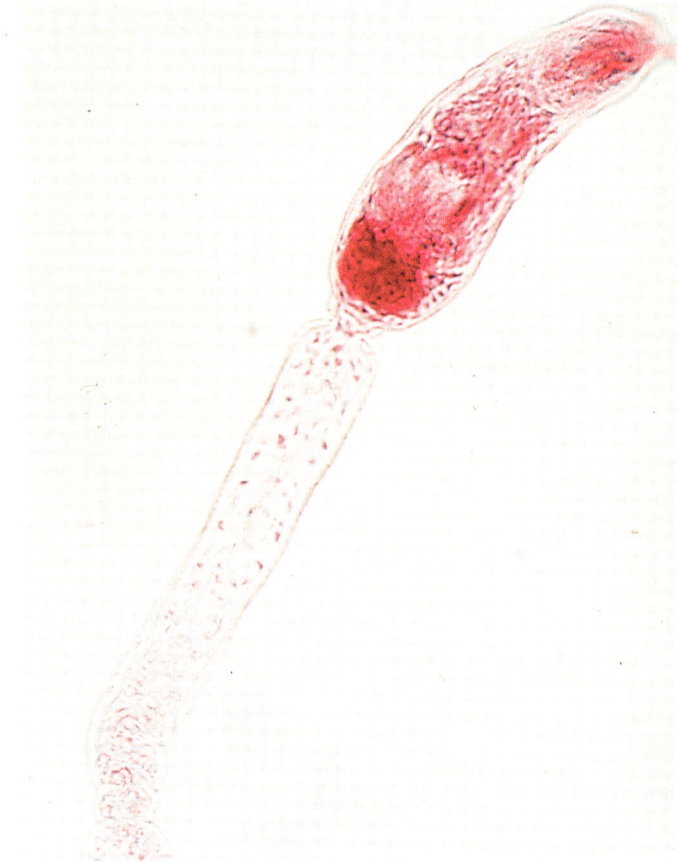

Fig. 44.3 Fork-tailed cercaria of *Schistosoma mansoni*. Carmine

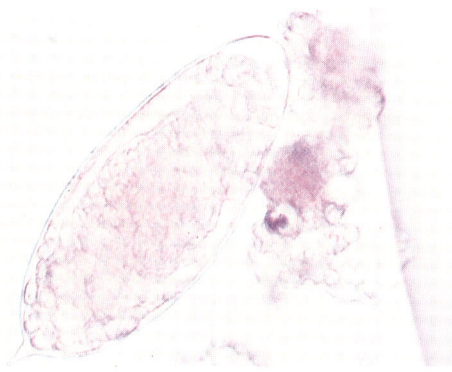

a.

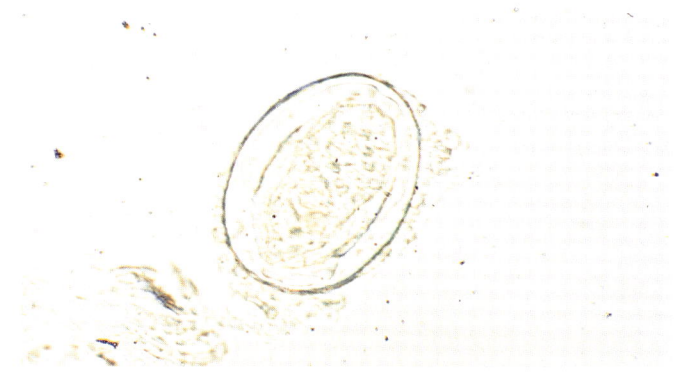

b.

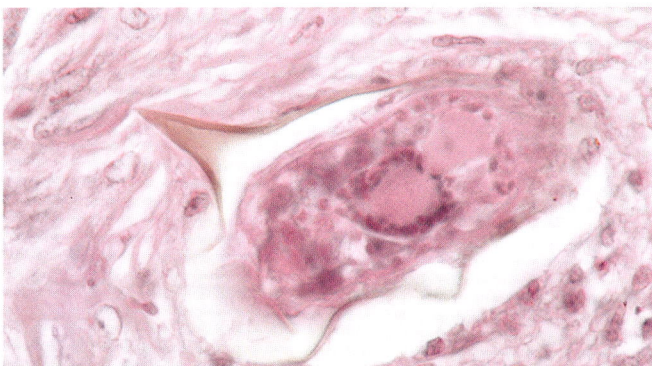

c.

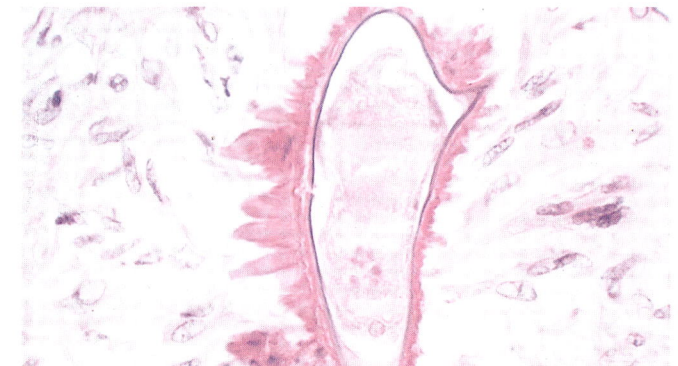

d.

Fig. 44.2 Eggs of the genus *Schistosoma*:
  a. *Schistosoma haematobium* (in urine) H&E;
  b. *Schistosoma japonicum* (in faeces);
  c. *Schistosoma mansoni* (in tissue with lateral spine) H&E;
  d. *Schistosoma mansoni* (in tissue with lateral spine and Hoeppli–Splendore phenomenon) H&E

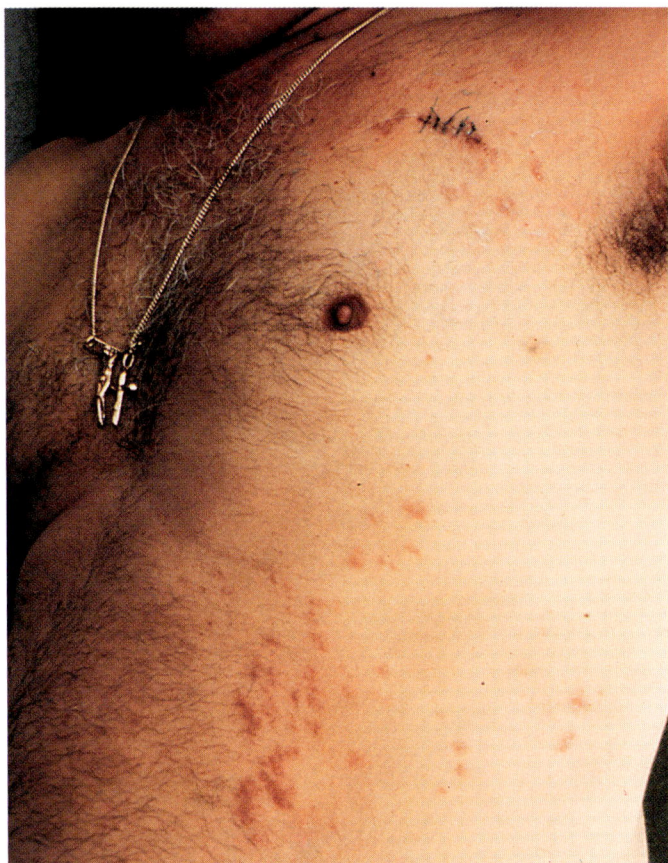

Fig. 44.4 Cercarial dermatitis in a 62-year-old male patient from Barinas, Venezuela

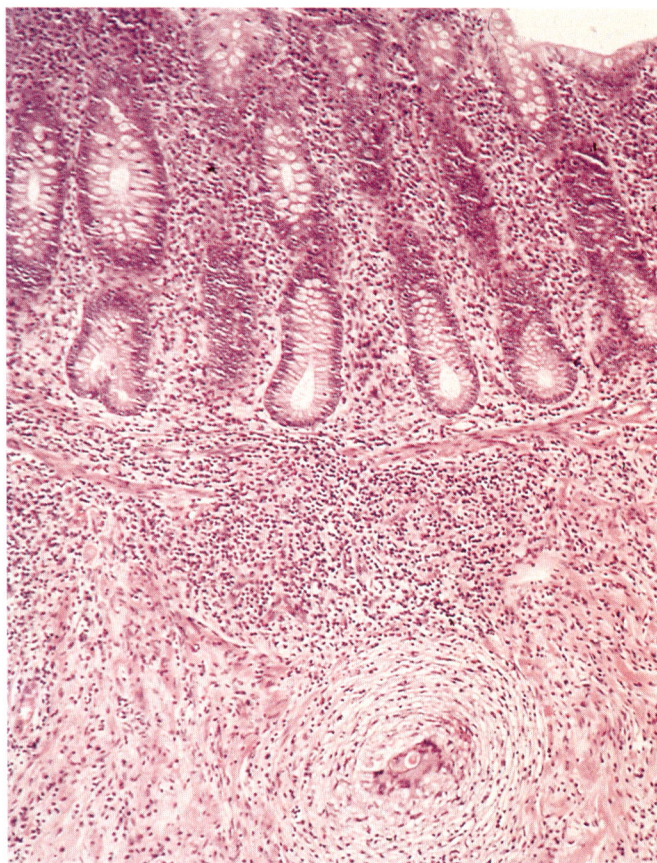

Fig. 44.5 *Schistosoma* granuloma in the submucosa of appendix. H&E

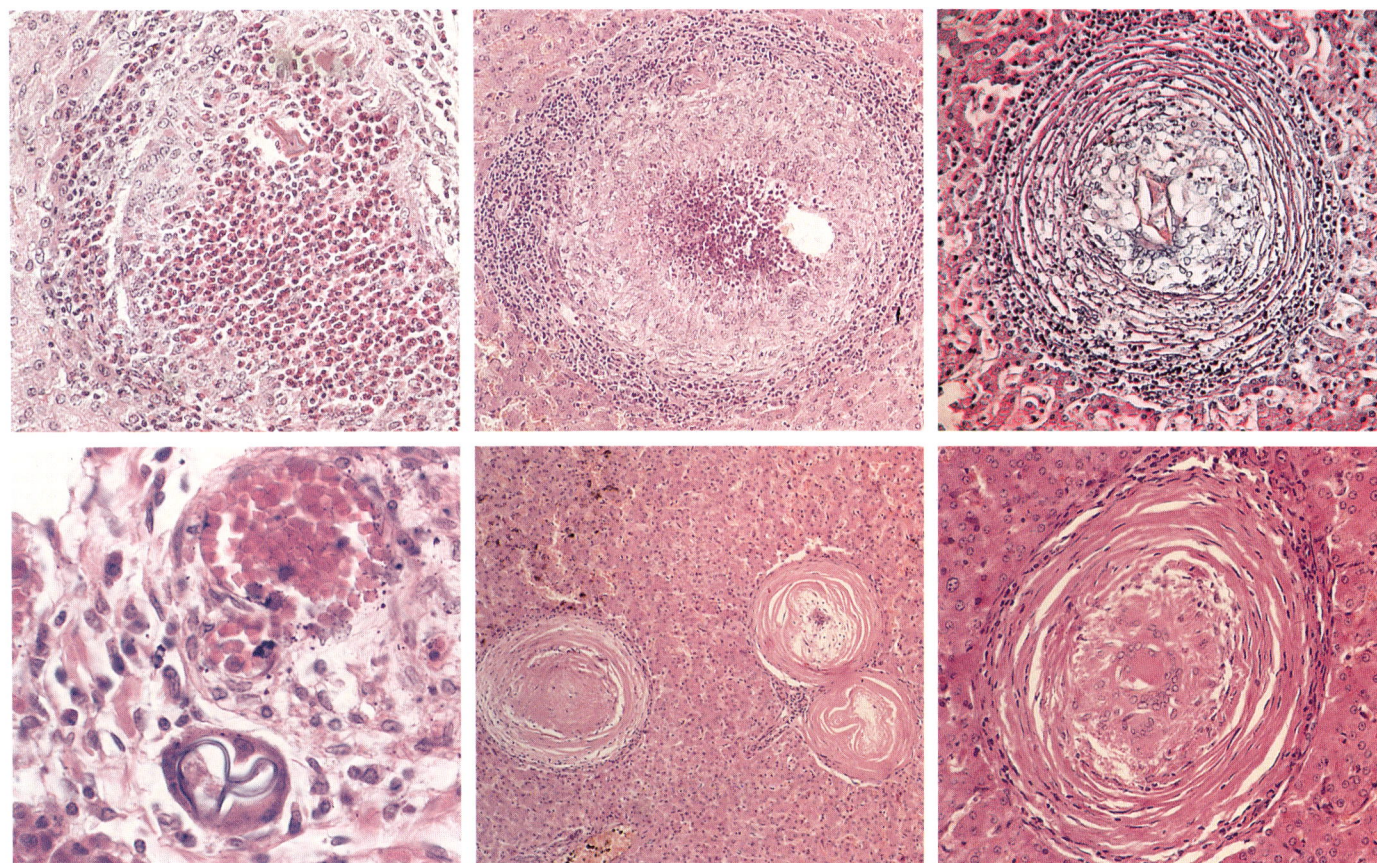

Fig. 44.6 *Schistosoma* granulomas in the liver in different stages of evolution with and without parasitic eggs. H&E

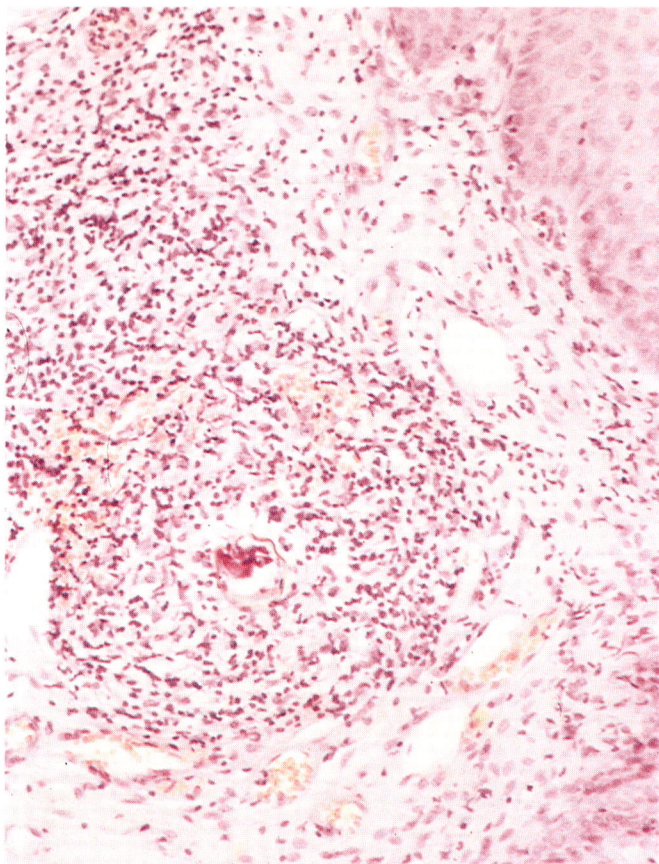

Fig. 44.7 *Schistosoma* granuloma at the uterine cervix. H&E

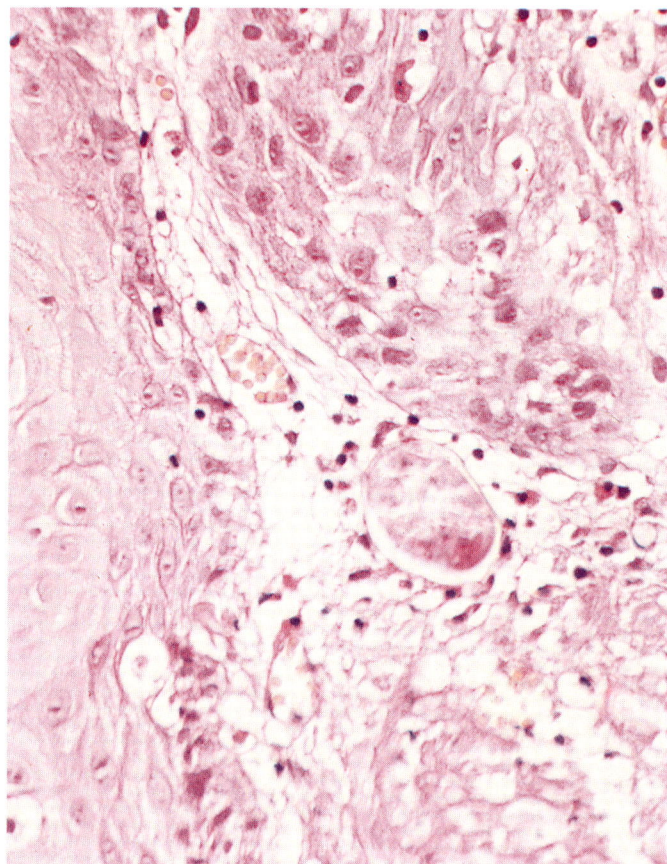

Fig. 44.8 Squamous cell carcinoma of the bladder with *Schistosoma* eggs. H&E

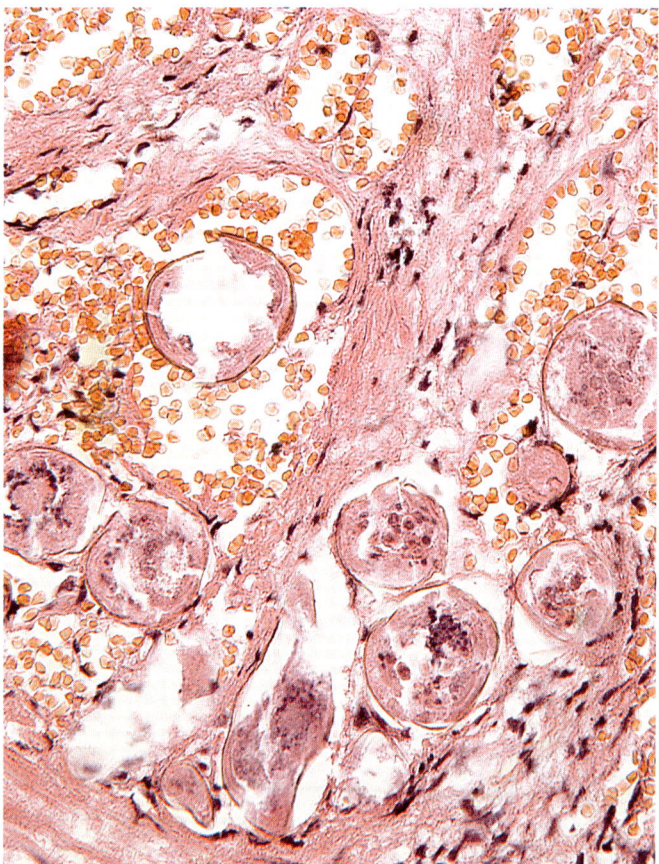

Fig. 44.9 Numerous deformed eggs of *Schistosoma haematobium* in the case of Fig. 44.8. H&E

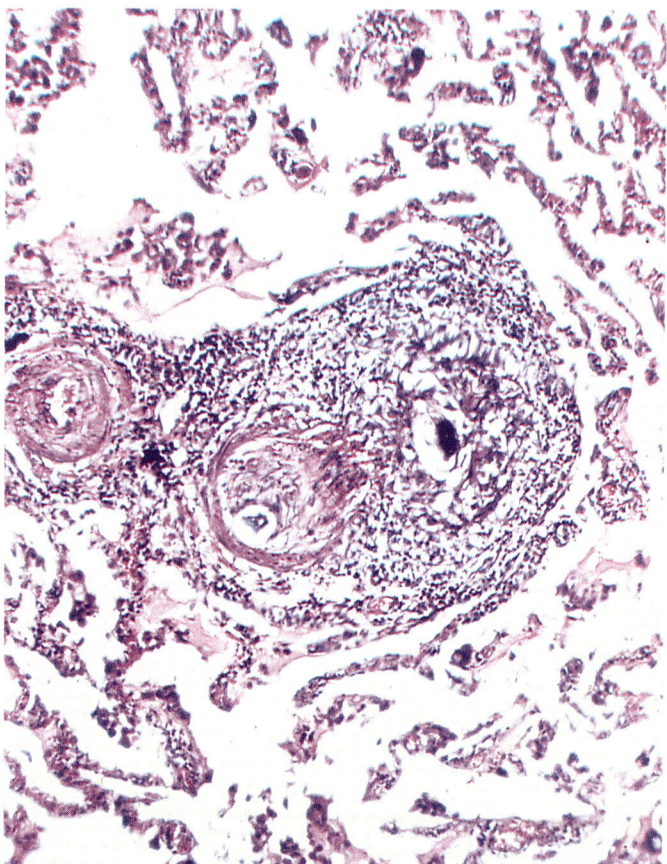

Fig. 44.10 *Schistosoma* granuloma in the lung near the pulmonary artery. A case with cor pulmonale. H&E

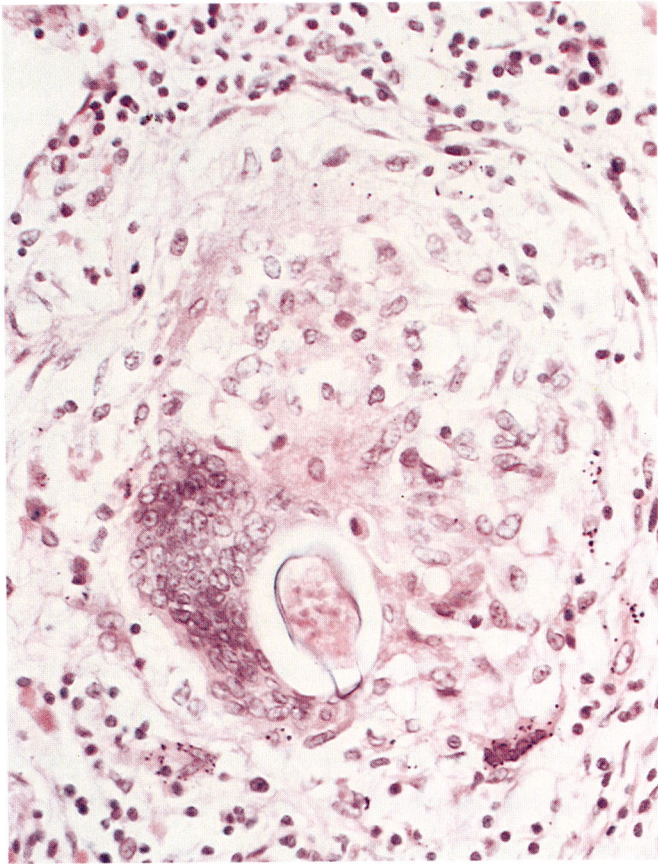

Fig. 44.11 Pulmonary *Schistosoma* granuloma with parasitic egg clearly visible. Same case as Fig. 44.10. H&E

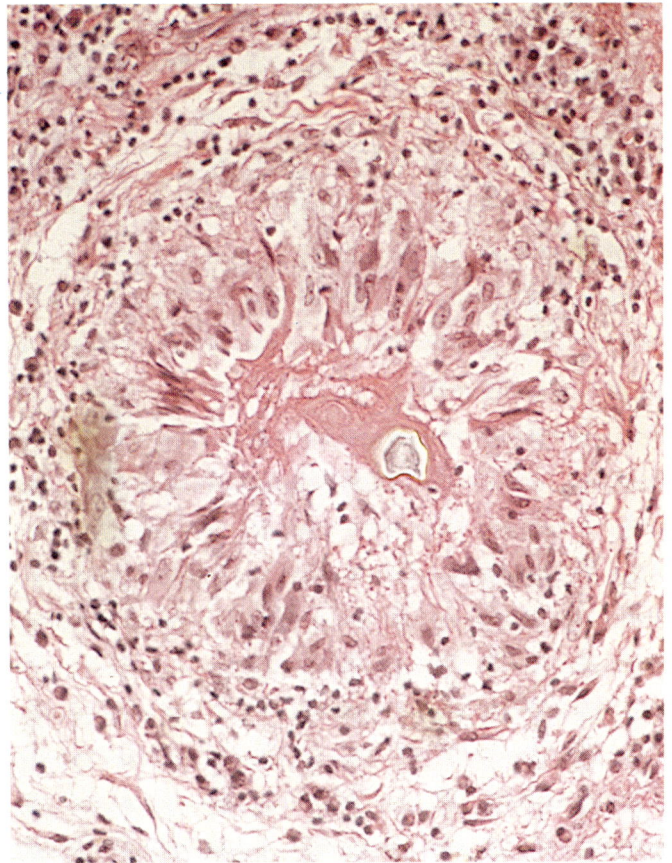

Fig. 44.12 *Schistosoma* meningo-myelitis with granuloma. Small deformed parasitic egg faintly visible in the centre of granuloma. H&E

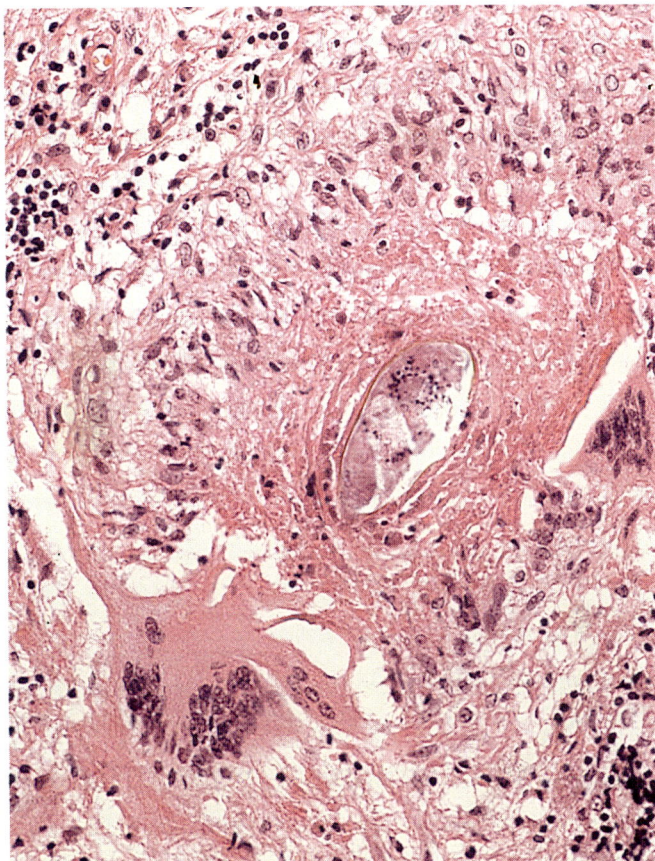

Fig. 44.13 Same case as Fig. 44.12 at higher power with *Schistosoma* egg clearly visible. H&E

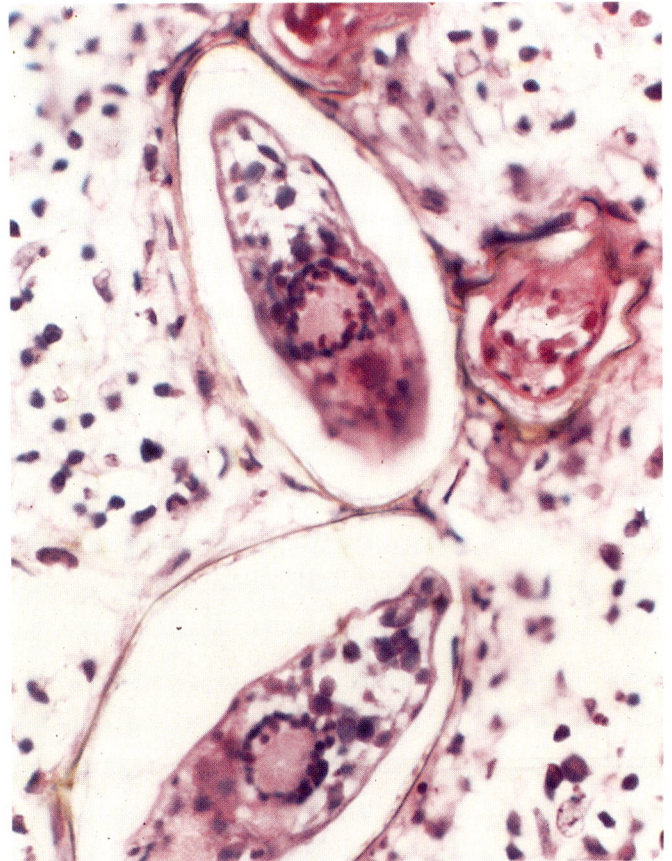

Fig. 44.14 Same case as Figs. 44.12 and 44.13. In two *Schistosoma* eggs miracidium structures are seen. The latter may be confused with multinuclear tissue giant cells. H&E

due to Schistosoma haematobium and its resolution following treatment with different doses of praziquantel. *Trans. R. Soc. Trop. Med. Hyg.*, **84**, 84

5. Obwolo, M. J. and Rogers, S. E. (1988). Schistosomal lesions in the bovine uterus. *J. Comp. Pathol.*, **98**, 501

6. Vignali, D. A. *et al.* (1989). Histological examination of the cellular reaction around schistosomula of Schistosoma mansoni in the lungs of sublethally irradiated and unirradiated immune and control rats. *Parasitology*, **98**, 57

7. Cheever, A. W. and Deb, S. (1989). Persistence of hepatic fibrosis and tissue eggs following treatment of Schistosoma japonicum infected mice. *Am. J. Trop. Med. Hyg.*, **40**, 620

8. Andrade, Z. A. and De Azevedo, T. M. (1987). A contribution to the study of acute schistosomiasis (an experimental trial). *Mem. Inst. Owaldo Cruz*, **82**, 311

9. Andrade, Z. A. (1987). Pathogenesis of pipe stem fibrosis of the liver (experimental observation on murine schistosomiasis). *Mem. Inst. Oswaldo Cruz*, **82**, 325

10. Melro, M. C. and Mariano, M. (1987). Extra-tissular Schistosoma mansoni egg granulomata in the peritoneal cavity of mice. *Mem. Inst. Oswaldo Cruz, 82* Suppl. **4**, 245

11. He, Y. X. *et al.* (1989). Dermal responses of various hosts to infection with Schistoma japonicum cercariae. *Chung. Kuo. Chi.*, **7**, 15

12. Meybehm, M. *et al.* (1989). Granulomatous colitis with pseudo-polyp in schistosomiasis. *Dtsch. Med. Wschr.*, **114**, 19

13. Yasawy, M. I. *et al.* (1989). Comparison between stool examination, serology and large bowel biopsy in diagnosing Schistosoma mansoni. *Trop. Doct.*, **19**, 132

14. Boros, D. L. (1989). Immunopathology of Schistosoma mansoni infection. *Clin. Microbiol. Rev.*, **2**, 250

15. Vercruysse, J. (1990). Schistosoma species in Senegal with special reference to the biology, epidemiology and pathology of Schistosoma curassoni Brumpt, 1931. *Verh. K. Akad. Geneeskd. Belg.*, **52**, 31

16. Al-Kraida, A. *et al.* (1988). Appendicitis and schistosomiasis. *Br. J. Surg.*, **75**, 58

17. Hamadto, H. A. *et al.* (1990). Correlation between intensity of infection and hepatic histopathological lesions in bilharzial patients. *J. Egypt. Soc. Parasitol.*, **20**, 147

18. Doehring-Schwerdtfeger, E. *et al.* (1990). Ultrasonographical investigation of periportal fibrosis in children with Schistosoma mansoni infection; evaluation of morbidity. *Am. J. Trop. Med. Hyg.*, **42**, 581

19. Adolphs, H.-D. *et al.* (1982). Manifestation der Bilharziose am Harntrakt. *Act. Urol.*, **13**, 277

20. Laurent, C. *et al.* (1990). Ultrasonographic assessment of urinary tract lesions due to Schistosoma haematobium in Nigeria after four consecutive years of treatment with praziquantel. *Trop. Med. Parasitol.*, **41**, 139

21. Mikhail, N. E. *et al.* (1988). Schistosomal orchitis simulating malignancy. *J. Urol.*, **140**, 147

22. Andrade, A. N. and Bastos, C. L. (1989). Cerebral schistosomiasis mansoni. *Arqu. Neuropsiquiatr.*, **47**, 100

23. Pitella, J. E. (1991). The relation between involvement of the central nervous system in schistosomiasis mansoni and the clinical forms of the parasitosis. A review. *J. Trop. Med. Hyg.*, **94**, 15

24. Selwa, L. M. *et al.* (1991). Spinal cord schistosomiasis: a pediatric case mimicking intrinsic cord neoplasm. *Neurology*, **41**, 755

25. Kephart, G. M. *et al.* (1988). Localization of eosinophil basic protein onto eggs of Schistosoma mansoni in human pathologic tissue. *Am. J. Pathol.*, **133**, 389

26. Sobh, M. A. *et al.* (1988). Characterization of kidney lesions in early schistosomal-specific nephropathy. *Nephrol. Dial. Transplant.*, **3**, 392

27. De Water, R. *et al.* (1988). Schistosoma mansoni: ultrastructural localization of the circulating anodic antigen and the circulating cathodic antigen in the mouse kidney glomerulus. *Am. J. Trop. Med. Hyg.*, **38**, 118

28. Sobh, M. W. *et al.* (1991). Schistosoma haematobium-induced glomerular disease: an experimental study in the golden hamster. *Neprhon*, **57**, 216

45.   LUNG TREMATODE INFECTION

Introduction

Autochthonous pulmonary fluke infection, or paragonimiasis, pulmonary distomiasis or endemic haemoptysis, is limited to certain geographical areas and practically found only in people with particular nutritional habits.

There are three species of the genus *Paragonimus* important for human infection:

1. *P. westermani* in the Far East, the Philippines and India,
2. *P. africanus* in the tropical countries of West Africa[1], and
3. *P. kellicotti* in North, Central and certain countries of South America, e.g. in Venezuela.

With their eggs, they may contribute to the contamination of water. The definitive hosts, in addition to man, are numerous species of domestic and fur-bearing animals[2,3]. The first intermediate hosts are water snails and the second intermediate hosts are crabs and crayfish. Each species of *Paragonimus* has its specific intermediate hosts. Experimentally, dogs and Rhesus monkeys, as well as cats, have been used[4].

Clinically, symptoms depend on the number of worms in the lungs and the other sites, where worms may be located eventually. Often, a chronic bronchitis with blood in sputum is present and differential diagnosis may be tuberculosis[5]. In China, some cases have been reported with no eggs in the sputum, but with heavy enlargement of the liver[6].

Clinical diagnosis is made by confirmation of golden-brown operculated eggs in the often blood-stained sputum and in stools. X-ray, tomography and sonography may lead to suspicion of pulmonary parasitic disease since the cysts may look like tumours (parasitic pseudotumours). In serological tests, cross-reactions with *Schistosoma* infection may occur.

The parasite

There are more than 20 species of lung trematodes and numerous ones of the genus *Paragonimus*[5]. The best-known pulmonary flukes in man are *Paragonimus westermani*, mostly in China, *P. africanus* and *P. kellicotti*.

The adult worms of *Paragonimus* measure 7–12 × 4–7 mm and are egg-shaped. They are reddish brown, like a roasted coffee bean, have two suckers and numerous prominent spines on the surface. Their lifespan in man may be more than 20 years.

The eggs are golden-brown, measure 90 × 60 μm and have an operculum at one end. They contain 5–10 yolk cells when immature, and, once laid, a miracidium larva grows within.

The eggs reach the exterior mostly with the sputum. In water, the hatched larval miracidia from the eggs penetrate into snails (the first intermediate host). There, cercariae with short tails and fine spines develop. They reach the water again, where they are eaten by crayfish and crabs. Inside these crustaceans (the second intermediate hosts), the cercaria encyst and transform into metacercariae which are situated in certain muscles.

Pathogenesis

Man is infected by consuming raw crab or crayfish meat. The metacercariae then reach the small intestine of the definitive host. Metacercariae are present too in the juice of crushed crustaceans and transmission may also take place, exceptionally, through handling infected crustaceans or eating raw pork meat[7,8].

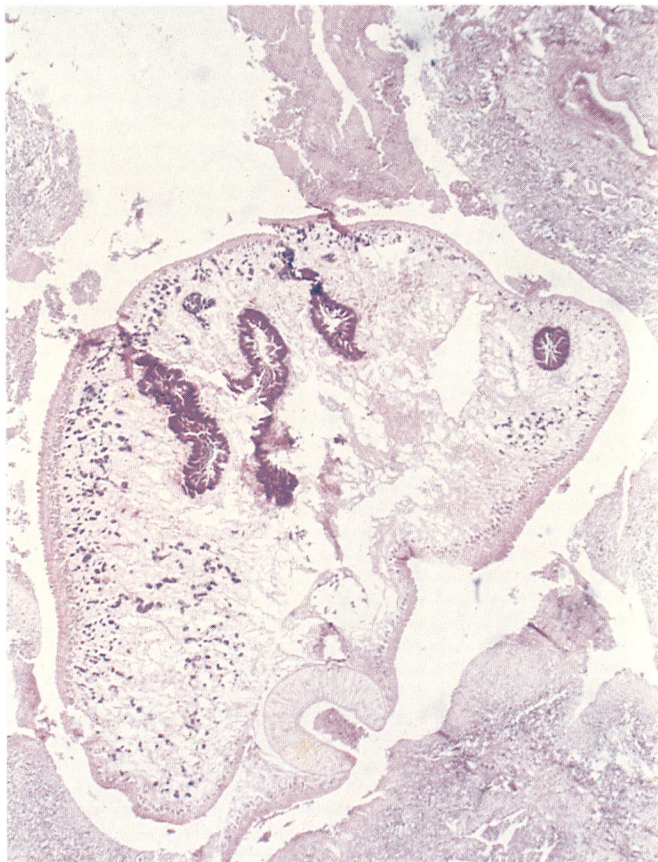

Fig. 45.1 *Paragonimus westermani* fluke in a pulmonary cyst. H&E

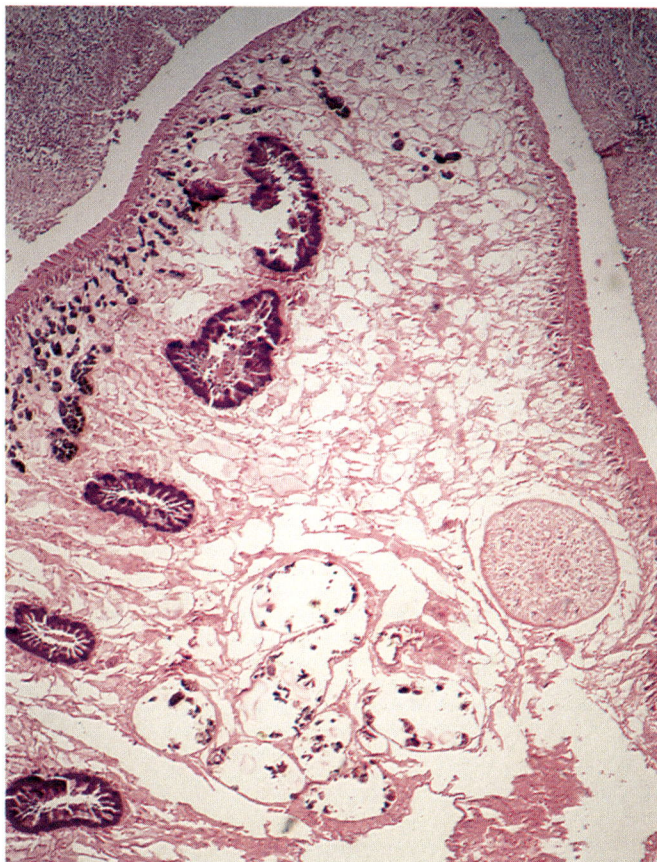

Fig. 45.2 Another large *Paragonimus westermani* fluke in a pulmonary cyst. H&E

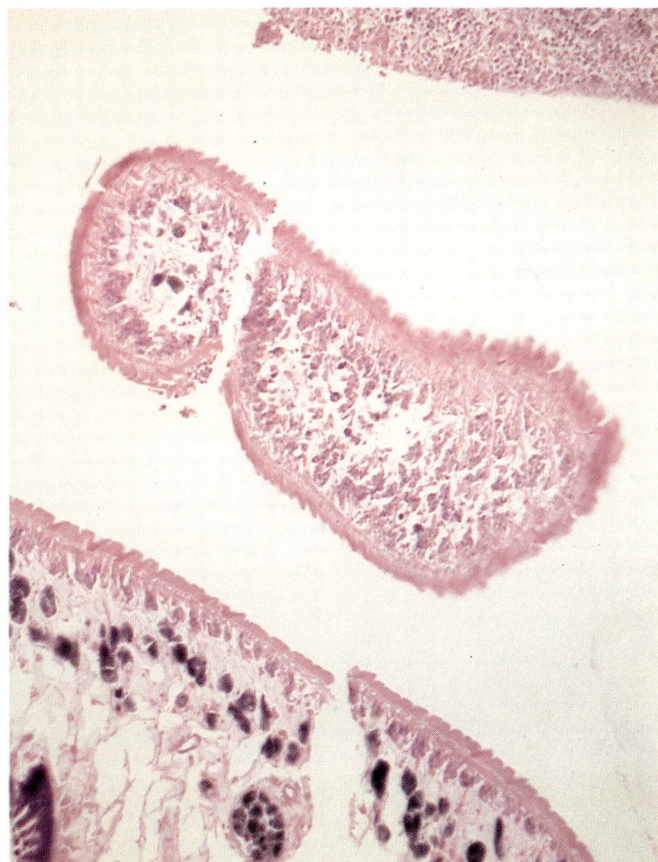

Fig. 45.3 The spines on the surface of these lung flukes are easily recognized. H&E

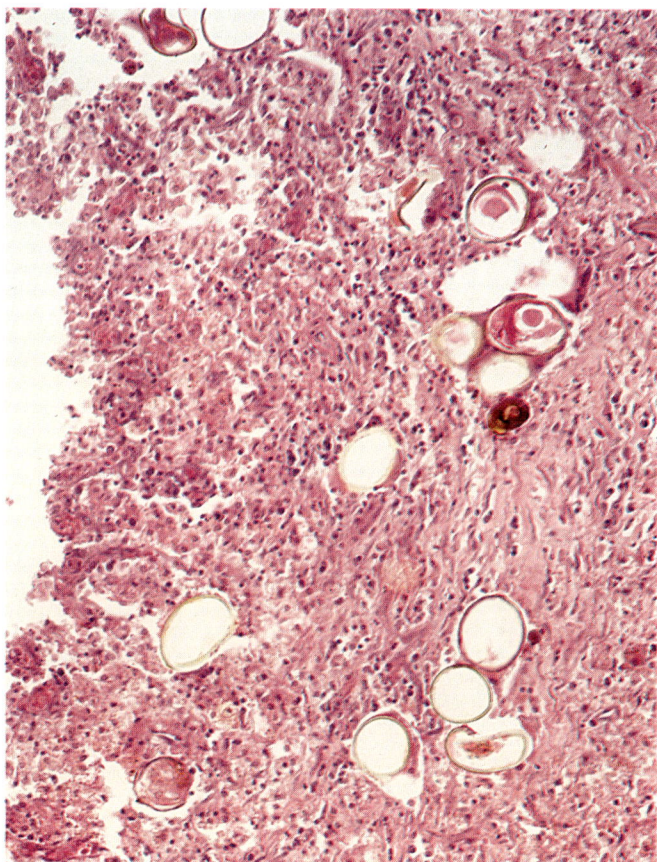

Fig. 45.4 Eggs of *Paragonimus westermani* in the granulation tissue around the flukes in the lung. H&E

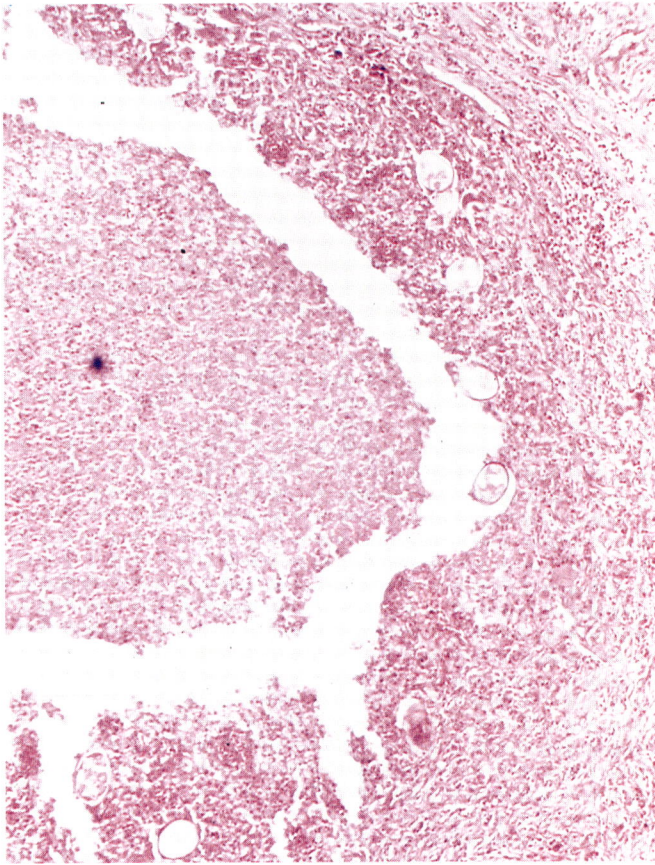

Fig. 45.5 Lung cyst in a case of paragonimiasis containing exudate with surrounding parasitic eggs. H&E

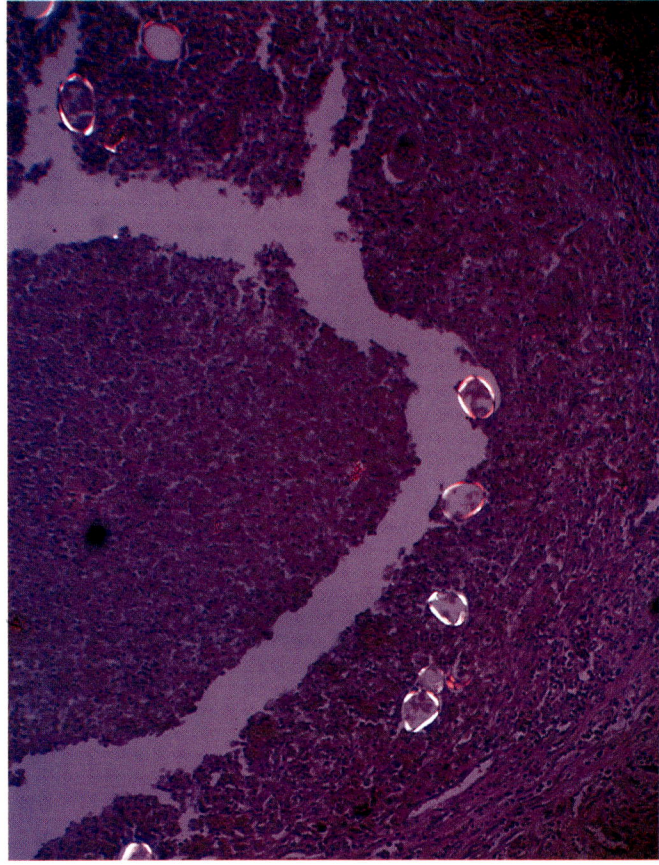

Fig. 45.6 The same cyst as Fig. 45.5 with polarized light. H&E

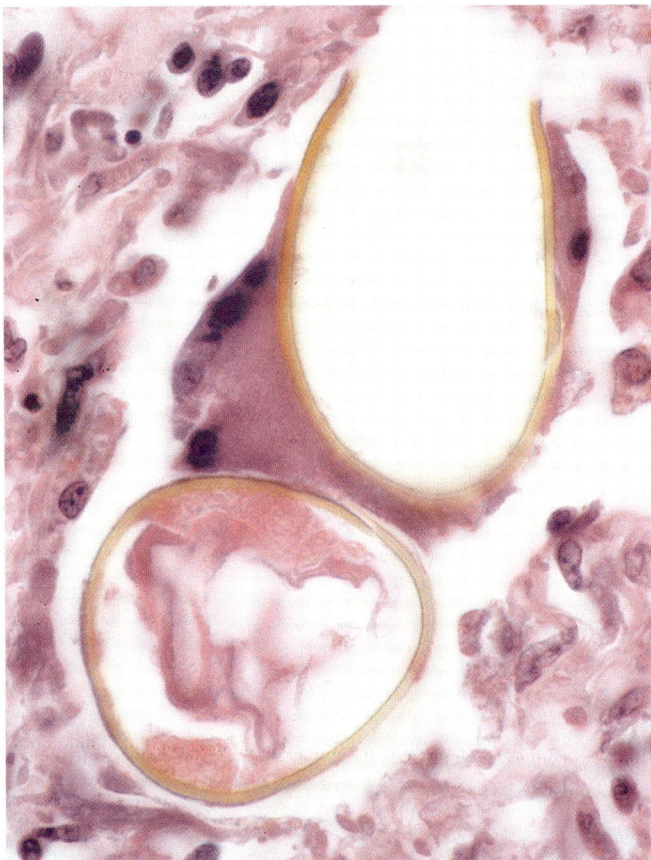

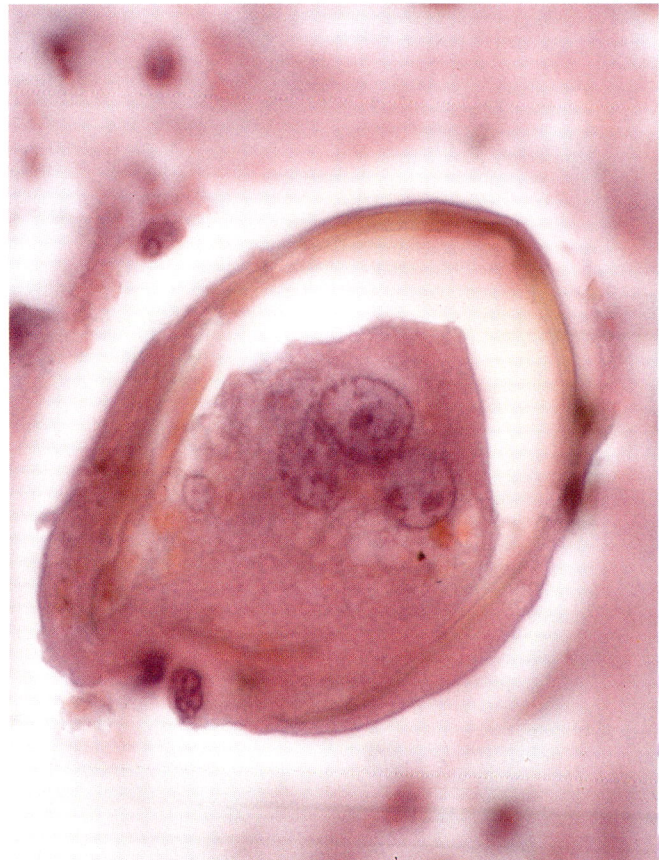

Figs. 45.7a and **b** Eggs of *Paragonimus westermani* in lung tissue. H&E

The metacercariae in the human small intestine hatch out of their shells as young flukes and penetrate the wall of the duodenum. Here, migration through the diaphragm into the thoracic cavity takes place, mostly with invasion of the lungs.

Pathology

Although the lungs are involved chiefly, aberrant flukes may reach extrapulmonary sites and remain there. Paragonimiasis lesions have been reported in the peritoneum, omentum, skin, liver[6], spleen, pancreas, kidneys, brain[9] and spinal cord.

In the lungs, young flukes are soon surrounded and enclosed by a fibrous wall, forming a cyst-like cavity, where they become sexually mature over the course of 2–3 months. These cysts are situated mostly in the vicinity of bronchi; they reach 1–2 cm in diameter. Several flukes may be present in a cyst, which also contains sanguineous and mucopurulent masses. In man, more than 10 flukes are seldom present in the lungs.

Histologically, the flukes are recognized by the spines on the surface and by their internal organs (Figs. 45.1–45.3). Typical eggs are present in mature flukes, around the parasites in the cysts, and in lung tissue outside the cysts. These eggs usually appear in H&E-stained sections of paraffin-embedded tissues as double refractile with polarized light (Figs. 45.4–45.7). Eggs of other parasitic helminths do not show this feature in tissues, a phen-omenon we are not able to explain. Around the cysts, and also the eggs, granulomas with giant cells and some eosinophilic granulocytes may be found.

References

1. Sachs, R. and Kern, P. (1982). Epidemiological investigations of human lung fluke infection in Gabon, Central Africa. *VII Intern. Congr. Inf. Paras. Diseases,* Stockholm
2. Van Rensburg, I. B. *et al.* (1987). Parasitic pneumonia in a dog by a lung fluke of the genus Paragonimus. *J. S. Afr. Vet. Assoc.,* **58**, 203
3. Duncan, R. B. Jr. *et al.* (1989). Fatal lungworm infection in an opossum. *J. Wildl. Dis.,* **25**, 266
4. Weina, P. J. and England, D. M. (1990). The American lung fluke, Paragonimus kellicotti, in a cat model. *J. Parasitol.,* **76**, 568
5. Kraus, A. *et al.* (1990). Paragonimiasis: an infrequent but treatable cause of hemoptysis in systemic lupus erythematosus. *J. Rheumatol.,* **17**, 244
6. Sachs, R. and Voelker, J. (1982). Human paragonimiasis caused by Paragonimus uterobilateralis in Liberia and Guinea, West Africa. *Tropenmed. Parasit.,* **33**, 15
7. Miyazaki, I. and Habe, S. (1976). A newly recognized mode of human infection with the lung fluke, Paragonimus westermani (Kerbert 1878). *J. Parasit.,* **62**, 646
8. Cheng, S. Z. *et al.* (1981). Hepatic lesions in 69 children infected with Paragonimus westermani in Southern Anhui. *WHO/Helm,* **82**, 5
9. Stefanko, S. and Zebrowski, S. (1961). The morphology of cerebral paragonimiasis. *Acta Med. Pol.,* **11**, 111

46. LIVER TREMATODE INFECTION

This is caused by numerous fluke species:

A by *Clonorchis sinensis* (liver fluke infection),
B by *Opisthorchis felineus* (cat liver fluke infection) or *Opisthorchis viverrini*[1],
C by *Dicrocoelium dentriticum* (small liver fluke infection), and
D by *Fasciola hepatica* (sheep liver fluke infection or fascioliasis).

A AND B, CHINESE AND CAT LIVER FLUKE INFECTION

Introduction

These infections are called also clonorchiasis and opisthorchiasis. **A** is closely related to **B**, practically the only difference being their occurrence in different geographical regions. Together they constitute a relatively important helminthic disease since it is estimated that 20 million people are infected, 7 million in Thailand alone (*O. viverrini*).

A is found in East Asia, mostly in China, and **B** in the temperate zones of Eastern Europe, the former USSR, India, South East Asia and Japan. Rural populations in river and lake regions are the main groups affected, men more than women. It has also been observed in three-month-old babies.

The definitive hosts are, in addition to man, cats, dogs and other domestic animals. The first intermediate hosts are water snails and the second intermediate hosts freshwater fishes.

Clinically, mild infections may be asymptomatic. In severe cases, symptoms of the bile duct and gallbladder with jaundice and cirrhosis may be noted. In chronic infections, unspecific gastrointestinal symptoms may prevail and carcinomas of liver and pancreas may develop.

Clinical diagnosis is made by confirmation of the presence of worm eggs, which are very small, in duodenal juice and faeces. In serological tests, cross-reactions with other trematode infections should be taken into consideration. Ultrasonographic and cholangiographic methods may be used[2–6].

The parasite

The three species, *Clonorchis sinensis*, also called *Opisthorchis sinensis* or the Chinese liver fluke, *Opisthorchis felineus*, the cat liver fluke, and *Opisthorchis viverrini* can be distinguished only by minimal details.

The adult flukes are up to 20 mm long and 1.5–5 mm wide; the *Opisthorchis* species are a little shorter. They have a lanceolate leaf-like structure and are almost transparent. Their lifespan is particularly long, up to 25 years in man (Figs. 46.1–46.4).

The eggs of these liver flukes are yellowish-brown, very small (30 μm) and jug-shaped (Fig. 46.5).

Miracidium larvae develop from the eggs in the uteri of mature worms. When they pass out into the bile duct, they reach (with the bile) the small intestine of the definitive host and, finally, the faeces. When water is contaminated by the faeces, the larvae are eaten by water snails (first intermediate hosts). Inside the snails, they transform into cercariae. When the cercariae are released from the snails, they penetrate, through the skin, into freshwater fish (second intermediate hosts). Within the fish, they move to the muscles where they transform into metacercariae.

Pathogenesis

Infection of the definitive host, including man, takes place by consuming raw fish with metacercariae. These structures, or young flukes, are released into the small

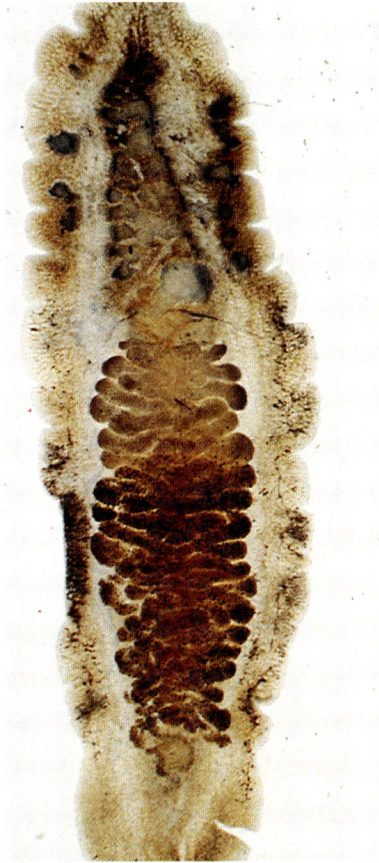

Fig. 46.1   Fluke of *Clonorchis sinensis*. H&E

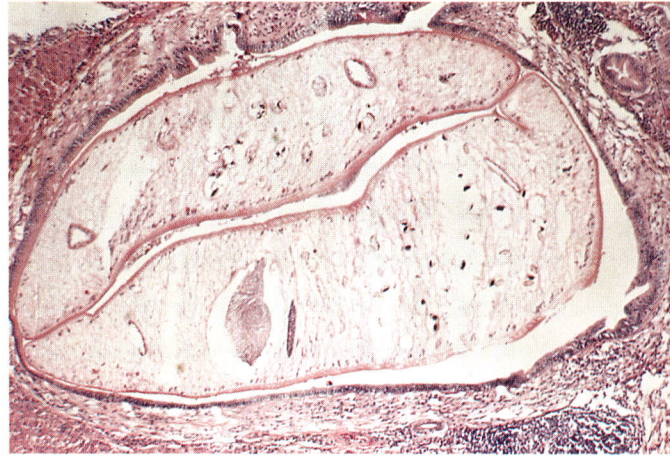

Fig. 46.2   Head of *Clonorchis sinensis* at higher power. H&E

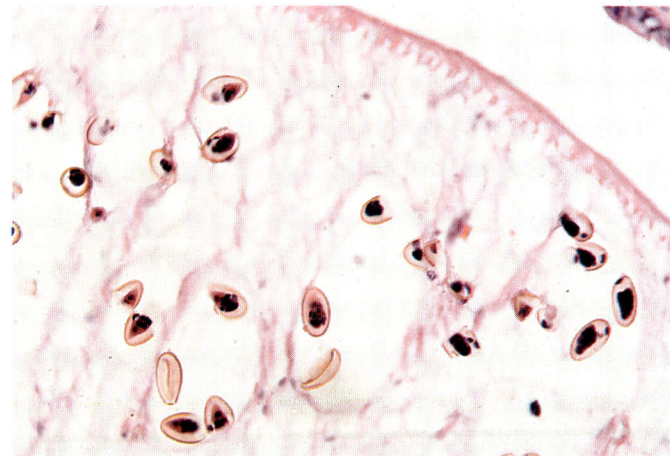

Fig. 46.3   *Opisthorchis viverrini* in the bile duct of a hamster. H&E

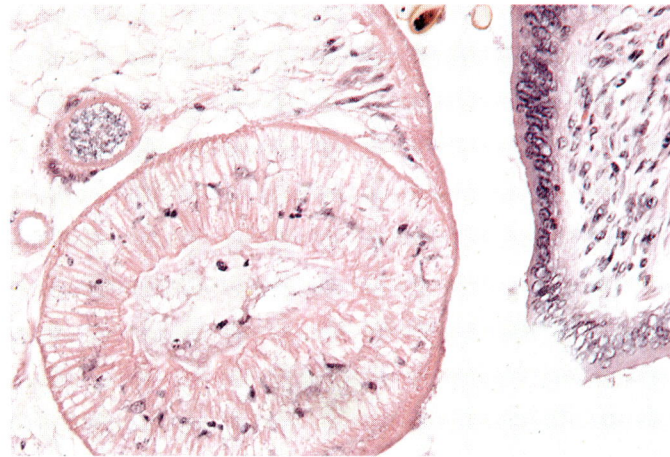

Fig. 46.4   Sucking apparatus of *Opisthorchis viverrini*. H&E

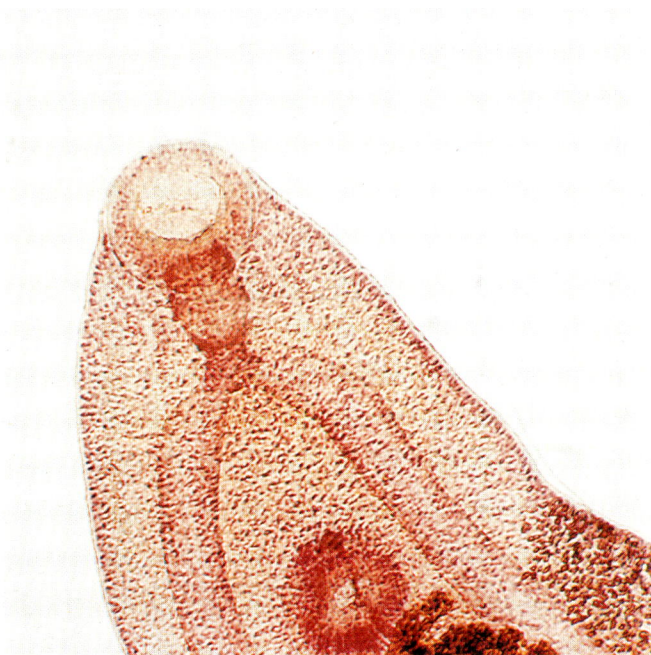

Fig. 46.5   Eggs of *Opisthorchis viverrini* inside the female fluke. H&E

intestine, from which they migrate actively into the bile ducts where they become sexually mature and may lay eggs. By obstructing the bile ducts and, eventually, also the pancreatic ducts, these flukes may cause damage which is different from that caused by other trematodes in the liver.

Pathology

Practically, only liver, and occasionally the pancreas, may be involved. The small worms can be detected with the naked eye in the bile ducts (Fig. 46.6). The obstruction of the bile ducts leads to cholangitis, cholangitic abscesses in the liver tissue, cholecystitis, cholelithiasis and hepatic fibrosis. In chronic infections, primary liver carcinomas, cholangiocarcinoma more frequently than hepatocellular carcinoma[7,8] may develop (Figs. 46.7–46.11). Pancreas carcinoma may also be associated with the lesions caused by this worm infection.

In contrast to the liver granulomas produced by the eggs of flukes like *Schistosoma* and, exceptionally, *Paragonimus*, the lesions in the liver produced by *Clonorchis* and *Opisthorchis*, are caused mostly by mature worms within the bile ducts and only rarely by eggs (Fig. 46.12).

C, SMALL LIVER FLUKE INFECTION

Introduction

This liver trematode infection is also called 'lancet liver fluke infection'. Primarily it is a parasitosis of ruminants and is only occasionally found in man, mainly in children. Recently, it has been observed in an AIDS patient[9].

It has been reported in North Africa, Siberia, Turkestan, South America and West Africa (here the species *D. hospes* occurs instead of *D. dentriticum*[10]).

The definitive principal hosts are sheep and cattle; man is only an 'accidental' secondary host. The intermediate hosts are completely different from those of **A** and **B**. The first intermediate hosts are land snails and the second intermediate hosts are ants.

The parasite

Dicrocoelium dentriticum is also called the small liver fluke. The adult worms are 5–12 mm long and pale reddish. The eggs measure 40 μm and are dark brown. Development takes place while passing through the intermediate hosts, see above.

Pathogenesis

Man is infected by inadvertent ingestion of ants. Otherwise, see **A** and **B**.

Pathology

See **A** and **B**.

D, SHEEP LIVER FLUKE INFECTION

Introduction

This infection is also called fascioliasis. It is mainly found in animals (herbivores). In man, infection is observed in Europe (France, Portugal, Corsica), North and South Africa, parts of Asia[11] and South America (Brazil, Peru, Chile).

The first intermediate hosts are, again, water snails, and second intermediate hosts, better described as passive intermediate carriers, watercress and other aquatic plants. Cattle, sheep and goats may be used for experimental studies[12-16].

The parasite

Fasciola hepatica is up to 40 mm long and 13 mm broad (Fig. 46.13). The large oval eggs measure 130–150 × 55–90 μm, have a small operculum and are yellow-brown (Figs. 46.14 and 46.15).

The eggs reach water in the same way as those of other liver flukes. The miracidium larvae hatch out and penetrate water snails. The cercariae (Fig. 46.16) leave the snails and attach to various water plants. There they encyst and become metacercariae.

Pathogenesis

The metacercariae from the ingested aquatic plants, once in the small intestine of the definitive host, penetrate the intestinal wall and reach the peritoneal cavity. Then, they penetrate the liver capsule and reach the bile ducts through the liver parenchyma (Fig. 46.17).

In contrast to the other liver flukes, **A**, **B** and **C**, which are ascending in the bile ducts, *Fasciola hepatica* worms, after maturing in the bile ducts, are descending in these hollow organs.

Pathology

See **A** and **B**. Primary hepatic carcinomas may be observed in chronic infections.

References

1. Sadun, E. H. (1955). Studies on Opisthorchis viverrini in Thailand. *Am. J. Hyg.*, **62**, 81
2. Bychkov, V. G. *et al.* (1990). A comparison of the count of Opisthorchis in the body of the host and of the eggs eliminated with the faeces. *Med. Parazitol. Mosk.*, **2**, 14
3. Pungpak, S. *et al.* (1989). Ultrasonographic study of the biliary system in opisthorchiasis patients after treatment with praziquantel. *Southeast Asian J. Trop. Med. Publ. Health*, **20**, 157
4. Al'perovich, B. I. *et al.* (1990). Opisthorchis of the liver. *Vestn. Khir.*, **144**, 27
5. Dao, A. H. *et al.* (1991). A case of opisthorchiasis diagnosed by cholangiography and bile examination. *Am. Surg.*, **57**, 206
6. Leung, J. W. *et al.* (1990). Endoscopic cholangiopancreatography in hepatic clonorchiasis – a follow-up study. *Gastrointest. Endosc.*, **36**, 360
7. Riganti, M. *et al.* (1989). Human pathology of Opisthorchis viverrini infection: a comparison of adults and children. *Southeast Asian J. Trop. Med. Publ. Health*, **20**, 95
8. Jang, J. J. *et al.* (1990). Enhancement of dimethylnitrosamine-induced glutathione S-transferase P-positive hepatic foci by Clonorchis sinensis infestation in F 344 rats. *Cancer Lett.*, **52**, 133
9. Drabick, J. J. *et al.* (1988). Dicroceliasis (lancet fluke disease) in an HIV seropositive man. *J. Am. Med. Assoc.*, **259**, 567
10. Lucius, R. and Frank, W. (1978). Beitrag zur Biologie von Dicrocoelium hospes Loos, 1907 (Trematodes, Dicrocoeliidae). *Acta Tropica*, **35**, 161
11. Kovalenko, V. L. *et al.* (1990). Fascioliasis of the liver. *Arkh. Patol.*, **52**, 59
12. Santiago, N. and Hillyer, G. V. (1988). Antibody profiles by EITB and ELISA of cattle and sheep infected with Fasciola hepatica. *J. Parasitol.*, **74**, 810
13. Foreyt, W. J. (1989). Efficacy of triclabendazole against experimentally induced Fascioloides magna infections in sheep. *Am. J. Vet. Res.*, **50**, 431

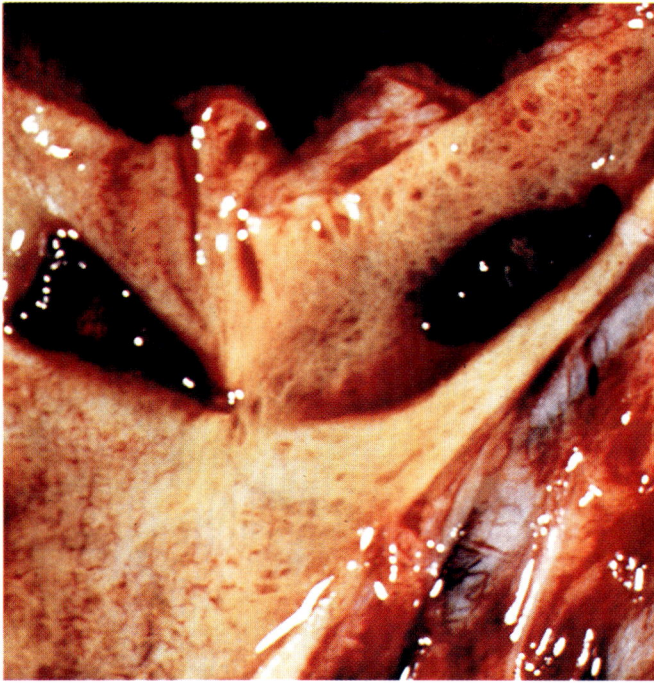

Fig. 46.6 Two worms of *Clonorchis sinensis* in the opened bile ducts near the hilar region of the liver in a 68-year-old patient. Autopsy material from Japan

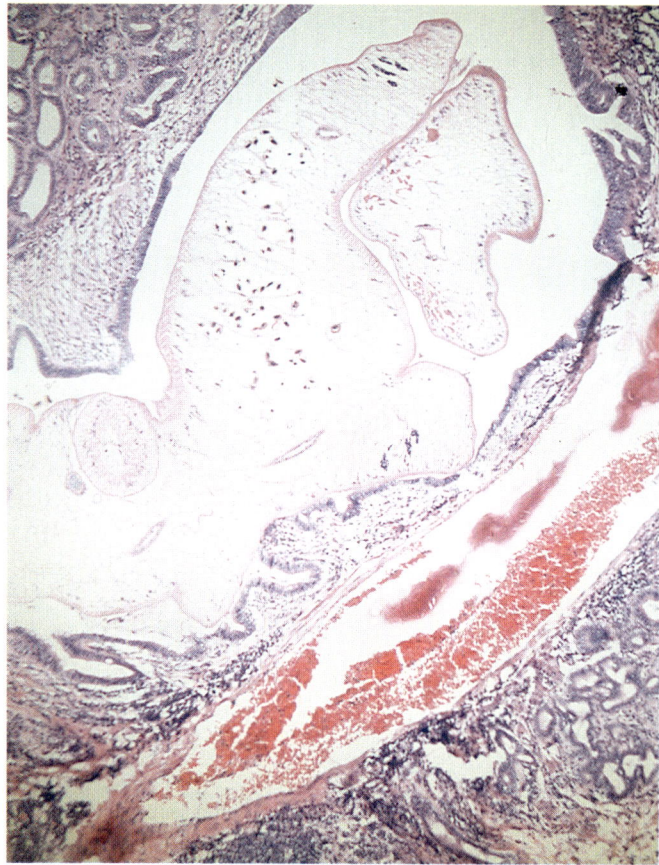

Fig. 46.7 *Opisthorchis viverrini* fluke inside hamster bile duct. Experiment to produce cancer. H&E

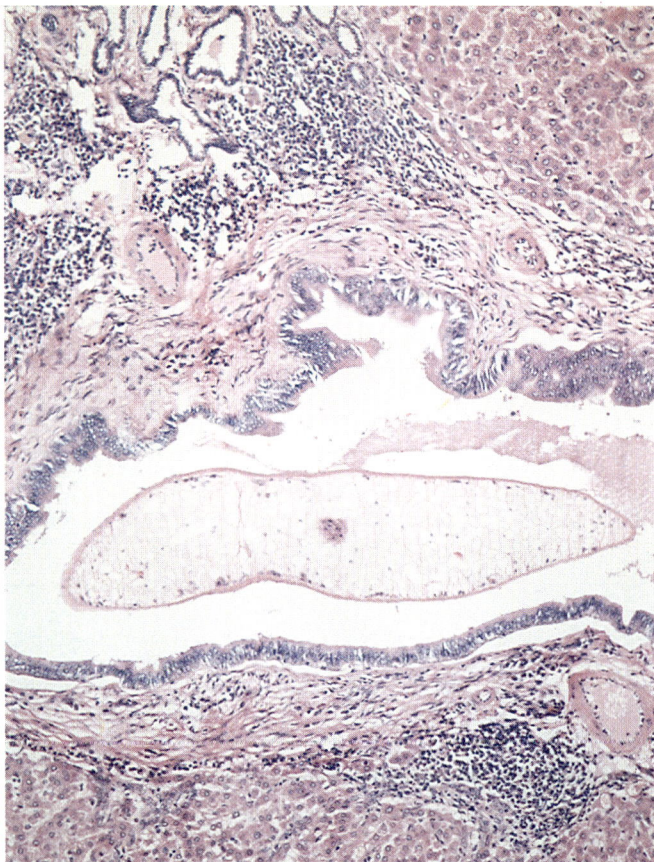

Fig. 46.8 Same case as Fig. 46.7. Fluke inside bile duct and carcinoma on one side. H&E

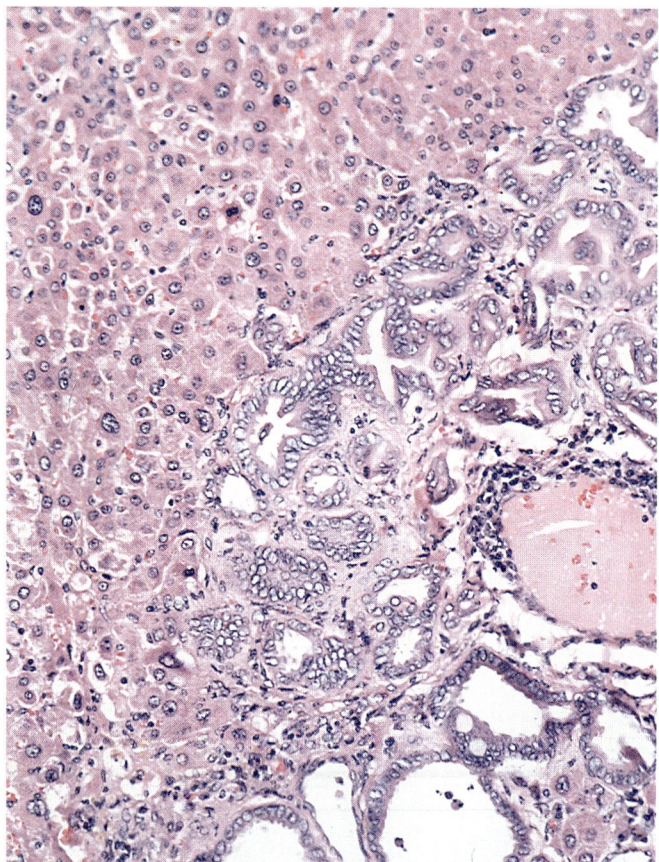

Fig. 46.9 Liver carcinoma (cholangiocarcinoma) produced experimentally in hamster by *Opisthorchis viverrini* and co-carcinogen. H&E

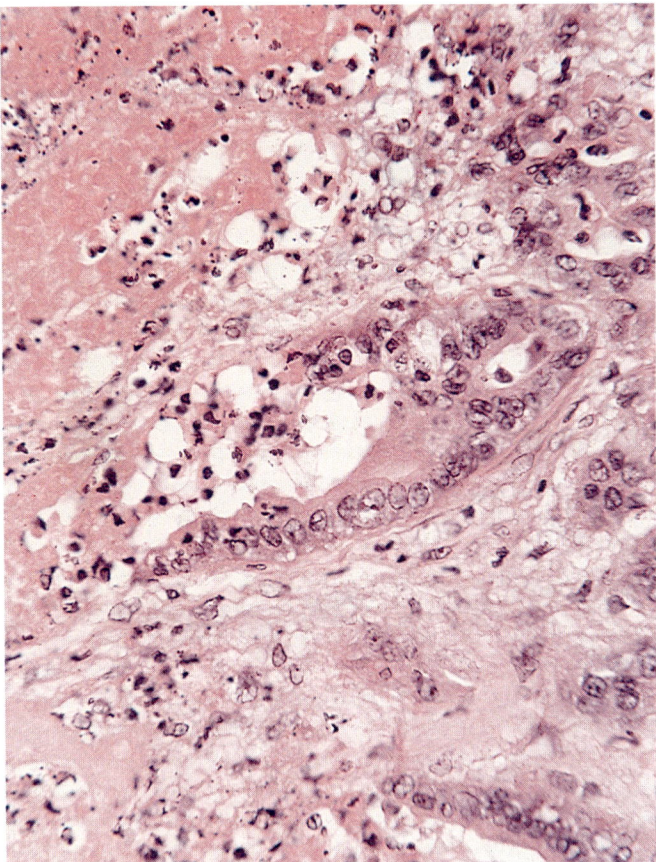

Fig. 46.10 Same case as Figs. 46.6–46.8. Cholangiocarcinoma with necrosis. H&E

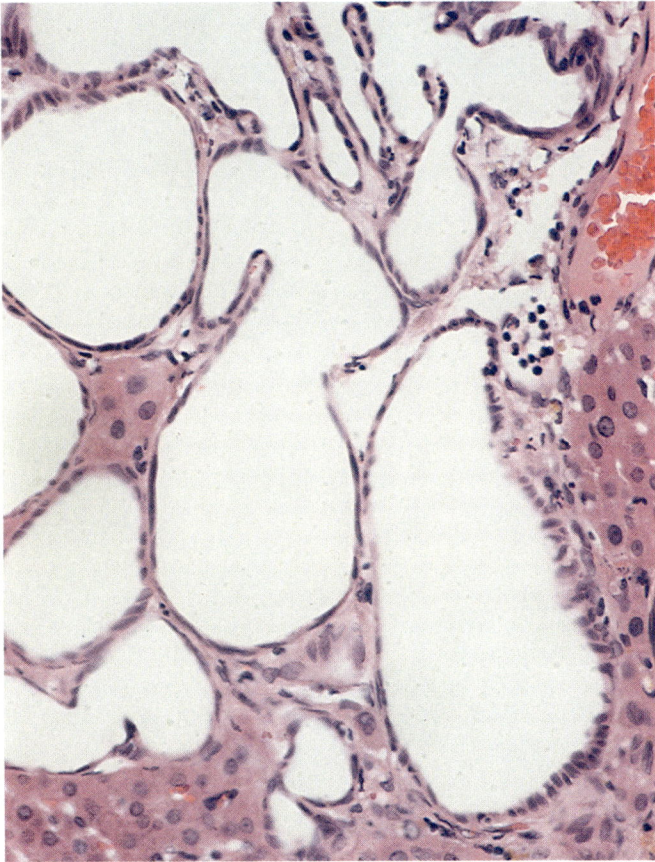

Fig. 46.11 Same case as Figs. 46.6–46.9. Another field of cholangiocarcinoma. H&E

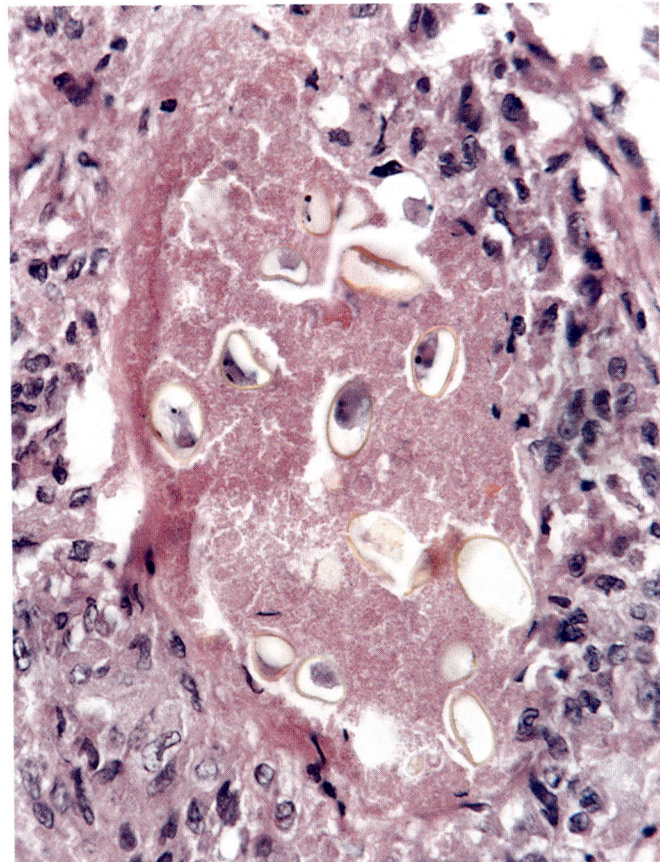

Fig. 46.12 Liver granuloma produced by eggs of *Opisthorchis viverrini*. Same case as Figs. 46.6–46.10. H&E

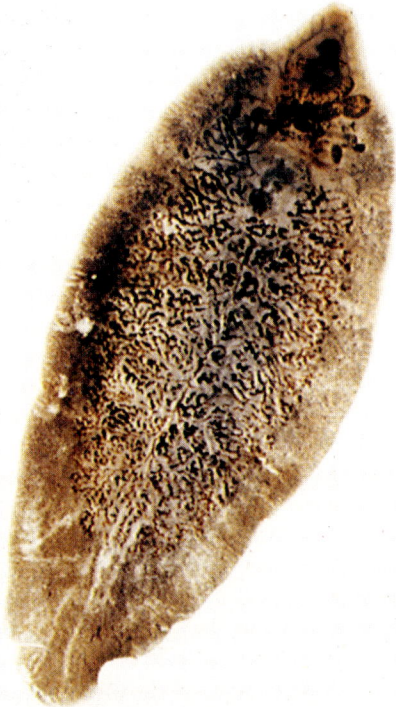

Fig. 46.13 *Fasciola hepatica* fluke. H&E

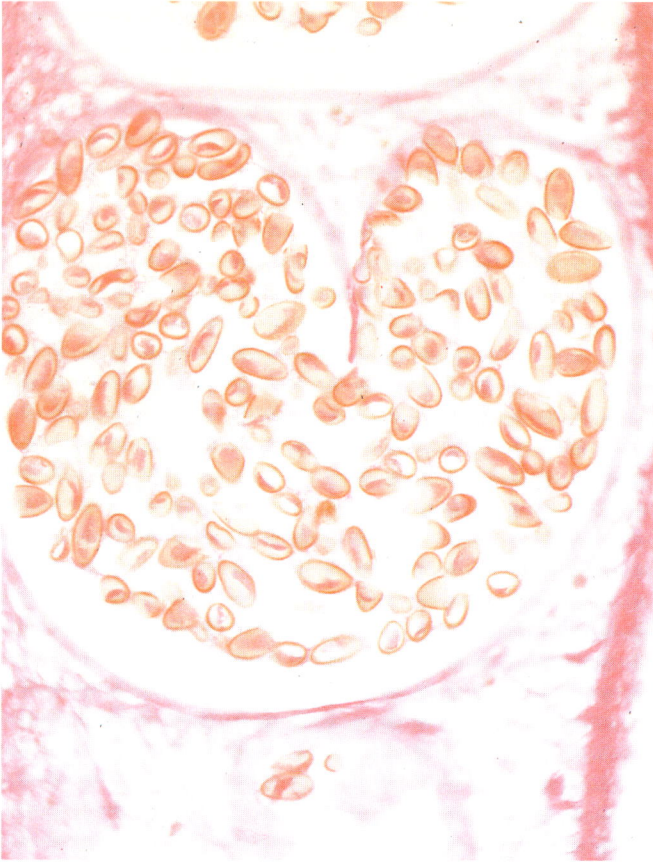

Fig. 46.14 *Fasciola hepatica* eggs inside the female fluke. H&E

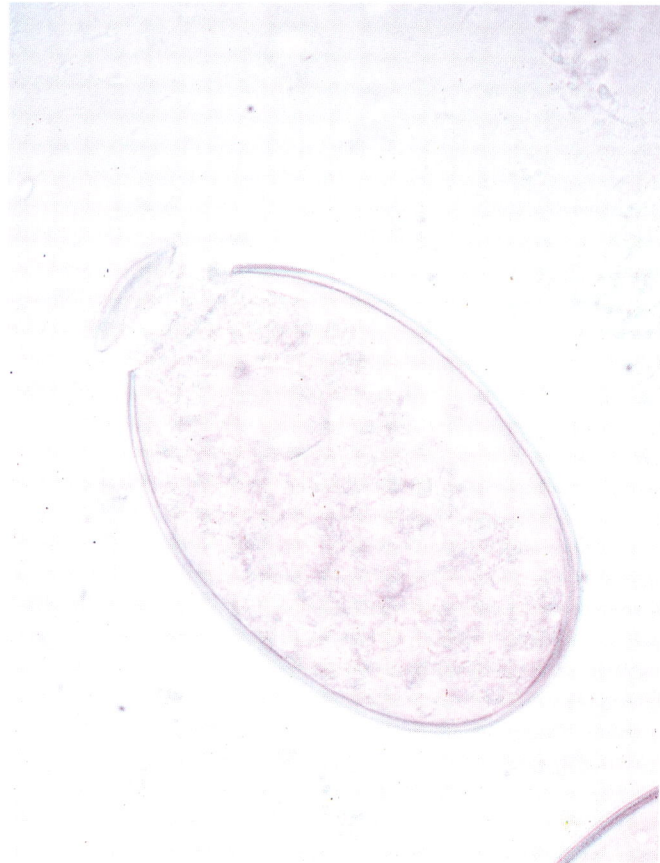

Fig. 46.15 Egg of *Fasciola hepatica* with operculum in the bile of cattle. H&E

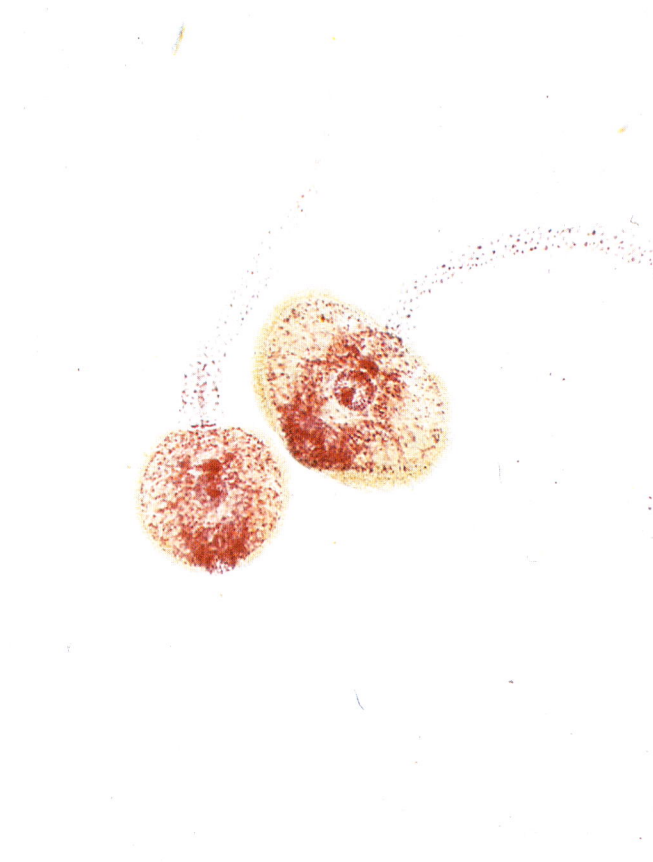

Fig. 46.16 Cercaria of *Fasciola hepatica* in the water. H&E

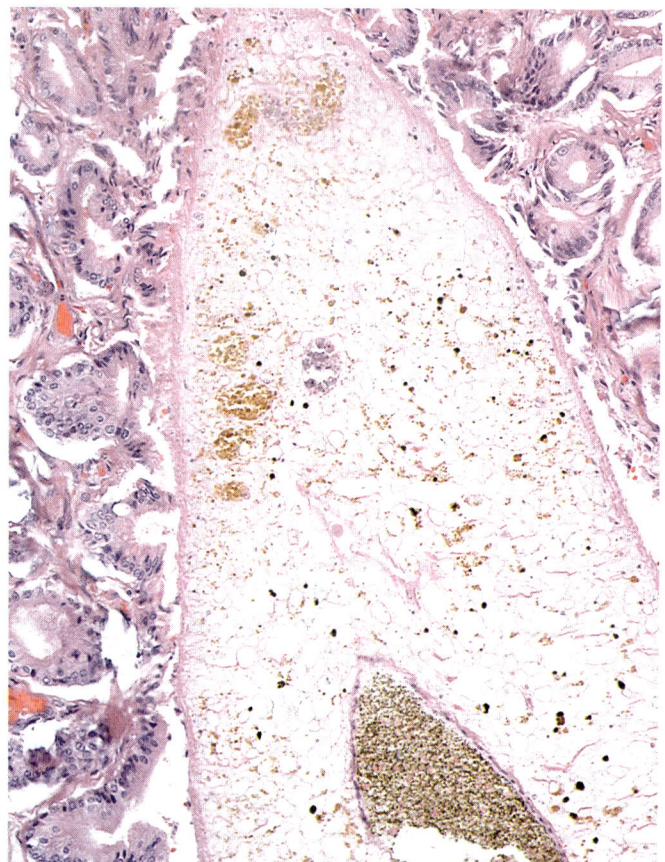

Fig. 46.17 Mature *Fasciola hepatica* fluke in the bile duct. H&E

14. Haroun, E. M. and Hillyer, G. V. (1988). Cross-resistance between Schistosoma mansoni and Fasciola hepatica in sheep. *J. Parasitol.*, **74**, 790
15. Haroun, E. M. *et al.* (1989). Responses of goats to repeated

infections with Fasciola gigantica. *Vet. Parasitol.*, **30**, 287
16. Foreyt, W. J. (1990). Domestic sheep as a rare definitive host of the large American liver fluke Fascioloides magna. *J. Parasitol.*, **76**, 736

47. INTESTINAL FLUKE INFECTIONS

Introduction

The two main intestinal fluke infections are caused by **A** *Fasciolopsis buski* and **B** species of *Echinostoma*. Infections caused by 5 other species are discussed briefly at the end of this section.

These trematode infections are of minor importance epidemiologically. They occur only due to particular nutritional habits.

A occurs in South East Asia and the Far East[1,2], in India, Bangladesh, Thailand[3–5], China and Taiwan, **B** occurs in India, the Philippines, Celebes and in Brazil.

The definitive hosts in both **A** and **B** are, in addition to man, pigs, dogs, cats, monkeys and rodents which act as animal reservoir hosts. Intermediate hosts in **A** are fresh water snails and water plants, and, in **B**, water snails, other snails and mussels. For experimental studies of **B**, the golden hamster may be used[6].

Clinically, infections with **A** and **B** are similar. Mild infection is asymptomatic. Severe infection, with hundreds of intestinal flukes, may cause unspecific intestinal symptoms, like pain and diarrhoea, oedema, ascites, anaemia and jaundice, and, but only exceptionally, death. The worms may produce toxic substances.

Clinical diagnosis is easily made by confirmation of worm eggs, which may be numerous in stools.

The parasite

A, *Fasciolopsis buski* or giant intestinal fluke, also called *Distoma buski*, is one of the largest flukes and up to 7 cm long. Eggs measure 130–40 × 80 μm.

The miracidium larvae penetrate the body surface of water snails, become cercariae, and, when again in water, become attached as metacercariae to water plants.

B, *Echinostoma ilocanum* and *Echinostoma echinatum* or small intestinal flukes, reach < 1 cm in length, are reddish-grey and covered by spines (Fig. 47.1). The eggs are operculated and measure 95 × 65 μm. The first and second intermediate hosts are snails and snails or mussels, respectively.

Pathogenesis

Uncooked water plants or fruits of water nuts with metacercariae, or raw snails and mussels containing metacercariae are ingested and develop into mature worms. In the bowel they may cause damage by their numbers.

Pathology

Intestinal flukes are found mainly in the duodenum or jejunum, or exceptionally, in the large intestine. Superficial erosion of the intestinal mucosa and hyperaemia of the small intestinal mucosa may be due to irritation by the flukes. There is no active tissue invasion by the worms.

Exceptionally, eggs of *Echinostoma* spp. (**B**) may be observed in the CNS and myocardium.

Other intestinal fluke infections

In addition to the *Echinostoma* infections discussed above, a few other *Echinostoma* species may be observed in man. Furthermore, five intestinal fluke species are found in man occasionally: *Heterophyes heterophyes*[7], *H. nocens*, *Metagonimus yokogawai* (Fig. 47.2), *Watsonius watsoni* and *Gastrodiscoides hominis*. They are reported in countries of East Asia and the Balkans, are small (1–10 mm long) and their presence in man is usually symptomless. Their first intermediate hosts are always snails and their second intermediate hosts may be water plants or fish.

References

1. Cross, J. H. (1969). Fasciolopsiasis in Southeast Asia and the Far East: a review. *4th South East Asia Seminar in Parasitology and Tropical Medicine*, Bangkok
2. Buckley, J. J. C. (1939). Observations on Gastrodiscoides hominis and Fasciolopsis buski in Assam. *J. Helminth.*, **17**, 1
3. Manning, G. S. and Ratanarat, C. (1970). Fasciolopsis buski in Central Thailand. *Am. J. Trop. Med. Hyg.*, **19**, 613
4. Plaut, A. G. *et al.* (1979). A clinical study of Fasciolopsis buski infection in Thailand. *Trans. R. Soc. Trop. Med. Hyg.*, **63**, 470
5. Sadun, E. H. and Maiphoom, C. (1953). Studies on the epidemiology of the human intestinal fluke. Fasciolopsis buski (Lankester) in Central Thailand. *Am. J. Trop. Med. Hyg.*, **2**, 1070
6. Fried, B. *et al.* (1990). Single and multiple worm infections of Echinostoma caproni (Trematoda) in the golden hamster. *J. Helminthol.*, **64**, 75
7. Mahmoud, L. H. *et al.* (1990). A preliminary study of liver functions in heterophiasis. *J. Egypt. Soc. Parasitol.*, **20**, 83

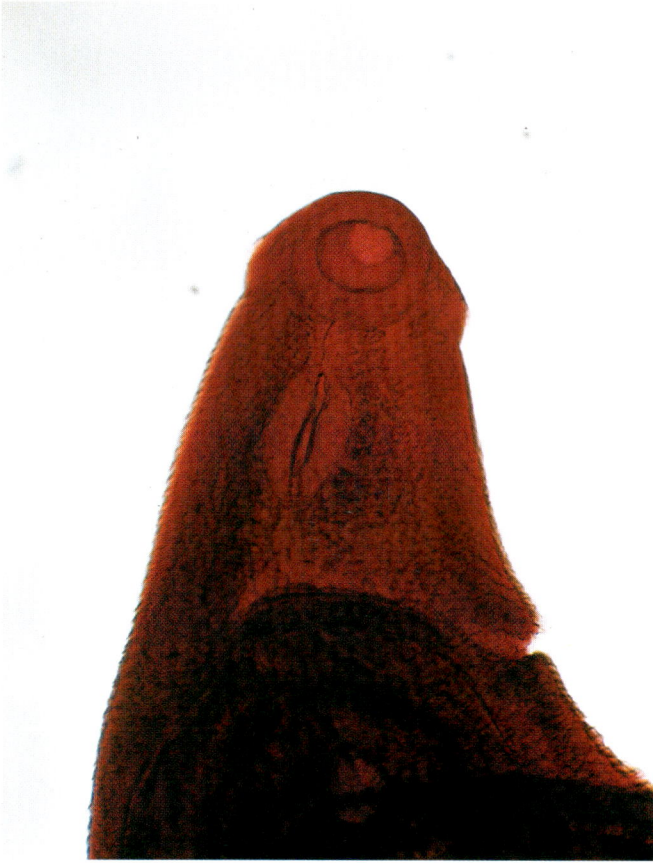

Fig. 47.1 *Echinostoma* sp. with anterior sucker. Carmine

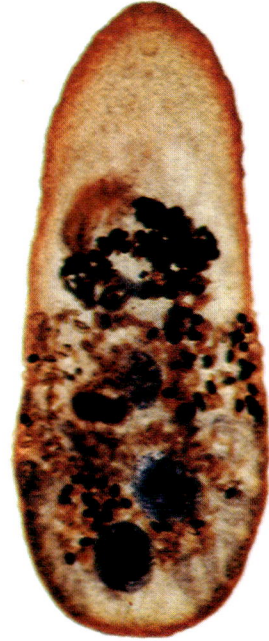

Fig. 47.2 *Metagonimus yokogawai* trematode. Carmine

D. WORM EGGS

Table 18 Nematodes

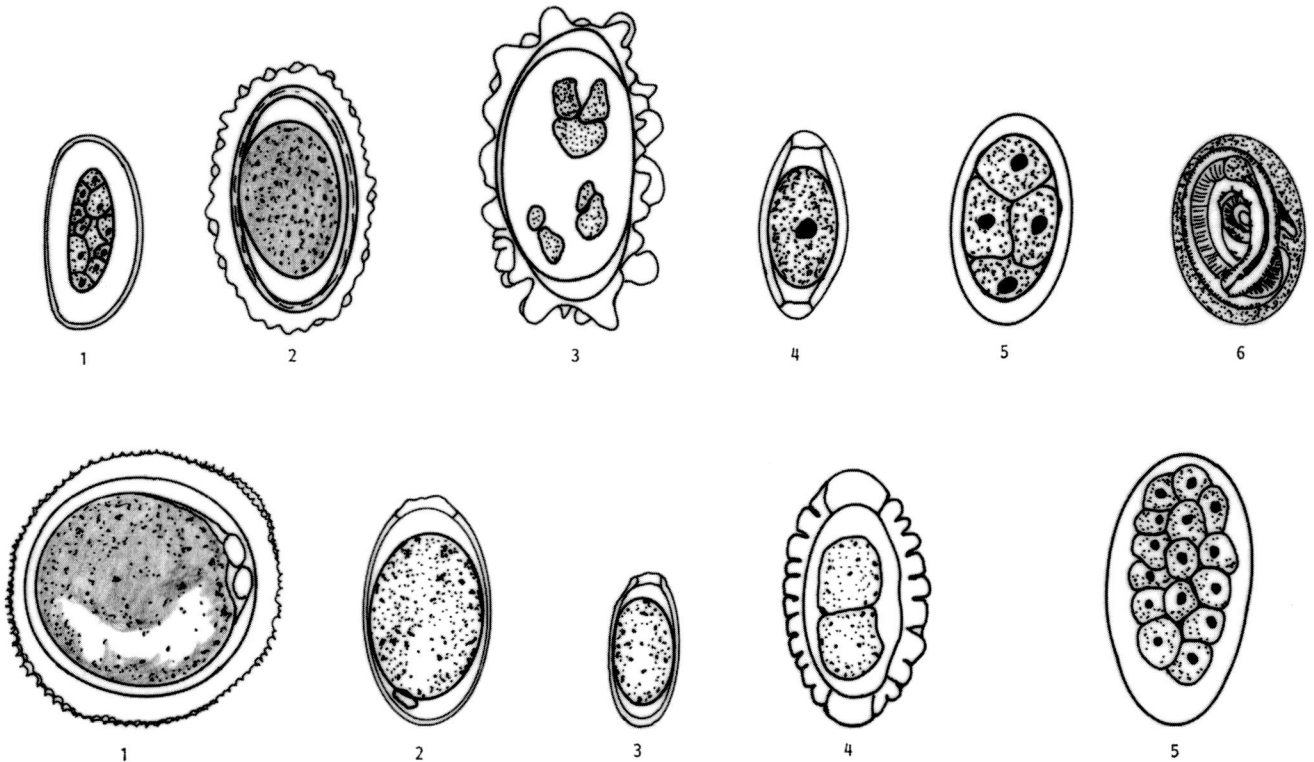

1. *Enterobius vermicularis*, 55 × 25 μm, colourless, ovoid, flattened on one side, thick membrane
2. *Ascaris lumbricoides*, 60–70 × 50 μm, yellowish, fertile, thick ondulated outer shell.
3. *Ascaris lumbricoides*, infertile.
4. *Trichuris trichiura*, 50 × 25 μm, pale to dark brown, two pale polar prominences.
5. Hookworm, *Necator* and *Ancylostoma* are identical, 60 × 40 μm, glass clear to pale yellowish, 4-cell stage.
6. *Strongyloides stercoralis*, 55 × 30 μm, egg with larva, seldom seen in stools.

7. *Toxocara canis*, 75–85 μm, not found in human faeces; however, similar eggs of *Toxocara cati* are found occasionally.
8. *Gnathostoma spinigerum*, 70 × 40 μm, yellowish, one-cell stage.
9. *Capillaria philippinensis*, 40 × 20 μm, flattened, bipolar plug at each end.
10. *Dioctophyma renale*, 66 × 42 μm, thick deeply pitted shell, two-cell stage.
11. *Trichostrongylus* sp., 75–100 × 30–50 μm, similar to hookworm egg, segmented ovum at morula stage.

Table 19 Cestodes

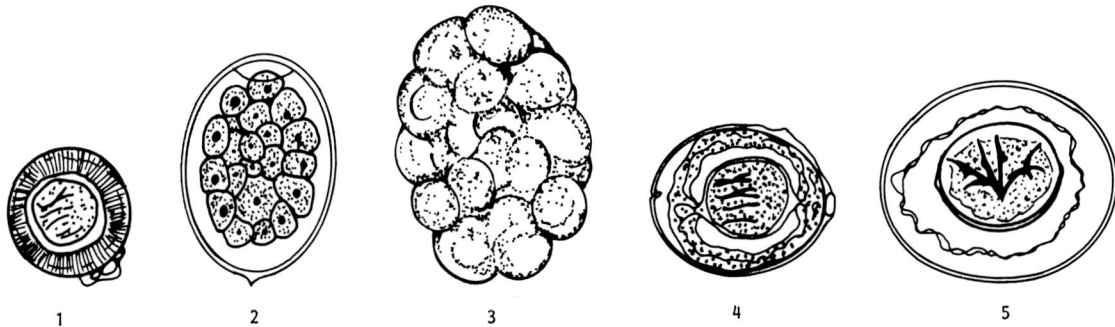

1. *Taenia* sp., *Taenia saginata* and *Taenia solium* are identical, 32 × 38 μm, the outer layer surrounds the yellow-brown radially striated embryophore around the larva with hooks, in the centre.
2. *Diphyllobothrium latum*, 50 × 70 μm, on one end a lid-like operculum, on the other, a small knob on the shell. Numerous yolk cells in addition to the egg cell.

3. *Dipylidium caninum*, individual egg 25 × 30 μm, contains larva with six hooks, in faeces, found in packets or masses of 30–40 eggs.
4. *Hymenolepsis nana*, 30 × 50 μm, colourless, occurs individually in faeces, hooks recognizable.
5. *Hymenolepis diminutum*, 65 × 75 μm, hooks are visible.

Table 20 Trematodes (blood, lung and liver flukes)

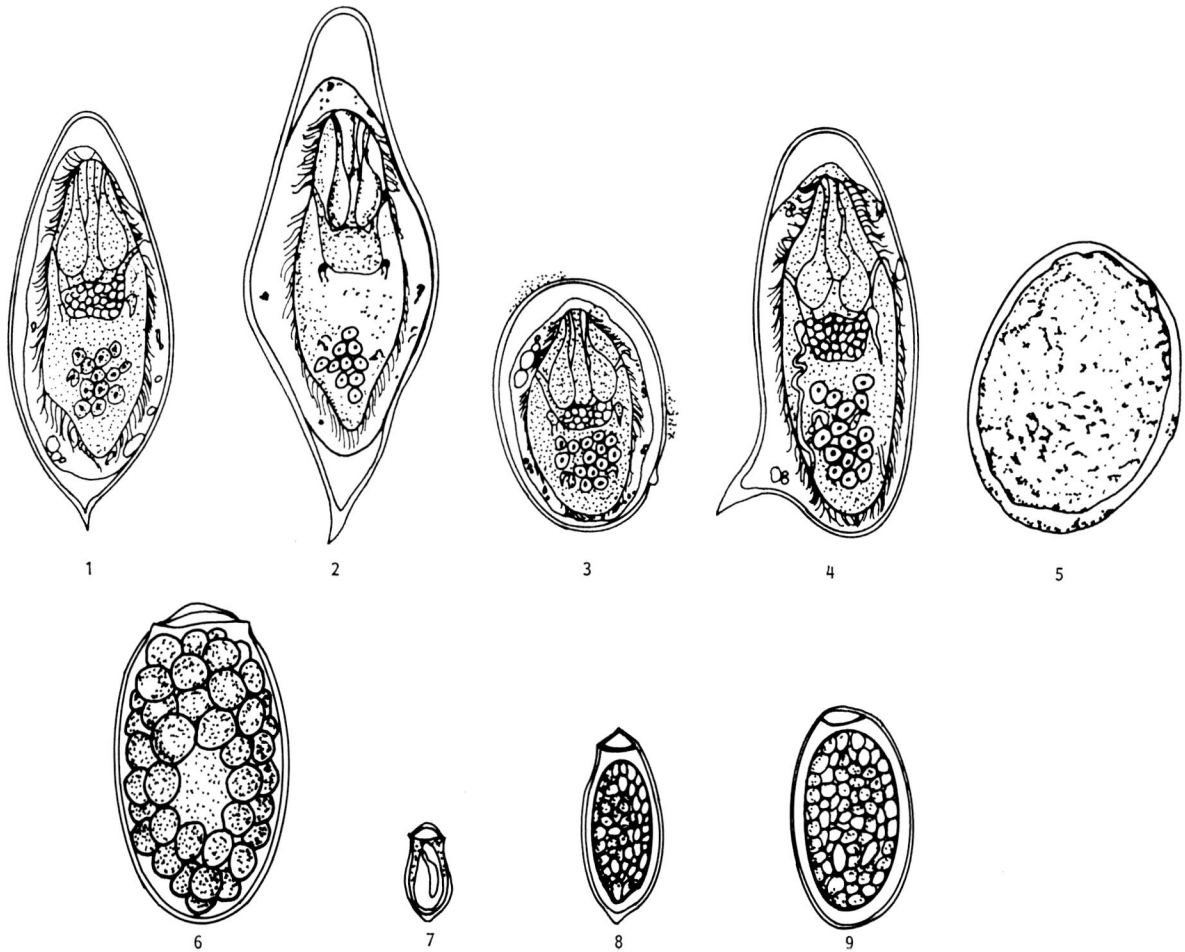

1. *Schistosoma haematobium*, 150 × 55 μm, almost colourless, terminal spine, only in urine, *Schistosoma* eggs do not have an operculatum.
2. *Schistosoma intercalatum*, 140 × 50 μm, terminal spine.
3. *Schistosoma japonicum*, 90 × 55 μm, almost spherical, small lateral knob.
4. *Schistosoma mansoni*, 150 × 60 μm, prominent lateral spine, young eggs already contain a miracidial larva.
5. *Schistosoma mekongi*, 40–50 μm, almost spherical, rudimentary knobbed lateral spine

6. *Paragonimus westermani*, 60 × 60 μm, golden brown, operculum, initially with 5–10 yolk cells.
7. *Clonorchis (Opisthorchis) sinensis*, 30 μm, yellowish-brownish, jug-shaped, 'lid' at the upper pole.
8. *Opisthorchis felineus*, 30 × 12 μm, yellowish-brown, jug-shaped (collar-like swelling).
9. *Dicrocoelium dentriticum*, 40 μm, dark brown, contain a fully developed larva when laid.

Table 21 Trematodes (intestinal flukes)

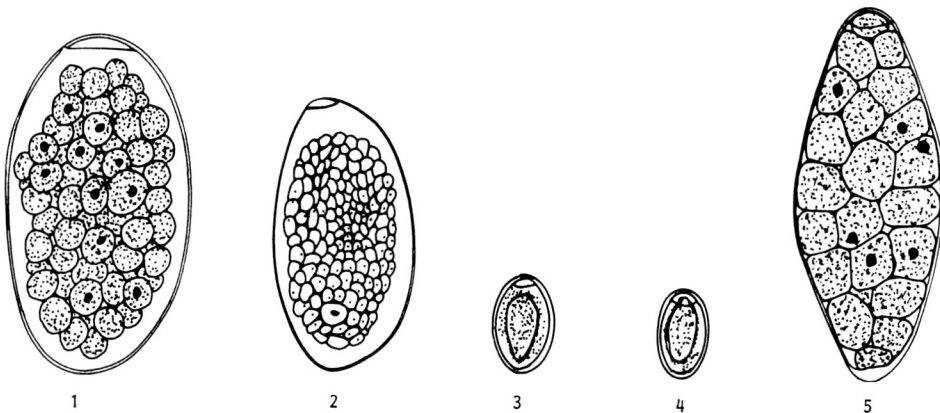

1. *Fasciolopsis buski*, 130–140 × 80 μm, eggs of *Fasciola hepatica* identical, always numerous in stools, operculate, numerous egg cells and yolk cells.
2. *Echinostoma ilocanum*, 65 × 95 μm, operculate.

3. *Heterophyes heterophyes*, 15 × 25 μm, operculate.
4. *Metagonimus yokogawai*, 16 × 28 μm, operculate.
5. *Gastrodiscoides hominis*, 160 × 70 μm, numerous yolk cells.

Disorders caused by Arthropods

Disorders in this group are common in man and often very unpleasant. However, in the great majority of cases, they are not true infections, diseases or parasitoses but only infestation. They are not normally discussed in the literature on parasitic diseases. However, to suffer from infestation of arthropods may be fatal in man.

The principal arthropods, and the disorders or diseases they produce or transmit, are listed summarily in Chapter I. As **ectoparasites**, they may: cause allergies, rarely involving circulatory collapse; act as vectors for viruses, bacteria and parasites; or serve as intermediate hosts. Some, however, such as certain insects and mites, may be completely inocuous and non-parasitic for man.

Those arthropods which produce **epizoonoses** may be pathogenic for man **permanently** (e.g. lice), **temporarily** (e.g. blood-sucking mosquitoes) or only **accidentally** (e.g. bees, wasps, etc.). The last situation leads only to local reactions, pruritus, oedema and pain, as the consequences of stings or bites. **Endozoonoses** result when arthropods (or other micro-organisms) penetrate the epidermis and remain for a time in the skin of man. Tables 22 and 23 show the most important arthropods and diptera (flies and mosquitoes).

The following five disorders are briefly discussed since some of their features may be of special interest for physicians and pathologists with an interest in morphology.

Table 22 Important arthropods

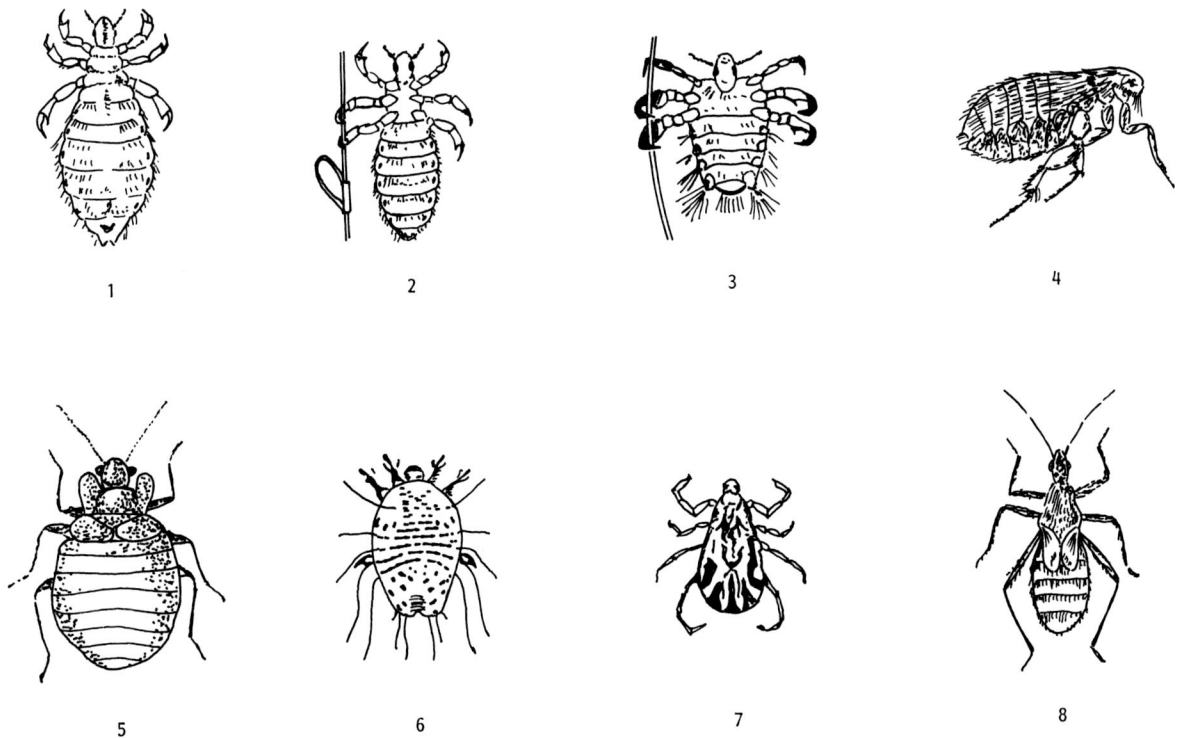

1. *Pediculus corporis*, body or clothing louse.
2. *Pediculis capitis*, head hair louse.
3. *Phthirius pubis*, crab louse.
4. *Ctenocephalides felis*, cat flea

5. *Cimex lectularius*, bed bug.
6. *Sarcoptes scabiei*, itch mite, causal agent of the itch.
7. *Acarina* sp., hard tick, vector of *Babesia* sp., etc.
8. *Reduviidae* sp., assasin bug, vector of *Trypanosoma cruzi.*

48. SCABIES

Introduction

This skin infection is also called 'the itch' and is produced by *Sarcoptes scabiei* or the itch mite. Together with demodicidosis, it is one of the most frequent ectoparasitoses in man. It occurs worldwide, mostly in poor hygienic conditions and recently, also in patients with immunodeficiencies[1,2]. Although it had almost completely disappeared after World War II, it is observed again now and may occur in epidemics[3–7]. It is considered as a kind of venereal disease and is well known in Venezuela.

Numerous animal species may be infected with varieties of the human *Sarcoptes* species[8]. These varieties of itch mite may infect man as a 'false host'. The disease in man is then named 'animal scabies'.

Table 23 Diptera (flies and mosquitos)

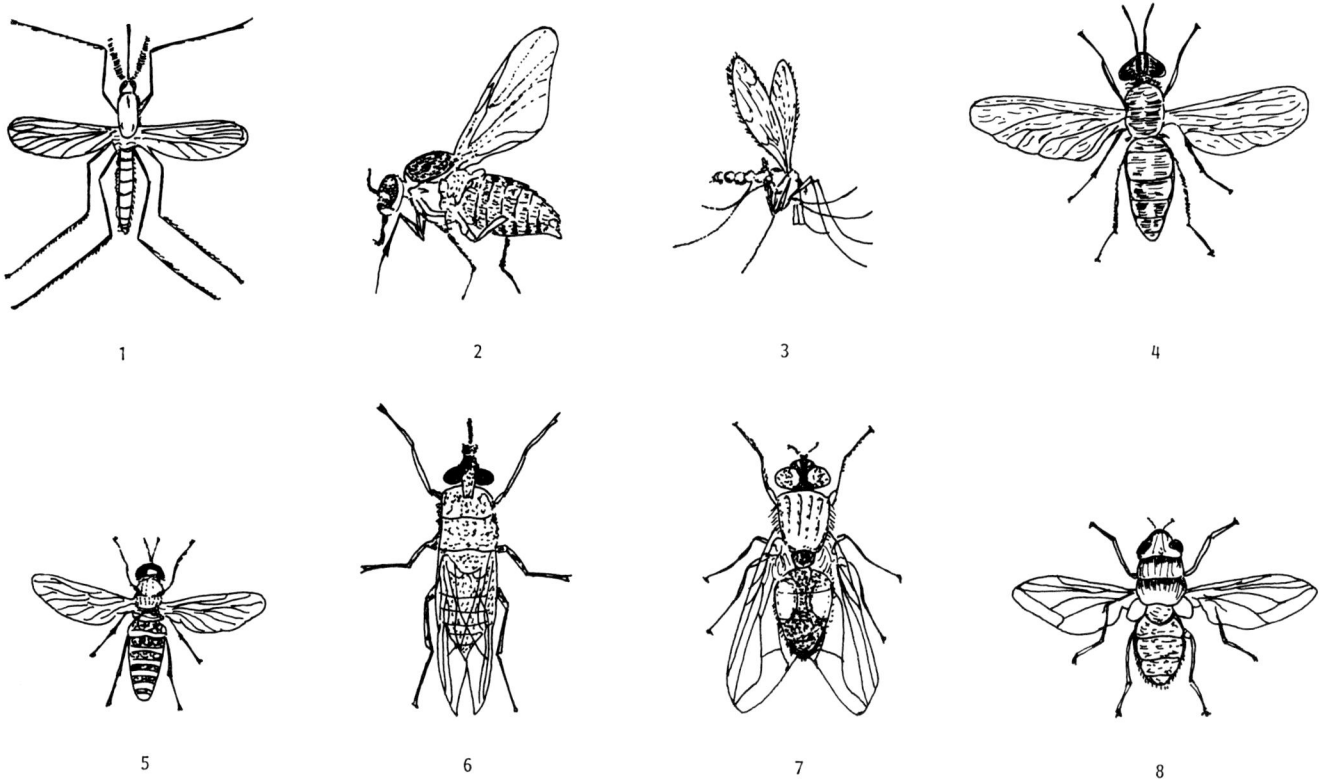

1. *Nematocera*, mosquitos or gnats. The suborder with long antennae comprises *Aedes, Anopheles, Culex, Simulium* and *Phlebotomus (Lutzomyia)*, transmit numerous diseases.
2. *Simulium* sp., black fly.
3. *Phlebotomus* sp., sand fly, transmit *Leishmaniae*.
4. *Brachycera*, horse fly with the genera *Chrysops, Tabanus*.
5. *Haematoporta pluvialis*, rain fly, passive transmission of numerous bacteria.
6. *Glossina* sp., tse-tse fly, vector of sleeping sickness.
7. *Musca domestica*, house fly, passive transmission of numerous agents.
8. *Dermatobia hominis*, tropical marble fly, larvae found in myiasis.

Table 24 Life cycle of *Sarcoptes scabiei*

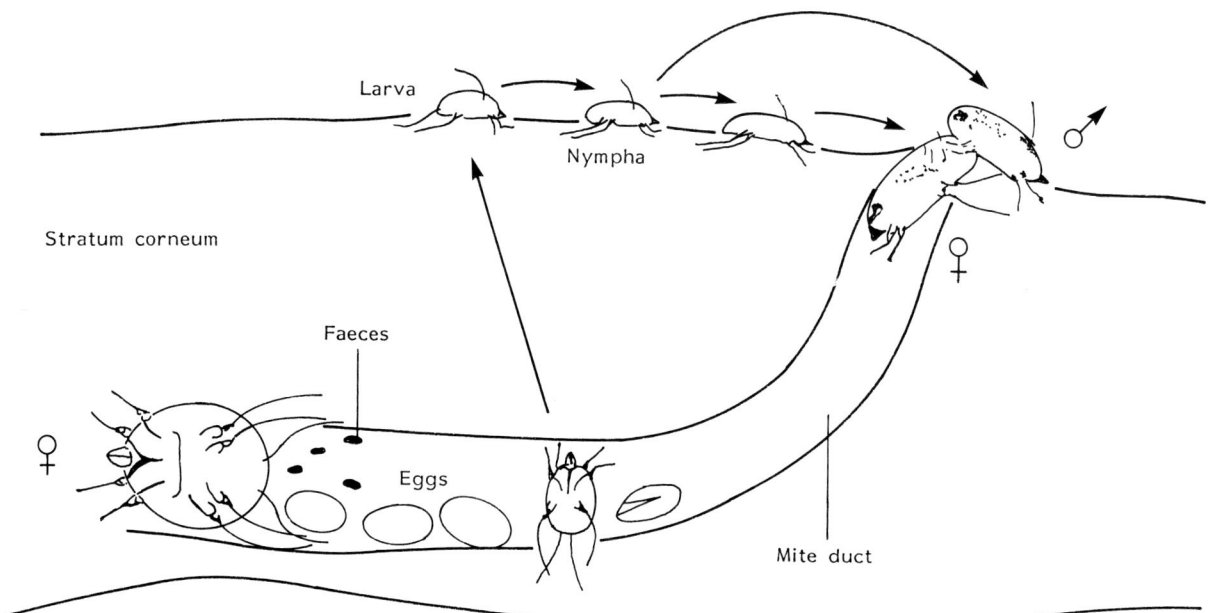

Clinically, pruritus, especially in the evenings, is typical. The intense scratching leads to exanthema and eczema. Folliculitis, furunculosis and superficial pyodermia may result in bacterial superinfections, also leading to glomerulonephritis. In patients with corticosteroid therapy, the lesions became atypical; there may be less pruritus and explosive reproduction of mites takes place. Several hundreds of scabies burrows have been found in this sort of case of infestation. Nodular[9–11] and crusty, or Norwegian[12–14], forms of scabies, already described in the last century, will be discussed under *Pathology*. 'Animal scabies' in man is characterized by rapid healing.

Clinical diagnosis is made by confirmation of the burrows, the mites themselves or their eggs. Anamnesis and data about the incubation period lead to suspicion of this mite infection.

The parasite

Sarcoptes scabiei var. *hominis*, or the itch mite, belongs to the subclass acari or mites. They may reach 0.3–0.5 mm in length, the males being a little shorter than the females. They have a grey-white ovoid body which is flattened dorsoventrally and four pairs of short legs. The eggs are whitish and measure 160–190 × 85–100 μm.

The entire developmental cycle occurs in man. For two months, the female lays 2–4 eggs each day. The larvae hatch out and develop within 9–10 days to male, or 12–15 days to female, mites. Outside the host, the mites soon die.

Pathogenesis

Infection takes place from man to man by direct close contact. The pregnant females of *Sarcoptes scabiei* reach the surface of the skin and dig cuniculi or burrows through the stratum corneum of epidermis, where they lay their eggs. The incubation period is 4 weeks. Table 24 shows the life cycle of the mite.

Pathology

With the exception of the back and face, all parts of the body may be affected (Figs. 48.1–48.4), preferentially, the interdigital spaces. Commonly, up to 15 mites may be found in one person. As a consequence of scratching, exanthema and eczema may be seen. Two other forms of scabies may be found: nodular and the so-called Norwegian, or crusty, forms. In the former, firm nodules with a smooth or scaling surface are found on covered sites, such as the gluteal and genital regions. Mites are

seldom present in the nodular form. The crusty form is characterized by thick hyperkeratotic papulomatous plaques.

The mites and eggs (Figs. 48.5–48.8) are located in burrows, which extend either obliquely or parallel to the skin surface and reach up to 1 cm long, in the stratum corneum of epidermis. They do not penetrate the dermis. Here, a non-specific cellular infiltrate with lymphocytes and histiocytes is seen, frequently with infiltrates consisting of eosinophilic leukocytes[15].

In the nodular form, there is a massive infiltrate of pleomorphic cells with numerous eosinophilic granulocytes. Often, the parasites themselves are no longer found in this form of the infection. The crusty material in the Norwegian form of scabies consists of laminar keratin masses with a sero-fibrinous exudate. It is crossed by numerous burrows with innumerable mites and eggs.

References

1. Anolik, M. A. and Rudolph, R. I. (1976). Scabies simulating Darier disease in an immunosuppressed host. *Arch. Dermatol.*, **112**, 73
2. Miller, D. A. and Weg, J. G. (1977). Epidemic scabies in respiratory intensive care unit. *Am. Rev. Respir. Dis.*, **115**, 267
3. Shrank, A. B. and Alexander, S. L. (1976). Scabies: another epidemic? *Br. Med. J.*, **1**, 669
4. Barthelmes, R. *et al.* (1970). Untersuchungen zur Zunahme der Scabieserkrankung. *Dermatol. Monatsschr.*, **156**, 881
5. Orkin, M. (1971). Resurgence of scabies. *J. Am. Med. Assoc.*, **217**, 593
6. Rutli, T. and Mumcuolglu, Y. (1975). Die häufigen übertragbaren Epizoonosen des Menschen. *Gynaekologe*, **8**, 153
7. Orkin, M. (1975). Today's scabies. *J. Am. Med. Assoc.*, **233**, 882
8. Hollanders, W. and Vercruyesse, J. (1990). Sarcoptic mite hypersensitivity: a cause of dermatitis in fattening pigs at slaughter. *Vet. Rec.*, **126**, 308
9. Barale, Th. *et al.* (1971). Nodule post-scabieux. *Bull. Soc. Franc. Dermatol. Syph.*, **78**, 449
10. Marghescu, S. and Ziethen, H. (1968). Über die nodöse Erscheinungsform der Scabies. *Dermatol. Wschr.*, **154**, 793
11. Thomson, J. *et al.* (1974). Histology simulating reticulosis in persistent nodular scabies. *Br. J. Dermatol.*, 421
12. Burks, J. W. *et al.* (1956). Norwegian scabies. *Arch. Dermatol.*, **74**, 131
13. Wishart, S. (1972). Norwegian scabies, a Christchurch epidemic. *Aust. J. Derm.*, **13**, 127
14. Nair, S. R. *et al.* (1978). Norwegian scabies in Hodgkin's disease. *Swiss Med. Dig. Dermatology*, 43
15. Head, E. S. *et al.* (1990). Sarcoptes scabiei in histopathologic sections of skin in human scabies. *Arch. Dermatol.*, **126**, 1475

49.   DEMODICIDOSIS

Introduction

Follicle mite infection by *Demodex folliculorum* and *D. brevis* is the most frequent permanent ectoparasitosis in man. It occurs worldwide, with a high prevalence in older people. It is called also pityriasis folliculorum.

Man is the exclusive host of these two species of *Demodex*. These mites could not be experimentally transmitted into laboratory animals. Ten of the 65 species of *Demodex* are pathogenic in man and various domestic and wild animals[1].

Clinical symptoms occur rarely. Only massive infections, with up to 1000 mites in one person, cause skin lesions and pruritus, almost only on the face. Since the clinical manifestations are similar to those of rosacea[2–4], perioral dermatitis, granulomatosis, pyodermia and blepharitis[5], the pathogenic role of *Demodex* infection in these morbid entities has been discussed, and there are controversial

opinions about this topic. Corticoids favour the infection with these mites[6,7].

Clinical diagnosis is made by finding mites in the smears of sebaceous material of hair follicles or sebaceous glands, as well as in scales or smears of pustular and vesicular material and the bases of hairs.

The parasite

Two species of mites, also called follicle mites, *Demodex folliculorum* and *Demodex brevis*, are pathogenic for man. They are morphologically very similar.

The 0.3–0.4 mm-long mites are elongated, cigar-like and have 4 pairs of very short clawed legs (Fig. 49.1).

There is controversy about whether *Demodex* mites may passively transmit micro-organisms.

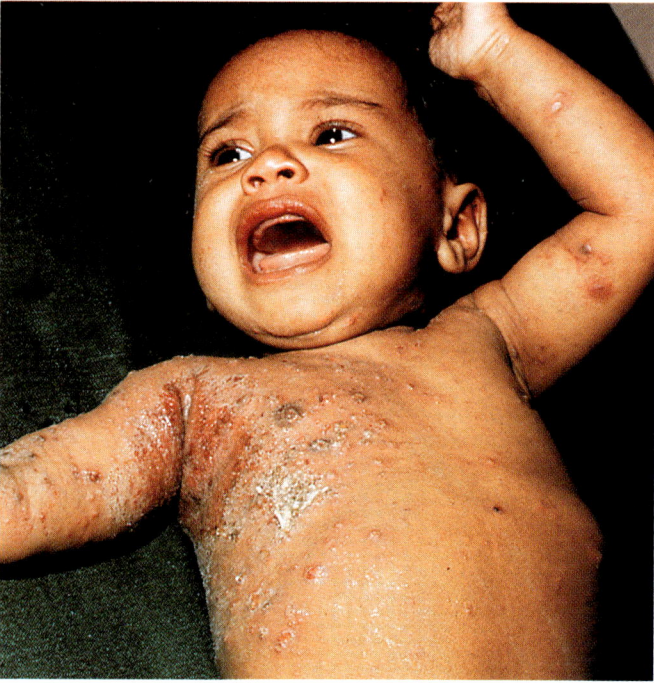

Fig. 48.1 Diffuse scabies in an infant. All gross pictures are patients from Barinas, Venezuela

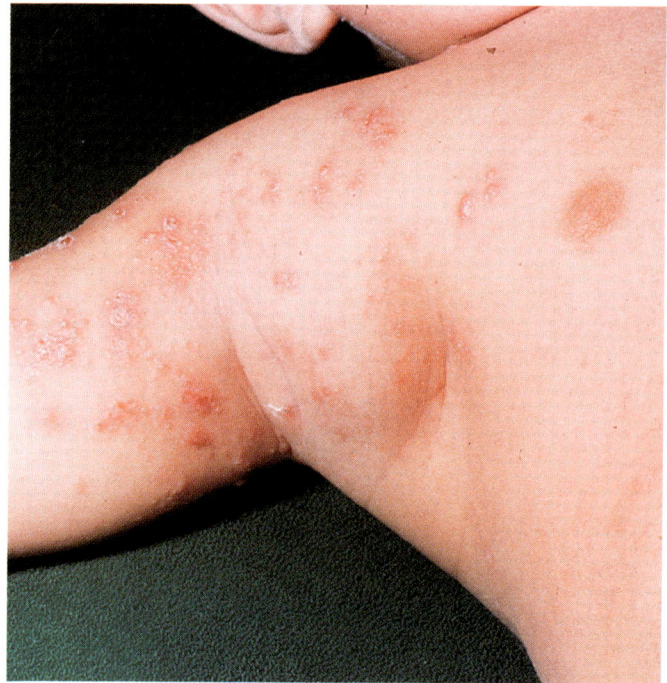

Fig. 48.2 Scabies in axillary region

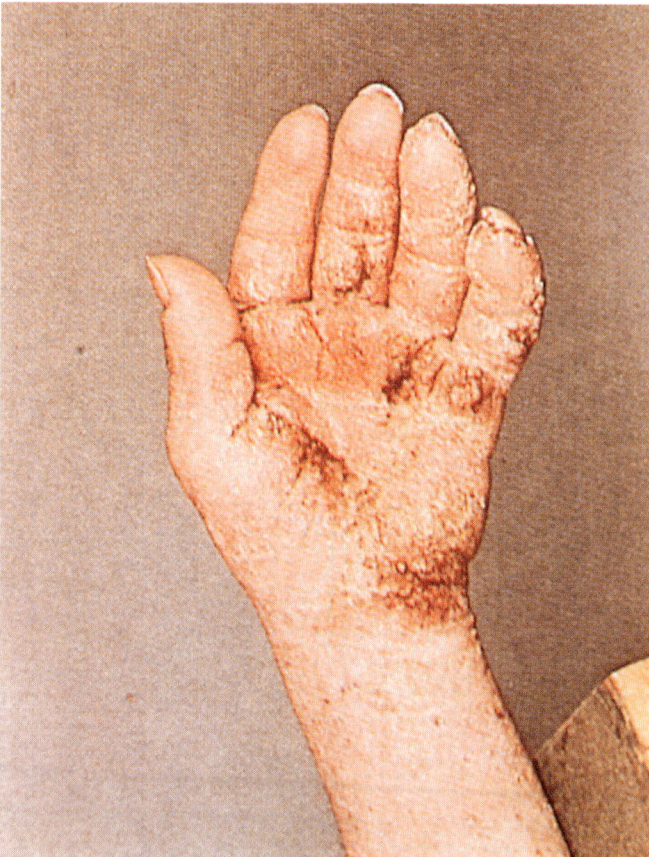

Fig. 48.3 'Norwegian form' of scabies

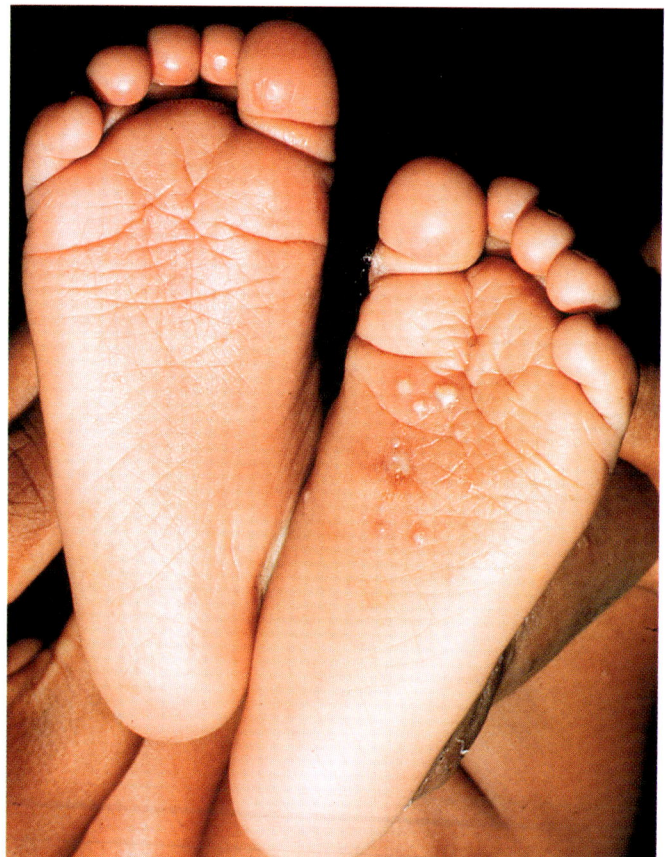

Fig. 48.4 Scabies on sole of foot

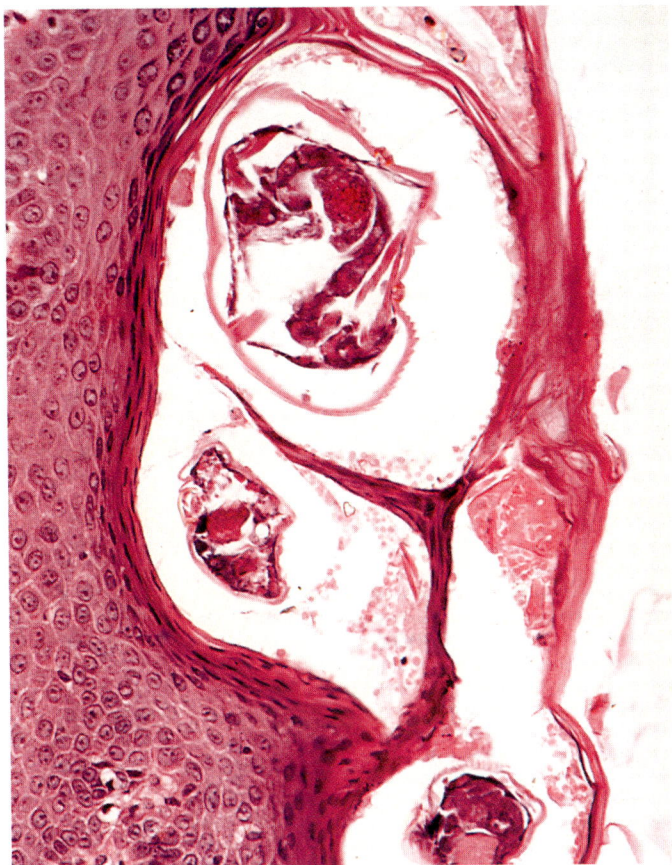

Fig. 48.5 Mites of *Sarcoptes scabiei* in the superior parts of human epidermis. H&E

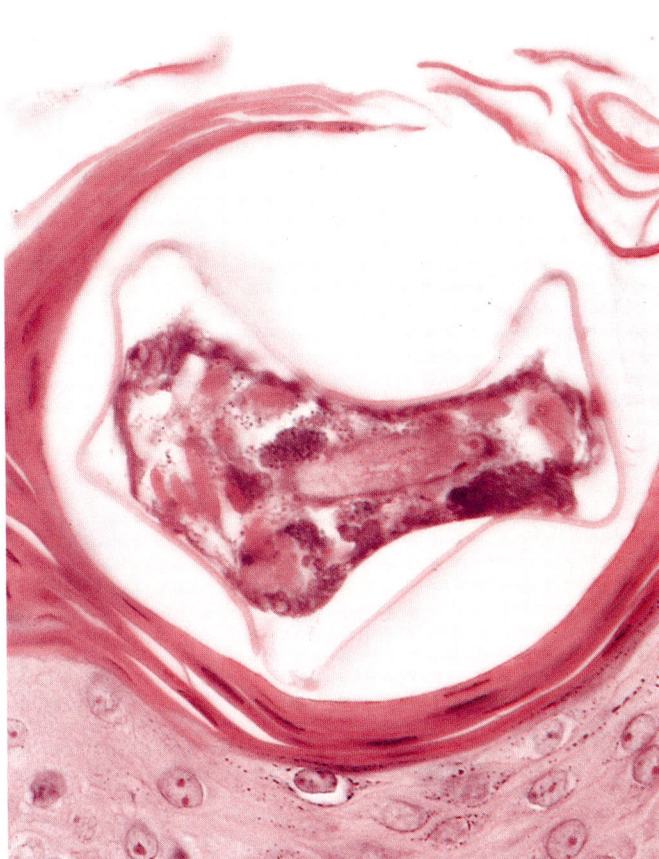

Fig. 48.6 Mite of *Sarcoptes scabiei* at higher power in the stratum corneum of epidermis. H&E

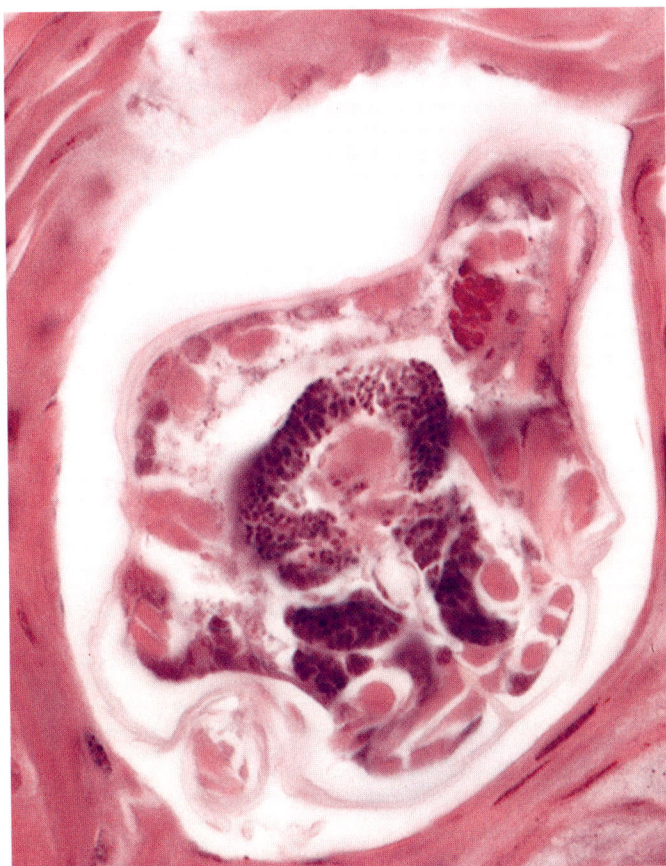

Fig. 48.7 Another mite of *Sarcoptes scabiei* with visible cuticula. H&E

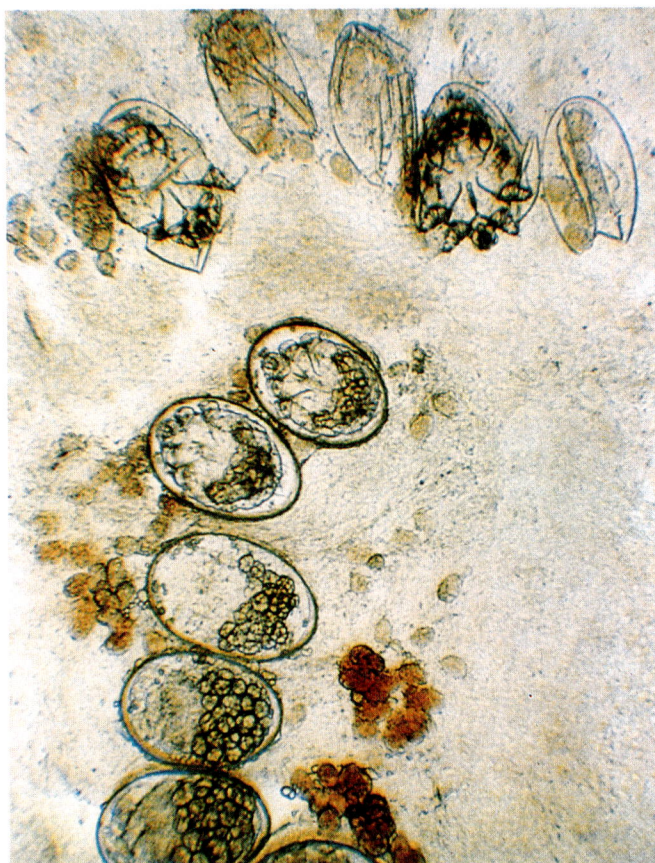

Fig. 48.8 Eggs of *Sarcoptes scabiei*, photographed with filter

Pathogenesis

Infection occurs by direct contact from man to man. The female *Demodex* mites are impregnated near the orifice of the hair follicle ducts. They migrate then into the sebaceous gland ducts. *Demodex folliculorum* mites remain in the glandular ducts, while the *Demodex brevis* mites invade the sebaceous glands themselves. After 12 hours inside the tissues, the females begin to lay eggs. Adult mites develop, through a larval stage, within 15 days.

Pathology

Mite infections with scarce lesions are commonly found at sites with numerous sebaceous glands, preferentially in the face (Fig. 49.2). The nasal region, the zone around the external auditory canal, the eyelids[8,9] and mamillae are the most affected sites. Rosacea-like and dermatitis-like lesions with papulo-pustular and vesicular manifestations are noted which may be confused easily with dermatoses of other origin. The pustules may contain numerous mites.

Histologically, the *Demodex* mites are found in the glandular ducts and in the sebaceous glands (Figs. 49.3–49.6). In the dermis, perifollicular non-specific cellular infiltrates are seen. Granulomas have been observed occasionally, and it is not clear whether they are due to the parasites or to the destroyed hair follicles[10,11]. Electron microscopic studies have also been performed on this type of lesion[12].

References

1. Bukva, V. *et al.* (1988). Pathological process induced by Demodex sp. (Acari: Demodicidae) in the skin of eland, Taurotragus oryx (Pallas). *Folia Parasitol. Praha*, **35**, 87
2. Beerman, H. and Stokes, J. (1934). Rosacea complex and Demodex folliculorum. *Arch. Dermatol. Syphilol.*, **29**, 874
3. Hojyo, T. and Dominguez, L. (1976). Demodicidosis y dermatitis rosaceiforme. *Med. Cut. I. L. A.*, **2**, 83
4. Rufli, Th., Mumcuoglu, Y. *et al.* (1981). Demodex folliuculorum: Zur Ätiopathogenese und Therapie der Rosacea und perioralen Dermatitis. *Dermatologica*, **162**, 12
5. Morgan, R. J. and Coston, T. O. (1964). Demodex blepharitis. *Southern Med. J.*, **57**, 694
6. Weber, G. (1976). Perioral dermatitis, an important side-effect of Corticosteroids. *Dermatologica*, **152** (Suppl. 1), 161
7. Ohtaki, N. and Irimajiri, T. (1977). Demodectic eruption following the use of topical corticosteroid (in Japanese). *Jpn. J. Dermatol.*, **31**, 465
8. Norn, M. S. (1970). Demodex folliculorum. Incidence and possible pathogenic role in the human eyelid. *Acta Ophthalmol. Suppl.*, **108**, 1
9. Roth, A. M. (1979). Demodex folliculorum in hair follicles of eyelid skin. *Ann. Ophthalmol.*, **11**, 37
10. Seifert, H. W. (1978). Demodex follicularum als Ursache eines solitären tuberkuloiden Granuloms. *Z. Hautkr.*, **53**, 540
11. Ramelet, A. A. and Perroulaz, G. (1988). Rosacea: histopathologic study of 75 cases. *Ann. Dermatol. Venereol.*, **115**, 801
12. English, F. P. *et al.* (1990). Electron microscopic study of acarine infestation of the eyelid margin. *Am. J. Ophthalmol.*, **109**, 139

50. TUNGIASIS

Introduction

Infection by sandfleas, chigoe or chigger, commonly limited to the skin of the feet, occurs only in determined geographical areas, such as Africa, the tropical Americas and China, mostly in people who walk bare footed. Tourists may bring this infection by insects back to their homelands[1]. This very unpleasant infection was well known in Venezuela when people went around without shoes. Now it occurs seldom. In Spanish, sandfleas are called niguas.

In addition to man, this infection is also observed in pigs, dogs, rats and other mammals.

Clinically, these fleas cause itching lesions, mostly on the feet. Scratching may lead to secondary infection and inflammation. Cases of tetanus and gas gangrene are known due to this flea infection.

Clinical diagnosis is made by squeezing out the lesions and looking in smears of the liquid for eggs of the fleas.

The parasite

Tunga penetrans is the scientific name for the sandflea, chigoe or chigger (Fig. 50.1). A synonymous term is *Dermatophilus penetrans*. The fleas belong to the insect orders, Siphonaptera or Aphaniptera. Nine species of sandfleas are known[2-5].

This is the smallest flea species, reaching only 1 mm in length and having a reddish-brownish colour. The males are temporary ectoparasites, while the female fleas are permanent, remaining in the host until they die. The ovaries of the females grow to several times their normal size, reaching the size of a pea. The eggs, when squeezed out, look like those in Fig. 50.2.

Pathogenesis

Infection occurs when walking bare-footed, either in houses or shacks or outside in sand or dust. The female fleas penetrate the skin but the posterior end stays outside for respiration and laying eggs. The latter transform into larvae and pupae, becoming adult fleas in 5–6 weeks. Infestation may occur also when lying naked on the floor or soil.

Pathology

Skin-penetrating female fleas are found mostly on the feet, plants, interdigital spaces and beneath the nails. Only occasionally are other parts of the body affected (Fig. 50.3–50.5).

Grossly, small hyperkeratotic wart-like foci are found covered by dark-brown crusts with a central brown–black dot. Scratching may lead to secondary bacterial infection, gangrenous inflammation, lymphangitis and tetanus or clostridial infections. The fleas have been studied ultrastructurally[6].

References

1. Pfister, R. (1977). Nehmen Sandfloh-Infektionen zu? *Fortschr. Med.*, **95**, 1373
2. Smith, K. G. V. (1973). *Insects and Other Arthropods of Medical Importance*. The Trustees of the British Museum (Nat. Hist.), London, p. 561
3. Smit, F. G. A. M. (1966). Siphonaptera. In *Insecta Helvetica*. Impr. La Concorde, Lausanne, p. 106
4. Rotschild, M. (1965). *Fleas*. Scientific American, p. 44
5. Cheng, T. C. (1973). *General Parasitology*. Academic Press, New York, London, p. 965
6. Fimiani, M. *et al.* (1990). Ultrastructural findings in tungiasis. *Int. J. Dermatol.*, **29**, 220

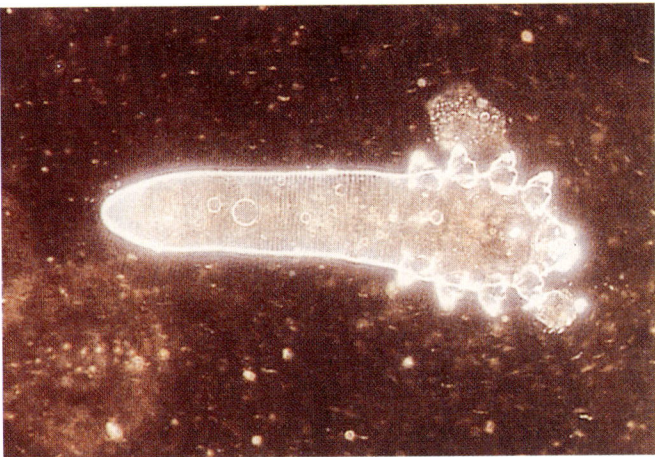

Fig. 49.1   Mite of *Demodex folliculorum* in dark field

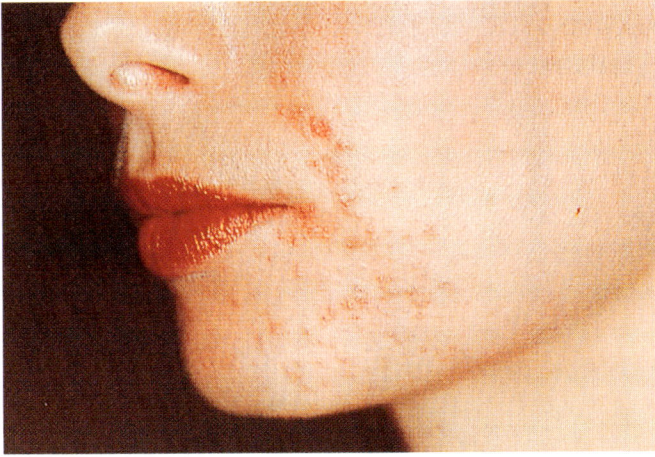

Fig. 49.2   Demodecitosis in the face

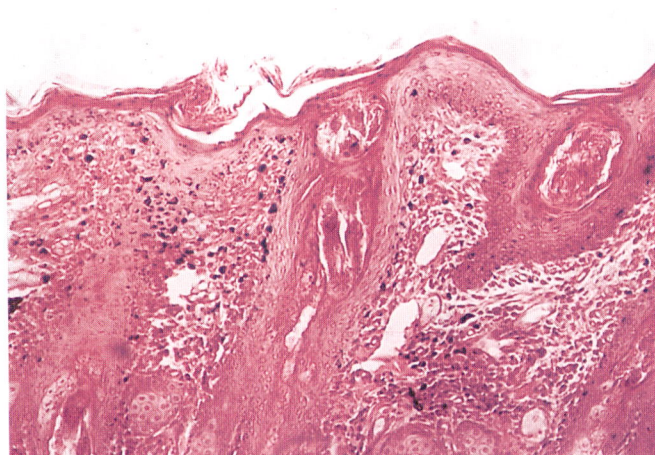

Fig. 49.3   *Demodex folliculorum* mites in ducts of sebaceous glands. H&E

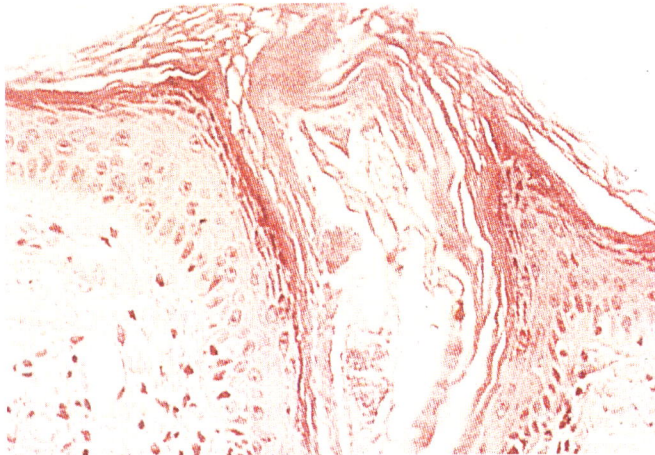

Fig. 49.4   Mite of *Demodex folliculorum* in duct of sebaceous gland at higher magnification. H&E

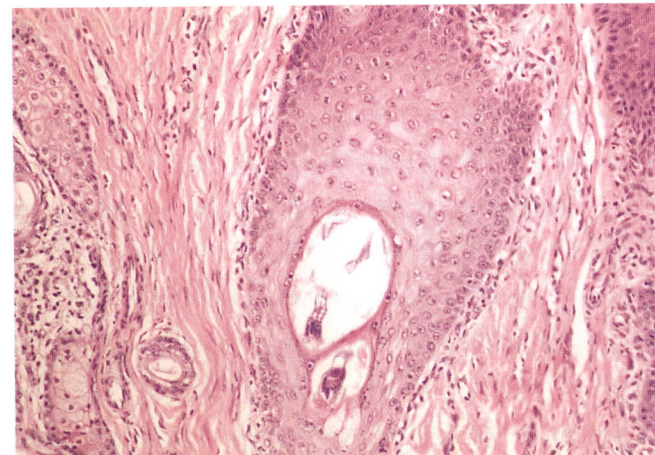

Fig. 49.5   Mite of *Demodex canii* in hair follicle. H&E

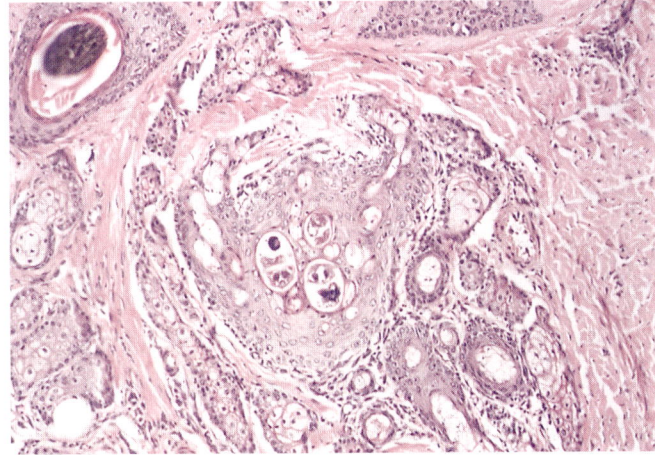

Fig. 49.6   *Demodex canii* fragments in hair follicle. H&E

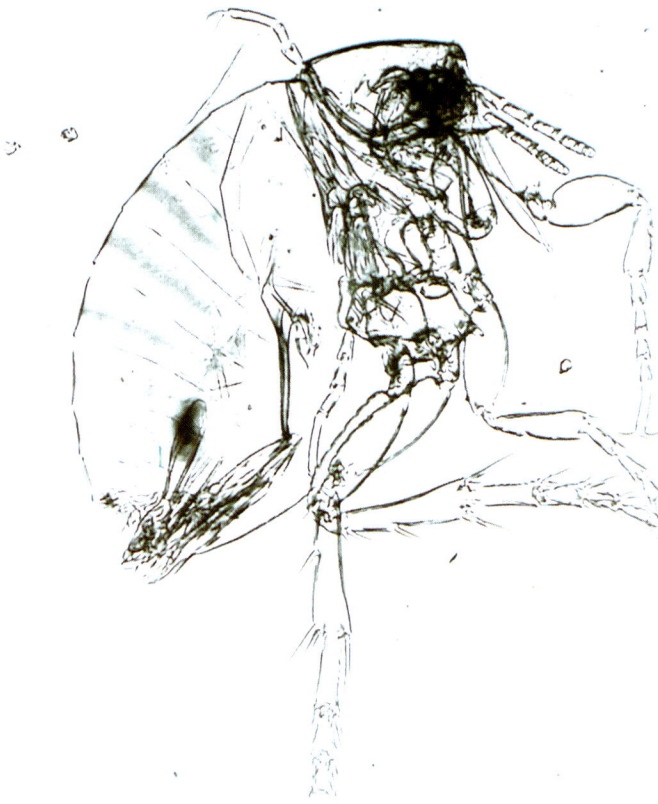

Fig. 50.1　The sandflea *Tunga penetrans*

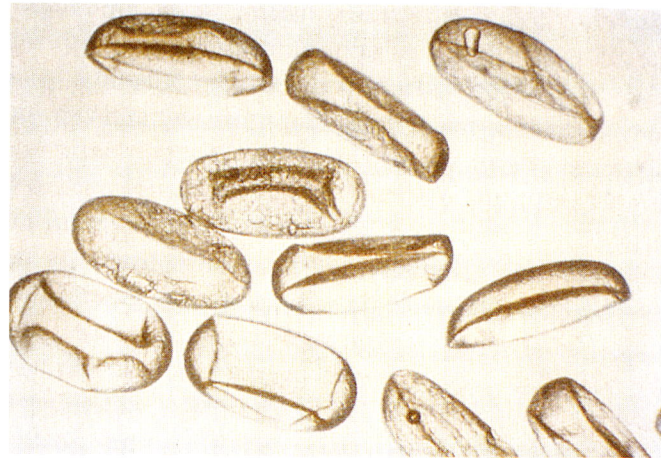

Fig. 50.2　Squeezed out eggs of *Tunga penetrans*

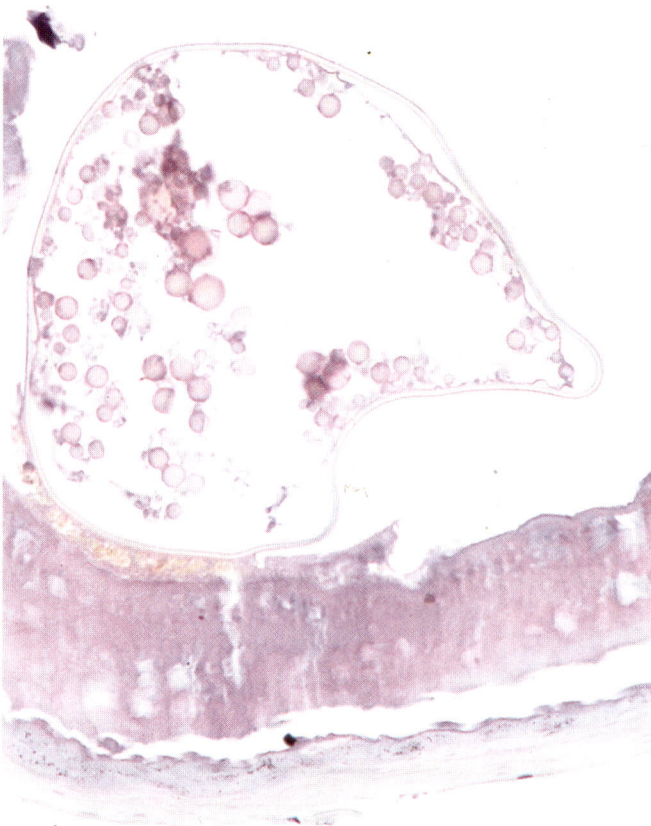

Fig. 50.4　Eggs of the sandflea in Fig. 50.3 at higher power. H&E

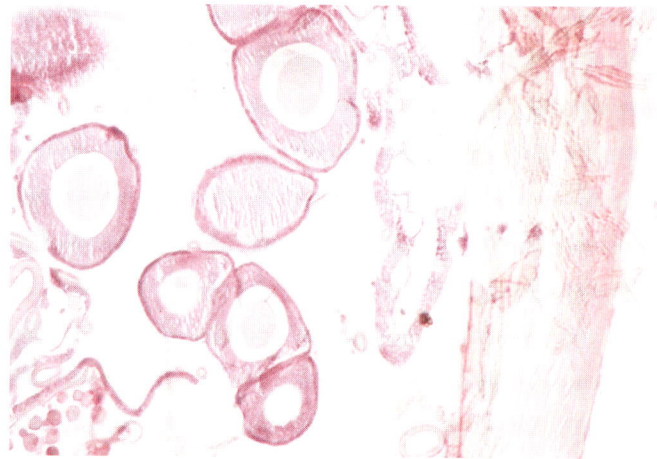

Fig. 50.3　Cut sandflea in an interdigital space of the foot. On the left side and beneath is the necrotic epidermis. The patient, a surgeon from München, Germany, went around bare-footed while on vacation in South America. H&E

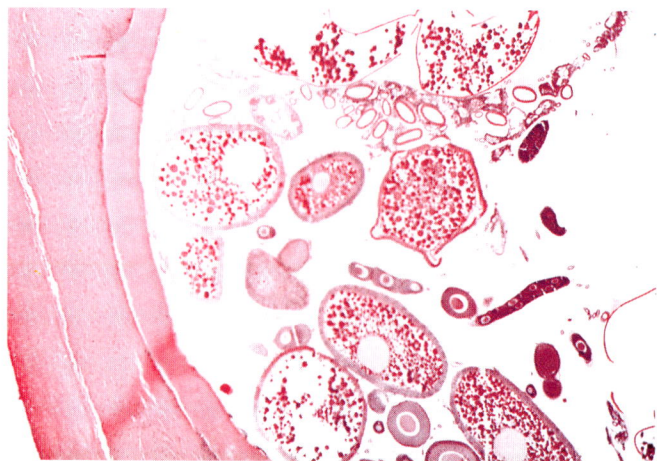

Fig. 50.5　Horizontal cut of *Tunga penetrans*. Numerous eggs are visible inside the sandflea. H&E

51. MYIASIS

Introduction

This entity, also called larval brachycerosis, may be defined as an infection due to maggots, i.e. larvae of flies or insects (*Diptera*) which live on tissues (alive or dead), in body fluids or in faecal material.

It seems to occur more frequently than commonly believed, since many cases in industrialized countries, apparently, are not reported. Distribution is worldwide; usually infants and old neglected people are affected. Frequently, the larval infestation befalls sick persons with chronic lesions. Myiasis is well known in Venezuela[1].

Man is a false host for the larvae of flies. Numerous domestic animals may be infected by the same insect species as man[2].

Clinically, six forms may be distinguished on the basis of the localization of the larvae in the human body: dermal myiasis[3-5]; wound myiasis, opthalmomyiasis[6-11], cavitary myiasis[12], intestinal myiasis[13] and ano-uro-genital myiasis[14,15]. The larvae produce variable symptoms. They may cause amazement or terror when discovered in the human body.

Clinical diagnosis is made by recognizing the larvae, dead or alive.

The parasite

About 80 species of flies (*Brachycera* or *Diptera*), 30 of them in Europe, may produce larvae which are found in man. Well-known species are *Dermatobia hominis, Musca domestica, Gasterophilus* spp., *Hypoderma bovis, Sarcophaga carnaria* and *Cordylobia anthropophaga*, also named tumbu fly. Certain species are observed preferentially in distinct geographical areas and in determined locations or diseases.

The larvae pass through three developmental stages, and measure from 1 mm up to 4 cm long. Commonly, they have no head and are segmented (with a head segment). They are covered by hairs and a whitish-grey colour (Fig. 51.1).

After the third larval stage, they become pupae and then adults which may fly and look like 2 cm-long bumble-bees. The developmental cycle from egg to adult fly takes about 2–3 weeks. Only exceptionally do the larvae grow into mature adult flies inside the human body. The eggs measure 1–2 mm. They are laid on dirty clothing, the floor, plants and, seldom, directly on the skin of man.

Pathogenesis

The portal of entrance for the eggs or larvae of flies are minor traumata, wounds or ulcers, stings or insect bites (of all kinds) on skin or mucosae. Once in the tissue, the larva moves by oral claws and stays alive, growing in tissues, for variable periods of time. They dig channels and may then either die or come out by perforation of skin.

Pathology

Dermal myiasis (synonyms: cutaneous m., dermato m., subdermal m., aureal m., furuncular m.): The areas of the head, back (Fig. 51.2) and extremities are mostly involved. There are three types: furuncular[16], migratory furuncular and creeping myiasis. The first begins with a small papule which itches and grows. The second shows furuncular swellings in a row, with periodic itching, because the larva moves along subdermally for months. Finally, it perforates as a mature larva, drops to the floor and becomes a pupa. The third type, creeping myiasis, is characterized by a young larva of the first stage, which, after penetration through skin, moves subdermally in a tortuous burrow and dies after a while, not reaching maturity.

The migratory furuncular and creeping myiases must be differentiated from cutaneous larva migrans or creeping eruption (Section 37).

Wound myiasis (synonym: traumatomyiasis): The female flies deposit their eggs on wounds or ulcers (Fig. 51.3); larvae being found preferentially in the crusts. Later, they also attack living tissues. Larvae of *Diptera* were or are still used for cleaning necrotic and gangrenous masses on superinfected ulcerated tumours.

Ophthalmomyiasis (synonym: ocular m.): External and internal types have been described. The first involves the conjunctivae, lids, lacrimal glands or periorbital tissues. Commonly, 5–10 small larvae may be found, sometimes up to 50.

The internal type is more dangerous and the consequence of a transcorneal or trans-scleral infestation. The moving larvae may be visible and cause destructive irreversible damage and ophthalmitis.

Cavitary myiasis (synonyms: nasopharyngeal m., nasal m., pharyngeal m., rhino-pharyngeal m., auricular m., oral m., oto m.): The synonyms point to the different locations of the larvae at the facial orifices and cavities, as well as in the upper respiratory and digestive tract. Tissues and organs in the vicinity may be involved (Figs. 51.4 and 51.5).

Intestinal myiasis (synonyms: entero m., pseudo m., gastro m., intestinal m.): This is the most frequent type of insect larval involvement in man and the most innocuous, often asymptomatic. Genuine intestinal myiasis is only present when migration of larvae occurs from the anus upwards. Oral infection with larvae, generally present in the food, is called pseudomyiasis.

The gastrointestinal mucosae are not attacked or invaded by the larvae. These are later, whether dead or alive, eliminated with the faeces.

Ano-uro-genital myiasis (synonyms: rectal m., uro-genital m., bladder m., urethro m., vulvo-rectal m., vaginal m., recto-vaginal m.): Again, the above mentioned synonyms point to the anatomical sites involved. Often, children and old neglected people suffer from this type of myiasis.

Tissue reaction against the fly larvae is a non-specific inflammation (Figs. 51.6 and 51.7). Often, bacterial superinfection with purulent inflammation is present. Larvae which migrate post-mortem into body orifices and hollow organs do not evoke an inflammatory reaction.

References

1. Soto, T. S. de and Soto Urribarri, R. (1989). Incidencia de miasis en pacientes de consulta externa. *Kasmera*, **17**, 31
2. Musa, M. T. (1989). Observations on Sudanese camel nasal myiasis caused by the larvae of Cephalopina titillator. *Rev. Elev. Med. Vet. Pays. Trop.*, **42**, 27
3. Alexis, J. B. and Mittleman, R. E. (1988). An unusual case of Phormia regina myiasis of the scalp. *Am. J. Clin. Pathol.*, **90**, 734
4. Nderagakura, F. *et al.* (1989). Myiasis: facial location. Apropos of a case of Dermatobia hominis infection. *Rev. Stomatol. Chir. Maxillofac.*, **90**, 7
5. Feuerstein, W. *et al.* (1969). Haut-Myiasis durch Cordylobia anthropophaga. *Wiener Klin. Wschr.*, **81**, 634

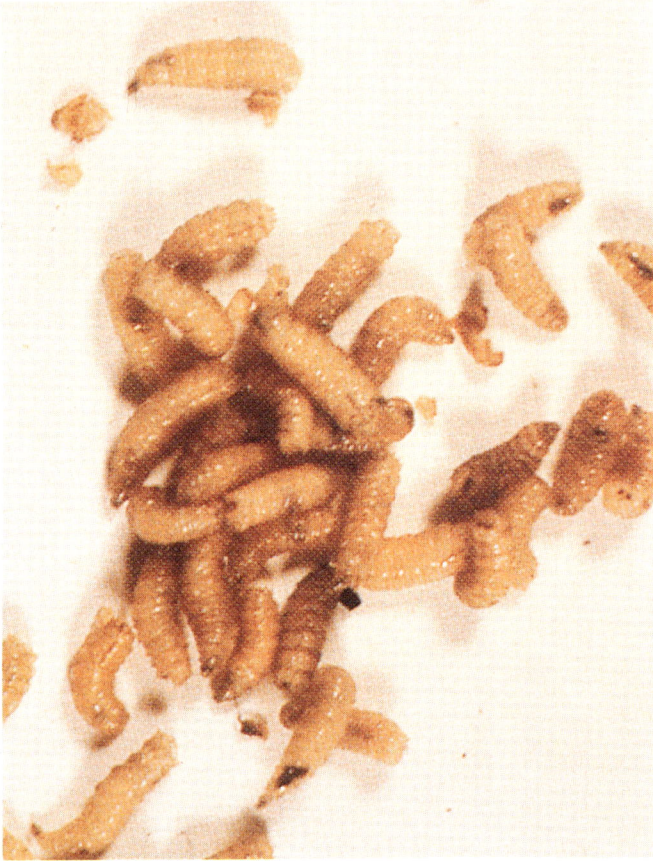

Fig. 51.1   Larvae of flies which may produce myiasis.

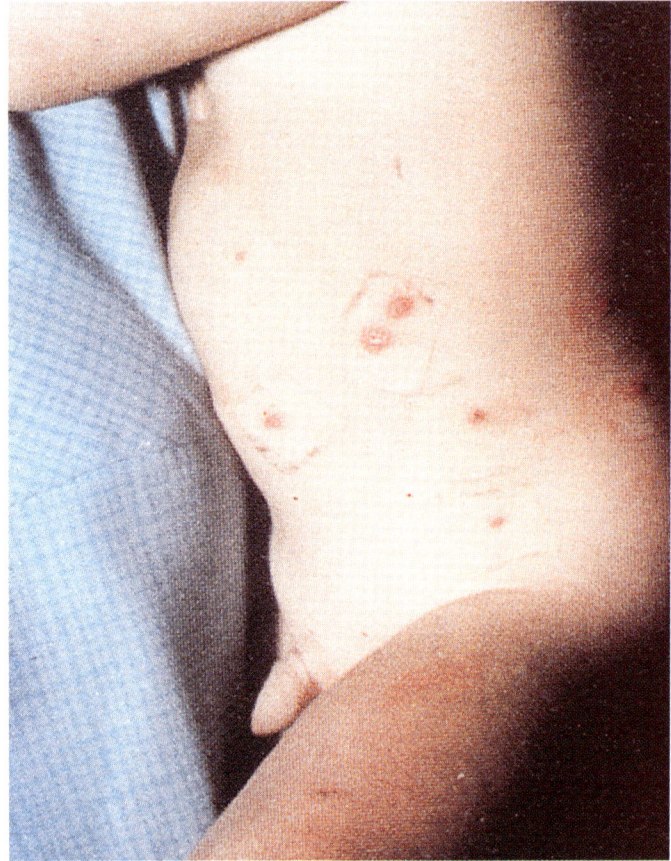

Fig. 51.2   Skin lesions of myiasis produced by larvae of *Cordyloba anthropophaga*

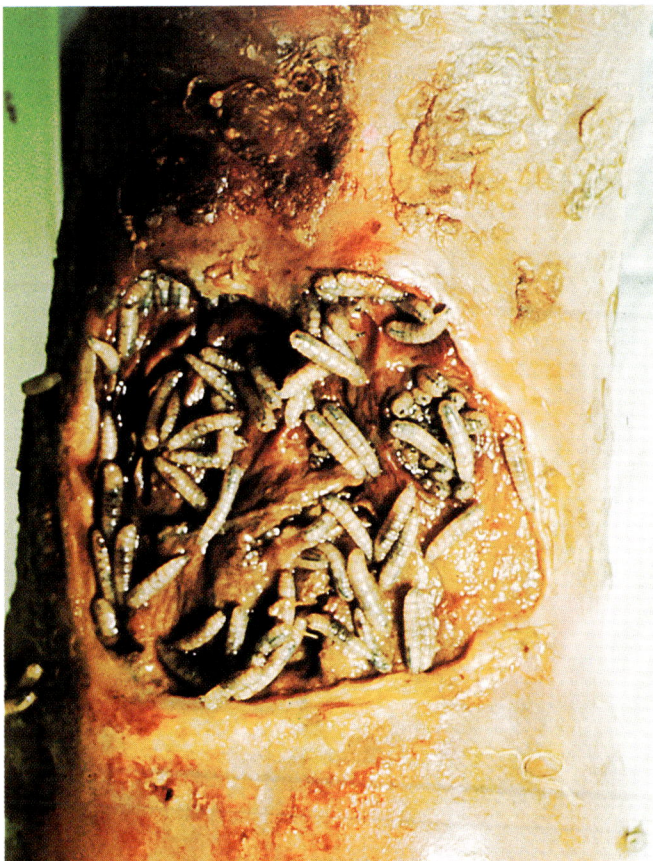

Fig. 51.3   Wound myiasis with numerous larvae

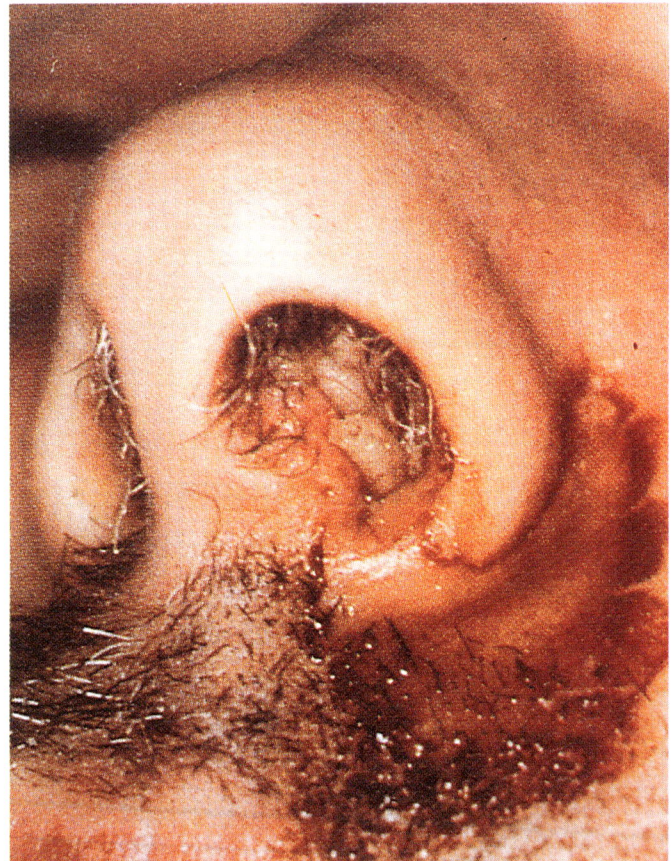

Fig. 51.4   Cavitary myasis produced by *Sarcophaga carnaria* larvae

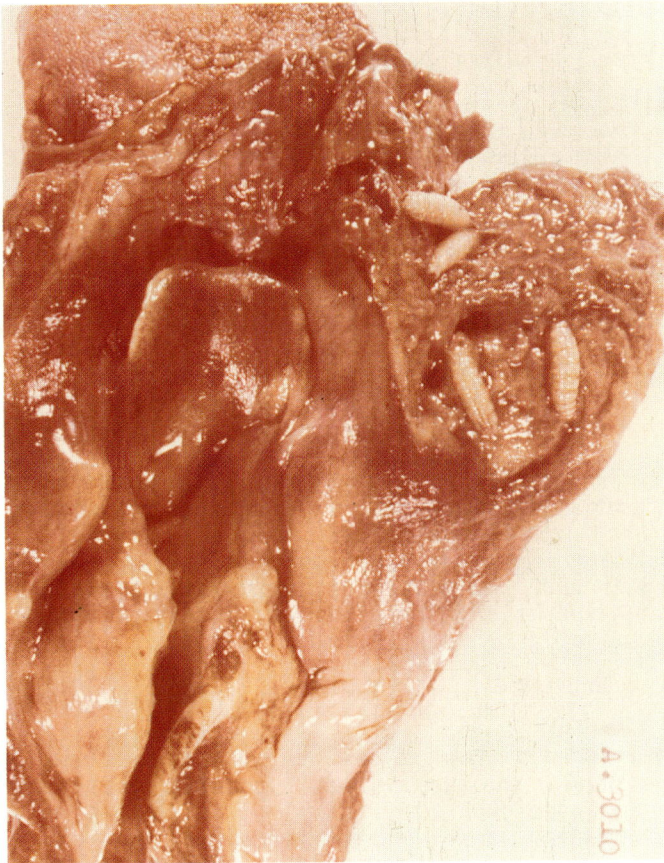

Fig. 51.5 Cavitary myiasis of the tonsillar region. H&E

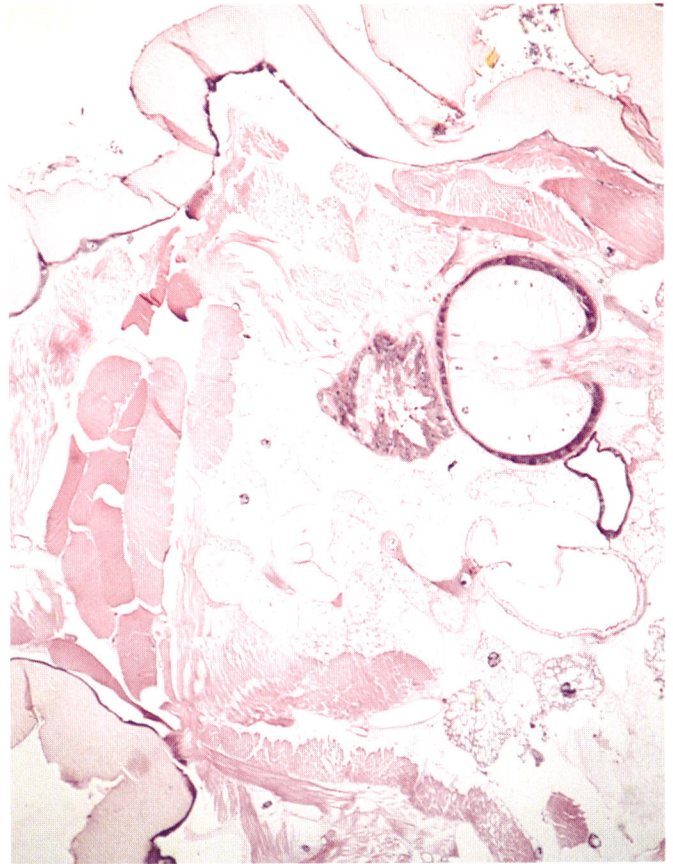

Fig. 51.6 Horizontal cut of larva of *Dermatoba hominis*. Note the thick cuticle. H&E

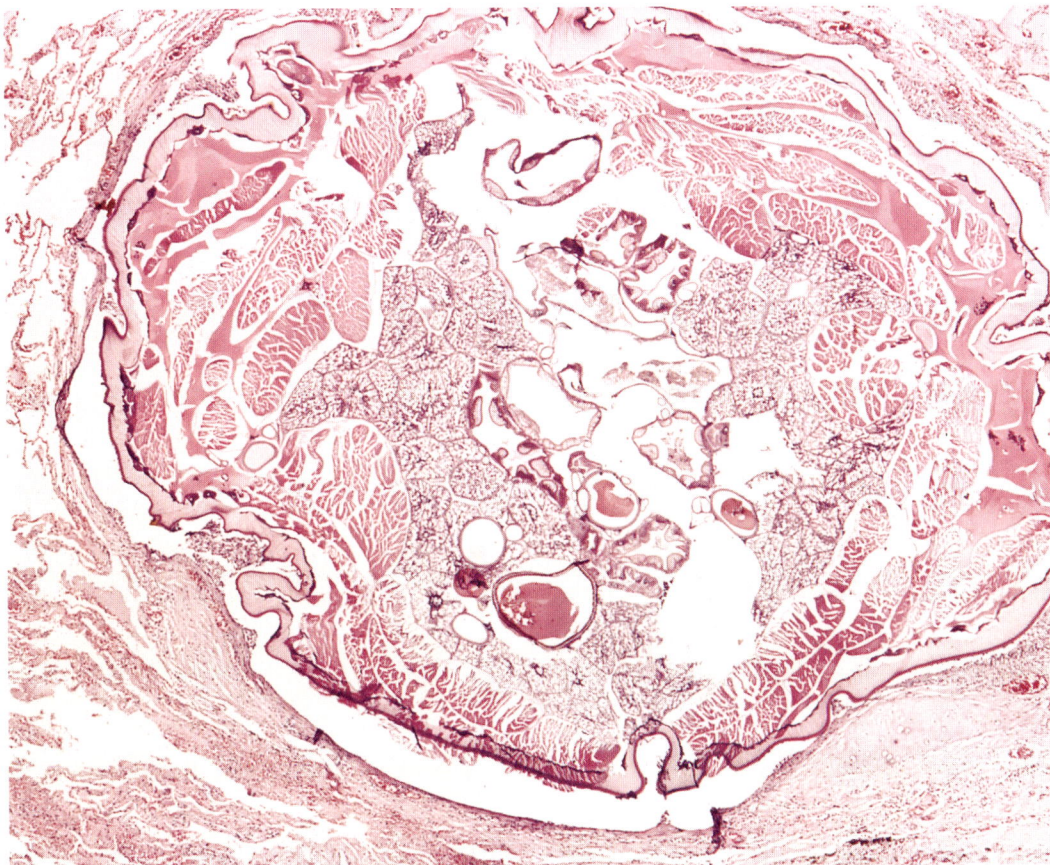

Fig. 51.7 Pulmonary myiasis. A minimal inflammatory reaction may be noted around the larva. This means there was an intravital aspiration of the larva. H&E

6. Hatvani, I. (1978). Durch Fliegenlarven verursachte Konjunktivitis. *Klin. Mbl. Augenheilk.* **172**, 783

7. Feigelson, J. *et al.* (1976). Un cas de myase oculaire 'Hypoderma bovis' chez un enfant atteint de mucoviscidose. *Pediatrie*, **31**, 77

8. Loewen, U. (1976). Die Ophthalmomyiasis. *Klin. Mbl. Augenheilk.*, **169**, 119

9. Zabroda, A. G. *et al.* (1990). The diagnosis of ophthalmomyiasis. *Oftalmol-Zh.*, **2**, 126

10. Agarwal, D. C. and Singh, B. (1990). Orbital myiasis – a case report. *Indian J. Ophthalmol.*, **38**, 187

11. Kearney, M. S. *et al.* (1991). Ophthalmomyiasis caused by the reindeer warble fly larva. *J. Clin. Pathol.*, **44**, 276

12. Sharma, H. (1989). Nasal myiasis: review of 10 years experience. *J. Laryngol. Otol.*, **103**, 489

13. Zumpt, F. (1963). The problem of intestinal myiasis in humans. *S. Afr. Med. J.*, **37**, 305

14. Aspoeck, H. *et al.* (1972). Urethrale Myiasis durch Fannia canicularis (L). *Wiener Kin. Wschr.*, **84**, 280

15. Aspoeck, H. and Leodolter, I. (1970). Vaginale Myiasis durch Sarcophaga argyrostoma (Rob-Desvoidy). *Wiener Klin. Wschr.*, **82**, 518

16. O'Rourke, F. J. (1968). Furuncular myiasis caused by warble fly (Hypoderma) larvae in patients from County Cork. *J. Irish Med. Assoc.*, **61**, 19

52. PENTASTOMIASIS

Introduction

This disease is also known as tongue-worm infection or porocephalosis. Nowadays, this entity is no longer observed but numerous cases were reported in Europe at the beginning of this century. It occurred worldwide, preferentially in tropical countries[1,2], the Far East and Malaysia[3]. In Venezuela, this disease is not known. In North America, a few cases have been reported[4].

Man and lower animals may be intermediate or definitive hosts. Natural infection occurs in numerous vertebrates[5,6] where the tongue-worms are permanent endoparasites or where larvae are harboured in viscera. Several species of laboratory animals may be used for experimental studies[7].

Clinically, in man as the intermediate host (infestation with larvae), rarely abdominal symptoms followed later by jaundice are noted. In man, as the definitive host, with worm-like adult parasites in the upper respiratory and digestive tract, several symptoms may be observed, but spontaneous cure occurs in 1–2 weeks.

Clinical diagnosis is made by detecting granulomas with larvae or nymphs in visceral biopsies or by recognition of worm-like parasites in the upper respiratory tract[8].

The parasite

The tongue-worms or pentastomids belong to the *Pentastomidae* or *Linguatulidae* with 60 known species. The taxonomic position of *Pentastomidae* is still controversial; most people consider that this parasite is an arthropod. Pathogenic to man are, above all, *Linguatula serrata* (syn. *L. rhinaria*) and some species of *Armillifer* (*Porocephalus*), e.g. *A. armillatus*, *A. moniliformis* and *A. grandii* which were described in the tropics.

The adult parasites are colourless worm-like annelids, without hairs or legs and a ring-like, but untrue, segmentation. Periorally, flour claws are present. The female pentastomata are up to 10 cm and the males 2 cm long. Their lifespan is said to be 2 years.

The larvae are microscopic in size up to 2.5 cm and have 4 rudimentary legs. The eggs measure 70–90 µm (Fig. 52.1).

Numerous eggs are laid by the female and reach the environment through nasal secretions or faeces. The eggs ar present in water and on plants. Intermediate hosts, hares, rabbits and goats (rarely man), become infected with eggs orally. The eggs become larvae which migrate through the intestinal wall and reach internal organs via the bloodstream. When larvae- or nymph-containing meat is eaten, man and lower animals become definitive hosts with the adult parasites.

Pathogenesis

Man (and animals) become infested as intermediate hosts when they consume parasitic eggs with water or unclean vegetables. The larvae develop from the eggs in the gastrointestinal tract and migrate, after penetrating the intestinal wall, into numerous organs. Later, they become nymphs and produce granulomas.

As the definitive host, man becomes infected by eating insufficiently cooked meat of rabbits, hares or goats. The adult parasites grow from the larvae or nymphs and remain in the region of the upper airways.

Pathology

In man, as intermediate host, the larvae or nymphs may be found in the intestinal wall, liver, spleen, mesenteral lymph nodes, kidneys and eyes[9–14]. The larvae (alive or dead) are situated in granulomas with necrotic tissue, which later have thick fibrotic capsules surrounded by infiltrates of lymphocytes. The granulomas may be similar to those of larva migrans (Figs. 52.2 and 52.3).

When man is the definitive host, the adult parasites produce practically no tissue lesions and are soon expelled.

References

1. Fain, A. and Salvo, G. (1966). Pentastomose humaine produite par les nymphes d'Armillifer grandis (Hett) au Republique democratique du Congo. *Ann. Soc. Belge. Med. Trop.*, **46**, 675

2. Self, J. T. *et al.* (1975). Pentastomiasis in Africans, a review. *Trop. Geogr. Pathol.*, **27**, 1

3. Prathap, K. *et al.* (1969). Pentastomiasis: A common finding at autopsy among Malaysian aborigines. *Am. J. Trop. Med. Hyg.*, **18**, 20

4. Guardia, S. N. *et al.* (1991). Pentastomiasis in Canada. *Arch. Path. Lab. Med.*, **115**, 515

5. Gill, H. S. *et al.* (1968). A note on the occurrence of Linguatula serrata (Froehlich, 1789) in domesticated animals. *Trans. R. Soc. Trop. Med. Hyg.*, **64**, 506

6. Basson, P. A. *et al.* (1971). Disease conditions of game in South Africa. Recent miscellaneous findings. *Vet. Med. Rev.*, **2**, 314

7. Boyce, W. M. and Kazacos, E. A. (1991). Histopathology of nymphal pentastomid infections (Sebekia mississippiensis) in paratenic hosts. *J. Parasitol.*, **77**, 104

8. Buslau, M. *et al.* (1990). Dermatological signs of nasopharyngeal linguatulosis (Halzoun, Marrara syndrome) – the possible role of major basic protein. *Dermatologica*, **181**, 327

9. Bouchaert, L. and Fain, A. (1959). Armillifer armillatus infection with fatal intestinal obstruction. *Ann. Soc. Belge Med. Trop.*, **39**, 393

10. Baird, J. K. (1988). Hepatic granuloma in a man from North America caused by a nymph of Linguatula serrata. *Pathology*, **20**, 198

11. Gratama, S. and von Thiel, P. H. (1958). Ocular Armillier armillatus in man. *Doc. Med. Geogr. Trop.*, **9**, 374

12. Rendtorff, R. C. *et al.* (1962). The occurrence of Linguatula serrata, a Pentastomid, within the human eye. *Am. J. Trop. Med. Hyg.*, **11**, 762

13. Deweese, M. W. *et al.* (1962). Case report of tongue worm (Linguatula serrata) in the anterior chamber. *Arch. Ophthalmol.*, **68**, 587

14. McKie Reid, A. and Ellis Jones, D. W. (1963). Porocephalus armillatus farrae presenting in the eye. *Br. J. Ophthalmol.*, **47**, 169

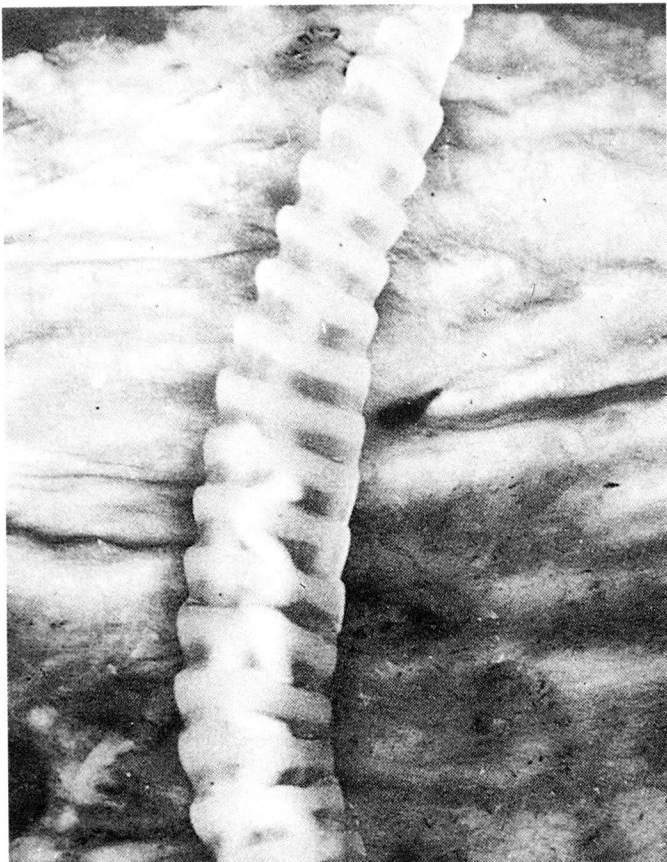

Fig. 52.1 Non-encysted larva of *Armillifer armillatus*

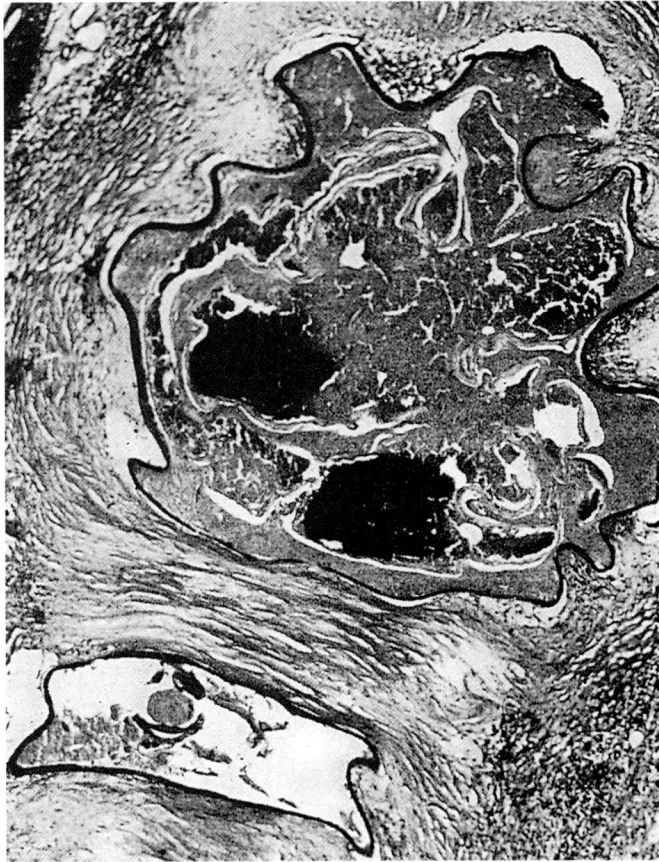

Fig. 52.2 Dead and calcified larva of *Armillifer armillatus* in human tissue. H&E

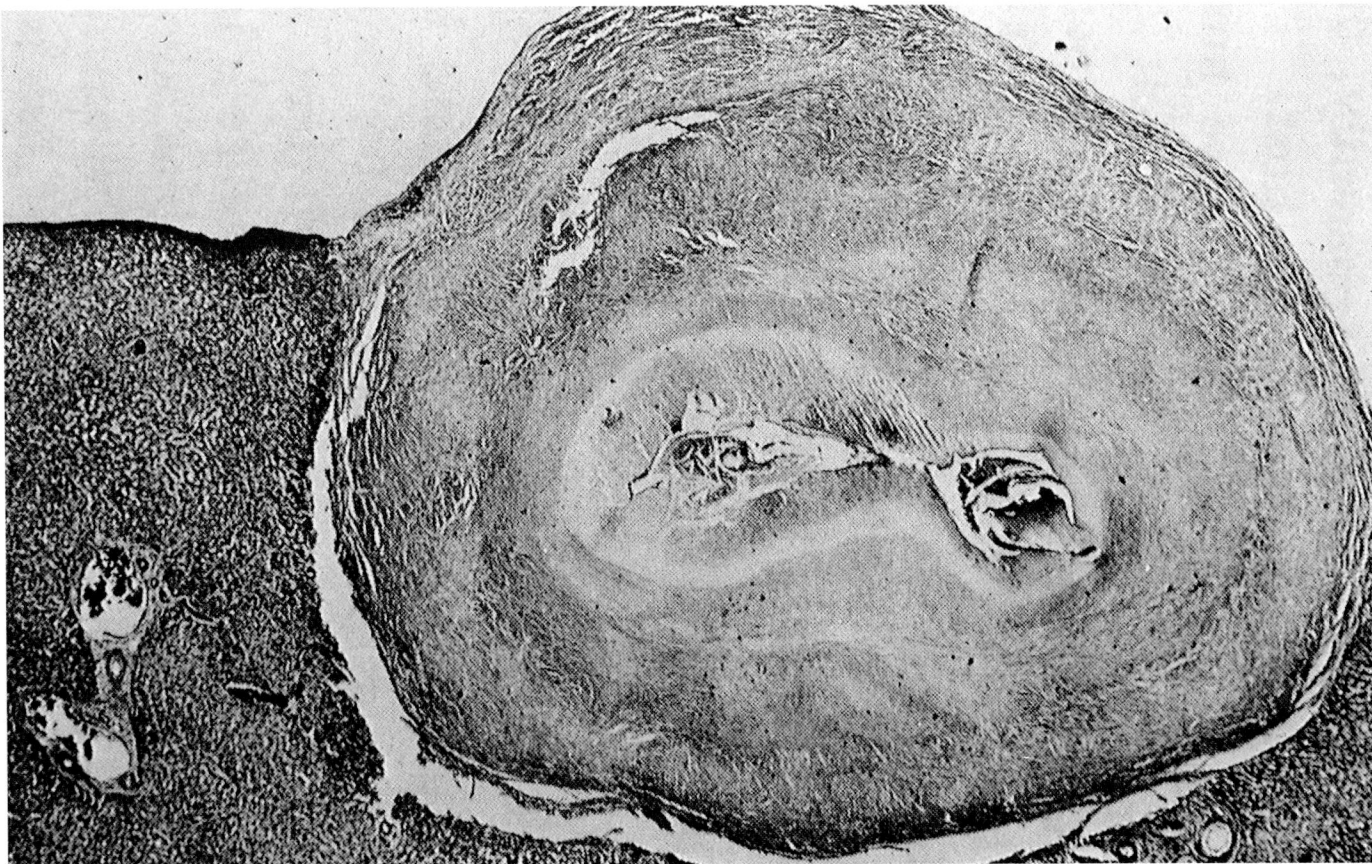

Fig. 52.3 Encysted necrobiotic and degenerated pentastomid larva in a fibrotic granuloma of the liver. H&E

Index

Italic page references are to figures

Acanthamoeba castallani 52
Acanthamoeba albertsoni 52
acanthamoebiasis 49–56
  clinical diagnosis 52
  differential diagnosis 52, 56
  epidemiology 49
  experimental infection 49
  gross pathology 52
  histology 53–5
    brain *9.3–9.8*
    Goldner's staining 52, *9.2*
    neuronophagy 52, *9.9*
    spinal fluid 53, *9.1*
  opportunistic infection 52
  parasite 52
    cytopathic effect 52
  pathogenesis 52
acari 174
Aedes aegypti 128, 134
AIDS 35, 52, 59, 62, 72, 73, 76, 77, 85, 87,
  95, 109, 165
acanthocephaliasis 137
Acanthocephala 137
allergic dermatitis 155
allergic reaction 11, 100, 112, 117, 124,
  126, 128
Alveococcus see Echinococcus multilocularis
Alzheimer nuclei type II 62
amastigotes 13, 15, 18, 23, 27, 29, 35
amoebae 91
amoebiasis 9, 43–9
  clinical diagnosis 43
  epidemiology 43
  gross pathology 43, 46
    chronic intestinal amoebiasis 46
    hepatic amoebiasis 46, *8.10, 8.11, 8.14*
    intestinal amoebiasis 43, 46, *8.3–8.6,*
      8.20, 8.21
    rare extraintestinal amoebiasis 46, 49,
      8.17, 8.25
  histology 44–51
    cervix 50, *8.23, 8.24*
    erythrophagia 49, *8.29*
    intestine 44–51, *8.3, 8.7, 8.8, 8.26–8.30*
    liver 47, 51, *8.12, 8.13, 8.31*
    lung 47, *8.16*
    lymph node 48, *8.18, 8.19*
    perianal lesion 48, *8.22*
    staining 49, *8.2b, c, d*
  pathogenesis 43
  X-ray, lung 47, *8.15*
amoebic appendicitis 46
amoebic colitis 46
amoebic dysentery *see* amoebiasis
amoebic granuloma 46, 49
amoeboma 46, 49, *8.9*
Ancylostoma braziliense 138
Ancylostoma caninum 138
Ancylostoma duodenale 106
anaemia 35, 96, 100, 106
anaemia, hypochromic microcytic 109
anaemia, iron deficiency type 109, 143
anaemia perniciosa 143
angiostrongylosis 119–23, 138
  american type 119
  asian type 119
  clinical diagnosis 119
  epidemiology 119
  experimental infection 119
  parasite 119, 120, *29.1, 29.4*
  pathogenesis 119

  pathology 119
    brain 120, *29.2*
    eggs 122, *29.13*
    experimental inoculation 121,
      29.7–29.10
    granulomatous reacting 123,
      29.16–29.18
    intestine 122, *29.11, 29.12*
    lung 120, *29.3–29.6*
    testicle 123, *29.15*
    vasculitis 123, *29.19*
Angiostrongylus cantonensis 119
Angiostrongylus costaricensis 119
anisakiasis 115–17, 138
  clinical diagnosis 115
  epidemiology 115
  parasite 115, 116, *27.1*
  pathogenesis 115
  pathology 116, 117, *27.2, 27.3*
Anisakis marina 117
anti-*Anopheles* campaigns 35, 77
Anopheles 81, 128, 134
Aphaniptera 178
Armillifer 184
Armillifer armillatus 184
Armillifer grandii 184
Armillifer moniliformis 184
arteritis, obstructive in schistosomiasis 155
arthropods, disorders by 173–84 (table 22)
arthropods in man, principal 11 (table 2)
ascaridiasis 100–4
  clinical diagnosis 100
  epidemiology 100
  parasite 100
    life cycle 100 (table 13)
  pathogenesis 100
  pathology 100, 101
    appendicitis 101
    ascaridioma 101
    cholangitis 101, 103, *21.8–21.10*
    intestinal 102, 103, *21.1–21.5*
    liver abscesses 101, 103, 104, *21.6,*
      21.7, 21.11–21.13
    pancreatitis 101
Ascaris 11
Ascaris lumbricoides 100, 138
ascaris roundworm 100
Ascaris suum 100
asthma 115, 138
autoinfection, in strongyloidiasis 109

Babesia bigemina 71, 74, *12.1*
Babesia bovis 69
Babesia divergens 69
Babesia microti 69
babesiosis 69–71
  blood transfusion 69
  clinical diagnosis 69
  differential diagnosis 70
  epidemiology 69
  parasite 70
    development cycle 70 (table 4)
    maltese cross 70
  pathogenesis 70
  pathology 70
    blood smear 71, *12.1*
    splenectomy 70
BAL (broncho-alveolar lavage) 85
balantidiasis 91–3
  clinical diagnosis 91
  epidemiology 91

  experimental infection 91
  gross pathology 91
    intestine 92, *18.3*
  histology 91, 92, 93
    exocervix 92, *18.5*
    intestine 93, *18.6–18.8*
    lymph node 92, *18.4*
  parasite 91
    cilia 92, *18.1, 18.2*
  pathogenesis 91
Balantidium coli 91
beef tapeworm 144, 147
bilharziosis *see* blood fluke infection
black water fever 175
black fly 131
bladder, carcinoma of the 155
blepharoblast 13, 41
Blastocystis hominis 56, 59
Blastocystis infection 56–9
  clinical diagnosis 56
  differential diagnosis 56
  experimental infection 56
  gross pathology 56, 59
  histology 59, *10.5–10.8*
  opportunistic infection 59
  parasite 56
    cell block section 57, *10.3, 10.4*
    iron haematoxylin 57, *10.2*
    signet ring appearance 57, *10.1*
  pathogenesis 56
blindness 116, 126, 128, 131, 138, 147
blood fluke infection 151–60
  clinical diagnosis 155
  epidemiology 155
  experimental infection 155
  gross pathology 155, 157
    cercarial dermatitis 157, *44.4*
  histology 155–9
    carcinoma of the bladder 158, *44.8,*
      44.9
    cervix 158, *44.7*
    eggs 156, *44.2*
    intestine, nodular lesion 157, *44.5*
    liver granulomas 157, *44.6*
    lung 158, 159, *44.10, 44.11*
    meningo-myelitis 158, *44.12–44.14*
  parasite 155, 156, *44.1–44.3*
  pathogenesis 155
blood transfusion, babesiosis 69
Bombyx mori 181
Brachycera 181
brachycerosis, larval 181
bradyzoites 59
brain resembling Swiss cheese 69
bronchitis, chronic, in lung fluke
  infection 160
broncho-alveolar lavage (BAL) 85
Brugia malayi 126
Brugia timori 126
buba *see* leishmaniasis, mucocutaneous
buffalo gnats 131
button hole ulcer 43, *8.7, 8.8*

Candida 32, 36
Capillaria hepatica 124, 138
Capillaria philippensis 124
capillariasis 124, 125
  clinical diagnosis 124
  epidemiology 124
  parasite 124, *30.2*
  pathogenesis 124

pathology 124, 125
    intestine 125, *30.1, 30.3*
carcinoma of the bladder 155
carcinoma of the cervix 41
carp spp. 143
cat liver fluke 163
cercaria 155, 160, 163, 165, 169
cercarial dermatitis 138, 155, 157
cestodiasis 141–51
Chagas disease *see* trypanosomiasis,
    American
chagoma of inoculation 15
Cheilospirura spp. 117
Chiclero ulcer *see* leishmaniasis,
    mucocutaneous
chigger 178
chigoe 178
Chinese liver fluke 163
cholangiocarcinoma 163
cholangitis 163
cholelithiasis 163
cholecystitis 163
Chrysops 128, 131
Ciliophora 91
clonorchiasis *see* liver fluke infection
Clonorchis sinensis 163, 165
chlorosis 109
Cnidosporidia 94
coccidian spp. 59, 72, 76
Coccidioides immitis 32
coccidiosis 72
codworm anisakiasis 115
coenurosis 141
colitis, balantidial 91
colitis, eosinophilic 124
complement fixation test, in anisakiasis 115
conjunctivitis 128
Cordylobia anthropophaga 181
cor pulmonale, in schistosomiasis 155
corticosteroid therapy, scabies 174
crayfish 160
creeping eruption 106, 109, 138, 181
creeping myiasis 181
crustaceans 143
crusty form, scabies 175
Cryptococcus neoformans 26
cryptosporidians 59
cryptosporidiosis 9, 76–8
    AIDS 76, 77
    clinical diagnosis 77
    epidemiology 76
    experimental infection 76
    histology 77
        intestine 78, *15.1–15.6*
    parasite 77
        evolution cycle 76 (table 6)
    faecal smear 78, *15.1–15.3*
Cryptosporidium 77
cryptozoites 82
cucumber tapeworm 145
Culex 128, 134
Culicoides 126
Cyclops 124, 126, 143
cyst, hydatid 148
cysticercoid stage 145, 147
cysticercosis 141, 143, 147–50
    clinical diagnosis 147
        computed tomography 147
        immunological methods 147
        MR (magnetic resonance) 147
        X-ray 149, *42.6*
    epidemiology 147
    experimental infection 147
    gross pathology 147, 149, 150
        brain 148, 149, *42.2–42.5*
        heart 150, *42.7*
    histology 148, 150
        meninges 150, *42.11*
    parasite 147, 149, *42.1, 42.11*
cysticercus 143, 147
Cysticercus cellulosae 147
Cysticercus bovis 147
Cysticercus racemosus 148
cystitis in schistosomiasis 155

cytomegaly 62, 87

Demodex brevis 175
Demodex canii 179, *49.5, 49.6*
Demodex folliculorum 175, 179
Demodex spp 175
demodicidosis 173, 175–8
    clinical diagnosis 175
    epidemiology 175
    parasite 175, 179, *49.1*
    pathogenesis 175, 178
    pathology 175
        face 179, *49.2*
        sebaceous glands *49.3, 49.4*
        hair follicle *49.5, 49.6*
Dermacentor reticulatus 70
dermatitis, cercarial 138, 155, 157
dermatitis, allergic 155
dermatitis, perioral, in demodicidosis 174
Dermatobia hominis 181
Dermatophilus penetrans 178
Dicrocoelium dendriticum 163, 165
Dicrocoelium hospes 165
Dictophyma renale 137
dictophymatosis 137
Dienthamoeba fragilis 43
Dipetalonema perstans 126
Dipetalonema streptocerca 126
diphyllobotriasis 143–5
    clinical diagnosis 143
    epidemiology 143
    parasite 145, *39.1–39.3*
    pathogenesis 143
    pathology 143, 145
    sparganosis 143, 145
    Spirometra spp. 144, *39.4, 39.5*
Diphyllobotrium 141
Diphyllobotrium latum 143
Diphyllobotrium pacificum 143
Diptera 173, 181
dipylidiasis 145
    clinical diagnosis 145
    epidemiology 145
    parasite 145, *40.1*
    pathogenesis 145
    pathology 145
Dipylidium 141
Dipylidium caninum 145
Dirofilaria 138
Dirofilaria conjunctivae 134
Dirofilaria immitis 126, 134
Dirofilaria repens 134
dirofilariasis 126, 134–7
    clinical diagnosis 134
    epidemiology 134
    parasite 134, *35.1*
    pathogenesis 134
    pathology 134
        Hoeppli–Splendore phenomenon *35.1*
        lung 135, *35.2, 35.3, 35.5, 35.7, 35.8*
        pulmonary artery 135, 136, *35.4, 35.6*
    reservoir hosts 134
Dirofilaria tenuis 134
Distoma buski *see* *Fasciolopsis buski*
distosomiasis, pulmonary *see* lung fluke
    infections
dog heartworm 134
dog tapeworm 145, 148
Donovan bodies 35
double refraction of polarized light, in lung
    fluke infection 163
dracontiasis *see* dracunculosis
dracunculiasis *see* dracunculosis
dracunculosis 124–6
    clinical diagnosis 124
    epidemiology 124
    parasite 124, *31.1*
    pathogenesis 124
    pathology 126
        skin 127, *31.2*
Dracunculus medinensis 96
dragon worm 124
Dürck's granulomas 81
dwarf tapeworm 145, 147

dwarf threadworm 109
dysenteric syndrome 43
dysentery, amoebic 91
dysentery, balantidial 91

earthworm 100
echinococcosis 141, 145, 148–54
    clinical diagnosis 148
        serology 148
        sonography 148
        X-ray 148
    differential diagnosis 148
    experimental infection 148
    epidemiology 148
    gross pathology 151
    histology 151–4
        brood capsule 152, *43.3–43.5*
        foreign body reaction 153, *43.9, 43.10*
        scolex 153, 154, *43.6–43.8,*
        43.11–43.13
    parasite 148, 152, *43.1, 43.2*
    pathogenesis 151
echinococcosis, alveolaris 148
Echinococcus 11, 145
Echinococcus alveolaris *see* *E. multilocularis*
Echinococcus cysticus *see* *E. granulosus*
Echinococcus hydaticus *see* *E. granulosus*
Echinococcus granulosus 148
Echinococcus multilocularis 148, 151
Echinococcus oligarthus 141
Echinococcus patagonicus 141
Echinococcus vogeli 141
Echinostoma echinatum 169
Echinostoma ilocanum 169
Echinostoma spp. 169
ectoparasite, general definition 173
eczema in scabies 174
elephantiasis, tropical 126, 128
ELISA 134
encephalitis, gnathostoma 117
Encephalitozoon 94
encephalopathy, hepatogenic, in
    toxoplasmosis 62
Endolimax nana 43
endometritis, in trichomoniasis 41
endozoonosis, general definition 173
Entamoeba coli 43
Entamoeba histolytica 43, 49
enterobiasis 97–100
    clinical diagnosis 98
    epidemiology 97
    parasite 98, 99, *20.1, 20.2*
        eggs 99, *20.2, 20.3*
    pathogenesis 98
    pathology 98
        appendix 99, *20.4*
        intestine 99, *20.5*
Enterobius vermicularis 98, 106
Enterocytozoon 94
enteritis, eosinophilic, in strongyloidiasis
    109
eosinophilia 100, 106, 109, 112, 115, 117,
    119, 124, 126, 128, 131, 138, 141
eosinophilia, tropical pulmonary 138
eosinophilic infiltrate 101, 106, 124, 138
eosinophilic syndrome 128
epilepsy 116, 138
epizoonosis, general definition 173
erythrophagia, in amoebiasis 119, *8.19*
espundia 27
exanthema, in scabies 117
exo-autoinfection, strongyloidiasis 109
eyeworm 128

Fasciola hepatica 163, 165
fasciolasis *see* sheep liver fluke infections
Fasciolopsis buski 169
fever, paratoses with fever 112
Fiedler's myocarditis, in American
    trypanosomiasis 15
Filaria infections 126–37
Filaria, migrating 128
filariasis 126–9
    clinical diagnosis 126, 128

epidemiology 126
experimental infections 126
parasite 128 (table 16), 129, *32.1, 32.3*
pathogenesis 128
pathology 128, 129
lymph node 129, *32.4, 32.5*
filariasis, human zoonotic 134
filariasis, lymphatic *see* filariasis
flagellates 39, 41
flagellum 13, 15, 41
flea larvae 145
flukes *see* trematodiasis
flukes, paired 155
folliculitis in scabies 174
foamy cells 62
fox tapeworm 148
fungal infection 87
furuncular myiasis 181
furunculosis, in scabies 174

GAE (granulomatous amoebic infection) 49,
52
gametocytes 80
gamont 70
gangrene, in tungiasis 178
Gastrodiscoides hominis 169
Gastrophilus spp. 181
gemistocytic transformation 26, 62
giant intestinal fluke *see* intestinal fluke
Giardia lamblia 39
giardiasis 9, 39–41
clinical diagnosis 39
epidemiology 39
histology 39
faecal smear 40, *6.1*
intestinal content 40, *6.4, 6.5*
staining 39
parasite 39
cysts 40, *6.2*
trophozoites 40, *6.2, 6.3*
pathogenesis 3
glial cell proliferation 81
glomerulonephritis in schistosomiasis 155
glomerulonephritis in scabies 174
Glossina palpalis 23
Glossina morsitans 23
Gnathostoma 138
Gnathostoma spinigerum 117
gnathostomiasis 117, 118
clinical diagnosis 117
epidemiology 117
experimental infection 117
parasite 117, 118, *28.1, 28.2*
pathogenesis 117
pathology 117
creeping eruption 118, *28.1, 28.3, 28.4*
Gongylonema pulchrum 117
Gram's staining, in microsporidiosis 94
granulomas, allergic 138
granuloma, eosinophilic 128, 131, 138, 155
granuloma of Dürck 81
granuloma of the liver in schistosomiasis
155
granuloma of the liver in liver fluke
infections 163
granulomatosis in demodicidosis 175
granulomatous reaction 11, 87, 119, 124,
143, 163, 184
green sickness 109
Grocott's method 85, 87, 94
ground itch 106
Guinea worm 124
gynaecophoric canal 155

haematin *see* malaria pigment
Haemoflagellate infections 13–26
haemolysis, intravasal, in malaria 81
haemoptysis, endemic, in lung fluke
infection 160
haemorrhages, annular, in malaria 81
Haemosporidia 80
haemozoin *see* malaria pigment
Haplosporidia 85
helminthic diseases 96–172

development stage 97 (table 10)
lifespan in man 97 (table 10)
prepatent period 97 (table 10)
source of infection 97 (table 10)
Hepaticola hepatica 124
hepatitis granulomatous 124
hepatitis in amoebiasis 46
hepatosplenomegaly in schistosomiasis 155
hermaphrodite 96, 141, 151
herring worm disease *see* anisakiasis
Heterophyes heterophyes 169
Heterophyes nocens 169
Hirudo medicinalis 151
HIV-1 43
Hodgkin's disease and toxoplasmosis 62
Hoeppli–Splendore phenomenon 136, *35.6,*
155, 156, *42.2d*
hookworms 100, 106
host, general definition 9
hydatid cyst, unilocular 151
hydatidosis *see* echinococcosis
hydatidosis, secondary 148
hydrocephalus, internal 147
hydronephrosis in schistosomiasis 155
Hymenolepis 141
Hymenolepis diminuta 145
Hymenolepis nana 145
hymenolepsiasis 145–7
clinical diagnosis 145
epidemiology 145
experimental infection 145
parasite 145, 147, *41.1*
pathogenesis 147
pathology 147
Hypoderma bovis 181
hypoproteinaemia, in uncinariasis 106

ileus, mechanical 101, 119
ileitis, eosinophilic 119
immunodeficiency 73, 85, 100, 106, 173
immunofluorescence, indirect, in
dracunculosis 124
immunodeficiency 73, 85, 100, 106
immunofluorescent staining in
pneumocystosis 85
immunological defects 62
immunosuppression 62, 109, 145
infiltration, eosinophilic 11
intestinal fluke infection 169–70
clinical diagnosis 169
epidemiology 169
experimental infection 169
parasite 169, 170, *47.1, 47.2*
pathogenesis 169
pathology 169
intrauterine infection in cysticercosis 147
Iodamoeba bütschlii 43
ISHAM congress, June 1991 85
Isospora belli 59, 63, 76
Isospora hominis 73
isosporosis 59, 73, 75, 76
AIDS 73
clinical diagnosis 73
epidemiology 73
parasite 73
faecal smear 75, *14.1–14.3*
pathogenesis 75, 76
pathology 76
itch mite *see* scabies
Ixodidae 70
Ixodes ricinus 70

jaundice, in pentastomiasis 184

kala-azar *see* leishmaniasis, visceral
kinetoplast 13, 15, 23, 29, 35, 62

lagochilascariasis 137
Lagochilascaris minor 137
lancet liver fluke 165
larvae, ciliate 143
larvae of pork tapeworm 147
larval stage 147, 151
larva migrans 100, 126, 128, 137–41

clinical diagnosis 138
epidemiology 137, 138
parasite 138, 139, *37.1*
pathogenesis 138
pathology 138
intestine 140, *37.5, 37.6*
liver granuloma 140, *37.7–37.9*
myocardium 139, *37.2–37.4*
larva migrans, cutaneous 106, 138
larva migrans, visceral 115, 117, 138
Leishmania 13, 15, 26
Leishmania braziliensis 27, 29
Leishmania donovani 29, 35
Leishmania donovani chagasi 35
Leishmania mexicana 29
Leishmania tropica 27, 29
Leishmania tropica aethiopica 27
Leishmania tropica major 27
Leishmania tropica minor 27
leishmaniases 9, 13, 26–39
leishmaniases, cutaneous 13, 27, 28
anergic disposition 27
clinical diagnosis 27
diffuse type 27
dry form 27
epidemiology 27
gross pathology 27, 28, *3.2, 3.3*
histology 27, 28, *3.4*
humid forms 27
parasite 27
pathogenesis 27
rural type 27
urban type 27
vector 27, 28, *3.1*
leishmaniasis, cutaneous post-kala-azar 35
leishmaniasis, diffuse tegumentary type 29
leishmaniasis, mucocutaneous 27–35
clinical diagnosis 29
differential diagnosis 32
leprosy 32
rhinoscleroma 32
histoplasmosis 32
diffuse tegumentary type 29, *4.10*
epidemiology 29, 32
gross pathology 29, 32
ear 30, *4.4*
mucosa of the upper respiration tract
31, *4.11*
nose 29, 30, *4.2, 4.3*
papulomatous lesion 29, 30, *4.5*
skin scar 31, *4.9*
skin ulcer 30, 31, *4.6–4.8*
histology 29, 30–4
amastigotes 29, 30, 33, *4.1, 4.12*
granulomatous reaction 32, 34, *4.17,*
4.18
Grocott's method 32
histiocytes 29, 32, 33, *4.13, 4.14*
kinetoplast 29
lymphadenitis, regional 32
phagocytosis 32, 33, *4.15*
tissue reaction 34, *4.16, 4.19*
parasite 29, *4.12*
parasitaemia 29
pathogenesis 29
leishmaniasis of the Old World *see*
leishmaniasis, cutaneous
leishmaniasis of the New World *see*
leishmaniasis, mucocutaneous
leishmaniasis, visceral 35–9
AIDS 35
clinical diagnosis 35
differential diagnosis 35
gross pathology 35
histology 35–8
liver 36, 38, *5.2, 5.9–5.11*
lymph node 36, 37, *5.3–5.6, 5.12*
Russell bodies 35, 38, *5.12*
small intestine 37, *5.7, 5.8*
spleen 38, *5.13*
parasite 35
kinetoplast 35
promastigote 35
pathogenesis 35

leishmanioma 35
lice, dog hair 145
Lieberkuhn's crypts 112
LM *see* larva migrans
Linguatula rhinaria 184
Linguatula serrata 184
Linguatulidae 184
linitis plastica, in strongyloidiasis 109
lipoproteinosis and pneumocystosis 87
liver carcinoma, primary, in liver fluke
      infection 163
liver fluke infection, chinese and cat 163–7
  clinical diagnosis 163
  epidemiology 163
  parasite 163, 164, *46.1, 46.2, 46.4, 46.5*
  pathogenesis 163, 165
  pathology 165
    bile duct (hamster) 164, *46.3, 46.7*
    bile duct (man) 164, *46.6*
    cholangiocarcinoma (hamster)
      46.8–46.11
    liver granuloma 164, 167, *46.12*
liver fluke infection, small 165
  AIDS 165
  epidemiology 165
  parasite 165
  pathogenesis 165
  pathology 165
liver fluke infection, sheep 165–9
  clinical diagnosis 165
  epidemiology 165
  experimental infection 165
  parasite 165, 168, *46.13*
    cercaria 168, *46.16*
    eggs 168, *46.14*
  pathogenesis 165
  pathology 165
    bile (cattle) 168, *46.15*
    bile duct 168, *46.17*
liver glia 62
liver granuloma, in schistosomiasis 155
liver trematode infection 163–9
Loa loa 126, 128
loa worm 128
loiasis 128–31
  clinical diagnosis 128
  epidemiology 128
  parasite 130, *33.1, 33.2*
  pathogenesis 131
  pathology 131
Löffler's syndrome 100, 101, 138
lung trematode infection 160–3
  clinical diagnosis 160
  differential diagnosis 160
  epidemiology 160
  experimental infection 160
  parasite 160
  pathogenesis 160, 163
  pathology 163
    eggs and granulation tissue 161, *45.4,*
      45.6
    eggs in polarized light 162, *45.7*
    pulmonary cyst 161, *45.1, 45.2, 45.3,*
      45.5
Lutzomyia 35
Lutzomyia longipalpis 29
lymphadenitis, eosinophilic 111, 129,
    24.10–24.12, 32.5
lymphadenitis, Piringer–Kuchinka 62

Macracanthorhyncus hirudinaceus 137
macrofilariae 126
maggots 181
malaria 9, 70, 77–85
  clinical diagnosis 79
  epidemiology 77
  experimental infection 77
  gross pathology 81
    bone marrow 83, *16.6*
    brain 83, *16.7*
    kidney 82, *16.5*
    spleen 83, *16.4*
  histology 81–4
    brain 83, 84, *16.8, 16.11*

    kidney 84, *16.12*
    liver 83, *16.10*
    placenta 83, *16.9*
  parasite 80, 81
    gametocytes 81, *16.1*
    intraerythrocytic structure 79 (table 7)
    trophozoites 81, *16.1*
    schizonts 81, *16.1, 16.2*
  pathogenesis 81
    evolutionary cycle 80 (table 8)
malaria, bovine 69
malaria, cerebral 81
malaria, congenital 81
malaria, imported 77
malaria, malignant 77
malaria, pernicious 77
malaria pigment 81, 83
malaria tropica 77
malabsorption syndrome, in strongyloidiasis
    109
maltese cross, in babesiosis 70
mango fly 128
Mansonella ozzardi 126
Mansonia 128
Medina worm 124
mega-organs, in American trypanosomiasis
    18
Meleney's synergistic gangrene, in
    amoebiasis 46
meningoencephalitis, eosinophilic, in
    angiostrongylosis 119
meningo-encephalomyelitis, in
    micronemiasis 137
merozoites 72, 73, 81
Mesocestoides spp. 141
metacercaria 160, 163, 165, 169
Metagonimus yokogawi 169, *47.2*
metastasis formation, in echinococcosis 151
Metazoa 96
Meyers–Koumenaar syndrome 138
Microfilaria bolivariensis 126
microfilaria, scheme of 126 (table 15)
Micronema deletrix 137
micronemiasis 137
Microspora 94
Microsporidia 85
microsporidiosis 94, 95
  AIDS 94
  clinical diagnosis 94
  differential diagnosis 94
  experimental infection 94
  histology 94, 95
    gastric carcinoma 95, *19.5, 19.6*
    halo 94, 95, *19.2*
    muscle 95, *19.1, 19.3, 19.4*
  parasite 94
  pathogenesis 94
Miescher's tubules 72
miracidium 155, 160, 163, 165
miscarriage 62, 81
Moniliformis moniliformis 137
mononucleosis, in toxoplasmosis 62
Montenegro skin test 27, 29
Morerastrongylus costaricensis 119
morula cell 25, *2.6, 2.8, 2.9*
Mott bodies 25, *2.6, 2.8, 2.9,* 26
MR (magnetic resonance) 147
Musca domestica 181
mussels 169
Mycobacterium tuberculosis 85
myiasis 138, 181–4
  clinical diagnosis 181
  epidemiology 181
  parasite 181
    larvae 182, *51.1, 51.6*
  pathogenesis 181
  pathology 181
    cavitary myiasis 182, 183, *51.4, 51.5*
    pulmonary myiasis 183, *51.7*
    skin 182, *51.2*
    wound myiasis 182, *51.3*
myocardial degneration, fatty, in uncinariasis
    109

Naegleri 49, 52
Naegleri australiensis 52
Naegleri fowleri 52
Necator americanus 106
necatoriasis *see* uncinariasis
Nemathelminthes *see* nematodiasis
nematodiases, rare and uncommon 137
nematodiasis 96–141
  anatomical features 97, 98 (tables 11, 12)
  evolutionary cycles 96, 97
    ascaris type 96
    enterobius type 96
    hookworm type 96
    trichinella type 97
nephrosis, haemoglobinuric, in malaria 81
neurocysticercosis 147
ngana 23
niguas 178
NNN medium 15, 26, 52
nodular form, scabies 175
Norwegian form, scabies 175
Nosema 94
Nosema connori 94
nosematosis *see* microsporidiosis

oesophageal bleeding, in schistosomiasis
    155
oesophagostomiasis 137
Oesophagostomum 106, 137
Onchocerca armillata 131
Onchocerca caecutiens 131
Onchocerca volvulus 126
onchocerciasis 126, 131–4
  clinical diagnosis 131
  epidemiology 131
  gross pathology 131
    onchocercoma 131
  histology 131
    skin lesion 132, 133, *34.2, 34.3,*
      34.6–34.8
  parasite 131, 132, *34.1, 34.4, 34.5*
  pathogenesis 131
Onchocercoma 131
oocysts 72, 76
operculum 143, 160, 165
ophthalmitis, granulomatous, in larva
    migrans 138
opistorchiasis *see* liver fluke infection
Opisthorchis felineus 163, 165
Opisthorchis sinensis 163
Opisthorchis viverrini 163
opportunistic infection 52, 59, 76, 85, 95,
    97
ovoviviparous 128
oxyuriasis *see* enterobiasis
Oxyuris vermicularis 98

Papanicolaou staining 41, 46
Pappenheimer bodies 70
paludism *see* malaria
PAME (primary amoebic meningo-
    encephalitis) 49, 52
pancreas carcinoma, in liver trematode
    infection 163, 165
Paracoccidioides brasiliensis 32
paragonimiasis *see* liver fluke infection
Paragonimus 160
Paragonimus africanus 160
Paragonimus kellicotti 160
Paragonimus westermanni 160
Parastrongylus cantonensis 119
Penicillium marneffi 32
pentastomiasis 184, 185
  clinical diagnosis 184
  epidemiology 184
  parasite 184
    larva 185, *52.1, 52.2*
  pathogenesis 184
  pathology 184
    granuloma of the liver 185, *52.3*
Pentastomidae 184
perforation, intestinal, in ascaridiasis 101
periodicity, day and night, in loiasis 128
peritonitis, granulomatous, in ascaridiasis
    101

Phlebotomus 27, 29, *3.1*, 35
Phlebotomus panamensis 29
pianbois *see* leishmaniasis, mucocutaneous
pinworm infection *see* enterobiasis
pipe stem fibrosis, in schistosomiasis 155
Piringer–Kuchinka lymphadenitis, in
    toxoplasmosis 62
Piroplasmia 70
piroplasmosis 69
pityriasis folliculorum *see* demodicidosis
Plasmodium 77, 79, 81
Plasmodium berghei 77
Plasmodium brazilianum 77
Plasmodium cynomolgi 77
Plasmodium knowlesi 77
Plasmodium malariae 77, 80
Plasmodium ovale 77, 80
Plasmodium vivax 77, 80
plerocercoids 143
Plysaloptera caucasica 117
PMS (phagocytic-mononuclear-system) 35,
    81
Pneumocystis carinii 62, 85
pneumocystosis 9, 85–90
   AIDS 85
   clinical diagnosis 85
   epidemiology 85
   experimental infection 85
   extrapulmonary lesions 85
   gross pathology 85, 87
     pneumocystoma 86, *17.5*
   histology 87–90
     alveolar content 88, 89, *17.10–17.13,*
      17.15
     granulomatous reaction 90,
      17.16–17.21
     liver 86, *17.4*
     lung 86, 88, *17.1–17.3, 17.7*
     lymph node 88, *17.6*
   parasite 85, 88, *17.8–17.9*
   pathogenesis 85
pneumonia, pneumocystis 85
pneumonia, interstitial plasma cell, in
    pneumocystosis 85
pneumonia, eosinophilic, in dirofilariasis 134
porocephalosis *see* pentastomiasis
pork tapeworm 141, 147
portal hypertension, in schistosomiasis 155
prepatent period 96, 97 (table 10)
proglottids 141, 143, 145, 148
promastigote 29
pseudocysts 59, 62
Pseudoterranova decipiens 117
pseudotumor, parasitic, in lung trematode
    infection 160
pulmonary hypertension, in schistosomiasis
    155
pyelonephritis, in schistosomiasis 155
pyodermia, in scabies 175
pyrexia, in larva migrans 138

quartana type of malaria 79

rat tapeworm 147
Reduviidae 23
refraction, double 81
renal insufficiency, in malaria 81
retinal detachment 116, 138
retroinfection, in *Taenia solium* 147
rhabditiform 96, 101, 110
rheumatic pain, in cysticercosis 147
rhodamine staining 85, 87
Rhodnius prolixus 16, *1.8*
river blindness 131
Romaňa sign 15, 16, *1.9*
rosacea, in demodicidosis 175
rostellum 145
round worms *see* nematodiasis
Russell bodies 26, 35

sandfleas 178
saprophyte 62, 85
Sarcocystis bovifelis 72
Sarcocystis bovihominis 59, 72, 73

Sarcocystis lindemanni 72
Sarcocystis spp. 94
Sarcocystis suicanis 73
Sarcocystis suihominis 59, 72, 73
Sarcophaga canaria 181
Sarcoptes scabiei var hominis 173, 174, 175
    (table 24)
Sarcoptes spp. 173
sarcosporidiosis 59, 72–4
   clinical diagnosis 72
   differential diagnosis 72
   epidemiology 72
   gross pathology 72
   histology 72, 74
     intestine 74, *13.3–13.6*
     myocardium 74, *13.1*
     oesophagus 74, *13.2*
   parasite 72
     development cycle 73 (table 5)
   pathogenesis 72
scabies 173–175
   clinical diagnosis 175
   epidemiology 173, 174
   parasite 174 (table 24), 175, 176,
     48.5–48.7
     eggs 177, *48.8*
   pathogenesis 175
   pathology 175, 176, *48.1–48.4*
Schistosoma 151, 155
Schistosoma curassoni 155
Schistosoma haematobium 151, 155
Schistosoma intercalatum 151, 155
Schistosoma japonicum 151, 155
Schistosoma mansoni 151, 155
Schistosoma mekongi 151, 155
schistosomes 151
schistosomiasis *see* blood fluke infections
schizont 70, 80
Schüffner's dots 80
scolex 141, 143, 145, 148, 151, 153
sheep liver fluke 163
shock, anaphylactic, in echinococcosis 148
Simulium flies 131
Siphonaptera 178
skin test 115, 124, 128
sleeping disease 9
sleeping sickness *see* African trypanosomiasis
small liver flukes 163
snails 163, 169
soil amoeba *see* acanthamoebiasis
sore of Aleppo, Biskra, Delhi, Jericho *see*
    leishmaniasis, cutaneous
sore, oriental *see* leishmaniasis, cutaneous
Spargana 143
sparganosis 138, 141, 143
Sparganum proliferum 141
spiruids 117
Spirometra spp. 138, 141, 144, *39.4, 39.5*
splenomegaly, in leishmaniasis 35
sporocysts 72, 73
sporozoa 59
Sporothrix schenckii 32
Sporozoa 59, 70, 76, 80, 85
sporozoites 76, 85
sporulation 59
status spongiosus 62
stool specimens, handling of 106
Strongyloides 138
Strongyloides stercoralis 96, 109
strongyloidiasis 9, 97, 109–12
   AIDS 109
   clinical diagnosis 109
   epidemiology 109
   gross pathology 109
   histology 109–111
     colitis 111, *24.7*
     gastric ulcer 110, *24.2*
     lung 111, *24.8, 24.9*
     lymph node 111, *24.10–24.12*
     intestine 110, *24.3–24.6*
suction disk 39
swamp fever *see* malaria
swimmer's itch 138

tachyzoites 56

Taenia 141
Taenia cysticercus 148
Taenia multiceps 141
taeniasis 141–3
   clinical diagnosis 141
   epidemiology 141
   parasite 141, 143, *38.1–38.5*
   pathology 143
Taenia saginata 141
Taenia solium 9, 141, 147
Taenia teniforme 141
tapeworm infection *see* cestodiasis
tertiana type of malaria 79
tetanus in tungiasis 174
Theileria spp. 69
Thelazia callipeda 117
Thelohania 94
threadworms *see* nematodiasis
ticks 69, 70
toluene blue staining 98
toluidine blue method 85, 87
tongue worm 184
Torulopsis glabrata 32
Toxocara 138
Toxocara canis 116
Toxocara cati 116
toxocariasis 115, 116
   clinical diagnosis 115
   epidemiology 115
   parasite 115, *26.1, 26.2*
   pathogenesis 115
Toxoplasma gondii 32, 59, 61, 62, 94
toxoplasmosis 9, 59–69, 72
   AIDS 59, 62
   clinical diagnosis 59
   differential diagnosis 62
   epidemiology 59
   experimental infection 59
   extrauterine infection 59, 61, 62
   gross pathology 62, 65, 66, 68
     lymphadenitis 62
     medulla oblongata 65, *11.22*
     ophthalmitis 62, 64, *11.11–11.13*
   histology 60, 63, 63–8
     bone marrow smear 60, *11.1*
     chorioretinitis, ophthalmitis 60, 62, 63,
      64, *11.7–11.13*
     cysts 60, 62, 65, *11.3–11.5, 11.16*
     encephalopathy 62, 65–7, *11.23–11.32*
     lung 64, 65, *11.16, 11.17*
     muscle 65, *11.19*
     myocardium 64, *11.14, 11.15*
     orchitis 65, *11.20, 21*
     pleural exudate 60, 65, *11.2, 11.18*
   intrauterine infection 59, 61, 62
     hydrocephalus 68, *11.38–11.39*
     miscarriage 62
     placentitis 62, 68, *11.33–11.37*
   opportunistic infection 59, 62
   parasite 59, 61
     evolutionary cycle 61 (table 3)
     sickle shaped feature 59, 60, *11.1–11.3*
   pathogenesis 59, 61
   serology 59, 62
TPE (tropical pulmonary eosinophilia) 138
transmission, general definition 11
trematode spp. 151
trematodiasis 151–69
Triatoma 23, *1.8*
Trichinella pseudospiralis 112
Trichinella spiralis 112
Trichinella spp. 124
trichinellosis *see* trichinosis
trichinosis 112–15
   clinical diagnosis 112
   epidemiology 112
   experimental infection 112
   parasite 112, 113, *25.1, 25.2*
   pathogenesis 112
   pathology 112–114
     intestine 113, *25.3*
     musculature 114, *25.4–25.8*
Trichocephalus trichuris 101
Trichomonas 11

Trichomonas vaginalis 41
trichomoniasis 41–3
    clinical diagnosis 41
    cytology 41, 42, *7.1, 7.2, 7.4*
    epidemiology 41
    histology 41, 42
        endocervix 42, *7.5, 7.6*
    pathogenesis 41
trichostrongyliasis 137
Trichostrongylus 106, 137
trichuriasis 101, 105
    clinical diagnostic 101
    epidemiology 101
    experimental infection 101
    parasite 101, 105, *22.1, 22.2*
    pathogenesis 101
    pathology 101
        appendix 105, *22.4*
        caecum 105, *22.3*
Trichuris trichuria 101, 106
Trichuris vulpis 138
trophozoites 39, 70, 72, 81, 91
tropism of cysticercosis 147, 148
trypanomastigotes 13, 15, 23, 26
Trypanosoma brucei 23
Trypanosoma brucei brucei 23
Trypanosoma brucei gambiense 23, 24, *2.2*
Trypanosoma brucei rhodesiense 23, 24, *2.1*
Trypanosoma cruzi 13, 15, 26, 29, 32, 94
Trypanosoma rangeli 13, 15, *1.5*
trypanosomiasis, African 23–6
    clinical diagnosis 23
    epidemiology 23
    histology 23, 24, 25
        blood smear 24, *2.2*
        choroid plexus (mouse) 24, *2.1*
        encephalitis 25, *2.5, 2.7*
        morula cell 25, *2.6, 2.8, 2.9*

inoculation chancre 23, 24, *2.4*
    parasite 23
    pathogenesis 23
    pathology 23
    vector 23, 24, *2.3*
trypanosomiasis, American 13–22
    clinical diagnosis 13
        Romaña sign 16, *1.9*
        xenodiagnosis 13
        X-ray 16, *1.11*
    epidemiology 13
    gross pathology 15, 18
        heart 17, *1.13–1.16*
    histology 15, 18–22
        blood smear 14, *1.4–1.5*
        central nervous system 16, 19, 20, *1.7, 1.19–1.23*
        intestine 20, *1.25, 1.26, 1.28*
        mediastinum 14, *1.2*
        myocardium 15, 18, 21, 22, *1.1, 1.6, 1.10, 1.12, 1.17, 1.18, 1.30–1.35*
        oesophagus 20, *2.4*
        orchitis 21, *1.29*
        placenta 20, *1.27*
        tongue 14, *1.3*
    parasite 13
    pathogenesis 15
    vector 15, 16, *1.8*
tsetse fly 23, 24, *2.3*
Tunga penetrans 178
tungiasis 178, 180
    clinical diagnosis 178
    epidemiology 178
    parasite 178, 180, *50.1, 50.5*
        eggs 180, *50.2*
    pathogenesis 178
    pathology 178
        interdigital space 180, *50.3, 50.4*

ulcer, tropical *see* leishmaniasis, cutaneous
uncinariasis 101, 106–9
    clinical diagnosis 106
    epidemiology 106
    experimental infection 106
    gross pathology 106
        intestine 107, *23.6*
        myocardium, fatty degeneration 108, *23.9*
    histology 109
        intestine 108, *23.7, 23.8*
    parasite 106
        life cycle 106 (table 14)
        worm 107, *23.1–23.5*
    pathogenesis 106
urolithiasis, in schistosomiasis 155
uta *see* leishmaniasis, mucocutaneous

vector, biological, general definition 11
Virchow–Robins spaces 18
volvulus, in ascariasis 101

water amoeba *see* acanthamoebae
water snail fever *see* blood fluke infection
water cress 165
waterplants 165, 169
waternuts 169
Watsonius watsoni 169
Whipple disease 62
whipworms 100
whipworm infection *see* trichuriasis
worm eggs 171, 172 (tables 18–21)
Wucheria bancrofti 126

xenodiagnosis, general definition 13

Ziehl–Neelsen method, in crytosporidiasis 77